Ischemic Stroke: Pathophysiology, Diagnosis and Management

Ischemic Stroke: Pathophysiology, Diagnosis and Management

Edited by Caroline West

hayle medical

New York

Hayle Medical,
750 Third Avenue, 9th Floor,
New York, NY 10017, USA

Visit us on the World Wide Web at:
www.haylemedical.com

ISBN: 978-1-63241-503-5

The publisher's policy is to use permanent paper from mills that operate a sustainable forestry policy. Furthermore, the publisher ensures that the text paper and cover boards used have met acceptable environmental accreditation standards.

Printed in China.

Cataloging-in-Publication Data

Ischemic stroke : pathophysiology, diagnosis and management / edited by Caroline West.
p. cm.
Includes bibliographical references and index.
ISBN 978-1-63241-503-5
1. Cerebral ischemia. 2. Cerebral ischemia--Pathophysiology. 3. Cerebral ischemia--Diagnosis.
4. Cerebral ischemia--Prevention. 5. Cerebrovascular disease.
6. Transient ischemic attack. I. West, Caroline.
RC388.5 .I83 2018
616.81--dc23

Table of Contents

Preface

Every book is initially just a concept; it takes months of research and hard work to give it the final shape in which the readers receive it. In its early stages, this book also went through rigorous reviewing. The notable contributions made by experts from across the globe were first molded into patterned chapters and then arranged in a sensibly sequential manner to bring out the best results.

Decreased blood supply to any part of the brain can lead to an ischemic stroke. Thrombosis, cerebral venous sinus thrombosis, embolism and systemic hypoperfusion are the four primary causes of ischemic stroke. The topics included in this book on ischemic stroke are of utmost significance and bound to provide incredible insights into its diagnosis and management. It will also provide interesting topics for research which readers can take up.

It has been my immense pleasure to be a part of this project and to contribute my years of learning in such a meaningful form. I would like to take this opportunity to thank all the people who have been associated with the completion of this book at any step.

Editor

Molecular Basis of Impaired Glycogen Metabolism during Ischemic Stroke and Hypoxia

Mohammed Iqbal Hossain[1]*, Carli Lorraine Roulston[2], David Ian Stapleton[1]

1 Department of Physiology, St. Vincent's Campus, The University of Melbourne, Melbourne, Victoria, Australia, **2** Department of Medicine, St. Vincent's Campus, The University of Melbourne, Melbourne, Victoria, Australia

Abstract

Background: Ischemic stroke is the combinatorial effect of many pathological processes including the loss of energy supplies, excessive intracellular calcium accumulation, oxidative stress, and inflammatory responses. The brain's ability to maintain energy demand through this process involves metabolism of glycogen, which is critical for release of stored glucose. However, regulation of glycogen metabolism in ischemic stroke remains unknown. In the present study, we investigate the role and regulation of glycogen metabolizing enzymes and their effects on the fate of glycogen during ischemic stroke.

Results: Ischemic stroke was induced in rats by peri-vascular application of the vasoconstrictor endothelin-1 and forebrains were collected at 1, 3, 6 and 24 hours post-stroke. Glycogen levels and the expression and activity of enzymes involved in glycogen metabolism were analyzed. We found elevated glycogen levels in the ipsilateral hemispheres compared with contralateral hemispheres at 6 and 24 hours (25% and 39% increase respectively; $P<0.05$). Glycogen synthase activity and glycogen branching enzyme expression were found to be similar between the ipsilateral, contralateral, and sham control hemispheres. In contrast, the rate-limiting enzyme for glycogen breakdown, glycogen phosphorylase, had 58% lower activity ($P<0.01$) in the ipsilateral hemisphere (24 hours post-stroke), which corresponded with a 48% reduction in cAMP-dependent protein kinase A (PKA) activity ($P<0.01$). In addition, glycogen debranching enzyme expression 24 hours post-stroke was 77% ($P<0.01$) and 72% lower ($P<0.01$) at the protein and mRNA level, respectively. In cultured rat primary cerebellar astrocytes, hypoxia and inhibition of PKA activity significantly reduced glycogen phosphorylase activity and increased glycogen accumulation but did not alter glycogen synthase activity. Furthermore, elevated glycogen levels provided metabolic support to astrocytes during hypoxia.

Conclusion: Our study has identified that glycogen breakdown is impaired during ischemic stroke, the molecular basis of which includes reduced glycogen debranching enzyme expression level together with reduced glycogen phosphorylase and PKA activity.

Editor: Jonathan A. Coles, Glasgow University, United Kingdom

Funding: This work was supported by a grant from the National Health and Medical Research Council (NHMRC-628698) to DIS. The funders had no role in study design, data collection and analysis, decision to publish, or preparation of the manuscript.

Competing Interests: The authors have declared that no competing interests exist.

* E-mail: mihos@unimelb.edu.au

Introduction

Stroke is the second most common cause of death and disability world-wide making it the most complex and devastating of all neurological diseases [1,2]. In spite of decades of intensive research in developing pharmacological interventions that prevent damage due to stroke, very few therapeutic options are currently available. Our lack of knowledge about cellular energy utilization during the excitotoxic phase of stroke is one of the many reasons for the lack of therapeutic success. The primary effect of ischemic stroke to neurons is a massive shortage of energy supply with rapid depletion of glucose and oxygen, which impairs the synthesis of ATP through glycolysis and oxidative phosphorylation [3].

The severity of the pathological consequences in stroke depends on the availability of alternative energy substrates and the rate of consumption of ATP by cells undergoing ischemic insults. Glycogen is the principal endogenous source of cellular energy alternative to blood-derived glucose during periods of energy-deficiency in the brain [4]. It is a complex branched polymer of glucose found predominantly in the liver and skeletal muscle where it maintains blood glucose homeostasis and provides energy for muscle contractions, respectively. It consists of glucose molecules covalently linked to α-1,4-glycosidic linkages attached to the polypeptide chain that are extended by the collaborative actions of glycogen synthase (GS) and glycogen branching enzyme (GBE) [5,6]. Glycogen degradation is mediated by the concerted action of glycogen phosphorylase (GP) and glycogen debranching enzyme (GDE) [5,6].

Brain glycogen storage plays a significant role in both physiological and pathological circumstances such as wakefulness [7], hypoglycemia [8], cerebral ischemia [4] and learning [9] by providing energy to adjacent neurons and axons [10,11]. It also provides protection against reactive oxygen species produced during cellular injury [12]. Studies using cell culture and optic nerve preparations have demonstrated that elevated glycogen improves neuronal survival and axonal function during glucose deprivation [13]. Glycogenolysis also supports the *de novo* synthesis of glutamate in astrocytes during glutamatergic activity [14]. Indeed glycogen-derived carbons are used for anaplerosis via pyruvate carboxyaltion in order to produce glutamate [14,15].

According to the Astrocyte-Neuron Lactate Shuttle Hypothesis (ANLSH), lactate or pyruvate derived from astrocytic glycogen upon stimulation of neurons by neurotransmitter glutamate, can be shuttled to neurons for oxidative metabolism to provide energy for maintaining ionic gradients and synaptic plasticity [4,13]. In contrast, based on the concentration and kinetic characteristics of the blood-brain barrier, neuronal and glial nutrient transporter proteins that specifically mediate brain glucose and lactate transport, Simpson et al. (2007) proposed that neurons metabolize glucose and export lactate to astrocytes [16]. This hypothesis is further supported by Mangia et al. (2009) who demonstrated shuttling of lactate from neurons to astrocytes (NALS) in the human brain during visual stimulation using proton Magnetic Resonance Spectroscopy (^{1}H MRS) [17]. An elegant mathematical modelling by DiNuzzo et al. (2010) suggests that glycogen can be used as a significant source of energy for astrocytes and can act as a regulator of astrocytic utilization of blood-born glucose [18,19]. According to the model, glycogenolysis regulates utilization of extracellular and blood-born glucose by astrocytes during brain stimulation by inhibition of astrocytic hexokinase and makes extracellular and blood-born glucose available for use by neurons to meet the immediate demand of energy during brain stimulation [18,20]. Glycogen in astrocytes also plays a significant role in the sequestration of excess extracellular K^+ released by neurons during action and synaptic potentials [21]. It is also used as a source of energy by astrocytes to scavenge excess glutamate during ischemic stroke-induced excitotoxicity [10]. For these reasons previous studies have reported that glycogen levels and metabolism is affected in pathological conditions such as cancer (gastric adenocarcinoma) and neurological disease (Alzheimer's disease and AIDS dementia) [22–25].

Little is known about the fate of glycogen and regulation of its metabolizing enzymes during ischemic stroke. Here, we report changes in the glycogen level and its associated metabolizing enzymes during stroke with reperfusion and investigate the signaling pathways involved in this energy-deficient pathology in the search for better treatments post-stroke.

Materials and Methods

Animals

All experiments involving animals were approved by the St. Vincent's Hospital Animal ethics committee, The University of Melbourne and were performed in accordance with the Prevention of Cruelty to Animals Act 1986 under the guidelines of the National Health and Medical Research Council Code of Practice for the Care and Use of Animals for Experimental Purposes in Australia. Male hooded Wistar rats were purchased from the University of Adelaide, Laboratory Animal Services, Australia. Rats were group-housed (4 rats to a cage) in the Biological Research Facility at The University of Melbourne until endothelin-1-induced (ET-1) middle cerebral artery constriction. Following stroke, they were housed in separate cages under diurnal lighting with ambient temperature maintained between 20 and 22°C and given free access to food and water.

Surgical implantation of ET-1 guide cannula

Male hooded Wistar rats, aged 10–12 weeks (n = 5/6 per groups, total 35/40) (300–340 g) were anesthetized with Ketamine/Xylazine (75 mg/kg Ketamine/10 mg/kg Xylazine *i.p.*) and maintained throughout surgery by inhalation isoflurane (95% oxygen and 2% isoflurane). A 23-gauge stainless-steel guide cannula was stereotaxically implanted into the piriform cortex 2 mm dorsal to the right middle cerebral artery (0.2 mm anterior, −5.2 mm lateral and −5.9 mm ventral) as described previously [26–28] for later delivery of ET-1 in conscious rats. Control rats underwent cannula implantation and saline infusion instead of ET-1 also described previously [26,27]. All surgery was performed under general anesthesia and all efforts were made to minimize suffering which included access to paracetomol (2 mg/kg in drinking water) 24 hours prior to and after surgery, as well as extensive monitoring of each rat throughout the duration of the study.

Stroke induction by ET-1 in conscious rats

Focal cerebral ischemia was induced in the conscious rats by constriction of the right middle cerebral artery with perivascular administration of ET-1 (60 pmol in 3 µl of saline over 10 min). Rats were placed in a clear Plexiglass box for observation during ET-1 injection. During stroke induction, counter-clockwise and/or clockwise circling, clenching, and dragging of the contralateral forepaw were observed, validating the correct placement of the cannula. Stroke severity was scored based on these responses, which have been shown to be a reliable prediction of stroke outcome [26]. Rats that did not display contralateral circling indicative of moderate to severe stroke were excluded from the study. Rectal temperatures were taken with a thermistor probe, prior to stroke and at 30 minutes intervals for 3 to 5 hours after stroke and maintained around 37°C (Figure S1 in Supporting Information S1) as described in previous studies [26,27]. Body weight was also recorded pre-surgery, pre-stroke and 24 hours post-stroke where appropriate.

Tissue collection

Rats were decapitated at 1, 3, 6 and 24 hours after stroke induction and forebrains were removed. Sham rats were also decapitated at these time points as control groups. The left and right hemispheres were separated and immediately snapped freeze in liquid nitrogen. Frozen tissues were powdered under liquid N_2 in a mortar kept on dry ice using a pestle precooled in liquid N_2 and proteins were extracted by homogenization with the ice-cold lysis buffer [50 mM Tris (pH 7.0), 1 mM EDTA, 5 mM EGTA, 1 mM dithiothreitol, 10% Glycerol, 0.1% Triton X-100, 150 mM NaCl, 50 mM NaF, 40 mM sodium pyrophosphate, 0.5 mM Na_3VO_4, 50 mM β-glycerophosphate, 0.2 mg/ml benzamidine, 0.1 mg/ml phenymethylsufonyl fluoride (PMSF), EDTA-free protease inhibitors and phosphatase inhibitors cocktail (Roche, Indianapolis, IN, USA)]. After centrifugation at 10,000×g for 10 minutes, supernatant was collected and total protein concentration was determined using Bradford assay (Bio-Rad, Hercules, CA, USA). The supernatant was stored at −20°C.

Rat primary cerebellar astrocyte culture

Rat primary astrocytes were cultured from the cerebellar hemispheres of 1- to 2-day old Wistar rat brains (n = 6/7 per culture) according to the methods described previously [29,30]. Briefly, cerebella were rapidly excised and transferred to an ice cold Ca^{2+}-free isotonic salt solution [29]. After removing meninges, the cerebella were digested using DMEM (Sigma-

Aldrich, USA) containing 0.1% trypsin for 5 minutes at room temperature in a sterile dish. Trypsin digestion was stopped by adding Eagle's Basal Medium (BME) supplemented with 10% fetal calf serum (FCS) (Sigma-Aldrich, USA). The tissue was then dissociated by triturating using successively decreasing bore sized fire-polished Pasteur pipettes. The cells were centrifuged at 600 rpm for 5 minutes and resuspended in DNAse containing solution. Centrifugation was repeated and the pellet was resuspended in DMEM (supplemented with 2.0 g of $NaHCO_3$, 2.0 g of glucose, 1000 U/L penicillin, 1 g/L streptomycin, and 5% FCS). The cells were plated in poly-D-lysine (PDL)-coated (0.001%) flasks (Invitrogen, USA) with DMEM and incubated at 37°C in a humidified atmosphere with 5% CO_2. The cells were maintained there for 7–8 days to allow for growth and proliferation to 60–70% confluency. The medium was changed at every three days until the cells were confluent at the desired level. The confluent cells were shaken overnight at 360 rpm at 37°C and washed with sterile PBS three times to remove oligodentrocytes. Fresh culture medium (DMEM supplemented with 10% FCS and 6 mM glucose) was then added to the pure astrocytes and the cultures were incubated for 24 hours. The next day astrocyte cultures were trypsinized and re-plated on to poly-D-lysine coated plates at a density of 2×10^4 cells per cm^2. With this method, the cells in the culture contained ≥95% astrocytes as revealed by immunocytochemistry using anti-GFAP antibody (1:300) (Figure S2 in Supporting Information S1). The medium was changed at every three days and all the experiments with astrocytes were performed at DIV 19–22.

Rat primary cortical neuronal culture

Rat primary cortical neuronal culture was performed based on the previously described method with modification [27]. Pregnant rats (n = 3) (gestational day 16–18) were euthanized by CO_2 aphyxiation and the embryos (n = 7/8 per rat) were collected by Cesarean section. Briefly, the cortical regions of the embryonic brains were aseptically dissected, freed of meninges and dissociated in Ca^{2+}-free Suspension Buffer [250 ml of Hanks balanced salt solution (HBSS) +1.94 ml of 150 mM $MgSO_4$+0.75 g BSA], subjected to trypsin digestion at 37°C for 5 minutes in Trypsin Digestion Buffer [20 ml Suspension Buffer +80 µl DNAse (10 µg/µl), +4 mg trypsin]. Tryptic digestion was stopped by the addition of Trypsin Inhibitor Buffer (16.8 ml of Suspension Buffer +80 µl DNAse, +200 µl of 150 mM $MgSO_4$+10.4 mg trypsin inhibitor) to the cell suspension and centrifuged at 1000×g for 5 minutes at 23°C. The pelleted sample was then subjected to mechanical trituration in Trypsin Inhibitor Buffer for 30 seconds. The cells were collected by centrifugation at 1000×g for 5 minutes at 23°C. Finally, the cells were re-suspended in pre-warmed (37°C) Neurobasal medium (GIBCO, USA) supplemented with 10% FCS, 0.25% GlutaMAX-I (GIBCO, USA) and 1% penicillin and streptomycin. The cells were plated to a density of 5×10^7cells in a petri dish (57 cm^2) (Nunc) previously coated with 0.1 mg/ml sterile poly-D-lysine. The cultures were maintained at 37°C in 5% CO_2 and 95% air in a humidified incubator. After 24 hours, the initial Neurobasal medium was replaced with the medium containing 2.5% B-27, (Invitrogen) 0.25% GlutaMAX-I and 1% penicillin and streptomycin. This medium supports long-term survival (several weeks) of neurons and suppresses the growth (< 2%) of glial cells in the total population. The old medium was replaced with new medium at every 4 days.

Induction of hypoxia

In vitro hypoxia/ischemia was induced by placing the cerebellar astrocyte cultures into a modular hypoxic incubator containing 2% O_2, 5% CO_2 and 93% N_2 gas mixture for 0 (control), 1, 3 6 and 24 hours. No decrease in pH below 7.2 was observed during hypoxia. Re-oxygenation was induced by returning the cultures to the normoxia incubator for 24 hours. The culture medium was replaced with glucose- and serum-free DMEM prior to hypoxia or normoxia.

PKA inhibitor treatment

Stock solutions (10x) of a cell permeable, potent and specific PKA inhibitors, H89 (*N*-[2-(*p*-bromo-cinnamylamino)-ethyl]-5-isoquinolinesulfonamide dihydrochloride) (Sigma-Aldrich, USA) and Rp-8-Cl-cAMPs (8-Chloroadenosine-3′, 5′-cyclic monophosphorothioate, Rp-isomer) (Calbiochem, USA) were prepared by dissolving in DMSO and milliQ water, respectively. Astrocytes were incubated in the culture medium (DMEM supplemented with 10% FCS and 6 mM glucose) containing H89 (1, 2, and 4 µM) or Rp-8-Cl-cAMPs (50, 100 and 150 µM) for 24 hours to monitor the effect of PKA inhibition.

Glycogen quantification

Total glycogen concentration was determined by colorimetric method based on the free glucose present in the lysates as previously described [23]. Briefly, 100 µl of brain/cell lysate was treated with 5 µl α-amyloglucosidase (10 µg/µl) in buffer containing 5 µl sodium acetate (pH 6.0). Samples without α-amyloglucosidase were used as negative controls. Both types of samples were incubated at 50°C for 20 minutes. After incubation samples were centrifuged at 14,000×g for 2 minutes and 50 µl of the supernatant were transferred to another microcentrifuge tube into which 350 µl PGO (Sigma-Aldrich, USA) reaction buffer containing O-dianisidine dihydrochloride was added. The mixture was further incubated for 20 minutes at 50°C to develop color. Standard curve was prepared using known concentration of glucose (5.56 mmol/l). Absorbance was taken at 450 nm using xMark micorplate absorbance spectrophotometer (Bio-Rad Inc. USA). Glucose content was calculated by plotting the absorbance values of the samples into standard curve and fitted with linear equation. Glycogen concentration was determined by subtracting values of negative assays (without α-amyloglucosidas), representing bound glucose to positive assays that represents free glucose. Glycogen concentration was expressed as µg glycogen per mg of protein in each sample.

Glycogen synthase (GS) activity assay

GS enzyme activity was determined by measuring the incorporation of [^{14}C]-glucose from (UDP-[^{14}C]-glucose) into glycogen [31]. The reaction was carried out in the absence or presence of the allosteric activator, glucose-6-phosphate (G6P). The enzyme (GS) is active (dephosphorylated form) when G6P is present and inactive when G6P is not present in the reaction. The ratio of (GS activity − G6P)/(GS activity + G6P), therefore provides the proportion of GS activation in the sample. To measure GS activity, 20 µl of brain/cell lysate was added to 40 µl of reaction buffer [50 mM Tris-HCl (pH 7.8), 25 mM potassium fluoride, 20 mM EDTA, 10 mg/ml glycogen, 6.7 mM UDP-[^{14}C]- glucose] either with or without 10.8 mM glucose-6-phosphate. The reaction is allowed to proceed for 30 minutes at 30°C and was terminated by precipitation of glycogen with cold (−20°C) ethanol (66%) and 50 µl of the reaction mix were put on small squares (2.5 cm×2.5 cm, approximately) of filter papers (Whatman 3031–915) and quickly put into cold ethanol (66%). The papers were washed three times in ethanol, one time with acetone and air dried. The reading was performed in scintillation liquid. GS activity was expressed as the ratio of (GS activity − G6P)/(GS activity + G6P), designated as I/T.

Table 1. Primary and secondary antibodies used in immunoblots.

Antibody	Immunogen	Host	Dilution	Source
Anti-GBE	GBE (189–202) RPKKPRSLRIYES	Rabbit	1:2000	Stapleton D et al.[60]
Anti-GDE	GDE (59–73) REKFRSLDWENPTE	Rabbit	1:1000	Stapleton D et al.[60]
Anti-GP	GP (804–818) NIATSGKFSSDRTI	Rabbit	1:500	Parker GJ et al.[61]
Anti-pGP	GP (9–21) phospho-S^{14} KRKQIS^{PO4}VRGL	Rabbit	1:500	Parker GJ et al.[61]
Anti-p-PKA substrate	Synthetic phospho-PKA substrate peptides	Rabbit	1:1000	Cell Signaling, USA
Anti-GFAP	Full length human GFAP	Rat	1:300	Abcam, USA
Anti -β-Actin	N-terminal residues of human β-actin	Mouse	1:1000	Cell Signaling, USA
Anti-rabbit	Whole IgG-HRP conjugated	Rabbit Fc	1:5000	GE Healthcare, UK
Anti-mouse	Whole IgG-HRP conjugated	Mouse Fc	1:5000	GE Healthcare, UK

Glycogen phosphorylase (GP) activity assay

GP activity assay was measured fluorometrically using coupled enzyme systems involving phosphoglucomutase and glucose-6-phosphate dehydrogenase that assist reduction of NAD^+ to NADH [32]. This assay measures enzyme activity in the glycogenolytic direction with the coupled enzyme reactions of phosphoglucomutase and glucose-6-phosphate dehydrogenase. The resulting reduction of NAD^+ to NADH is then measured. The reaction was started by adding 10 µl of brain/cell lysate into the reaction buffer [50 mM sodium glycerol-phosphate (pH 7.1), 10 mM potassium phosphate, 5 mM $MgCl_2$, 0.5 mM NAD^+, 1 mM DTT, 1.6 unit phosphoglucomutase, 1.6 unit glucose-6-phosphate dehydrogenase, and 0.2% glycogen] in a total volume of 300 µl of reaction mixture. The reaction was monitored by measuring the increase of fluorescence (NADH generation) (excitation 350 nm, emission 470 nm) in a Fluorskan Ascent fluorescence spectrophotometer (Thermo Electron corp.) and fluorescence was measured at every 2 minutes for 1 hour. The results were plotted into a fluorescence (FLU) vs time graph. The slope of the curve representing the reaction velocity was calculated by linear equation and normalized to protein concentration and time.

Immunoblot

Equal amounts of protein were loaded in each well of 4–15% SDS-PAGE gel and separated using running buffer [25 mM Tris-HCl (pH 7.4), 192 mM glycine, 10% (w/v) SDS] for approximately 60 minutes at 150 V, and then transferred onto PVDF membrane by Turbo Trans blot system (Bio- Rad). The membrane was then blocked with 5% (w/v) non-fat dry milk/ BSA in Tris buffered saline with Tween 20 (TBST) [0.2 M Tris-HCl (pH 7.4), 1.5 M NaCl, and 0.1% Tween 20]. After blocking and washing with TBST, the membrane was probed with respective primary antibodies (Table 1) for overnight at 4°C. The membrane was again washed with TBST three times before probing with horseradish peroxidase-conjugated secondary antibodies for 1 hour at 25°C. Protein bands were visualized using chemiluminescence (ECL, Amersham Biosciences) according to the manufacturer's instruction. Images were taken using Chemi-Doc MP analyzer using the Image Lab 4.0 software (Bio-Rad).

PKA activity assay

PKA activity assay was performed using ProFluro PKA assay kit (Promega, USA) according to the manufacturer's instruction (Details have been described in Supporting Information S1).

Real-time RT-PCR

The mRNA expressions of genes for GBE (*Gbe1*), GS (*Gys1*), GDE (*Agl*) and GP (*Pygb*) were determined by real-time RT-PCR. Total RNA was extracted from 15 to 20 µg of contralateral and ipsilateral hemispheres of sham and stroke-induced rat brains (n = 5 for each group) using a commercially available kit (PureLink RNA Mini Kit, Invitrogen, Carlsbad, CA, USA), according to the manufacturer's instructions. RNA integrity was evaluated on Agilent 2100 Bioanalyzer (Agilent Technologies, Santa Clara, CA) and quantification of RNA was determined using Nanodrop ND-2000 spectrophotometer (Thermo Fisher Scientific). All of the samples showed 260/280 ratio values around 2, which corresponds to pure RNA. RNA Integrity Number (RIN) values were between 9.6 and 10, suggesting RNA samples with high integrity. The RNA samples were stored at −80°C. Complementary DNA (cDNA) was prepared from 1 µg of RNA using the iScript cDNA Synthesis Kit (Bio-Rad Laboratories, Hercules, CA) according to the manufacturer's instructions and was stored at −20°C for subsequent analysis. Real-Time PCR was performed using the Bio-Rad iCycler Thermal Cycler (Bio-Rad Laboratories, Hercules, CA). Primers' sequences are shown in Table 2. The reaction consisted of 4 minutes at 95°C (one cycle) and then 50 cycles of 95°C for 15 sec, 65°C for 15sec, 72°C for 30 sec. PCR was

Table 2. Primers used in real-time RT-PCR.

Gene	Forward (5-3)	Reverse (5-3)
Glycogen Phosphorylase (*Pygb*)	TCAGGGATGTAGCCAAGGTC	AGCCATGTGGTAACCAGGAG
Glycogen Debranching Enzyme (*Agl*)	CTCACCAGCTGTCATCAGGA	GTGGAGCAGGGACTCTTCTG
Glycogen Branching Enzyme (*Gbe1*)	TTTTCAACTTCCACCCAAGC	CAAAAGCCTCGGCAAAGTAG
Glycogen Synthase (*Gys1*)	CCCCCAATGGACTAAATGTG	AGCGTCCAGCGATAAAGAAA

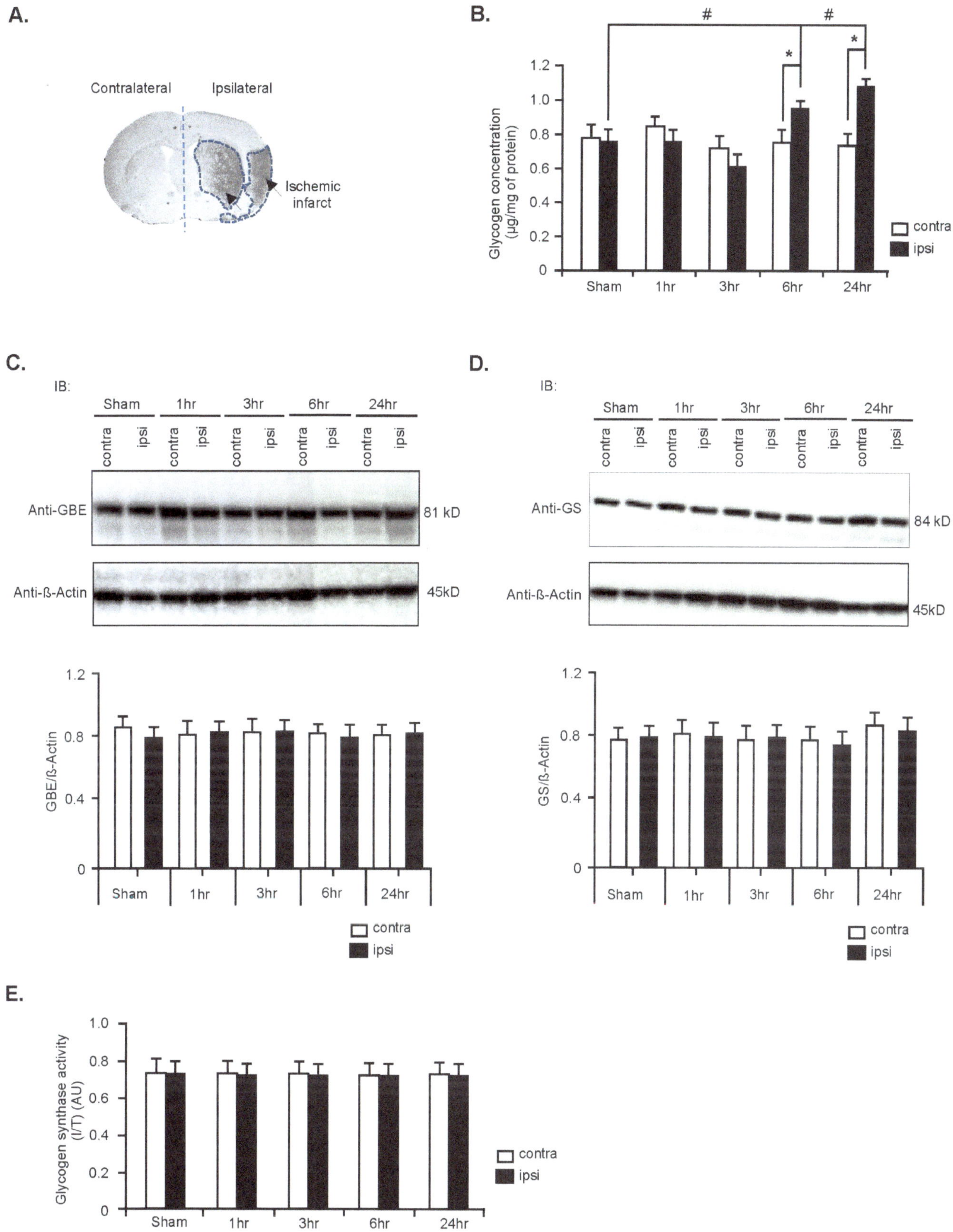

Figure 1. Glycogen is accumulated in stroke-affected brain. (**A**) A representative sample image generated from an unstained section collected between 1.2 mm to −2.8 mm bregma from an ET-1-induced stroke rat brain. Stroke-induced damage is shown to be located predominately around the site of ET-1-induced vasoconstriction, referred to as the 'core' ischemic infarct (arrow sign) in the ipsilateral hemisphere. (**B**) Glycogen concentration in contralateral and ipsilateral hemispheres of control (sham) and stroke brains. Values are expressed as mean ±SD, n = 5 rats for each

group. $^{\#}P$ and $^{*}P<0.05$ compared to sham ipsilateral and stroke contralateral hemispheres, respectively. Expression levels of GBE (**C**) and GS (**D**) in contralateral and ipsilateral hemispheres of sham and stroke rat brains between 1 hr and 24 hr. Expression levels were normalized against β-Actin (middle panel). Quantification of this data is shown in the lower panel. Data are mean ±SD, n = 5. (**E**) GS activity in sham and stroke rat brains at different time points post-stroke. Data are represented as mean ±SD; n = 5. ($^{*}P$ = Student's t-test and $^{\#}P$ = one-way ANOVA followed by Tukey's *post hoc* test).

conducted in a reaction mixure containing SYBR Green (iQ SYBR Green Supermix, Bio-Rad), forward and reverse primers (0.5 μM), and cDNA template (5 ng). Measurements included a no-template control as well as an RT (reverse transcription) negative control. For each cDNA sample, three technical replicates were averaged and dissociation curves were routinely performed to check for the presence of a single peak corresponding to the required amplicon. The content of single stranded DNA (ssDNA) in each sample was determined using the Quanti-iT OliGreen ssDNA Assay Kit (Molecular Probes, Eugene, OR, USA), according to the manufacturer's instruction. Gene expression was quantified by normalizing to the cDNA content of each sample and expressed as arbitrary units (AU).

Treatment of astrocytes with GP inhibitors

To monitor the effect of glycogen during hypoxia, astrocytes were treated with the GP inhibitors, CP-316819 (5-Chloro-N-[(1S, 2R)-2-hydroxy-3-(methoxymethylamino)-3-oxo-1-(phenylmethyl) propyl]-1H-indole-2-carboxamide) or DAB (1,4-dideoxy-1,4-imino-D-arabinitol hydrochloride) (Sigma-Aldrich, USA) based on previous studies [8,33]. DMSO (vehicle) and milliQ water were used to make a 10× stock concentrations of CP-316819 and DAB, respectively. The cerebellar astrocytes (DIV 18–19, 2×10^{4} cells per well) were incubated in the culture medium (DMEM supplemented with 10% FCS and 6 mM glucose) containing either DMSO, or CP-316819 (10 μM) or DAB (1 mM) separately for 24 hours. After incubation the astrocyte cultures were washed twice with fresh culture medium. These cultures along with untreated cultures were then incubated in serum- and glucose-free DMEM and placed in the hypoxic incubator for 0 (control), 1, 3, 6 and 24 hours for induction of hypoxia.

MTT assay

The cells in each well were monitored for viability by the MTT assay. Briefly, MTT reagent was dissolved in RPMI 1640 medium (without phenol red) at a stock concentration of 5 mg/ml and filtered using 0.22 μm to remove insoluble residues as described previously [34]. After induction of hypoxia for different time points, MTT solution equal to 10% (v/v) of the volume of culture medium (0.5 mg/ml final concentration) was added to each well containing astrocytes. The culture plates were then incubated at 37°C in a 5% CO_2 incubator for 30 minutes. The culture medium was removed by aspiration and dried for 10 minutes. An aliquot of 200 μl DMSO was added to dissolve the formazan crystals formed from the reduction of MTT reagent by the mitochondrial reductase of live cells. To determine the amount of formazan formed, three aliquots (100 μl each) of the mixture from each well of cells were transferred in three separate wells of a 96-well microtiter plate (Falcon) and the absorbance at 570 nm was measured using Envision Multilabel plate reader (PerkinElmer, USA). The cell viability was compared as a percentage of DMSO treated and untreated astrocytes (0 hr) for CP-316819 and DAB treated astrocyte cultures, respectively.

LDH assay

The LDH assay was performed in dark according to the manufacturer's protocol (Promega, USA). Briefly, after induction of hypoxia for different time points, 50 μl of culture medium from each well of the culture plate containing astrocytes was transferred to 96 well-micro titre plates (Falcon). A 100 μl of LDH assay mixture containing equal volume of LDH Assay Substrate solution, LDH Assay Dye solution and LDH Assay Cofactor was then added to each well. The reaction was allowed to proceed at room temperature for 30 minutes in dark and was stopped by adding 50 μl of 1 mM acetic acid. The absorbance of whole mixture was measured in triplicate at a wavelength of 490 nm using Envision Multilabel plate reader (PerkinElmer, USA). The release of LDH was calculated as a percentage of DMSO treated and untreated astrocytes (0 hr) for CP-316819 and DAB treated astrocyte cultures, respectively.

Monitoring live and dead cells by calcein-AM and EthD-1 staining

Calcein acetoxymethyl (calcein-AM) and ethidium homodimer-1 (EthD-1) were used to visualize live and damaged astrocyte respectively after induction of hypoxia. The disrupted cell membranes of damaged astrocytes allow entry of EthD-1, which upon binding to nucleic acids, produces red fluorescence (excitation wavelength, ~528 nm; emission wavelength, ~617 nm). While the membrane-permeable calcein-AM is converted by the intracellular esterases of live cells only to form intensely fluorescent calcein (excitation wavelength, ~494 nm; emission wavelength, ~517 nm).

In brief, after induction of hypoxia, the astrocyte cultures were washed twice with 1× PBS and stained with calcein-AM and EthD-1 (final concentrations: 2 μM and 5 μM respectively) (Invitrogen, USA) dissolved in DMEM without phenol red and incubated at 37°C for 30 minutes in a 5% CO_2 incubator. After staining, the cells were washed twice with 1× PBS. Live and dead cells were visualized (5–6 images for each well) using a fluorescence microscope (Leica DMI6000B) and the number of viable and dead cells was counted using the image J software. The ratios of live to dead cells obtained from each of the groups were compared.

Statistical analysis

Densitometry analyses for the quantification of the bands on immunoblots were performed using Image J software. Statistical analyses were performed with the Statistical Package for Social Sciences for Windows, version 16 (SPSS, Inc, Chicago, Illinois, USA). The data were reported as the mean ±SD and the statistical significance were determined by parametric procedure as student's t-test (two-tailed) and one-way analysis of variance (ANOVA) followed by Tukey's *post hoc* test (for multiple comparisons). $p<0.05$ was considered statistically significant for all experiments.

Results

Stroke induction

Among the rats used in the current study, 4 were excluded from the analysis due to lack of observed behavioral changes during stroke induction. Total mortality was 1/28 due to severe stroke. Some post-stroke weight loss was observed in the 24 hours recovery groups.

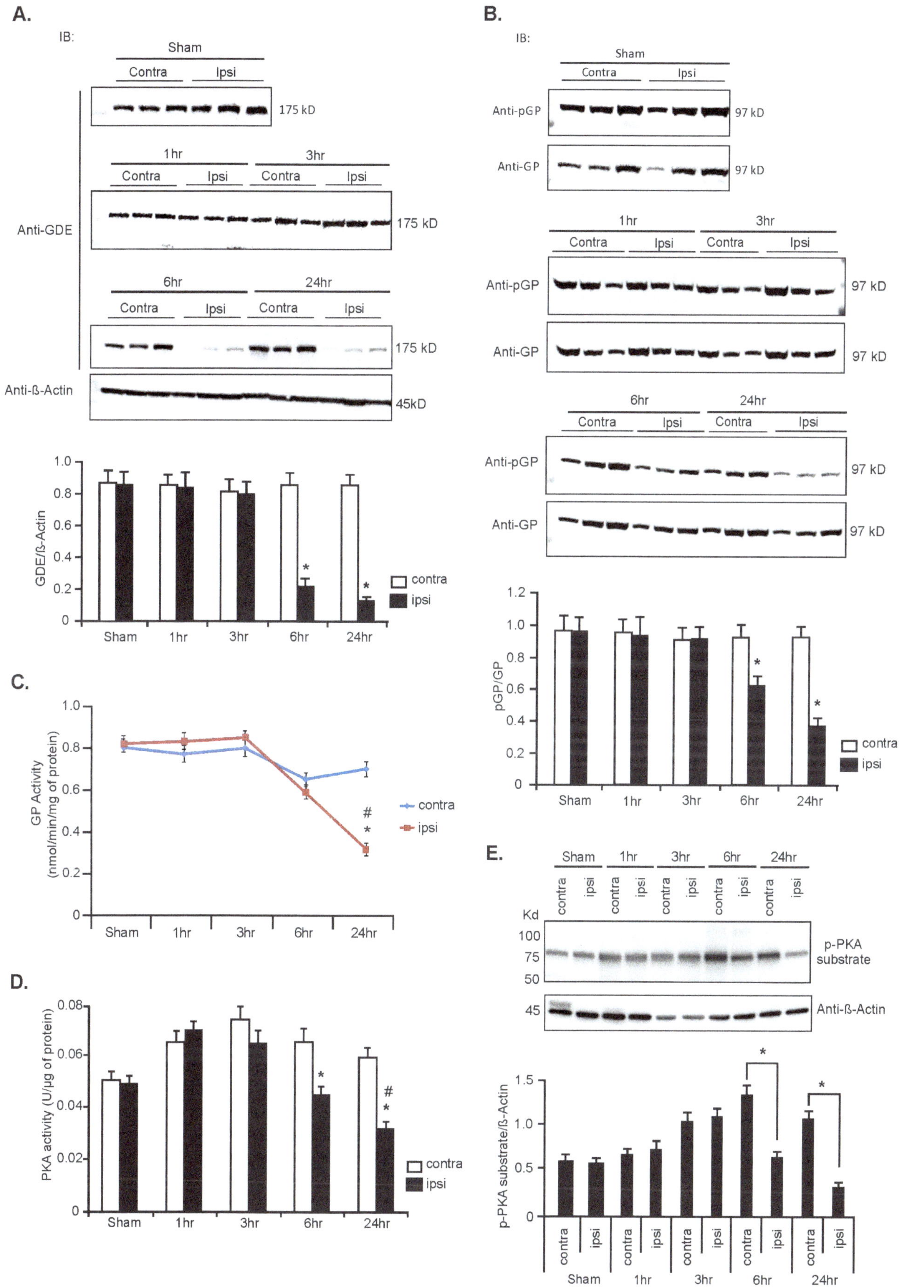
A.
IB:
Sham
Contra
Ipsi
175 kD
1hr
3hr
Contra
Ipsi
Contra
Ipsi
Anti-GDE
175 kD
6hr
24hr
Contra
Ipsi
Contra
Ipsi
175 kD
Anti-ß-Actin
45kD
GDE/ß-Actin
1.0
0.8
0.6
0.4
0.2
0
Sham
1hr
3hr
6hr
24hr
contra
ipsi
B.
IB:
Sham
Contra
Ipsi
Anti-pGP
97 kD
Anti-GP
97 kD
1hr
3hr
Contra
Ipsi
Contra
Ipsi
Anti-pGP
97 kD
Anti-GP
97 kD
6hr
24hr
Contra
Ipsi
Contra
Ipsi
Anti-pGP
97 kD
Anti-GP
97 kD
pGP/GP
1.2
1.0
0.8
0.6
0.4
0.2
0
Sham
1hr
3hr
6hr
24hr
contra
ipsi
C.
GP Activity (nmol/min/mg of protein)
1.0
0.8
0.6
0.4
0.2
0
Sham
1hr
3hr
6hr
24hr
contra
ipsi
D.
PKA activity (U/µg of protein)
0.08
0.06
0.04
0.02
0
Sham
1hr
3hr
6hr
24hr
contra
ipsi
E.
Sham
1hr
3hr
6hr
24hr
contra
ipsi
Kd
100
75
50
45
p-PKA substrate
Anti-ß-Actin
p-PKA substrate/ß-Actin
1.5
1.0
0.5
0

Figure 2. Expression levels of GDE, and activity of GP and PKA are decreased during ischemic stroke. (**A**) Representative immunoblot showing expression levels of GDE in contralateral and ipsilateral hemispheres of sham and stroke brains at different time points following stroke induction. Expression level of GDE was normalized against β-Actin protein. Lower panel: Quantification data of GDE expression level. Data are represented as mean ±SD, n = 6; $^{*}P<0.05$ vs contralateral hemispheres (6 hr and 24 hr). (**B**) Representative immunoblot of phosphorylation level of GP in sham and stroke rat brains. Immunoblot analysis data (lower panel) as mean ±SD, n = 6, $^{*}P<0.05$ vs contralateral hemispheres of stroke brains (6 hr and 24 hr). (**C**) GP enzyme activity in sham and stroke rat brains. Data are mean ±SD, n = 6 rats for each group. $^{\#}P = 0.001$ vs sham ipsilateral and $^{*}P = 0.003$ vs stroke contralateral hemisphere (24 hr). (**D**) PKA activity in sham and stroke brains [mean ±SD, n = 6; $^{\#}P = 0.003$ (24 hr) vs sham ipsilateral and $^{*}P = 0.004$ (6 hr) and 0.003 (24 hr) vs stroke contralateral hemispheres]. (**E**) Representative immunoblot of p-PKA substrate of sham and stroke brains. Phosphorylation level was normalized against β-Actin protein [mean ±SD, n = 5; $^{*}P = 0.003$ (6 hr) and 0.002 (24 hr)]. ($^{*}P$ = Student's t-test and $^{\#}P$ = one-way ANOVA followed by Tukey's *post hoc* test).

Glycogen is accumulated in contralateral hemisphere during ischemic stroke

We first assessed the metabolic fate of glycogen in ischemic stroke-affected rat brains. For this, we measured the level of glycogen in control (sham) and ischemic stroke brains in both the contralateral and ipsilateral hemispheres that underwent ET-1-induced stroke after 1, 3, 6 and 24 hours of recovery. We found that glycogen levels were increased in the ipsilateral (stroke-affected) hemispheres compared with that of the contralateral hemispheres between 6 and 24 hours after stroke induction (25% and 39% increase, respectively; n = 5, $^{*}P<0.05$; Figure 1B) as well ipsilateral hemisphere of sham operated controls (23% and 34% increase, respectively; n = 5, $^{\#}P<0.05$; Figure 1B).

The two key enzymes involved in glycogen synthesis are GBE and GS. We therefore monitored the expression level of these two enzymes after stroke at different time intervals. We found that the expression levels of both enzymes remained unchanged in the contralateral and ipsilateral hemispheres of stroke brains in

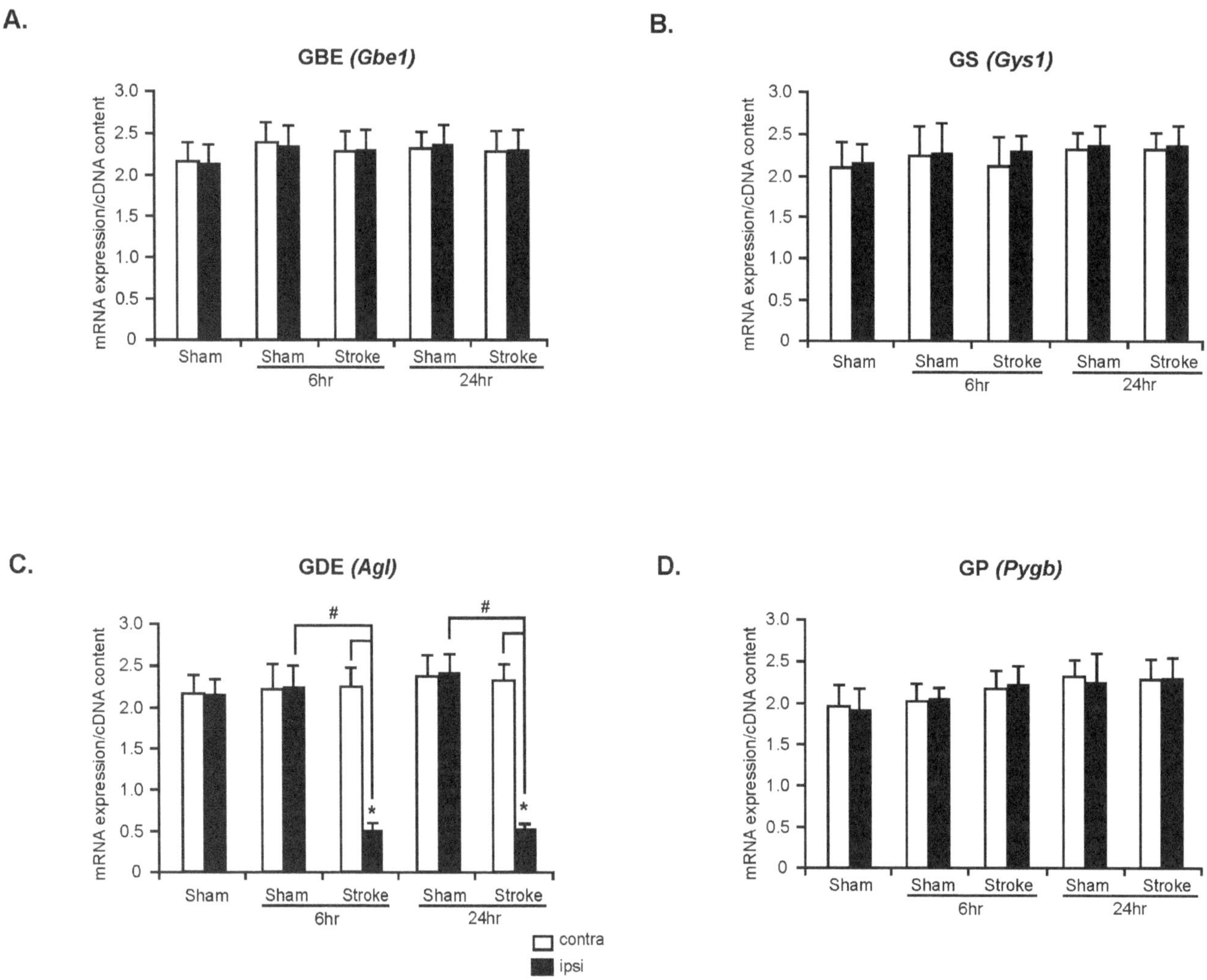

Figure 3. Reduced GDE mRNA expression in ischemic stroke. mRNA expression of GBE (*Gbe1*) (**A**), GS (*Gys1*) (**B**), GDE (*Agl*) (**C**) and GP (*Pygb*) (**D**) in contralateral and ipsilateral hemispheres of sham and stroke rat brains. Data are presented as mean ±SD, n = 5 for each group. *Agl* analysis: $^{*}P<0.05$ vs contralateral hemispheres of stroke rat brains (6 and 24 hr) and $^{\#}P<0.05$ vs ipsilateral hemispheres of sham rat brains of 6 hr and 24 hr groups. ($^{*}P$ = Student's t-test and $^{\#}P$ = one-way ANOVA followed by Tukey's *post hoc* test).

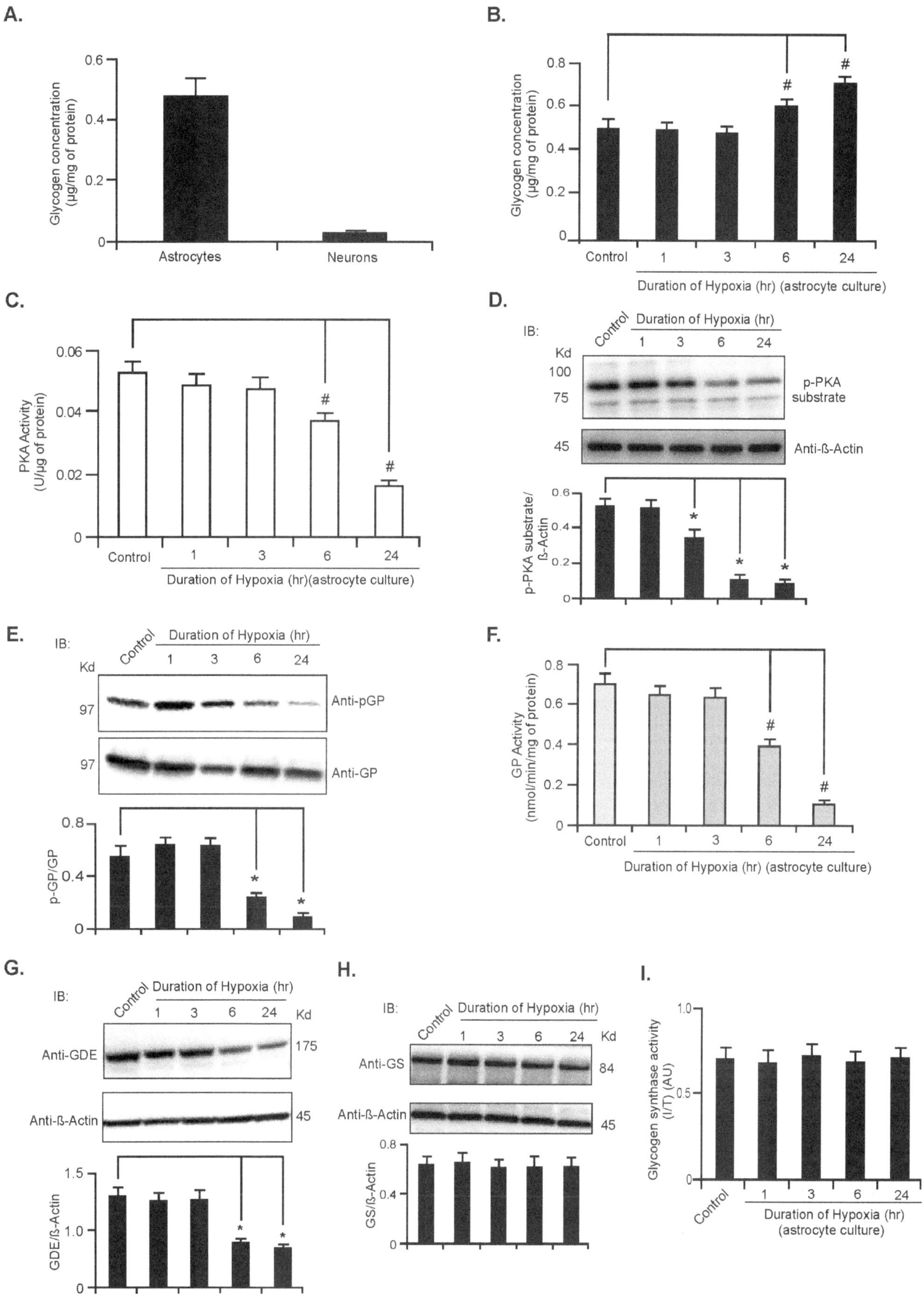
A.
Glycogen concentration (µg/mg of protein)
0.6
0.4
0.2
0
Astrocytes
Neurons
B.
Glycogen concentration (µg/mg of protein)
0.8
0.6
0.4
0.2
0
#
#
Control
1
3
6
24
Duration of Hypoxia (hr) (astrocyte culture)
C.
PKA Activity (U/µg of protein)
0.06
0.04
0.02
0
#
#
Control
1
3
6
24
Duration of Hypoxia (hr)(astrocyte culture)
D.
IB:
Control
Duration of Hypoxia (hr)
1
3
6
24
Kd
100
75
p-PKA substrate
45
Anti-ß-Actin
p-PKA substrate/ ß-Actin
0.6
0.4
0.2
0
*
*
*
E.
IB:
Control
Duration of Hypoxia (hr)
1
3
6
24
Kd
97
Anti-pGP
97
Anti-GP
p-GP/GP
0.8
0.4
0
*
*
F.
GP Activity (nmol/min/mg of protein)
0.8
0.6
0.4
0.2
0
#
#
Control
1
3
6
24
Duration of Hypoxia (hr) (astrocyte culture)
G.
IB:
Control
Duration of Hypoxia (hr)
1
3
6
24
Kd
Anti-GDE
175
Anti-ß-Actin
45
GDE/ß-Actin
1.5
1.0
0
*
*
H.
IB:
Control
Duration of Hypoxia (hr)
1
3
6
24
Kd
Anti-GS
84
Anti-ß-Actin
45
GS/ß-Actin
0.8
0.4
0
I.
Glycogen synthase activity (I/T) (AU)
1.0
0.5
0
Control
1
3
6
24
Duration of Hypoxia (hr) (astrocyte culture)

Figure 4. Glycogen is accumulated in astrocytes during hypoxia. (**A**) Glycogen levels in rat primary cerebellar astrocytes and cortical neurons. Data are expressed as mean ±SD of 5 independent cultures. (**B**) Glycogen levels in rat cerebellar astrocytes kept under hypoxic conditions for 0 (control), 1, 3, 6 and 24 hr as described in the Materials and Methods section. Glycogen levels were measured following 24 hr incubation in normoxic condition. Values are expressed as mean ±SD, n = 5; $^{\#}P<0.05$ vs control astrocytes. (**C**) PKA activity in astrocytes exposed to hypoxic conditions. (Data are mean ±SD, n = 5; $^{\#}P<0.05$ compared with control astrocytes). (**D**) Representative immunoblot of p-PKA substrate immunoblot analysis in astrocytes maintained in hypoxic conditions for the indicated time periods. Phosphorylation levels were normalized against β-Actin protein, the analysis is shown in the lower panel (mean ±SD, n = 5; $^{*}P<0.05$). (**E**) Representative immunoblot of pGP in astrocytes incubated under hypoxic conditions. Quantification of phosphorylation levels was performed using the total level of GP protein. Quantification data (lower panel) are represented as mean ±SD, n = 5; $^{*}P<0.05$. (**F**) GP activity in astrocytes during hypoxia. Data are mean ±SD, n = 5; $^{\#}P<0.05$ vs control astrocytes. (**G**) Representative immunoblot showing expression level of GDE in astrocytes exposed to hypoxic condition for indicated time points. Expression of GDE was normalized against β-Actin protein. Data are represented as mean ±SD, n = 5; $^{*}P<0.05$ vs control astrocytes. GS protein expression (**H**) and GS enzymatic activity (**I**) in hypoxic astrocytes. Data are represented as mean ±SD, n = 5. ($^{*}P$ = Student's t-test and $^{\#}P$ = one-way ANOVA followed by Tukey's *post hoc* test).

comparison to sham controls (Figure 1C and D respectively, n = 5). In addition, the activity of GS was unaltered in the stroke-affected rat brains in comparison to sham controls (Figure 1E, n = 5).

Expression of GDE, and activity of GP and PKA are suppressed in ischemic stroke

The enzymes essential for glycogen degradation are GDE and the brain isoform of GP. GDE converts α-1,6-glycosidic linkages in glycogen to α-1,4-glycosidic linkages for further breakdown by GP [35]. We therefore investigated the expression level of GDE and activity of GP various times following initiation of the stroke. Immunoblot analyses of sham and stroke- affected rat brains were performed at 1, 3, 6 and 24 hours after stroke induction. Immunoblot analyses revealed that the expressions of GDE in the stroke-affected brain at early time points (1 and 3 hr) were similar to that of the sham controls (Figure 2A). GDE expression, however, was significantly lower in the ipsilateral hemispheres compared with that of the contralateral and sham controls (67% and 77% decrease in stroke contralateral hemisphere, respectively, Figure 2A, lower panel; n = 6, $^{*}P<0.05$) at later time points. Analysis of GP phosphorylation level at Ser-14 (pGP) by immunoblot revealed a significant decrease of phosphorylation in the stroke ipsilateral hemispheres compared with that of the contralateral hemispheres and sham controls at 6 and 24 hours time points (Figure 2B and lower panel; n = 6, $^{*}P<0.05$). Measurement of GP activity further confirmed a decrease in phosphorylase activity in the ipsilateral hemispheres 2 hours post-stroke compared with that of the contralateral hemispheres (58% reduction, n = 6, $^{*}P = 0.003$; Figure 2C) and ipsilateral hemispheres of sham operated controls (61.5% reduction, n = 6, $^{\#}P = 0.001$; Figure 2C). GP is primarily regulated by phosphorylation at Ser-14 by phosphorylase kinase (PhK) which is activated by cAMP-dependent protein kinase A (PKA) [6,36]. We therefore measured PKA activity in sham and stroke-induced rat brains. PKA activity was significantly reduced in the ipsilateral hemisphere compared with that of the contralateral hemisphere in stroke rat brains at 6 and 24 hours post-stroke [32% and 48.3% reduction, respectively, n = 6; $^{*}P = 0.004$ (6 h) and 0.003 (24 h); Figure 2D] and sham controls [36% reduction vs sham ipsilateral hemisphere, n = 6; $^{\#}P = 0.003$ (24 h); Figure 2D]. Immunoblot data with a p-PKA substrate antibody that detects all PKA-phosphorylated motifs in sham and stroke rat brain homogenates further indicated a down-regulation of p-PKA immunoreactivity (p-PKA substrate blot) in the ipsilateral hemispheres in comparison to the contralateral hemispheres in stroke brains [Figure 2E, n = 5, $^{*}P = 0.003$ (6 h) and 0.002 (24 h)]. We further noticed that the contralateral hemispheres of stroke rat brains (3, 6 and 24 hr) showed increased PKA activity and p-PKA substrate immunoreactivity compared with either hemispheres of the sham rat brains (Figure 2D and E), therefore, we further analyzed PKA activity of contralateral and ipsilateral regions of sham rat brains after saline infusion at different time points. Though, we found increased p-PKA substrate immunoreactivity and PKA activity in both hemispheres of sham rat brains at later time points compared with that of the earlier time points, the changes were statistically not significant among the groups (Figure S3 A and B in Supporting Information S1).

The mRNA expression level of glycogen metabolizing enzymes in sham and ischemic stroke rat brains

To assess whether ischemic insult alters the mRNA expression level of genes involved in glycogen metabolism we measured mRNA expression level of *Gbe1*, *Gys1*, *Agl* and *Pygb* in the contralateral and ipsilateral hemispheres of sham and stroke-affected rat brains. Real-Time RT-PCR data revealed that mRNA expression levels of *Gbe1*, *Gys1*, and *Pygb* remained unchanged in contralateral and ipsilateral hemispheres of both sham and stroke rat brains at 6 and 24 hours time points (Figure 3A, B and D, n = 5). However, the level of mRNA expression of *Agl* was significantly decreased in the ipsilateral hemispheres compared with that of the contralateral hemispheres and sham controls at 6 and 24 hours (73% and 72% reduction, respectively, Figure 3C, n = 5; $^{*}P$ and $^{\#}P<0.05$).

Hypoxia induces accumulation of glycogen in astrocytes

To investigate the effect of hypoxia on glycogen metabolism *in vitro* we cultured rat primary cerebeller astrocytes and cortical neurons and measured total amount of glycogen present in these two types of cells. Glycogen was mainly localized to astrocytes while neurons contained very little or no glycogen (Figure 4A, n = 5) confirming previous studies [37]. Next, we induced hypoxia in rat cerebeller astrocytes for 1, 3, 6 and 24 hours and monitored its effect on glycogen level. The cerebellar astrocyte cultures exposed to hypoxia for 6 and 24 hours showed significantly higher amounts of accumulated glycogen compared with that of the control (0 hr) astrocytes (Figure 4B, n = 5; $^{*}P<0.05$) suggesting decreased breakdown of astrocytic glycogen during hypoxia. To explore the potential effect of PKA in this pathway we further investigated PKA's activity in hypoxic astrocytes by enzymatic assay and by immunoblot using an anti-p-PKA substrate antibody. As shown in Figure 4C and D PKA activity was significantly reduced in astrocytes exposed to hypoxic condition for 6 and 24 hours (n = 5; $^{*}P<0.05$). Since GP is essential to glycogen metabolism and is also an indirect downstream target of PKA, we therefore measured GP activity by both phosphoimmunoblot and enzymatically in hypoxic astrocytes. These experiments showed a significant decrease in GP activity in hypoxic astrocytes at 6 and 24 hours periods in comparison to that of the control astrocytes (Figure 4E and F, respectively, n = 5; $^{*}P<0.05$). The expression

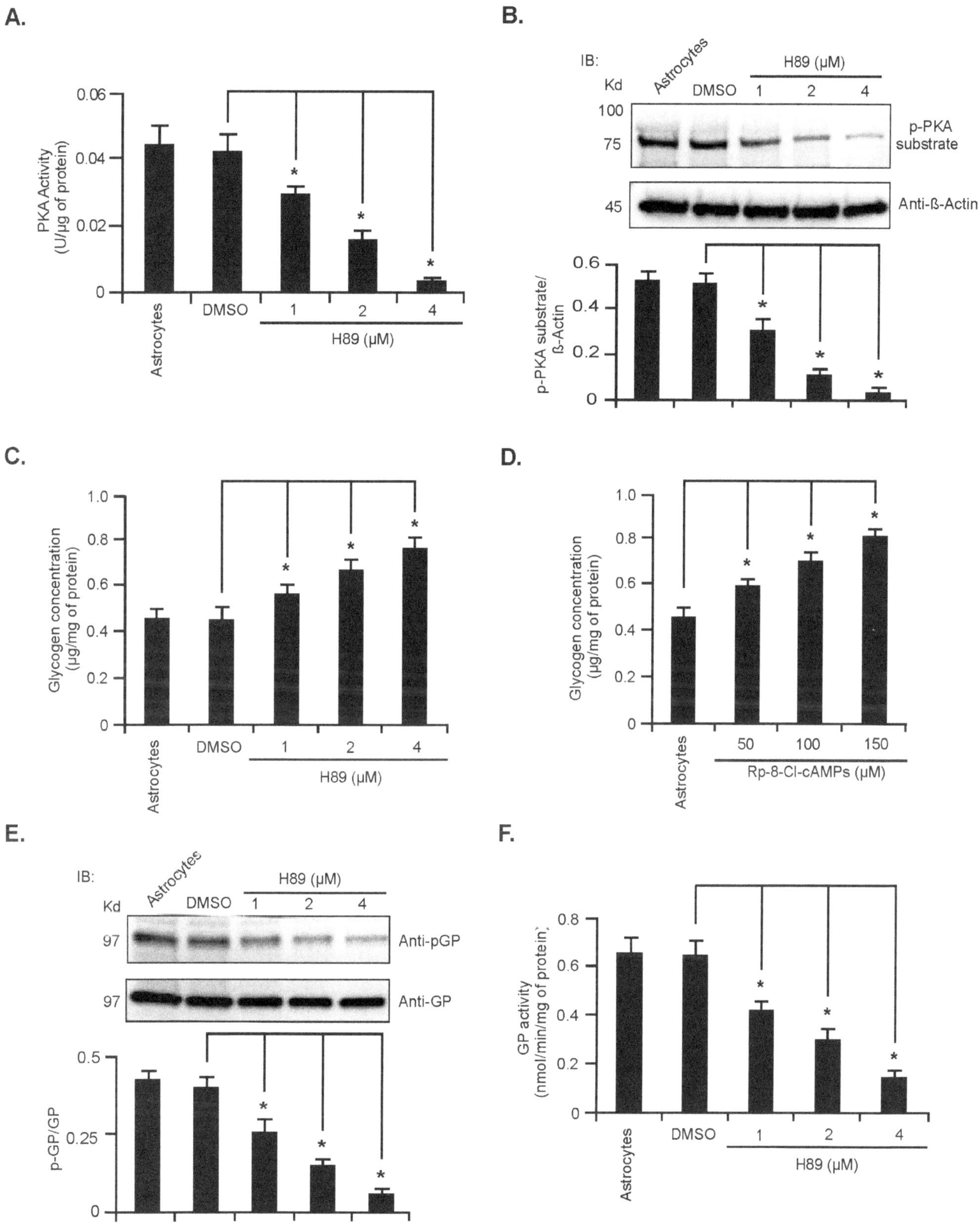

Figure 5. Inhibition of PKA activity in cultured cerebellar astrocytes increases glycogen accumulation. (**A**) PKA activity in cerebellar astrocytes treated with different concentrations of H89 for 24 hr [mean ±SD, n = 5; $^*P<0.05$ compared with DMSO (vehicle) treated astrocytes]. (**B**) Representative immunoblot of p-PKA substrate in astrocytes treated with either DMSO or H89 for 24 hr. Phosphorylation level was normalized against β-Actin protein, the analysis is shown in the lower panel (n = 5; $^*P<0.05$). Glycogen levels in astrocytes treated with H89 (**C**) and Rp-8-Cl-cAMPs (**D**) (mean ±SD, n = 5; $^*P<0.05$). (**E**) Immunoblot of pGP in H89 treated astrocytes. Quantification, shown in the lower panel, was performed using total GP protein. Data are represented as mean ±SD, n = 5; $^*P<0.05$. (**F**) GP activity in H89 treated astrocytes. Data are mean ±SD, n = 5; $^*P<0.05$ vs DMSO treated astrocytes. ($^*P=$ Student's t-test).

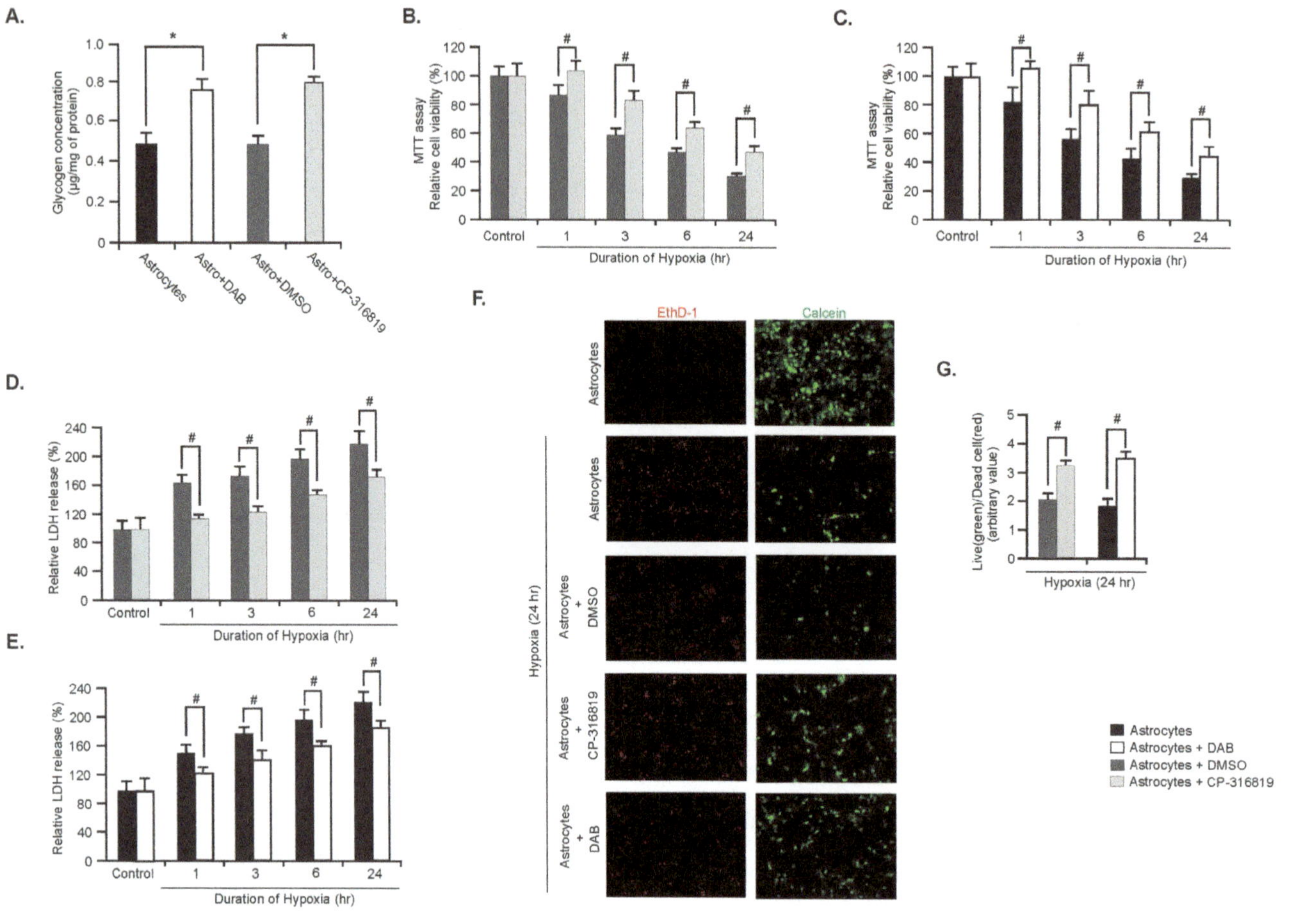

Figure 6. Elevated glycogen levels protect astrocytes during hypoxia. (**A**) Glycogen levels in astrocytes treated with either DAB (1 mM) or CP-316819 (10 µM) or DMSO for 24 hr. Data are presented as mean ±SD, n = 5; $^*P<0.05$. MTT assay showing cell viability in astrocytes treated with either CP-316819 (**B**) or DAB (**C**) for 24 hr and exposed to hypoxia for indicated time points. (Data are mean ±SD, n = 5; $^\#P<0.05$). LDH assay in astrocytes treated with either CP-316819 (**D**) or DAB (**E**) for 24 hr and exposed to hypoxia. (Data are mean ±SD, n = 5; $^\#P<0.05$). (**F**) Representative images of live (green) and dead (red) cells in astrocytes exposed to hypoxia for 24 hr. Astrocytes were treated with CP-316819, DMSO or DAB for 24 hr prior to hypoxia. (**G**) Ratio of live to dead cells in astrocytes treated with either CP-316819 or DAB and exposed to hypoxia for 241hr. Data are mean ±SD, n = 5; $^\#P<0.05$. ($^*P$ = Student's t-test and $^\#P$ = one-way ANOVA followed by Tukey's *post hoc* test).

level of GDE was decreased in hypoxic astrocytes (Figure 4G, n = 5; $^*P<0.05$) while both expression and activity of GS remained unchanged (Figure 4H and I, respectively, n = 5).

Inhibition of PKA activity leads to increase glycogen accumulation in cultured astrocytes

To confirm the direct involvement of PKA in the regulation of glycogen metabolism, rat primary cerebellar astrocytes were treated with 1, 2 and 4 µM of the PKA inhibitor H89 for 24 hours. Both PKA activity measurements demonstrated that PKA activity was decreased in a dose dependant manner upon H89 treatment (Figure 5A & B respectively, n = 5; $^*P<0.05$). Next, we measured the level of glycogen in astrocytes treated with H89. As shown in Figure 5C astrocytes treated with H89 contained significantly increased amounts of glycogen in comparison to that of the vehicle (DMSO) treated astrocytes (Figure 5C, n = 5; $^*P<0.05$). For further confirmation, we determined the glycogen level in astrocytes treated with a different PKA inhibitor, Rp-8-Cl-cAMPs using concentrations ranging from 50 to 150 µM for 24 hours, and similarly found that the level of glycogen was increased significantly in astrocytes upon treatment with the PKA inhibitor in a dose dependent manner (Figure 5D, n = 5; $^*P<0.05$).

We next investigated whether decreased PKA activity could also decrease GP enzyme activity. As shown in Figures 5E and F, treatment of astrocytes with H89 resulted in decreased GP phosphorylation (Ser-14) and enzyme activity, respectively (n = 5; $^*P<0.05$). Decreased PKA or GP activity however, did not alter the expression of GDE or the activity of GS (Figure S4A and B in Supporting Information S1). Taken together, these data suggest that inhibition of PKA activity leads to the accumulation of glycogen in astrocytes by decreasing GP activity but has no effect on the activity of GS or expression of GDE.

Effects of elevated glycogen on the viability of astrocytes during hypoxia

In the final experiments we assessed the effect of elevated glycogen in astrocytes during hypoxic insults. For this astrocyte cultures were treated with GP inhibitors, CP-316819 or DAB to increase glycogen content. Glycogen levels in astrocytes were significantly increased following incubation of the astrocytes with the two different GP inhibitors for 24 hours (Figure 6A, n = 5; $^*P<0.05$). Astrocyte viability following GP inhibitors treatment and hypoxia induction were monitored by MTT and LDH assay, and by the live/dead cell staining method.

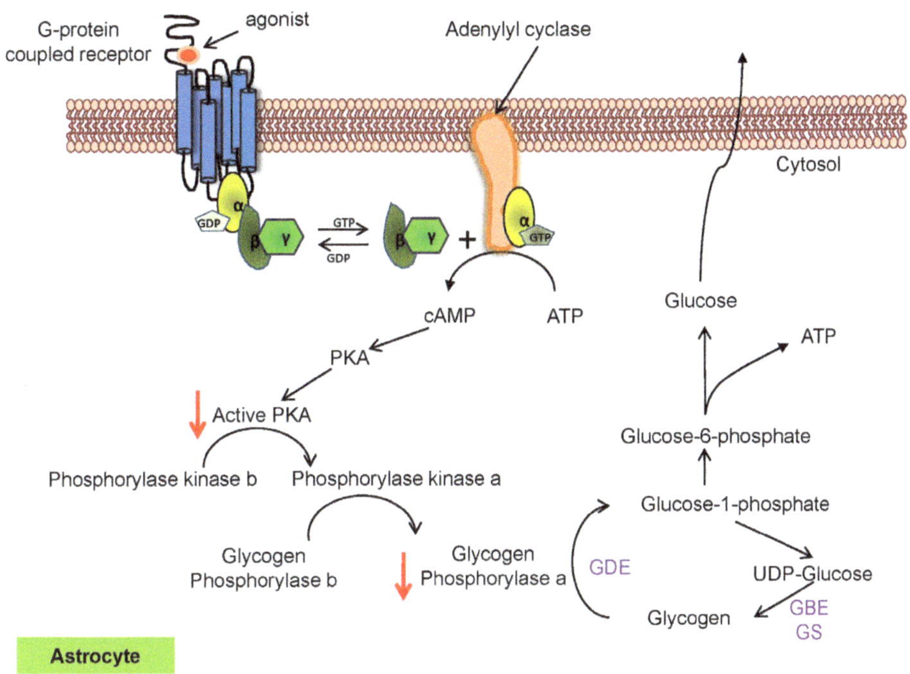

Figure 7. Signaling model of PKA's involvement in impaired glycogen metabolism during ischemic stroke. Within astrocytes under physiological conditions, the binding of an agonist to its receptor leads to the activation of G-proteins (α, β and γ subunits), which in turn activate adenylyl cyclase (AC). Active AC then converts ATP to cAMP that binds to the regulatory subunits of tetrameric PKA. This releases free catalytic subunits that phosphorylate phosphorylase kinase b to convert it to active phosphorylase kinase a. Active phosphorylase kinase then phosphorylates GP*b* to GP*a* initiating glycogen breakdown to provide energy for associating neurons [4,59]. Inhibition of PKA activity during ischemic conditions, however suppresses this downstream signaling cascade that is essential for glycogen metabolism leading to the accumulation of glycogen in astrocytes in the stroke-affected brain.

The MTT assay data showed that cell viability was significantly higher in either CP-316819 or DAB treated astrocytes compared with that of the DMSO treated or control astrocytes (untreated) respectively at each time points of hypoxia (Figure 6B and C, respectively n = 5; $^{\#}P<0.05$). The LDH assay revealed that CP-316819 or DAB treated astrocytes had significantly decreased level of LDH released in the culture medium compared with that of the DMSO treated or control (untreated) astrocytes under hypoxic conditions (Figure 6D and E, respectively, n = 5; $^{\#}P<0.05$). Viability of the astrocytes following 24 hours of hypoxia by calcein AM and EthD-1 showed that both CP-316819 and DAB treated astrocytes contained more viable cells (green) compared with DMSO treated or untreated astrocytes, respectively (Figure 6F). Moreover, the live to dead cell ratios revealed that CP-316819 or DAB treated astrocytes had significantly higher number of live cells compared with the control groups of astrocytes (Figure 6G, n = 5; $^{\#}P<0.05$).

Discussion

During ischemic stroke extracellular potassium levels rise within a few seconds of ischemic insults, which is preceded by rapid Ca^{2+} influx and a fall in ATP levels, triggering cascades of numerous ionic and biochemical events that initiate cellular demise [2,20,38]. The ability of ischemic tissue to recover normal functions requires a sustained supply of energy to re-establish the electrolyte imbalances between the intracellular and extracellular compartments that arise during the insult [2,4]. Brain glycogen has been reported to serve as an endogenous source of metabolic energy during periods of ischemia and can be targeted as a therapeutic approach to cerebral ischemia [39,40].

In the present study, we found an increase in the level of glycogen in the stroke-affected brain between 6 and 24 hours post-stroke (Figure 1B) suggesting impaired glycogen metabolism. To determine the signaling pathways involved in this process, we measured the expression level and activity of glycogen synthesizing enzymes GBE and GS. These enzymes are responsible for elongation of newly synthesized glycogen molecules by forming α-1,4-glycosidic linkages with UDP-glucose as the glucosyl donor and α-1,6-glycosidic linkages. We found no changes in the expression level of GBE, nor changes in the expression and activity of GS (Figure 1C, D and E), suggesting that these enzymes are not of the direct cause for glycogen accumulation in the ischemic brain.

Enzymatic cleavage of glycogen to generate glucose-1-phosphate during scarcity of glucose is exclusively catalyzed by GP in conjunction with GDE, the enzyme essential for removing branched glucose chains in the glycogen particle. Decreased activity and expression level of these enzymes would contribute to the accumulation of glycogen. We clearly showed a decreased GP activity in stroke-affected rat brains at 6 and 24 hours post-stroke (Figure 2B and C) that would contribute to the increased glycogen amount. In addition, we unexpectedly found significantly reduced expression of GDE in the ischemic stroke brain at these time points (Figure 2A). Reduced GDE expression was further validated by reduced mRNA level of GDE gene, *Agl* in the stroke brain (Figure 3C). The mechanism behind this reduced GDE mRNA expression has never been reported but suggests that the stroke-induced cellular environment includes a negative regulator of GDE gene expression. This observed GDE expression, would lead to incomplete glycogen breakdown since GP cannot degrade glycogen beyond the α-1,6 branch points. Therefore, only 30% of the glycogen particle could be degraded by GP [41] before resynthesis could take over again. Furthermore, given that GP is also partially inactive, the amount of available glucose derived from glycogen breakdown would be significantly blunted in the stroke-affected brain.

Our investigation in hypoxic astrocytes confirmed these data with increased glycogen (Figure 4B), decreased PKA and GP activity (Figure 4C, D, E and F) and decreased GDE expression (Figure 4G), suggesting similar signaling pathways are involved in the regulation of glycogen metabolism during ischemic stroke and hypoxia. During a shortage of cellular ATP, β_1 and/or β_2 adrenergic receptors are activated and trigger a cascade of signal transduction activating adenylyl cyclase (AC) [42]. Active AC converts ATP to cAMP leading to PKA activation. Active PKA phosphorylates and activates PhK, which in turn, activates GP by phosphorylating Ser-14 leading to glycogen breakdown [43]. PhK can also be activated by intracellular Ca^{2+} and directly phophorylates GP, converting it from inactive (GP*b*) to active (GP*a*) form [36]. The decreased PKA activity in the stroke-affected brain between 6 and 24 hours (Figure 2D and E) suggests insensitivity of the adrenoreceptors to the energy-deficient state. This insensitivity might be the result of increased expression of β-arrestin-1 during cerebral ischemia [44], which binds G-protein receptor kinase (GRK)-mediated phosphorylated form of the adrenoreceptors, preventing coupling of the receptor with G-protein, and also recruits phosphodiesterases that mediate degradation of cAMP [45–47]. Uncoupling of the receptor also causes receptor internalization through β-arrestin and clarithin depended pathway and reduces the number of functional receptors available in the cell membrane [47–49]. Low levels of cAMP might also be responsible for decreased PKA and adrenoreceptor activity as both are regulated by cAMP [42,50,51]. We hypothesized that the decreased activity of PKA contributes to the accumulation of glycogen in stroke brain and in the primary cerebellar astrocytes (Figure 5C and D), possibly by suppressing activity of GP (Figure 5E and F).

Increased glycogen accumulation following induction of stroke could also be caused by glycogen supercompensation, a phenomenon that has been observed in the skeletal muscle following exercise and in the brain [52]. The mechanism, in muscle at least, is caused by activation of GS and inactivation of GP [53] but the mechanism in the brain is unknown. Glycogen supercompensation may be a protective measure taken by the affected tissue in preparation for the next bout of metabolic stress [23]. Therefore, the increased glycogen observed during hypoglycaemia and also in this study of ischemia/hypoxia could be considered similar, as they both occur following metabolic stress. Furthermore, elevated glycogen can also protect astrocytes during hypoxia as we demonstrated (Figure 6) and as shown previously [13,54].

A schematic diagram (Figure 7) based on the data we found indicates that inhibition of PKA activity decreases GP activity resulting in impaired breakdown of glycogen. Manipulation of these pathways may be a beneficial strategy for optimization of brain glycogen metabolism and maintenance of glucose homeostasis during ischemic stroke. Beneficial effects of pharmacological manipulation of cAMP/PKA-mediated pathways have been recently documented in other diseases including diabetes and cancer [55,56], suggesting that this approach should be investigated in animal models of ischemic stroke to test the efficacy as a therapeutic intervention. Furthermore, compounds that increase cAMP generation in astrocytes might be useful in providing metabolic support to neurons during conditions such as glucose deprivation and intense neuronal activity by mobilizing glycogen content in astrocytes. In support of this, soluble adenylyl cyclase (sAC) has been reported to propagate cellular cascades to meet metabolic demands by initiating breakdown of glycogen. HCO_3^- mediated activation of sAC increases cAMP concentration [57], leading to the breakdown of glycogen [58] thereby providing an alternative energy source to neurons. Recently, it has been demonstrated that sAC is highly expressed in astrocytes and activation of this enzyme increases glycogen breakdown via increased intracellular cAMP to provide energy to neurons [42].

In summary, we demonstrate that decreased PKA activity along with decreased GP activity and GDE expression induce impaired glycogen metabolism in ischemic stroke rat brain. To the best of our knowledge this is the first comprehensive study of the regulation of metabolic enzymes in the ischemic stroke brain projecting new light in glycogen metabolism and may provide new therapeutic intervention strategies to prolong cellular activity and minimize post-ischemic damage.

Supporting Information

Supporting Information S1 Supplement information and supporting figures.

Acknowledgments

We thank Dr Heung-Chin Cheng and Ashfaqul Hoque for rat brain sample lysates, Jian Zheng for helping during rat primary astrocyte and cortical neuron culture and Daniel Ham for statistical analysis.

Author Contributions

Conceived and designed the experiments: MIH CLR DIS. Performed the experiments: MIH. Wrote the paper: MIH CLR DIS. Read and approved final manuscript: MIH CLR DIS.

References

1. Lo EH (2010) Degeneration and repair in central nervous system disease. Nat Med 16: 1205–1209.
2. Moskowitz MA, Lo EH, Iadecola C (2010) The science of stroke: mechanisms in search of treatments. Neuron 67: 181–198.
3. Lipton P (1999) Ischemic cell death in brain neurons. Physiol Rev 79: 1431–1568.
4. Rossi DJ, Brady JD, Mohr C (2007) Astrocyte metabolism and signaling during brain ischemia. Nat Neurosci 10: 1377–1386.
5. Roach PJ (2002) Glycogen and its metabolism. Curr Mol Med 2: 101–120.
6. Roach PJ, Depaoli-Roach AA, Hurley TD, Tagliabracci VS (2012) Glycogen and its metabolism: some new developments and old themes. Biochem J 441: 763–787.
7. Kong J, Shepel PN, Holden CP, Mackiewicz M, Pack AI, et al. (2002) Brain glycogen decreases with increased periods of wakefulness: implications for homeostatic drive to sleep. J Neurosci 22: 5581–5587.
8. Suh SW, Bergher JP, Anderson CM, Treadway JL, Fosgerau K, et al. (2007) Astrocyte glycogen sustains neuronal activity during hypoglycemia: studies with the glycogen phosphorylase inhibitor CP-316,819 ([R-R*,S*]-5-chloro-N-[2-hydroxy-3-(methoxymethylamino)-3-oxo-1-(phenylmethyl)pro pyl]-1H-indole-2-carboxamide). J Pharmacol Exp Ther 321: 45–50.
9. Gibbs ME, Anderson DG, Hertz L (2006) Inhibition of glycogenolysis in astrocytes interrupts memory consolidation in young chickens. Glia 54: 214–222.
10. Shulman RG, Hyder F, Rothman DL (2001) Cerebral energetics and the glycogen shunt: neurochemical basis of functional imaging. Proc Natl Acad Sci U S A 98: 6417–6422.
11. Tekkok SB, Brown AM, Westenbroek R, Pellerin L, Ransom BR (2005) Transfer of glycogen-derived lactate from astrocytes to axons via specific monocarboxylate transporters supports mouse optic nerve activity. J Neurosci Res 81: 644–652.

12. Rahman B, Kussmaul L, Hamprecht B, Dringen R (2000) Glycogen is mobilized during the disposal of peroxides by cultured astroglial cells from rat brain. Neurosci Lett 290: 169–172.
13. Brown AM, Sickmann HM, Fosgerau K, Lund TM, Schousboe A, et al. (2005) Astrocyte glycogen metabolism is required for neural activity during aglycemia or intense stimulation in mouse white matter. J Neurosci Res 79: 74–80.
14. Hertz L, Gibbs ME (2009) What learning in day-old chickens can teach a neurochemist: focus on astrocyte metabolism. J Neurochem 109 Suppl 1: 10–16.
15. Hertz L, O'Dowd BS, Ng KT, Gibbs ME (2003) Reciprocal changes in forebrain contents of glycogen and of glutamate/glutamine during early memory consolidation in the day-old chick. Brain Res 994: 226–233.
16. Simpson IA, Carruthers A, Vannucci SJ (2007) Supply and demand in cerebral energy metabolism: the role of nutrient transporters. J Cereb Blood Flow Metab 27: 1766–1791.
17. Mangia S, Simpson IA, Vannucci SJ, Carruthers A (2009) The in vivo neuron-to-astrocyte lactate shuttle in human brain: evidence from modeling of measured lactate levels during visual stimulation. J Neurochem 109 Suppl 1: 55–62.
18. DiNuzzo M, Mangia S, Maraviglia B, Giove F (2010) Glycogenolysis in astrocytes supports blood-borne glucose channeling not glycogen-derived lactate shuttling to neurons: evidence from mathematical modeling. J Cereb Blood Flow Metab 30: 1895–1904.
19. DiNuzzo M, Mangia S, Maraviglia B, Giove F (2010) Changes in glucose uptake rather than lactate shuttle take center stage in subserving neuroenergetics: evidence from mathematical modeling. J Cereb Blood Flow Metab 30: 586–602.
20. Dinuzzo M, Mangia S, Maraviglia B, Giove F (2012) The role of astrocytic glycogen in supporting the energetics of neuronal activity. Neurochem Res 37: 2432–2438.
21. Xu J, Song D, Xue Z, Gu L, Hertz L, et al. (2013) Requirement of glycogenolysis for uptake of increased extracellular K+ in astrocytes: potential implications for K+ homeostasis and glycogen usage in brain. Neurochem Res 38: 472–485.
22. Govender D, Ramdial PK, Clarke B, Chetty R (2004) Clear cell (glycogen-rich) gastric adenocarcinoma. Ann Diagn Pathol 8: 69–73.
23. Brucklacher RM, Vannucci RC, Vannucci SJ (2002) Hypoxic preconditioning increases brain glycogen and delays energy depletion from hypoxia-ischemia in the immature rat. Dev Neurosci 24: 411–417.
24. Lau X, Zhang Y, Kelly DJ, Stapleton DI (2013) Attenuation of Armanni-Ebstein lesions in a rat model of diabetes by a new anti-fibrotic, anti-inflammatory agent, FT011. Diabetologia 56: 675–679.
25. Vesce S, Rossi D, Brambilla L, Volterra A (2007) Glutamate release from astrocytes in physiological conditions and in neurodegenerative disorders characterized by neuroinflammation. Int Rev Neurobiol 82: 57–71.
26. Roulston CL, Callaway JK, Jarrott B, Woodman OL, Dusting GJ (2008) Using behaviour to predict stroke severity in conscious rats: post-stroke treatment with 3′, 4′-dihydroxyflavonol improves recovery. Eur J Pharmacol 584: 100–110.
27. Hossain MI, Roulston CL, Kamaruddin MA, Chu PW, Ng DC, et al. (2013) A truncated fragment of Src protein kinase generated by calpain-mediated cleavage is a mediator of neuronal death in excitotoxicity. J Biol Chem 288: 9696–9709.
28. Weston RM, Lin B, Dusting GJ, Roulston CL (2013) Targeting oxidative stress injury after ischemic stroke in conscious rats: limited benefits with apocynin highlight the need to incorporate long term recovery. Stroke Res Treat 2013: 648061.
29. Singaravelu K, Lohr C, Deitmer JW (2006) Regulation of store-operated calcium entry by calcium-independent phospholipase A2 in rat cerebellar astrocytes. J Neurosci 26: 9579–9592.
30. Paquet M, Ribeiro FM, Guadagno J, Esseltine JL, Ferguson SS, et al. (2013) Role of metabotropic glutamate receptor 5 signaling and homer in oxygen glucose deprivation-mediated astrocyte apoptosis. Mol Brain 6: 9.
31. Thomas JA, Schlender KK, Larner J (1968) A rapid filter paper assay for UDPglucose-glycogen glucosyltransferase, including an improved biosynthesis of UDP-14C-glucose. Anal Biochem 25: 486–499.
32. Zhang T, Wang S, Lin Y, Xu W, Ye D, et al. (2012) Acetylation negatively regulates glycogen phosphorylase by recruiting protein phosphatase 1. Cell Metab 15: 75–87.
33. Walls AB, Sickmann HM, Brown A, Bouman SD, Ransom B, et al. (2008) Characterization of 1,4-dideoxy-1,4-imino-d-arabinitol (DAB) as an inhibitor of brain glycogen shunt activity. J Neurochem 105: 1462–1470.
34. Shioda N, Han F, Moriguchi S, Fukunaga K (2007) Constitutively active calcineurin mediates delayed neuronal death through Fas-ligand expression via activation of NFAT and FKHR transcriptional activities in mouse brain ischemia. J Neurochem 102: 1506–1517.
35. Villar-Palasi C, Larner J (1970) Glycogen metabolism and glycolytic enzymes. Annu Rev Biochem 39: 639–672.
36. DiNuzzo M, Mangia S, Maraviglia B, Giove F (2013) Regulatory mechanisms for glycogenolysis and K+ uptake in brain astrocytes. Neurochem Int 63: 458–464.
37. Cataldo AM, Broadwell RD (1986) Cytochemical identification of cerebral glycogen and glucose-6-phosphatase activity under normal and experimental conditions. II. Choroid plexus and ependymal epithelia, endothelia and pericytes. J Neurocytol 15: 511–524.
38. Lo EH, Dalkara T, Moskowitz MA (2003) Mechanisms, challenges and opportunities in stroke. Nat Rev Neurosci 4: 399–415.
39. Otori T, Friedland JC, Sinson G, McIntosh TK, Raghupathi R, et al. (2004) Traumatic brain injury elevates glycogen and induces tolerance to ischemia in rat brain. J Neurotrauma 21: 707–718.
40. Xu L, Sun H (2010) Pharmacological manipulation of brain glycogenolysis as a therapeutic approach to cerebral ischemia. Mini Rev Med Chem 10: 1188–1193.
41. Shearer J, Graham TE (2004) Novel aspects of skeletal muscle glycogen and its regulation during rest and exercise. Exerc Sport Sci Rev 32: 120–126.
42. Choi HB, Gordon GR, Zhou N, Tai C, Rungta RL, et al. (2012) Metabolic communication between astrocytes and neurons via bicarbonate-responsive soluble adenylyl cyclase. Neuron 75: 1094–1104.
43. Newgard CB, Hwang PK, Fletterick RJ (1989) The family of glycogen phosphorylases: structure and function. Crit Rev Biochem Mol Biol 24: 69–99.
44. Lombardi MS, van den Tweel E, Kavelaars A, Groenendaal F, van Bel F, et al. (2004) Hypoxia/ischemia modulates G protein-coupled receptor kinase 2 and beta-arrestin-1 levels in the neonatal rat brain. Stroke 35: 981–986.
45. Gurevich VV, Benovic JL (1993) Visual arrestin interaction with rhodopsin. Sequential multisite binding ensures strict selectivity toward light-activated phosphorylated rhodopsin. J Biol Chem 268: 11628–11638.
46. Baillie GS, Sood A, McPhee I, Gall I, Perry SJ, et al. (2003) beta-Arrestin-mediated PDE4 cAMP phosphodiesterase recruitment regulates beta-adrenoceptor switching from Gs to Gi. Proc Natl Acad Sci U S A 100: 940–945.
47. Premont RT, Inglese J, Lefkowitz RJ (1995) Protein kinases that phosphorylate activated G protein-coupled receptors. FASEB J 9: 175–182.
48. Moore CA, Milano SK, Benovic JL (2007) Regulation of receptor trafficking by GRKs and arrestins. Annu Rev Physiol 69: 451–482.
49. Pierce KL, Lefkowitz RJ (2001) Classical and new roles of beta-arrestins in the regulation of G-protein-coupled receptors. Nat Rev Neurosci 2: 727–733.
50. Laureys G, Clinckers R, Gerlo S, Spooren A, Wilczak N, et al. (2010) Astrocytic beta(2)-adrenergic receptors: from physiology to pathology. Prog Neurobiol 91: 189–199.
51. Dong JH, Chen X, Cui M, Yu X, Pang Q, et al. (2012) beta2-adrenergic receptor and astrocyte glucose metabolism. J Mol Neurosci 48: 456–463.
52. Oz G, Kumar A, Rao JP, Kodl CT, Chow L, et al. (2009) Human brain glycogen metabolism during and after hypoglycemia. Diabetes 58: 1978–1985.
53. Mamedova LK, Shneyvays V, Katz A, Shainberg A (2003) Mechanism of glycogen supercompensation in rat skeletal muscle cultures. Mol Cell Biochem 250: 11–19.
54. Wender R, Brown AM, Fern R, Swanson RA, Farrell K, et al. (2000) Astrocytic glycogen influences axon function and survival during glucose deprivation in central white matter. J Neurosci 20: 6804–6810.
55. Wang D, Luo P, Wang Y, Li W, Wang C, et al. (2013) Glucagon-like peptide-1 protects against cardiac microvascular injury in diabetes via a cAMP/PKA/Rho-dependent mechanism. Diabetes 62: 1697–1708.
56. Gold MG, Gonen T, Scott JD (2013) Local cAMP signaling in disease at a glance. J Cell Sci 126: 4537–4543.
57. Chen Y, Cann MJ, Litvin TN, Iourgenko V, Sinclair ML, et al. (2000) Soluble adenylyl cyclase as an evolutionarily conserved bicarbonate sensor. Science 289: 625–628.
58. Sorg O, Magistretti PJ (1992) Vasoactive intestinal peptide and noradrenaline exert long-term control on glycogen levels in astrocytes: blockade by protein synthesis inhibition. J Neurosci 12: 4923–4931.
59. Brown AM, Baltan Tekkok S, Ransom BR (2004) Energy transfer from astrocytes to axons: the role of CNS glycogen. Neurochem Int 45: 529–536.
60. Stapleton D, Nelson C, Parsawar K, McClain D, Gilbert-Wilson R, et al. (2010) Analysis of hepatic glycogen-associated proteins. Proteomics 10: 2320–2329.
61. Parker GJ, Koay A, Gilbert-Wilson R, Waddington LJ, Stapleton D (2007) AMP-activated protein kinase does not associate with glycogen alpha-particles from rat liver. Biochem Biophys Res Commun 362: 811–815.

2

Dynamic Cerebral Autoregulation Is Heterogeneous in Different Subtypes of Acute Ischemic Stroke

Zhen-Ni Guo[1]⁹, Jia Liu[2]⁹, Yingqi Xing[3], Shuo Yan[1], Cunling Lv[1], Hang Jin[1], Yi Yang[1]*

1 Neuroscience Center, Department of Neurology, the First Norman Bethune Hospital of Jilin University, Chang Chun, China, **2** Shenzhen Institutes of Advanced Technology, Chinese Academy of Sciences, Xueyuan Avenue, Shenzhen University Town, Shenzhen, China, **3** Center for Neurovascular ultrasound, the First Norman Bethune Hospital of Jilin University, Chang Chun, China

Abstract

Background and Purpose: Stroke of large-artery atherosclerosis and small-artery occlusion are two main subtypes of stroke according to TOAST classification. The underlying mechanisms of how these two subtypes affect dynamic cerebral autoregulation (dCA) might be heterogeneous, resulting in varied clinical conditions and outcomes. We therefore studied the pattern of dCA in these two subtypes.

Methods: Forty-one patients with acute unilateral middle cerebral artery (MCA) territory stroke (15 with ipsilateral large-artery atherosclerosis and 26 with small-artery occlusion) and 20 healthy volunteers were enrolled. Non-invasive continuous cerebral blood flow velocity and arterial blood pressure were recorded simultaneously from each subject in supine position using transcranial Doppler on MCA bilaterally and servo-controlled plethysmograph on the middle finger, respectively. Transfer function analysis was applied to derive autoregulatory parameters, gain, phase difference (PD), and slope of step response.

Results: In the large-artery atherosclerosis group, PD in affected hemisphere was 42.9±18.5 degree, which is significantly lower than the unaffected hemisphere (72.4±29.9 degree, $P<0.01$), and the healthy group ($P<0.01$). However, PD is similar in the unaffected hemisphere and healthy group ($P>0.1$). In the small-artery occlusion group, PD in the affected hemisphere was similar to that in the contralateral hemisphere (33.8±17.9 vs. 32.6±21.1 degree, $P>0.1$), both sides were significantly lower than the healthy group (all $P<0.001$).The results of the slope of step response agree with the findings in PD.

Conclusions: DCA in different subtypes of acute ischemic stroke is heterogeneous, which might be attributed to the varied pathologic changes of cerebral blood vessels.

Editor: Mathias Gelderblom, University Hospital-Eppendorf, Germany

Funding: The authors have no funding or support to report.

Competing Interests: The authors have declared that no competing interests exist.

* E-mail: doctor_yangyi@hotmail.com

⁹ These authors contributed equally to this work.

Introduction

Dynamic cerebral autoregulation (dCA) is likely affected in acute ischemic stroke[1,2,3]. Large-artery atherosclerosis and small-artery occlusion (lacune) are considered as the most common subtypes of acute ischemic stroke[4]. However, the underlying mechanisms of how these cerebrovascular diseases affect cerebral hemodynamics might be heterogeneous, resulting in varied clinical conditions and outcomes. The understanding of the pattern of dCA in these subtypes may help in stroke prevention, early treatment, and outcome predictions.

In large-artery stenosis, previous studies suggested that hemodynamics in ipsilateral side is altered due to the reduction of the effectiveness of vasodilation as the related vessels may have already dilated in compromise of hypoperfusion[5,6]. The contralateral side is, however, unlikely to be affected due to the patency of the intracranial anastomoses[6] and other unknown reasons. Whereas, in small-artery occlusion, the changes of hemodynamics are more diffuse as the causes of cerebral small vessel diseases, such as hypertension, diabetes, and etc[7,8], are normally chronic, which might affect dCA bilaterally.

We thus hypothesized that, in large-artery atherosclerosis, the dCA on the ischemic side is more likely impaired than the unaffected side, whilst in unilateral small-artery occlusion, dCA is impaired bilaterally. In the present study, we attempt to investigate this hypothesis by assessing the dCA in large-artery atherosclerosis and small-artery occlusion using transfer function analysis (TFA).

Methods

Participants

All participants gave their written informed consent prior to the investigation. The study protocol and written informed consent form was approved by the ethics committee of the First Norman Bethune Hospital of Jilin University. We carried out a prospective study of consecutive admissions to the Department of Neurology at the First Hospital of Jilin University during April 2013 to October

2013. Patients were included in this study if they (1) a first occurrence of acute ischemic stroke; (2) unilateral middle cerebral artery territory stroke with/without middle cerebral artery (MCA) stenosis; no other intracranial or/and extracranial major vascular stenosis/occlusion; (3) did not receive thrombolytic, interventional or surgical treatment; (4) a sufficient bilateral temporal bone window for insonation of the MCA. Patients with consciousness disorders or inability to cooperate sufficiently to complete the dCA examination, and insufficient quality of dCA signals were excluded. Also, patients were excluded if they had a history of atrial fibrillation, myocardial infarction, unstable angina, diabetes mellitus, visible leukoencephalopathy and dilated perivascular space shown in magnetic resonance imaging (MRI), impaired renal function, autonomic disturbance, or were taking any medication known to affect the cardiovascular or autonomic nervous system at the time of the study. Extracranial and intracranial artery stenosis or occlusion was diagnosed by transcranial Doppler (TCD, MultiDop X2, DWL, Sipplingen, Germany), carotid ultrasound (IU22, Phillips, Andover, Massachusetts, USA) and magnetic resonance angiography (MRA). Stenosis ≥50% of the MCA was determined by a mean velocity> 100 cm/s; stenosis ≥70% of the MCA was determined by a mean velocity >120 cm/s in TCD[9], the results of MRA was used as a reference. Atrial fibrillation, myocardial infarction and/or unstable angina were excluded by cardiologists. Stroke patients were divided into two groups: large-artery atherosclerosis and small-artery occlusion according to TOAST classification[4]. The lacunar on MRI was shown as lesion with a diameter of less than 1.5 cm demonstrated. The large-artery atherosclerosis was diagnosed as infarcts greater than 1.5 cm in diameter on MRI, and a stenosis of greater than 50% in ipsilateral MCA. Patients were excluded if they are not in these two types. Each patient was diagnosed with stroke and classified by two neurologists according to clinical symptoms, MRI, MRA and TCD. Twenty medically and psychiatrically healthy volunteers were recruited as normal controls.

Study Protocol

DCA examination was carried out during 5–10 days of symptom onset. Subjects avoided alcohol, caffeine and nicotine for at least 12 hours before the dCA examination, which were made in a quiet, dedicated research laboratory, at controlled temperature of 20–24 °C with external stimuli minimized. Subjects were asked to adopt a relaxed supine position for 10 minutes, and then the baseline blood pressure was measured at the brachial artery (automatic blood pressure monitor, Omron 711). Continuous cerebral blood flow velocity (CBFV) and arterial blood pressure (ABP) were recorded simultaneously from each subject in supine position for 10 minutes. The recorded data were then used to assess cerebral autoregulation.

The continuous ABP was measured non-invasively using servo-controlled plethysmograph (Finometer Pro, Netherlands) on the middle finger. Endtidal CO2 (EtCO2) was monitored using a capnograph (MultiDop X2, DWL, Sipplingen, Germany) with face mask attached to the nasal cannula. TCD was used to measure CBFV in MCA bilaterally at a depth of 45–60 mm. The probes were fixed with a custom made head frame.

Data Analysis

The recorded data was processed by a personal computer using MATLAB (a suite of commercial software for data processing). Beat-to-beat alignment of the data was achieved using cross-correlation function to remove the possible time lags. A 3rd order Butterworth low-pass filter (cutoff at 0.5 Hz) was then applied as an anti-alias filter before down sampling the data to 1 Hz. The dynamic cerebral autoregulation was evaluated using TFA[10]. Transfer function between ABP and CBFV is calculated as the quotient of the cross-spectrum of the two signals and the autospectrum of ABP in frequency domain. Impulse and frequency responses are derived from TFA. In time domain, step response was calculated by convolution between impulse response and a normalized step to show how CBFV responses to a step change of ABP. A linear regression of the first 4 seconds of the step response was performed and the slope of the regression line was used to quantify how quick CBFV may return to the baseline level, where a steeper slope indicate a faster return[11]. In frequency domain, we estimated phase difference (PD), gain, and coherence function within low frequency range, 0.06–0.12 Hz, to evaluate cerebral autoregulation, where the derived parameters are considered most relevant to this hemodynamics[12]. We only used the autoregulatory parameters for the later statistical analysis if the coherence within 0.06–0.12 Hz is > 0.5.

Statistical Analysis

The statistical program for social sciences version 17.0 (SPSS, IBM, West Grove, PA, USA) was used to analyze all data. The measurement data are expressed as the mean ± SD, and the count data are expressed as the rate (percentage). Student's *t*-test used to identify measurement data. The chi-square test and fisher exact test were used to identify count data. The level of significance was set at $P<0.05$

Results

Demographic information

In total, 41 patients (50.7±12.0 years; 33 males and 8 females) were enrolled in the study. Fifteen patients were the large-artery atherosclerosis group (44.7±13.1 years; 12 males and 3 females) and twenty-six patients were the small-artery occlusion (54.1±9.7 years; 21 males and 5 females). In the large-artery atherosclerosis group, seven patients (46.7%) had impairment in movement alone, two (13.3%) presented with loss of speech alone, and six (40.0%) had loss of function in both movement and speech; ten patients with MCA stenosis ≥50% and 5 patients with MCA stenosis ≥ 70%. In the small-artery occlusion group, fourteen patients (53.8%) were pure motor stroke, two (7.7%) were pure sensory stroke and ten (38.5%) were sensorimotor stroke. Twenty medically and psychiatrically healthy volunteers (42.2±13.7 years; 16 males and 4 females) served as controls. We did not find any significant differences in sex, heart rate and $EtCO_2$ in the three groups. The patients in the small-artery occlusion group were approximately 10 years older in average than those in the healthy group ($t = 3.4$, $P = 0.001$) and large-artery atherosclerosis group ($t = -2.6$, $P = 0.012$). Simultaneously, the mean blood pressure in the small-artery occlusion group was higher than that in the healthy group ($t = 2.2$, $P = 0.031$). Baseline characteristics of the data are given in Table 1.

Dynamic cerebral autoregulation

Three autoregulatory parameters, gain, PD, and step response, were derived from the transfer function. The valid frequency range for dCA (PD and gain) is 0.06–0.12 Hz and the first 4 seconds of step response was used to calculate the slope. Graphical results are shown in Figure 1 and the statistical analysis of the parameters is given in Table 2 and Figure 2.

Table 1. Baseline characteristics.

	Large-artery atherosclerosis group (n = 15)	Small-artery occlusion group (n = 26)	Controls (n = 20)
Male	12 (80.0%)	21 (80.8%)	16 (80.0%)
Age (years)	44.7±13.1	54.1±9.7	42.2±13.7
Hypertension	7 (46.7%)	19 (73.1%)	0 (0%)
Mean blood pressure (mmHg)	90.0±17.0	101.5±19.7	89.5±16.0
Heart rate (beats/min)	71.7±6.4	71.2±8.8	74.3±7.4
$EtCO_2$ (mm Hg)	36.2±2.6	37.2±2.9	36.4±2.4
NIHSS score	7.1±4.7	3.8±2.8	

Phase difference

In the healthy group, PD (0.06–0.12) between ABP and CBFV was 65.8±24.1 degree in the left hemisphere and 67.4±24.2 degree in the right hemisphere, which is no difference ($t = 0.4$, $P > 0.1$, Table 2, Figure 1 and 2).The overall PD in this group was 66.6±23.8 degree.

In the large-artery atherosclerosis group, PD in affected hemisphere was 42.9±18.5 degree, which is significantly lower than the unaffected hemisphere (72.4±29.9 degree, $t = -4.2$, $P < 0.01$), and the healthy group ($t = -3.4$, $P < 0.01$). However, PD is similar in the unaffected hemisphere and healthy group ($t = -0.74$, $P > 0.1$; Table 2, Figure 1 and 2).

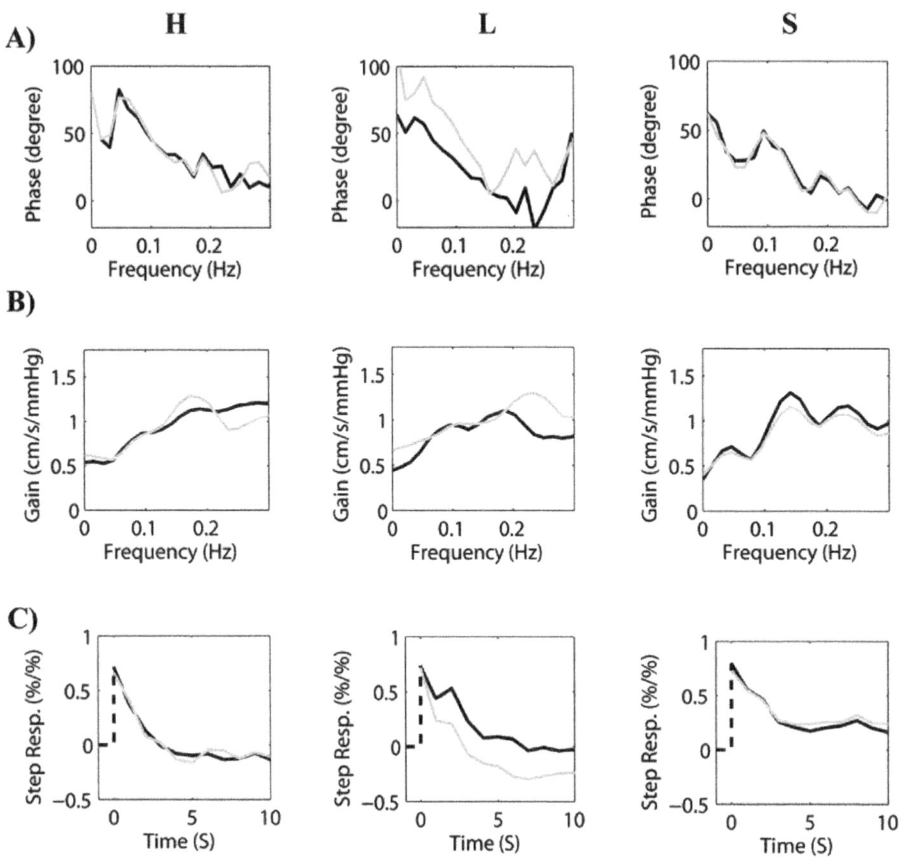

Figure 1. Three autoregulatory parameters, A) phase difference, B) gain, and C) step response, derived from the transfer function are plotted. H (—: right side and —: left side), L (—: affected side and —: unaffected side), and S (same legends as L) denote healthy controls, large-artery atherosclerosis group, and small-artery occlusion group, respectively. The first column shows that all parameters in the healthy group from both sides indicate that autoregulation is intact. There is evident positive phase difference. The shape of high-pass filter can also be speculated. The step response, H-C), shows that cerebral blood flow velocity quickly returns to the baseline level within approximately 4 seconds if a unit step change of arterial blood pressure is induced. In the second column, the parameters changes asymmetrically. Dynamic cerebral autoregulation on the affected side is substantially reduced than the unaffected side with decreased phase difference, flattened gain, and slower return of cerebral blood flow velocity in response to a step change of arterial blood pressure. In the last column, this series of subplots show that autoregulation is worsen bilaterally when comparing with the healthy controls.

Table 2. Phase difference (PD), gain and slope of step response in patients and controls.

		PD (degree)	Gain (cm/s/mmHg)	Slope of step response (%/%)
Healthy group	Left	65.8±24.1	0.72±0.26	−0.24±0.14
	Right	67.4±24.2	0.71± 0.35	−0.23±0.15
	Overall	66.6±23.8	0.71±0.30	−0.23±0.14
Large-artery atherosclerosis	Affected hemisphere	42.9±18.5*†	0.81±0.53	−0.14±0.15 *†
	Unaffected hemisphere	72.4±29.9	0.83±0.32	−0.24±0.11
Small-artery occlusion	Affected hemisphere	33.8±17.9†	0.66±0.31	−0.17±0.09†
	Unaffected hemisphere	32.6±21.1†	0.62±0.26	−0.15±0.08†

*and †denote the same statistical meaning as Figure 2.

In the small-artery occlusion group, PD in the affected hemisphere was similar to that in the contralateral hemisphere (33.8±17.9 vs. 32.6±21.1 degree, t = 0.60, $P>0.1$), both sides were significantly lower than the healthy group (all $P<0.001$, Table2, Figure 1 and 2).

Gain

There was no difference between groups and two sides in each group (all $P>0.05$, Table 2, Figure 1 and 2).

Step response

In the healthy group and the small-artery occlusion group, there is no significant difference between the two sides within these groups for the slopes of the step response. However, the overall slope of the healthy group (−0.23±0.14) is steeper (larger absolute value) than the affected and unaffected sides of the small-artery occlusion group (affected: −0.17±0.09, t = 2.1, $P<0.05$; unaffected: −0.15±0.08, t = 2.8, $P<0.01$; Table 2, Figure 1 and 2), respectively.

The characteristics of step response in the large-artery atherosclerosis group are asymmetric. The slope on the unaffected side is significantly steeper than the affected side (−0.24±0.11 vs. 0.14±0.15, t = 3.1, $P<0.01$; Table 2, Figure 1 and 2). Furthermore, there is no difference between the unaffected side and the healthy group (t = −0.17, $P>0.1$), whereas the slope on the affected side is flatter than the controls (t = 2.0, $P<0.05$).

Discussion

The main findings of this study are that, in stroke patients: 1) dCA is impaired at the affected side in the patients with large-artery atherosclerosis, whereas dCA on the unaffected contralateral side remains intact; 2) the dCA is impaired bilaterally in patients with unilateral small-artery occlusion. These agree with our hypothesis and suggest that cerebral hemodynamics is varied in different stroke subtypes, indicating that the underlying mechanisms of how dCA is altered in these clinical conditions are different.

It has been reported that in the patients with severe unilateral carotid and MCA stenosis, dCA is impaired ipsilaterally when compared with the contralateral sides[5,13,14]. Immink *et al* found that dCA is impaired ipsilaterally on the ischemic side in the patients with unilateral large MCA territory infarcts[7]. However, these authors did not link acute ischemic stroke with artery stenosis. In this study, we considered the underlying relationship of these two and focused on this specific subtype of ischemic stroke (large-artery atherosclerosis in TOAST classification). This can eliminate the influence of other subtypes of stroke, such as cardioembolism, small artery occlusion and unexplained stroke.

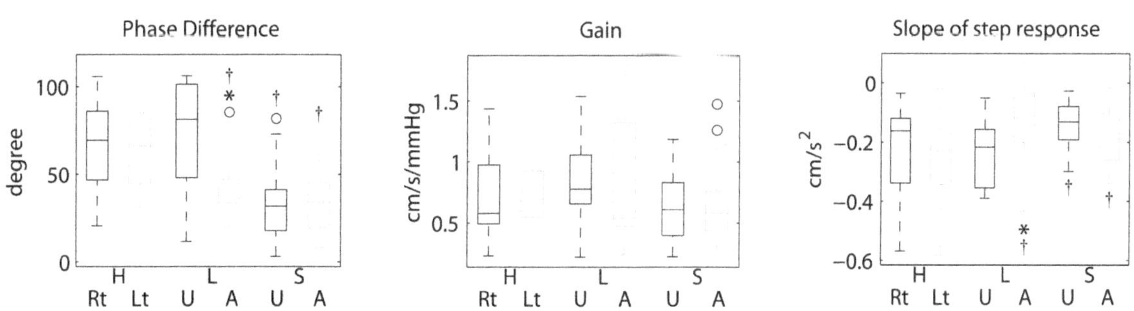

Figure 2. Statistical distributions of the autoregulatory parameters for each category are shown above. A) Phase difference (PD) from the affected side in the large-artery atherosclerosis group is significantly lower than the contralateral side as well the healthy group. PD from the small-artery occlusion group is bilaterally lower than those in the healthy group but there is no difference within the group. B) No statistical difference is detected using gain. C) The results of the slope of step response agree with the findings in PD. Flatter slope (the value of the slope of step response is closer to zero) is observed within the affected side in large-artery atherosclerosis group than in other conditions. The slope in the small-artery occlusion group is also flatter than the healthy controls only. H, L, and S denote the three groups as Figure 1. Rt and Lt stand for right and left side, respectively, for the healthy controls. U and A denote unaffected and affected sides, respectively, for the patients. For each box plot, the central mark is the median and the edges of the box are the 25th and 75th percentiles, the whiskers extend to the most extreme data points which are not outliers, and the outliers are plotted individually as 'o'. *denotes $P<0.05$ for comparing between two sides within the same group. † denotes $P<0.05$ for comparing with the overall of healthy group.

We thus consider that the ipsilateral change of dCA is mainly attributed to the large-artery stenosis, causing vasodilatation of the vessels in ipsilateral MCA territory in compromise of hypoperfusion. The relatively high mean value (42.9±18.5 degree, Table 2) of PD on the affected side may be contributed by collateral circulation, which is developed with progressive artery stenosis[15]. However, there is a limitation when analyzing this subtype as we cannot answer whether acute large-artery stroke additionally impairs autoregulation, because a moderate or severe upstream stenosis can cause impairment of dCA[5,13,14] and there was lack of control group with asymptomatic stenosis of the same degree and same collateral capacity for comparison.

We also noted that there were other studies showing that the impairment of dCA may spread to the contralateral side, which is manifested in 5–14 days after onset[2,16,17]. In order to achieve comparable results, we recorded the data during 5–10 days after onset and our results however did not agree with these studies. We considered the difference is mainly due to the more strict inclusion criteria, with lacunar infarction, cardioembolism and unexplained stroke excluded.

In small-artery occlusion, we included unilateral middle cerebral artery territory acute lacunar infarction and our results are consistent with Immink *et al*'s group that dCA is impaired bilaterally in lacunar stroke patients[7]. Some authors attributed this to cerebral small vessel disease[7,8] caused by chronic diseases such as hypertension, diabetes, and etc. Though the real mechanisms of cerebral small vessel diseases remain uncertain, one of the main explanations of these pathological vascular abnormalities is arteriolosclerosis[8,18], which increases stiffness of small vessels and decreases the systolic and diastolic function. Therefore dCA is impaired and the function of clearance of embolus decreased followed by uncontrolled CBF, eventually leading to embolism[19,20]. It should be emphasized that cerebral small vessel disease is diffuse. The impairment of dCA in MCA may therefore represent the impairment of the whole cerebral small vessels. We thus believe that it is more likely that dCA is an important risk factor that leads to acute lacunar rather than caused by acute lacunar, because the infarcts are small, and less likely to cause global impairment. Impaired dCA can decrease the function of clearance of embolus followed by uncontrolled CBF, eventually leading to embolism and resulting in lacunar infarcts. It is however unknown if acute lacunar can aggravate dCA.

There are a few limitations of the data collection, addressed as follows. Monitoring CBFV in stenotic MCA was difficult in the patients with large-artery atherosclerosis. Data were discarded if signal-to-noise ratio is low, resulting in less data in large-artery atherosclerosis. Male subjects are more than female in our study, as prevalence of stroke in China is higher in men than women[21] and female subjects are more likely to have insufficient bilateral temporal bone window for insonation due to the low density of the temporal bone[22]. We noted that the age and ABP in small-artery occlusion are different from other groups, the differences are one of our limitations in our study. However, as previous studies suggested that small-artery occlusion is likely caused by chronic pathology from hypertension, diabetes, and etc. [7,8], it might be difficult to control these factors which are possibly the risk factors or causes of small-artery occlusion. In addition, we selected patients with mild to moderate symptoms, as they can cooperate with the study, this may however bias the statistical analysis as possible characteristics of dCA of the severe patients might have been ignored.

Conclusions

The current study shows that dCA in different subtypes of acute ischemic stroke is heterogeneous, which might be in association with the varied pathologic changes of cerebral blood vessels. Large artery atheroselerosis affects dCA ipsilaterally, whereas small artery disease is more likely to impair dCA globally.

Acknowledgments

This study was supported by Shuang Wang, YangYang Zhou and Jie Zhang from the Center for Neurovascular ultrasound, the First Norman Bethune Hospital of Jilin University.

Author Contributions

Conceived and designed the experiments: YY. Performed the experiments: ZNG JL YX SY CL. Analyzed the data: ZNG JL HJ. Contributed reagents/materials/analysis tools: ZNG JL YX. Wrote the paper: ZNG JL.

References

1. Eames PJ, Blake MJ, Dawson SL, Panerai RB, Potter JF (2002) Dynamic cerebral autoregulation and beat to beat blood pressure control are impaired in acute ischaemic stroke. J Neurol Neurosurg Psychiatry 72: 467–472.
2. Dawson SL, Panerai RB, Potter JF (2003) Serial changes in static and dynamic cerebral autoregulation after acute ischaemic stroke. Cerebrovascular diseases 16: 69–75.
3. Saeed NP, Panerai RB, Horsfield MA, Robinson TG (2013) Does stroke subtype and measurement technique influence estimation of cerebral autoregulation in acute ischaemic stroke? Cerebrovasc Dis 35: 257–261.
4. Adams HP, Bendixen BH, Kappelle LJ, Biller J, Love BB, et al. (1993) Classification of Subtype of Acute Ischemic Stroke - Definitions for Use in a Multicenter Clinical-Trial. Stroke 24: 35–41.
5. White RP, Markus HS (1997) Impaired dynamic cerebral autoregulation in carotid artery stenosis. Stroke 28: 1340–1344.
6. Kleiser B, Widder B (1992) Course of Carotid-Artery Occlusions with Impaired Cerebrovascular Reactivity. Stroke 23: 171–174.
7. Immink RV, van Montfrans GA, Stam J, Karemaker JM, Diamant M, et al. (2005) Dynamic cerebral autoregulation in acute lacunar and middle cerebral artery territory ischemic stroke. Stroke 36: 2595–2600.
8. Khan U, Porteous L, Hassan A, Markus HS (2007) Risk factor profile of cerebral small vessel disease and its subtypes. Journal of Neurology Neurosurgery and Psychiatry 78: 702–706.
9. Zhao L, Barlinn K, Sharma VK, Tsivgoulis G, Cava LF, et al. (2011) Velocity criteria for intracranial stenosis revisited: an international multicenter study of transcranial Doppler and digital subtraction angiography. Stroke; a journal of cerebral circulation 42: 3429–3434.
10. Zhang R, Zuckerman JH, Giller CA, Levine BD (1998) Transfer function analysis of dynamic cerebral autoregulation in humans. Am J Physiol 274: H233–241.
11. Liu Y, Birch AA, Allen R (2003) Dynamic cerebral autoregulation assessment using an ARX model: comparative study using step response and phase shift analysis. Medical engineering & physics 25: 647–653.
12. Haubrich C, Wendt A, Diehl RR, Klotzsch C (2004) Dynamic autoregulation testing in the posterior cerebral artery. Stroke 35: 848–852.
13. Reinhard M, Roth M, Muller T, Guschlbauer B, Timmer J, et al. (2004) Effect of carotid endarterectomy or stenting on impairment of dynamic cerebral autoregulation. Stroke 35: 1381–1387.
14. Gong XP, Li Y, Jiang WJ, Wang YJ (2006) Impaired dynamic cerebral autoregulation in middle cerebral artery stenosis. Neurological Research 28: 76–81.
15. Henderson RD, Eliasziw M, Fox AJ, Rothwell PM, Barnett HJ (2000) Angiographically defined collateral circulation and risk of stroke in patients with severe carotid artery stenosis. North American Symptomatic Carotid Endarterectomy Trial (NASCET) Group. Stroke 31: 128–132.
16. Reinhard M, Rutsch S, Lambeck J, Wihler C, Czosnyka M, et al. (2012) Dynamic cerebral autoregulation associates with infarct size and outcome after ischemic stroke. Acta Neurologica Scandinavica 125: 156–162.
17. Reinhard M, Roth M, Guschlbauer B, Harloff A, Timmer J, et al. (2005) Dynamic cerebral autoregulation in acute ischemic stroke assessed from spontaneous blood pressure fluctuations. Stroke 36: 1684–1689.
18. Pantoni L (2010) Cerebral small vessel disease: from pathogenesis and clinical characteristics to therapeutic challenges. Lancet Neurology 9: 689–701.

19. Caplan LR, Hennerici M (1998) Impaired clearance of emboli (washout) is an important link between hypoperfusion, embolism, and ischemic stroke. Archives of neurology 55: 1475–1482.
20. Diehl RR (2002) Cerebral autoregulation studies in clinical practice. Eur J Ultrasound 16: 31–36.
21. Liu M, Wu B, Wang WZ, Lee LM, Zhang SH, et al. (2007) Stroke in China: epidemiology, prevention, and management strategies. Lancet Neurology 6: 456–464.
22. Wijnhoud AD, Franckena M, Van Der Lugt A, Koudstaal PJ, Dippel EDWJ (2008) Inadequate acoustical temporal bone window in patients with a transient ischemic attack or minor stroke: Role of skull thickness and bone density. Ultrasound in Medicine and Biology 34: 923–929.

Protective Effect of Glycyrrhizin, a Direct HMGB1 Inhibitor, on Focal Cerebral Ischemia/Reperfusion-Induced Inflammation, Oxidative Stress, and Apoptosis in Rats

Gu Gong[1,¶], Lei Xiang[2,¶], Libang Yuan[3], Ling Hu[1], Wei Wu[1], Lin Cai[1], Liang Yin[1], Hailong Dong[3]*

1 Department of Anaesthesiology, General Hospital of the People's Liberation Army, Chengdu, Sichuan, China, **2** Department of Neurology, Tianjin Huanhu Hospital, Tianjin, China, **3** Department of Anaesthesiology, Xijing Hospital, Fourth Military Medical University, Xi'an, Shaanxi, China

Abstract

Aim: Glycyrrhizin (GL) has been reported to protect against ischemia and reperfusion (I/R)-induced injury by inhibiting the cytokine activity of high mobility group box 1 (HMGB1). In the present study, the protective effects of GL against I/R injury, as well as the related molecular mechanisms, were investigated in rat brains.

Methods: Focal cerebral I/R injury was induced by intraluminal filamentous occlusion of the middle cerebral artery (MCA) in Male Sprague-Dawley rats. GL alone or GL and rHMGB1 were administered intravenously at the time of reperfusion. Serum levels of HMGB1 and inflammatory mediators were quantified via enzyme-linked immunosorbent assay (ELISA). Histopathological examination, immunofluorescence, RT-PCR and western blotting analyses were performed to investigate the protective and anti-apoptotic effects and related molecular mechanisms of GL against I/R injury in rat brains.

Results: Pre-treatment with GL significantly reduced infarct volume and improved the accompanying neurological deficits in locomotor function. The release of HMGB1 from the cerebral cortex into the serum was inhibited by GL administration. Moreover, pre-treatment with GL alleviated apoptotic injury resulting from cerebral I/R through the inhibition of cytochrome C release and caspase 3 activity. The expression levels of inflammation- and oxidative stress-related molecules including TNF-α, iNOS, IL-1β, and IL-6, which were over-expressed in I/R, were decreased by GL. P38 and P-JNK signalling were involved in this process. All of the protective effects of GL could be reversed by rHMGB1 administration.

Conclusions: GL has a protective effect on ischemia-reperfusion injury in rat brains through the inhibition of inflammation, oxidative stress and apoptotic injury by antagonising the cytokine activity of HMGB1.

Editor: Ronald J. Korthuis, University of Missouri, United States of America

Funding: This study was supported by the State Key Program of the National Natural Science Foundation of China (Grant NO. 110469), Sichuan Province and Chengdu military area command general hospital Awards Fund (2011YG-A06). The funders had no role in study design, data collection and analysis, decision to publish, or preparation of the manuscript.

Competing Interests: The authors have declared that no competing interests exist.

* E-mail: hldong2012_12@163.com

¶ These authors contributed equally to this work.

Introduction

Ischemic stroke remains one of the leading cause of death and disability worldwide. Recent insight into the basic mechanism involved in ischemic stroke indicates that endothelial dysfunctions along with oxidative stress and neuroinflammation represent key elements in the occurrence and development of ischemic brain damage that results in cell damage and death [1,2]. Within hours of the ischemic insult, infiltrating leukocytes, as well as resident brain cells including neurons and glia, may release pro-inflammatory mediators such as cytokines, chemokines, and oxygen/nitrogen free radicals that contribute to the evolution of tissue damage [3]. Furthermore, the cerebral ischemia that occurs in brain cells affected by a stroke triggers a complex array of molecular and cellular alterations including the activation of signalling pathways that may either contribute to neuronal damage or protect neurons. Mitogen-activated protein kinases (MAPKs) have crucial roles in signal transduction from the cell surface to the nucleus and regulate cell death and survival processes. Among the MAPK pathways known to be activated in neurons in response to ischemia are the JNK, ERK, and p38 MAPK pathways [4,5].

High mobility group box 1 (HMGB1), a ubiquitous and abundant nuclear protein, can either be passively released into the extracellular milieu in response to necrotic signals or actively secreted in response to inflammatory signals [6–8]. Recently, HMGB1 has been reported to be a potent pro-inflammatory cytokine-like factor that contributes to the pathogenesis of vasculature and connects excitotoxicity-induced acute damage processes with delayed inflammatory processes in the post-ischemic brain [9,10]. The receptor for advanced glycation end products (RAGE), one of the most important receptors for HMGB1, functions as a sensor of necrotic cell death, and the HMGB1–RAGE signalling axis contributes to inflammation and ischemic brain damage [11]. Intravenous injection of neutralising anti-HMGB1 mAb or intranasal delivery of HMGB1 siRNA conferred robust neuroprotection in the post-ischemic brain by antagonising the pro-inflammatory function of HMGB1 [12,13].

Glycyrrhizin (GL) is a major active constituent of *Glycyrrhiza glabra* root and is composed of a molecule of glycyrrhizic acid and two molecules of glucuronic acid. This compound has been associated with numerous pharmacological effects, including anti-inflammatory, anti-viral, anti-tumour, and hepatoprotective activities, and is commonly used in Asia to treat patients with chronic hepatitis [14–17]. It was reported by Sitia et al [18] that, as an HMGB1 inhibitor, GL binds directly to HMGB1 (Kd ~150 μM), interacting with two shallow concave surfaces formed by the two arms of both HMG boxes. GL has been reported to protect from I/R-induced injury in many organs, including the liver [19], spinal cord [20] and heart [21], by inhibiting the chemoattractant and mitogenic functions of HMGB1. Recently, a robust neuroprotective effect of Stronger Neo-Minophagen C (SNMC), a GL-containing preparation, has been reported in the post-ischemic brain, and this neuroprotective effect is due, at least in part, to an anti-inflammatory effect [22]. However, it is not known if the neuroprotective effect of GL occurs through the antagonism of HMGB1 and the ensuing molecular signalling events. Therefore, the aim of this study was to investigate the potential protective effect of GL, as well as the related mechanisms, against I/R injury in the rat brain, mainly in relation to the following aspects: (1) the neuroprotective effects of GL on focal cerebral ischemia; (2) the release of HMGB1 in rat serum and brain; (3) the effect of GL on the alleviation of apoptosis caused by I/R injury; (4) the expression of HMGB1-dependent inflammation- and oxidative stress-related molecules; (5) the involvement of certain MAPK pathways that are modulated by GL.

Materials and Methods

Animals and groups

All experiments were performed in accordance with the "Guide for the Care and Use of Laboratory Animals" published by the US NIH (National Institutes of Health Publication No. 85-23, revised 1996) and were approved by the Committee on Animal Experiments of the Sichuan Neurosurgical Institute. Male Sprague-Dawley rats weighing 325±25 g were obtained from the Experimental Animal Centre of the Sichuan Neurosurgical Institute (China) and were allowed free access to laboratory chow and tap water in day-night quarters at 25°C. Rats were randomly divided into the following four experimental groups of 8 animals each: (1) healthy control, sham-operated rats (the sham group); (2) I/R rats pre-treated with saline (the NS group); (3,4,5) I/R rats pre-treated with GL separately at doses of 2 mg/kg, 4 mg/kg and 10 mg/kg (the 2 mg/kg, 4 mg/kg and 10 mg/kg GL groups); (6) I/R rats pre-treated with GL and recombinant HMGB1 (100 μg per rat) (the GL+rHMGB1 group). In the pre-treatment groups, after 30 min ischemia and before reperfusion, NS, GL or GL plus rHMGB1 was administered intravenously in the tail vein in a volume of 0.5 ml followed by a 48 h reperfusion.

Focal cerebral I/R

Focal cerebral ischemia was induced by performing intraluminal filamentous occlusion of the middle cerebral artery (MCA) for 60 min, according to methods that have been described previously [23]. After 60 min of MCA occlusion, reperfusion of the MCA was initiated by removing the MCA-occlusive filament. The right femoral artery was cannulated to monitor mean arterial blood pressure, arterial blood gases, and pH. Regional cerebral blood flow was monitored using a laser Doppler flowmeter (Periflux System 5000; Perimed, Jarfalla, Sweden). A thermoregulated heating pad and an overhead heating lamp were used to maintain a rectal temperature of 37±0.5°C. In sham-operated rats, an incision was made over the MCA, but the artery was not occluded. The cerebral I/R injury model was developed with 60 min of MCA occlusion followed by 48 h reperfusion.

Triphenyltetrazolium chloride (TTC) staining and infarct volume assessments

Coronal brain sections (2-mm thickness) were incubated with 2% TTC at 37°C for 30 min with gentle shaking and then fixed with 10% formalin in PBS. The stained slices were photographed, and the size of the infarct was quantified using NIH image software.

TTC staining was used to measure infarction volumes two days after I/R (n = 8 per group) and whole brains were dissected coronally into 2-mm brain slices. Two investigators blinded to the study protocol measured the infarct sizes with a computerised image analyser. To account for cerebral oedema and differential shrinkage resulting from tissue processing, the areas of ischemic lesions were determined by subtracting the areas in ipsilateral hemispheres from those of contralateral hemispheres. Infarct volumes were calculated (in mm^3) by multiplying the summed section infarct areas by the section thickness.

Evaluation of neurological deficits

Neurological deficits were evaluated by two methods. In the rota-rod test, rats were conditioned for 3 days before MCA occlusion on an accelerating rota-rod cylinder at 5 to 15 rpm. Rats that could stay on the rotating rod at 15 rpm for 180 s were subjected to MCA occlusion. After MCA occlusion, each rat was subjected to trials conducted at 3 different speeds (5, 10 and 15 rpm), and the mean duration of three trials at each speed on the rota-rod was recorded. The other test was a neurological scoring method, which was performed essentially as described by Bederson et al [24]. The scores were categorised according to four grades (0, normal; 1, moderate; 2, considerable; 3, severe). The modified Neurological Severity Scores system consists of motor, sensory, balance, and reflex tests, all of which are graded using a scale of 0–18 (normal: 0, maximal deficit: 18). The neurological evaluation was performed by an investigator who was blind to the treatment condition.

Serum ELISA detection

Blood samples (0.5 ml) were collected from the femoral vein at 6, 12, 24 and 48 h after reperfusion. Serum was isolated from the blood after centrifugation at 14 000 rpm for 20 min at 4°C. After centrifugation, serum was frozen at −80°C until enzyme-linked immunosorbent assay (ELISA) analyses were performed. HMGB1 concentrations and the levels of inflammatory mediators (TNF-α, iNOS,IL-1β, COX-2 and IL-6) in the serum samples were quantified using specific ELISA kits for rats according to the manufacturer's instructions (Biosource International Inc., Camarillo, CA, USA).

Western blot

Total protein extracts or detached subcellular fractions from rat cerebral tissue were prepared as described previously [25]. The antibodies and the dilutions were as follows: p-JNK No. 9255 (1:2000), t-JNK No. 9252 (1:1000), p-ERK [1/2] No. 9101 (1:1000), t-ERK [1/2] No. 4695 (1:1000), p-p38 No. 9211(1:1000), t-p38 No. 9212 (1:1000) (Cell Signaling Technology, Danvers, Mass), Cytochrome c (1 μg/ml, No. ab90529, Abcam Plc., Cambridge, UK) and HMGB1 (1 μg/ml, No. ab18256, Abcam Plc., Cambridge, UK). Horseradish peroxidase-coupled rabbit and mouse IgG (1:2000) were used as secondary antibodies. Proteins were separated on 10–20% SDS polyacrylamide gels and electrophoretically transferred to polyvinylidene difluoride membranes, which were then incubated overnight at 4°C with the primary antibody diluted in blocking solution. After washing, membranes were treated with horseradish peroxidase-conjugated secondary antibodies and then with enhanced chemiluminescence reagent (Amersham Biosciences, Piscataway, NJ). The film was scanned with a GS-700 imaging densitometer (Bio-Rad Laboratories, Hercules, CA), and the results were quantified with Multi-Analyst software (Bio-Rad Laboratories).

RNA preparation and reverse transcription-PCR

Total RNA was prepared using Trizol reagent (Invitrogen, Gaithersburg, MD) according to the manufacturer's instructions, and 1 μg RNA samples were used for cDNA synthesis. First-strand cDNA synthesis was primed with random hexamers and conducted according to the manufacturer's specifications (RT-PCR kit; Roche, Mannheim, Germany). cDNA equivalent to 200 ng of total RNA was subjected to PCR using the manufacturer's protocol (PCR core kit; Roche). The sense and antisense primers used for the analysis of rat HMGB1, TNF-α, IL-1β, iNOS, COX-2, IL-6 and GAPDH expression were as follows. HMGB1: 5′-CTGATGCAGCTTA TACGAAG-3′ and 5′-TCAGGTAAGGAGCAGAACAT- 3′ (460 bp). TNF-α: 5′-CC-C CTTTATCGTCTACTCCTC-3′ and 5′-GCTGGTAGTT-TAGCTCCGTTT-3′ (553 bp). IL-1β: 5′-TCATTGTGGCTG-TGGAGAAG-3′ and 5′-CTATGTCCCGACCATTGCTG-3′ (579 bp). iNOS: 5′-GCATCCCAAGTACGAGTGGT-3′ and 5′-GAAGGCGTAG CTGAACAAGG-3′ (700 bp). COX-2: 5′-GTGGGATGACGAGCGACTGT-3′ and 5′ -TTTCAGGGAG-AAGCGTTTGC-3′ (454 bp). IL-6: 5′-GGATACCACCCA-CAACAGAC-3′ and 5′-TTGCCGAGTAGACCTCATAG-3′ (520 bp). GAPDH: 5′-CCATCAC TGCCACTCAGAAGA-3′ and 5′-CATGAGGTCCACCACCCTGT- 3′ (446 bp). The annealing temperature was 55°C for all primer pairs.

Immunofluorescence and TUNEL staining

Brains were isolated and fixed with 4% paraformaldehyde by transcardial perfusion and post-fixed in the same solution overnight at 4°C. Coronal brain sections (20 μm) from the ischemic core region were prepared using a vibratome (Leica, Solms, Germany), and immunological staining was performed using a previously described floating method [26]. Rabbit anti-HMGB1 (ab18956; Abcam, Cambridge, UK) antibody was used at a 1:500 dilution. FITC-labelled anti-rabbit IgG (Jackson ImmunoResearch Laboratories, West Grove, PA) was used as a secondary antibody for anti-HMGB1.

The terminal deoxynucleotidyl transferase-mediated dUTP-biotin nick end labelling (TUNEL) assay was carried out with a commercial TUNEL kit (Roche, Switzerland) according to the manufacturer's instructions. Apoptotic cells in the rat heart after I/R in each group were counted separately using Image J software.

Analysis of superoxide and peroxynitrite formation

The oxidative fluorescent dye dihydroethidium (DHE; Sigma-Aldrich) was used to evaluate in situ superoxide production [27]. Frozen, enzymatically intact brains from the ischemic core region were cut into 30-μm thick sections and placed on glass slides. The sections were simultaneously incubated with DHE (10 μmol/L) in phosphate-buffered saline for 30 min at 37°C, in a humidified chamber that was shielded from light. We also monitored peroxynitrite formation by detecting nitrosylated tyrosine residues on proteins. We performed immunostaining with an anti-3-nitrotyrosine (3-NT) antibody (1:1000; Upstate Biotechnology). Coronal sections cut through the striatum (3 sections per brain, 1 mm in width) were imaged in parallel. Superoxide or 3-NT–positive cells were manually counted in the eight regions around the striatum under ×100 magnification using a laser scanning confocal microscope equipped with a Bio-Rad MRC 1024 (argon and krypton).

Measurement of lipid peroxidation

Malondialdehyde (MDA) was estimated as an indicator of lipid peroxidation (n = 8 per group). Brain tissues were homogenised with sodium phosphate buffer (pH 7.4). The reagents (1.5 ml acetic acid, 1.5 ml thiobarbituric acid, and 0.2 ml sodium dodecyl sulphate) were added to 0.1 ml of processed tissue sample. The mixture was then heated at 100°C for 60 min. The mixture was cooled with tap water and 5 ml of n-butanol:pyridine (15:1), and 1 ml of distilled water was added. After centrifugation at 4000 rpm for 10 min, the organic layer was withdrawn and the absorbance was measured at 532 nm using a spectrophotometer.

Statistical analysis

All data were expressed as the means±SEM (standard error of the mean). SPSS 17.0 was used for statistical analysis of the data. The concentrations of serum HMGB1 and inflammatory mediators were analysed using two-way repeated measures (time and group) analysis of variance followed by the post hoc Student-Newman-Keuls test. The significance level was set at $p<0.05$.

Results

Neuroprotective effects of GL on focal cerebral ischemia

No damage was observed upon TTC staining in the cerebrums of sham-group rats, whereas MCA occlusion for 60 min in rats produced massive infarction 48 h after reperfusion. Pre-treatment with different concentrations of GL significantly reduced the infarct volumes in a dose-dependent manner in focal cerebral I/R rats. There were no significant differences between the infarct volumes of the 4 mg/kg and 10 mg/kg GL-pre-treatment groups. Hence, a dose of 4 mg/kg of GL was selected for subsequent experiments, considering the potential for drug toxicity (Figure 1A).

High Neurological Severity Scores in the NS rats persisted for up to 48 h. Consistent with the reduced infarct volumes, when 4 mg/kg GL was administered at 30 min after ischemia and before reperfusion, the mean modified Neurological Severity Scores were significantly lower than those of rats in the PBS-treated NS group from 6 h to 48 h. From 6 h to 24 h, the Neurological Severity Scores declined slowly and reached the minimum value at 48 h after reperfusion in the GL group (Figure 1B). Motor activities were assessed using the rota-rod test at 5, 10 or 15 rpm speed loads. Pre-treatment with 4 mg/kg GL markedly improved the neurological deficits observed on the rota-rod test from 6 h to 48 h, regardless of whether the 5, 10 or 15 rpm speed load was used (Figure 1C). These results showed that pre-treatment with GL had neuroprotective effects on the

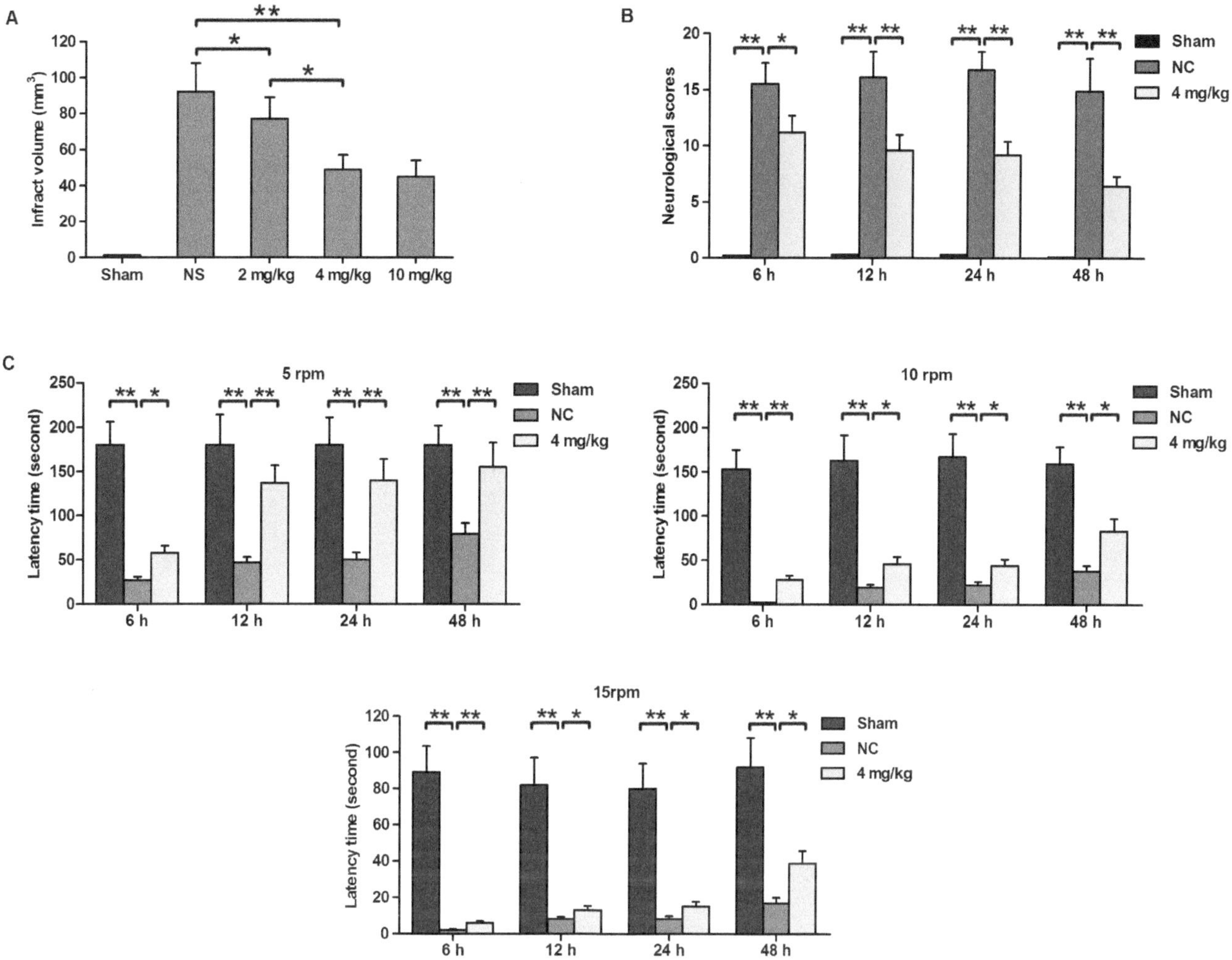

Figure 1. The neuroprotective effect of GL against cerebral I/R injury in rats. A) Cerebral infarction induced by MCA occlusion was evaluated 48 h after reperfusion by TTC staining of brain slices from rats treated with different doses of GL or NS. Sham-operated rats showed no infarction or TTC staining. The infarct volumes were quantified using computerised image analysis. B) Neurological scoring was carried out according to the categories described in the Materials and Methods. C) Neurological deficits in rats after MCA occlusion were examined using the rota-rod test. In the rota-rod test, trials were performed at 3 different speeds, and the time intervals running on the rod were determined for each rat after reperfusion. Values are means±SEM, n = 8 for each group. *P<0.05, **P<0.01 (t test).

post-ischemic brain, which were manifested as improvements in motor impairments and neurological deficits scores.

Inhibition of HMGB1 release by GL in rats that underwent MCAO

We observed that plasma HMGB1 levels rapidly increased starting 6 h after MCAO for 1 h, peaked at 24 h after reperfusion, and then declined slowly (Figure 2A–B). When rats were pre-treated with 4 mg/kg GL, the plasma HMGB1 level was significantly decreased compared with that observed in the NS group at any time during the experimental procedure (Figure 2A–B). At 12 h after MCA occlusion (MCAO)/reperfusion, brain HMGB1 levels in the infarct area declined significantly to below the basal level and reached a minimum value at 24 h after MCAO/reperfusion. Moreover, at each time point from 12 h to 48 h after MCAO/reperfusion, brain HMGB1 levels after treatment with GL were significantly higher than those observed in the NS group (Figure 2C).

Immunofluorescence staining of nuclear HMGB1 was observed in the cerebral cortex in rats from the sham group (Figure 2D). However, the staining almost disappeared in the core of the infarct in the NS group 48 h after reperfusion, and markedly increased HMGB1 staining was observed in the extracellular space. The number of nuclear HMGB1-positive cells significantly increased upon pre-treatment with 4 mg/kg GL, and this was accompanied by a decrease in extracellular HMGB1 staining. These data suggested that increased serum levels of HMGB1 are probably attributable to spill-over from necrotic neural cells during cerebral ischemia and that GL may have a protective effect against MCAO/reperfusion-mediated cell death in neural cells, thereby decreasing the amount of HMGB1 released from the cerebral cortex into the serum.

GL inhibits HMGB1-dependent apoptotic injury

To further demonstrate that the protective effect of GL against brain I/R injury occurs via antagonism of HMGB1 function, we determined the infarct volumes of rat brains under conditions in

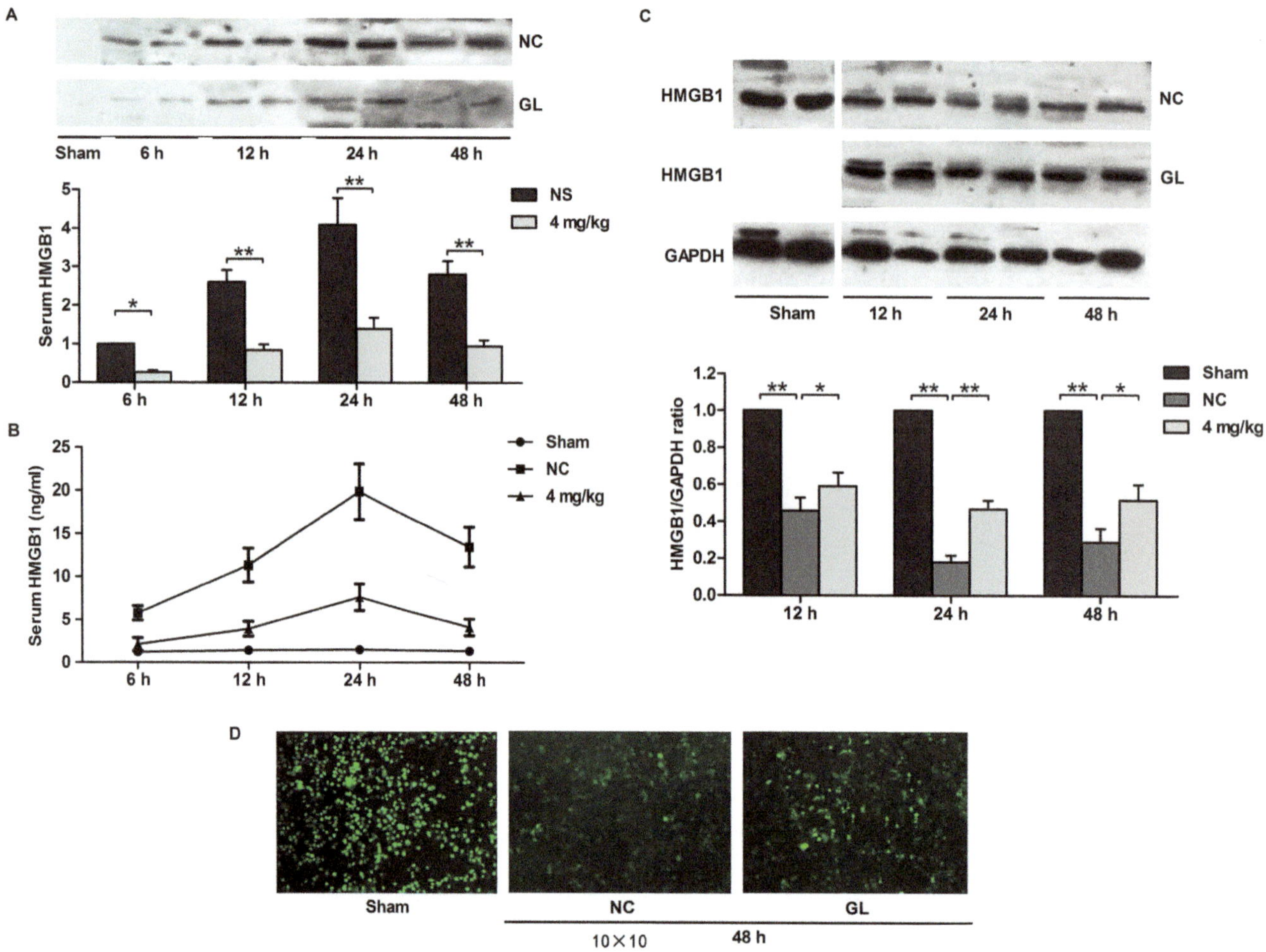

Figure 2. Inhibition of HMGB1 release by GL in the I/R brain. A) The serum HMGB1 concentrations of 4 mg/kg GL-pre-treated rats were determined by immunoblot at the indicated times after 1 h of MCAO. B) Serum HMGB1 concentrations were also determined by ELISA. Values are means±SEM, n=8. **P<0.01 (t test). C) HMGB1 levels in I/R hemispheres were determined by immunoblot at various times after 1 h of MCAO. GAPDH was used as a loading control. D) Immunofluorescence staining showing different extracellular and intracellular distributions of HMGB1 in the I/R hemispheres after 48 h reperfusion. Values are means±SEM, n=8 for each group. *P<0.05, **P<0.01 (t test).

which rHMGB1 was included. As shown in Figure 3A, although the infarct volume was significantly decreased in the 4 mg/kg GL group compared with the NS group, co-treatment with 4 mg/kg GL and 100 μg rHMGB1 30 min before ischemia significantly alleviated these changes, resulting in infarct volumes similar those observed in the NS group.

Next, we investigated whether the anti-inflammatory effect of GL can alleviate I/R-induced, HMGB1-dependent apoptosis and whether cytochrome C and caspase 3, the two most important players, are involved in this process. As depicted in Figure 3B, a large number of TUNEL-positive cells was observed in the right cortex of rats subjected to I/R injury, whereas TUNEL positive cells were not detected in the right cortex of sham-operated rats. Upon pre-treatment with 4 mg/kg GL, the number of TUNEL-positive cells was significantly reduced in the right cortex compared with the NS group. Moreover, co-treatment with rHMGB1 increased the number of TUNEL-positive cells, as expected.

In the sham group, under basal conditions, cytochrome C was predominantly expressed in the mitochondrial fraction (Figure 3C). The NS group exhibited a significant decrease in cytochrome C expression in the mitochondrial fraction when compared with the sham group, whereas an increase was observed in the cytosolic fraction. Pre-treatment with GL resulted in a significant increase in cytochrome C expression in the mitochondrial fraction and a decrease in the cytosolic fraction compared with the NS group. However, expression still did not reach the level observed in the sham group. Moreover, co-treatment with rHMGB1 can partly abolish the effect of GL on the subcellular distribution of cytochrome C proteins between the cytosolic and mitochondrial fractions. There was no significant difference in the total expression of cytochrome C protein between each group (Figure 3C). As an executioner caspase, the change in caspase 3 activity was similar to that observed with cytochrome C expression in the cytosolic fraction (Figure 3D). These results demonstrate that the administration of GL significantly alleviates the cerebral cell apoptotic injury caused by I/R through the antagonism of HMGB1 function and that the mechanism involved regulation of cytochrome C release and caspase 3 activation.

GL inhibits HMGB1-dependent inflammatory molecule expression and oxidative stress

The expression of mRNA encoding inflammation- and oxidative stress-related molecules was determined by RT-PCR. As

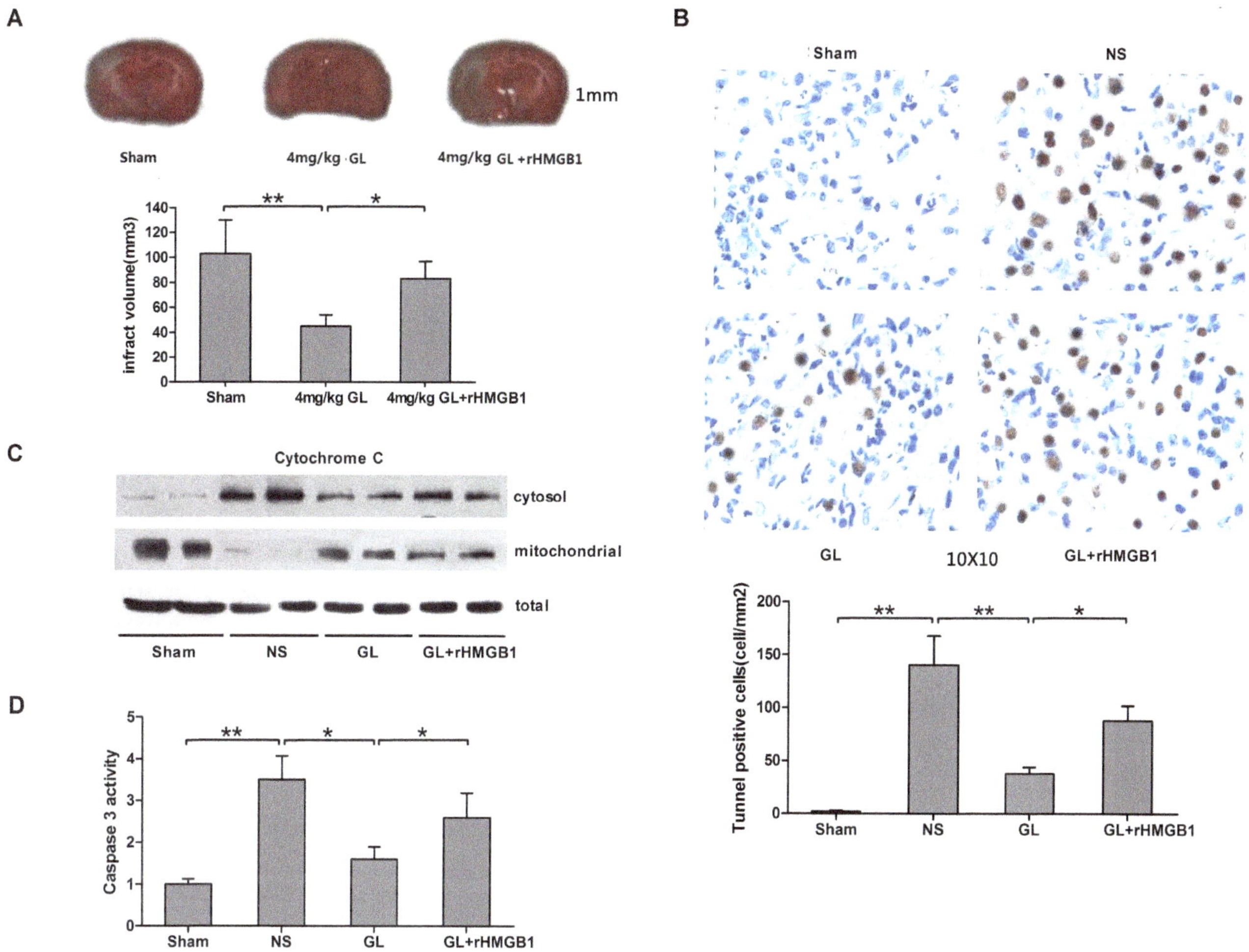

Figure 3. The protective effect of GL on I/R-induced infarct volume and apoptosis injury is HMGB1 dependent. A) Brain infarction induced by right MCA occlusion was evaluated by TTC staining from rats pre-treated with 4 mg/kg GL with or without 100 μg recombinant HMGB1, and the infarct volumes 48 h after reperfusion were quantified using NIH image software. B) Representative photomicrographs show TUNEL staining for apoptotic cells in rat brains at 48 h after reperfusion in the sham, NS, GL and GL+rHMGB1 groups. Effects on the severity of cerebral apoptosis are shown in an average quantitative analysis of the number of TUNEL-positive cells. C) Representative blots showing the effects of GL with or without rHMGB1 treatment on Cytochrome c translocation between the mitochondrial and cytosolic fractions. D) Effects of GL with or without rHMGB1 treatment on caspase-3 activity in areas at the risk zone of cerebral tissues at 48 h after reperfusion. Values are means±SEM, n = 8 for each group. *P<0.05, **P<0.01 (t test).

showed in Figure 4A, MCA occlusion/reperfusion significantly up-regulated the expression of TNF-α, iNOS, IL-1β, COX-2 and IL-6 in the cerebral cortex compared with the non-ischemic side in the sham group. Treatment with GL significantly inhibited the expression of TNF-α, iNOS, IL-1β and IL-6 but had no apparent effect on the expression of COX-2. In contrast, co-treatment with rHMGB1 and GL again enhanced the expression of TNF-α, iNOS, IL-1β and IL-6 compared with the GL-pre-treatment alone group ($P<0.01$). The serum concentrations of TNF-α, iNOS, IL-1β and IL-6 in each group showed a similar trend to that of the mRNA expression levels, as determined by ELISA (Figure 4B). These results indicated that GL can inhibit the I/R-induced expression of HMGB1-dependent inflammation- and oxidative stress-related molecules in rat brains.

In the sham group, little DHE-induced EtBr fluorescence or 3-NT immunoreactivity was observed. The relative fluorescence intensities of superoxide-generating cells and 3-NT–positive cells were significantly increased in the NS-treated I/R hemisphere (Figure 5A–B). When rats were pre-treated with 4 mg/kg GL, the fluorescence intensity caused by superoxide and 3-NT production was significantly reduced compared with the NS group. In contrast, co-treatment with 4 mg/kg GL and 100 μg rHMGB1 enhanced the fluorescence intensity of superoxide and 3-NT production compared with the GL group, though the intensity was still lower than that in the NS group (Figure 5A–B). These histological results were further supported by a biochemical assay for MDA, a lipid peroxidation product. Pre-treatment with 4 mg/kg GL significantly decreased the level of MDA, compared with the NS group, while co-treatment with 100 μg rHMGB1 again increased the level of MDA, though this was still lower than that in the NS group (Figure 5C).

GL modulates P38 and P-JNK but not p-ERK signalling

The mitochondrial-dependent apoptosis pathway is tightly regulated by the mitogen_activated protein (MAP) kinase family, and among these, JNK, ERK1/2, and p38 have been demonstrated to be activated during I/R injury [28,29]. To study whether GL can modulate MAP kinase activity, we analysed these

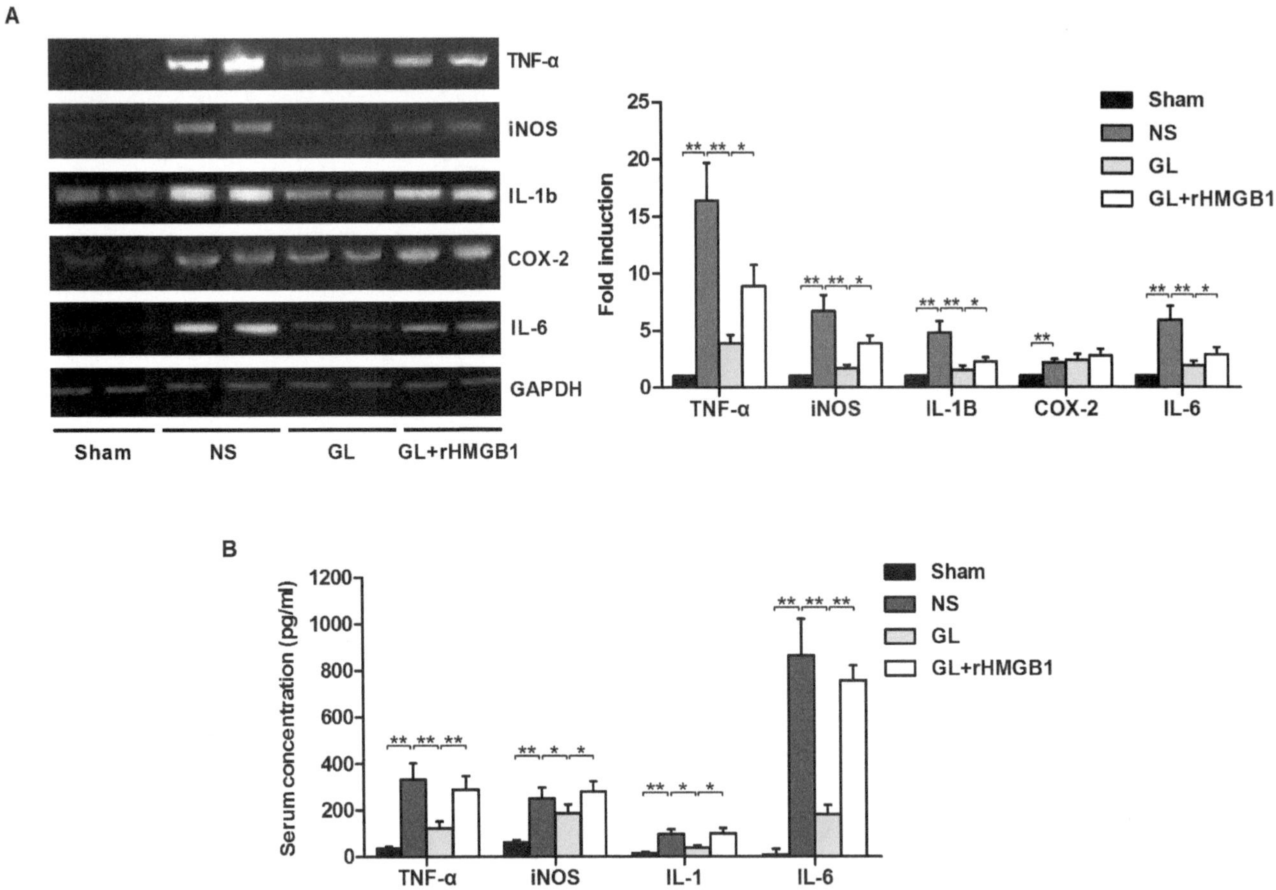

Figure 4. Expression of inflammation- and oxidative stress-related molecules in the brain and serum of MCA-occluded rats at 48 h after reperfusion. A) Representative blots showing the effects of GL with or without rHMGB1 treatment on mRNA expression levels of pro-inflammatory and oxidative stress markers: TNF-α, iNOS, IL-1β, COX-2 and IL-6. GAPDH was used as a loading control. The bar graph showing semi-quantitative densitometric analysis summarises the fold change of TNF-α, iNOS, IL-1β, COX-2 and IL-6 expression in each group. B) Serum concentrations of TNF-α, iNOS, IL-1β, COX-2 and IL-6 at 48 h after I/R in each groups are determined. Values are means±SEM, n = 8 for each group. *$P<0.05$, **$P<0.01$ (t test).

MAP kinases by immunoblotting. As shown in Figure 6, I/R induced phosphorylation of JNK, ERK, and p38 in isolated rat brain cerebral cortex. In GL-pre-treated rats, the phosphorylation levels of p38 and p-JNK were decreased compared with the NS-treated group, whereas p-ERK1/2 was not affected. Co-treatment with rHMGB1 enhanced the phosphorylation of p38 and JNK compared with the GL group, but the levels were still lower than those observed in the NS group. Pre-treatment with GL alone or with rHMGB1 did not affect the total levels of the JNK, ERK1/2, and p38 proteins. These results demonstrated that GL can modulate the p38 and JNK signalling pathways, but not the ERK signalling pathway, in the brains of MCA-occluded rats and that this effect is HMGB1 dependent.

Discussion

Traditional Chinese medicine has become increasingly important in the treatment of cardiovascular ischemia/reperfusion injury. GL is a natural anti-inflammatory compound that is commonly used in Japan to treat patients with chronic hepatitis [14–17]. In the present study, we demonstrated that intravenous pre-treatment with a wide range of concentrations of GL, from 2 mg/kg to 10 mg/kg, reduced cerebral infarct volumes and ameliorated the neurological deficits of rat cerebral I/R injury. The use of a medium concentration of 4 mg/kg yielded considerable improvements, similar to those found at the high concentration of 10 mg/kg GL. Furthermore, this neuroprotective effect was accompanied by a reduction in the release of HMGB1 into the extracellular space and in the related inflammatory factors TNF-α, iNOS, IL-1β, and IL-6, both in the brain and serum of rats (Figure 2 and 4). Using this dose, no significant toxicities were observed in the effects investigated, including changes in the baseline hemodynamic values, cardiac electrophysiology, and in histopathological analysis of vital organs including liver, spleen, lung, kidney, and brain (data not shown).

HMGB1 is a nonhistone DNA-binding protein that possesses two HMG boxes that are DNA binding domains [30]. As a chromosomal protein, it has been implicated in diverse intracellular functions including stabilising nucleosomal structure and facilitating of gene transcription [31]. Moreover, HMGB1 is massively released extracellularly and plays a cytokine-like function in the post-ischemic brain [26,32]. HMGB1 is actively secreted by macrophages and monocytes or released by necrotic cells into the extracellular milieu, where it might be involved in triggering inflammation [33–36]. The present study demonstrated that the predominantly nuclear HMGB1 staining of neurons in rats from the sham group weakened and disappeared during

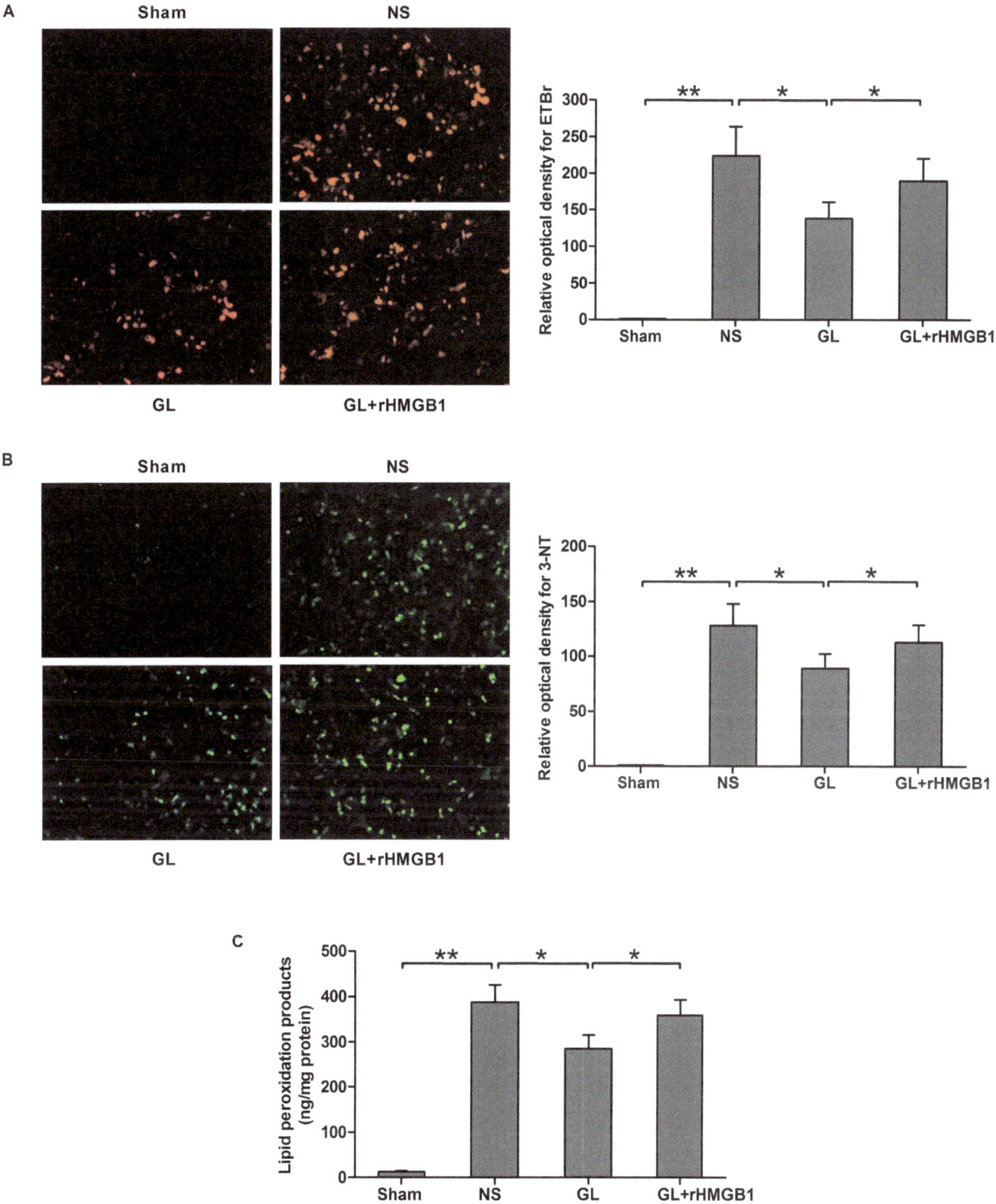

Figure 5. The antioxidant effects of GL are HMGB1 dependent. A) Fluorescent images after incubation with DHE showing superoxide levels in the I/R brain (red). Quantitative measurements of the fluorescence intensity indicated a significant change in the 4 mg/kg GL-treated group with or without rHMGB1, compared with the saline-treated I/R (NS) group. B) Representative photomicrographs showing 3-NT formation in the ischemic brain (green). Data from image analysis also indicated a significant change in the 4 mg/kg GL-treated group with or without rHMGB1, compared with the saline-treated I/R (NS) group. Bar = 50 μm. C) The effects of 4 mg/kg GL with or without rHMGB1 on MDA content in rat brains after I/R. Values are means±SEM, n = 8 for each group. *$P<0.05$, **$P<0.01$ (t test).

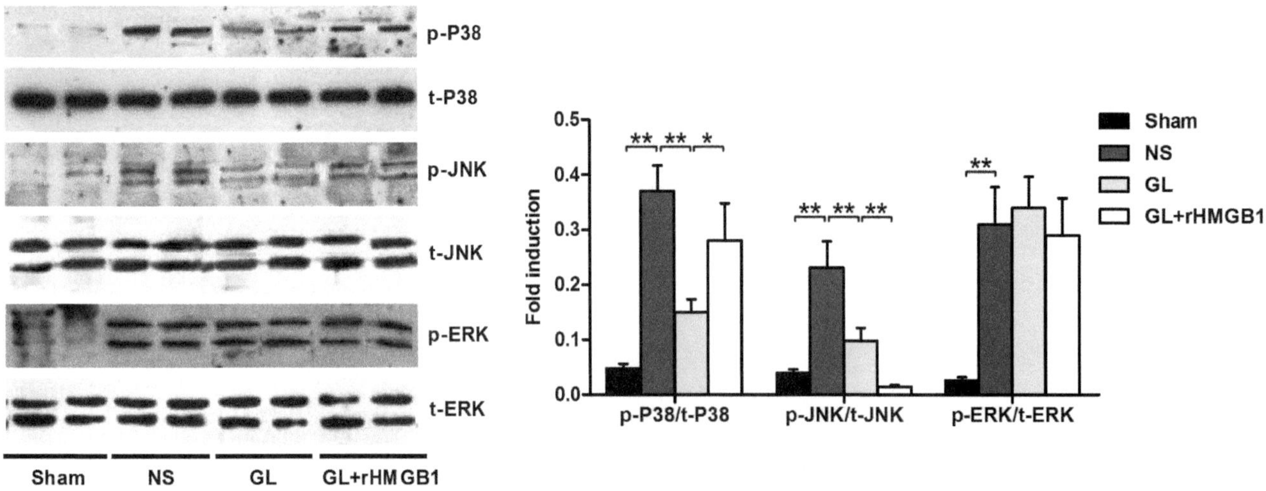

Figure 6. Representative blots showing the effects of GL with or without rHMGB1 treatment on phosphorylated (p) and total (t) p38, JNK, and ERK expression. Each blot shown is representative of 3 experiments with similar results. The bar graph showing semi-quantitative densitometric analysis summarises the fold change in phosphorylated to total p38, JNK and ERK in each group. Values are means±SEM, n = 8 for each group. *P<0.05, **P<0.01 (t test).

cerebral ischemia (Figure 2D). Thus, release from necrotic neural cells is the most likely source of elevated HMGB1 concentrations in the serum, which were further determined by immunoblot analysis in rats subjected to focal cerebral ischemia. A recent report of elevated serum concentrations of HMGB1 in stroke patients confirmed our findings [37]. Antagonising the pro-inflammatory function or blocking the expression of HMGB1 by a neutralising antibody [11,12], HMGB1 box A [11], or a short hairpin RNA [10,13] ameliorated brain damage. In particular, the expression of TNF-α, iNOS and IL-1β, which were all up-regulated in the post-ischemic brain, was reduced when HMGB1 was inhibited [10,11], consistent with our results. HMGB1 has been reported to stimulate the production of IL-1, TNF-α, IL-6, and IL-8 and to induce iNOS expression [38,39]. In the present study, we demonstrated that the ischemia-induced up-regulation of iNOS, IL-1β, IL-6 and TNF-α was inhibited by treatment with GL. Co-treatment with rHMGB1 can partially reverse this effect (Figure 4). The induction of iNOS and TNF-α following an ischemic insult was reported to occur mainly in microglia. Thus, it is likely that HMGB1 activates microglia in the brain, leading to the up-regulation of iNOS and TNF-α expression. In fact, the induction of iNOS and TNF-α has been reported to be involved in the inflammatory response and the disruption of the blood-brain barrier, leading to the aggravation of brain infarction [40,41]. The regulation of any one of these factors has been postulated to reduce ischemic injury. Therefore, it is reasonable that GL, which has the ability to substantially reduce the expression of pro-inflammatory factors, exerted profound therapeutic effects on brain infarction.

In this study, pre-treatment with GL alleviated apoptosis injury resulting from cerebral I/R, and this was at least partly due to the inhibition of cytochrome C release and caspase 3 activity. Similarly, GL exhibited an anti-apoptotic effect by preventing HMGB1-induced cytochrome C release and caspase 3 activation in vitro in Huh-BAT cells [42]. Though the anti-apoptotic effect of GL has been linked with HMGB1 inhibition and caspase-dependent cytochrome c release, the question remains how GL regulates caspase-dependent cytochrome c release through the inhibition of HMGB1. The exact answer is not known at the present time, but we speculate that GL may modulate the activity of a particular kinase that contributes to cytochrome c transloca-tion and is involved in I/R-induced HMGB1-dependent apopto-sis.

Apoptosis is tightly regulated by the mitogen-activated protein (MAP) kinase family, and the JNK, ERK1/2, and p38 members of this family have been demonstrated to be activated in I/R injury. MAPKs play important roles in transducing signals by phosphor-ylating intracellular enzymes, transcription factors and cytosolic proteins involved in apoptosis and inflammatory cytokine produc-tion. Sustained MAPK activation has been shown to be associated with neuronal cell death/apoptosis following ischemic stroke, and the inhibition of this pathway is neuroprotective. In a Huh-BAT cell model, GL prevented HMGB1_induced cytochrome c release and p38 activation but had no effect on phospho_JNK and ERK1/2 [42]. In I/R-induced myocardial injury of rat heart, treatment with HMGB1 box A significantly reduced ERK1/2 and JNK phosphorylation, but did not affect the level of phospho-p38 [43]. However, in another similar study, treatment with GL significantly decreased JNK phosphorylation, but did not affect the level of phospho-p38 and ERK1/2[21]. Interestingly, in our studies, GL could modulate the p38 and JNK signalling pathways, but did not affect the ERK signalling pathway in the brains of MCA-occluded rats, and rHMGB1 could reverse this effect (Figure 6). This ambiguity regarding which single class of MAPK can be modulated by GL appears to primarily depend on the cell and tissue types used and differences in MAPK levels in vivo and in vitro.

In conclusion, our results demonstrated that pre-treatment with GL blocked and inhibited the extracellular cytokine activity of HMGB1 and explored the protective effect on I/R-induced apoptosis through the blockage of the JNK and p38-mediated pathways in rats in vivo. These data suggest a new therapeutic possibility for the treatment of ischemic stroke with GL. Considering the biological differences between species that may influence drug adsorption, metabolism, distribution, and toxicity in rats and humans, it is not clear whether GL has similar protective effects in humans. Hence, future research should be performed to evaluate the beneficial protective effect of GL in clinical settings with humans, as this might ultimately lead to a new therapeutic strategy for ischemic stroke.

Author Contributions

Conceived and designed the experiments: GG LX HD. Performed the experiments: LY LH WW LC LY. Analyzed the data: GG LX HD. Contributed reagents/materials/analysis tools: LY LH WW LC LY. Wrote the paper: GG LX HD.

References

1. Ceulemans AG, Zgavc T, Kooijman R, Hachimi-Idrissi S, Sarre S, et al. (2010) The dual role of the neuroinflammatory response after ischemic stroke: modulatory effects of hypothermia. J Neuroinflammation 7: 74.
2. Gursoy-Ozdemir Y, Can A, Dalkara T (2004) Reperfusion-induced oxidative/nitrative injury to neurovascular unit after focal cerebral ischemia. Stroke 35: 1449–1453.
3. Amantea D, Nappi G, Bernardi G, Bagetta G, Corasaniti MT (2009) Post-ischemic brain damage: pathophysiology and role of inflammatory mediators. FEBS J 276: 13–26.
4. Li J, Zeng Z, Viollet B, Ronnett GV, McCullough LD (2007) Neuroprotective effects of adenosine monophosphate-activated protein kinase inhibition and gene deletion in stroke. Stroke 38: 2992–2999.
5. Piao CS, Kim JB, Han PL, Lee JK (2003) Administration of the p38 MAPK inhibitor SB203580 affords brain protection with a wide therapeutic window against focal ischemic insult. J Neurosci Res 73: 537–544.
6. Lotze MT, Tracey KJ (2005) High-mobility group box 1 protein (HMGB1): nuclear weapon in the immune arsenal. Nat Rev Immunol 5: 331–342.
7. Oozawa S, Mori S, Kanke T, Takahashi H, Liu KY, et al. (2008) Effects of HMGB1 on ischemia-reperfusion injury in the rat heart. Circ J 72: 1178–1184.
8. Lakhan SE, Kirchgessner A, Hofer M (2009) Inflammatory mechanisms in ischemic stroke: therapeutic approaches. J Transl Med 7: 97.
9. Yang QW, Wang JZ, Li JC, Zhou Y, Zhong Q, et al. (2010) High-mobility group protein box-1 and its relevance to cerebral ischemia. J Cereb Blood Flow Metab 30: 243–254.
10. Kim JB, Sig Choi J, Yu YM, Nam K, Piao CS, et al. (2006) HMGB1, a novel cytokine-like mediator linking acute neuronal death and delayed neuroinflammation in the postischemic brain. J Neurosci 26: 6413–6421.
11. Muhammad S, Barakat W, Stoyanov S, Murikinati S, Yang H, et al. (2008) The HMGB1 receptor RAGE mediates ischemic brain damage. J Neurosci 28: 12023–12031.
12. Liu K, Mori S, Takahashi HK, Tomono Y, Wake H, et al. (2007) Anti-highmobility group box 1 monoclonal antibody ameliorates brain infarction induced by transient ischemia in rats. FASEB J 21: 3904–3916.
13. Kim ID, Shin JH, Kim SW, Choi S, Ahn J, et al. (2012) Intranasal delivery of HMGB1 siRNA confers target gene knockdown and robust neuroprotection in the postischemic brain. Mol Ther 20: 829–839.
14. Arase Y, Ikeda K, Murashima N, Chayama K, Tsubota A, et al. (1997) The long term efficacy of glycyrrhizin in chronic hepatitis C patients. Cancer 79: 1494–1500.
15. van Rossum TG, Vulto AG, Hop WC, Schalm SW (2001) Glycyrrhizin-induced reduction of ALT in European patients with chronic hepatitis C. Am J Gastroenterol 96: 2432–2437.
16. Yoshida T, Abe K, Ikeda T, Matsushita T, Wake K, et al. (2007) Inhibitory effect of glycyrrhizin on lipopolysaccharide and d-galactosamine-induced mouse liver injury. Eur J Pharmacol 576: 136–142.
17. Sato H, Goto W, Yamamura J, Kurokawa M, Kageyama S, et al. (1996) Therapeutic basis of glycyrrhizin on chronic hepatitis B. Antiviral Res 30: 171–177.
18. Sitia G, Iannacone M, Müller S, Bianchi ME, Guidotti LG (2007) Treatment with HMGB1 inhibitors diminishes CTL-induced liver disease in HBV transgenic mice. J Leukoc Biol 81: 100–107.
19. Ogiku M, Kono H, Hara M, Tsuchiya M, Fujii H (2011) Glycyrrhizin prevents liver injury by inhibition of high-mobility group box 1 production by Kupffer cells after ischemia-reperfusion in rats. J Pharmacol Exp Ther 339: 93–98.
20. Gong G, Yuan LB, Hu L, Wu W, Yin L, et al. (2012) Glycyrrhizin attenuates ischemic spinal cord injury by suppressing HMGB1 in rats. Acta Pharmacol Sin 33: 11–18.
21. Zhai C, Zhang M, Zhang Y, Xu H, Wang J, et al. (2012) Glycyrrhizin protects rat heart against ischemia-reperfusion injury through blockade of HMGB1-dependent phospho-JNK/Bax pathway. Acta Pharmacol Sin 10: 1–11.
22. Kim SW, Lim CM, Lee HK, Lee JK (2011) The use of Stronger Neo-Minophagen C, a glycyrrhizin-containing preparation, in robust neuroprotection in the postischemic brain. Anat Cell Biol 44: 304–313.
23. Lee ST, Chu K, Jung KH, Ko SY, Kim EH, et al. (2005) Granulocyte colony-stimulating factor enhances angiogenesis after focal cerebral ischemia. Brain Res 1058: 120–128.
24. Bederson JB, Pitts LH, Tsuji M, Nishimura MC, Davis RL, et al. (1986) Rat middle cerebral artery occlusion: evaluation of the model and development of a neurologic examination. Stroke 17: 472–476.
25. Okuno S, Saito A, Hayashi T, Chan PH (2004) The c-Jun N-terminal protein kinase signaling pathway mediates Bax activation and subsequent neuronal apoptosis through interaction with Bim after transient focal cerebral ischemia. J Neurosci 24: 7879–7887.
26. Kim JB, Lim CM, Yu YM, Lee JK (2008) Induction and subcellular localization of high-mobility group box-1 (HMGB1) in the postischemic rat brain. J Neurosci Res 86: 1125–1131.
27. Bindokas VP, Jordan J, Lee CC, Miller RJ (1996) Superoxide production in rat hippocampal neurons: selective imaging with hydroethidine. J Neurosci 16: 1324–1336.
28. Frangogiannis NG, Smith CW, Entman ML (2002) The inflammatory response in myocardial infarction. Cardiovasc Res 53: 31–47.
29. Kaiser RA, Bueno OF, Lips DJ, Doevendans PA, Jones F, et al. (2004) Targeted inhibition of p38 mitogen-activated protein kinase antagonizes cardiac injury and cell death following ischemia-reperfusion in vivo. J Biol Chem 279: 15524–15530.
30. Landsman D, Bustin M (1993) A Signature for the HMG-1 box DNA-binding proteins. Bioessays 15: 539–546.
31. Bustin M (1999) Regulation of DNA-dependent activities by the functional motifs of the high-mobility-group chromosomal proteins. Mol Cell Biol 19: 5237–5246.
32. Faraco G, Fossati S, Bianchi ME, Patrone M, Pedrazzi M, et al. (2007) High mobility group box 1 protein is released by neural cells upon different stresses and worsens ischemic neurodegeneration in vitro and in vivo. J Neurochem 103: 590–603.
33. Wang H, Bloom O, Zhang M, Vishnubhakat JM, Ombrellino M, et al. (1999) HMG-1 as a late mediator of endotoxin lethality in mice. Science 285: 248–251.
34. Abraham E, Arcaroli J, Carmody A, Wang H, Tracey KJ (2000) HMG-1 as a mediator of acute lung inflammation. J Immunol 165: 2950–2954.
35. Scaffidi P, Misteli T, Bianchi ME (2002) Release of chromatin protein HMGB1 by necrotic cells triggers inflammation. Nature 418: 191–195.
36. Bonaldi T, Talamo F, Scaffidi P, Ferrera D, Porto A, et al. (2003) Monocytic cells hyperacetylate chromatin protein HMGB1 to redirect it towards secretion. EMBO J 22: 5551–5560.
37. Goldstein RS, Gallowitsch-Puerta M, Yang L, Rosas-Ballina M, Huston JM, et al. (2006) Elevated high-mobility group box 1 levels in patients with cerebral and myocardial ischemia. Shock 25: 571–574.
38. Andersson U, Wang H, Palmblad K, Aveberger AC, Bloom O, et al. (2000) High mobility group 1 protein (HMG-1) stimulates proinflammatory cytokine synthesis in human monocytes. J Exp Med 192: 565–570.
39. Ren D, Sun R, Wang S (2006) Role of inducible nitric oxide synthase expressed by alveolar macrophages in high mobility group box 1-induced acute lung injury. Inflamm Res 55: 207–215.
40. Iadecola C, Zhang F, Xu X (1995) Inhibition of inducible nitric oxide synthase ameliorates cerebral ischemic damage. Am J Physiol 268: R286–R292.
41. Barone FC, Arvin B, White RF, Miller A, Webb CL, et al. (1997) Tumor necrosis factor-alpha. A mediator of focal ischemic brain injury. Stroke 28: 1233–1244.
42. Gwak GY, Moon TG, Lee DH, Yoo BC (2012) Glycyrrhizin attenuates HMGB1-induced hepatocyte apoptosis by inhibiting the p38-dependent mitochondrial pathway. World J Gastroenterol 18: 679–684.
43. Andrassy M, Volz HC, Igwe JC, Funke B, Eichberger SN, et al. (2008) High-mobility group box-1 in ischemia-reperfusion injury of the heart. Circulation 117: 3216–3226.

4

Association between Hypoxia and Perinatal Arterial Ischemic Stroke

Lili Luo[1,2,3], Dapeng Chen[1], Yi Qu[1,2], Jinlin Wu[1], Xihong Li[3], Dezhi Mu[1,2*]

1 Department of Pediatrics, West China Second University Hospital, Sichuan University, Sichuan, China, 2 Key Laboratory of Obstetric & Gynecologic and Pediatric Diseases and Birth Defects of Ministry of Education, Sichuan University, Sichuan, China, 3 Department of Emergency, West China Second University Hospital, Sichuan University, Sichuan, China.

Abstract

Background: Perinatal arterial ischemic stroke (AIS) occurs in an estimated 17 to 93 per 100000 live births, yet the etiology is poorly understood. Although investigators have implicated hypoxia as a potential cause of AIS, the role of hypoxia in AIS remains controversial. The aim of this study was to estimate the association between perinatal hypoxia factors and perinatal arterial ischemic stroke through a meta-analysis of published observational studies.

Patients and methods: A systematic search of electronically available studies published through July 2013 was conducted. Publication bias and heterogeneity across studies were evaluated and summary odds ratios (ORs) and 95% confidence intervals (CIs) were calculated with fixed-effects or random-effects models.

Results: A total of 8 studies describing the association between perinatal hypoxia factors and neonatal arterial ischemic stroke (AIS) met inclusion criteria, and 550 newborns with AIS were enrolled. The associations were found for AIS: preeclampsia (OR 2.14; 95% CI, 1.25 to 3.66), ventouse delivery (OR 2.23; 95% CI, 1.26 to 3.97), fetal heart rate abnormalities (OR 6.30; 95% CI, 3.84 to 10.34), reduced fetal movement (OR 5.35; 95% CI, 2.17 to 13.23), meconium-stained liquor (OR 3.05; 95% CI, 2.02 to 4.60), low Apgar score (OR 5.77; 95% CI, 1.66 to 20.04) and resuscitation at birth (OR 4.59; 95% CI, 3.23 to 6.52). Our data did not show any significant change of the mean risk estimate for oxytocin induction (OR 1.33; 95% CI, 0.84 to 2.11) and low arterial umbilical cord ph (OR 4.63; 95% CI 2.14 to 9.98).

Conclusions: There is a significant association between perinatal hypoxia factors and AIS. The result indicates that perinatal hypoxia maybe one of causes of AIS. Large scale prospective clinical studies are still warranted.

Editor: Graham R. Wallace, University of Birmingham, United Kingdom

Funding: All phases of this study were supported by the National Science Foundation of China (No. 81330016 and No. 31171020 to Dezhi Mu; No. 81172174 and 81270724 to Yi Qu), and the Grant of clinical discipline program (neonatology) from the Ministry of Health of China. The funders had no role in study design, data collection and analysis, decision to publish, or preparation of the manuscript.

Competing Interests: The authors have declared that no competing interests exist.

* E-mail: mudz@scu.edu.cn

These authors contributed equally to this work.

Introduction

Neonatal stroke is classified as either ischemic or hemorrhagic stroke, and ischemic stroke is further divided into arterial ischemic stroke (AIS) and cerebral sinovenous thrombosis (CSVT) [1]. Perinatal ischemic stroke (PAIS) is defined as a group of heterogeneous conditions in which there is a focal disruption of cerebral blood flow secondary to arterial or venous thrombosis or embolization [2], which occurred from birth up until 28 days postnatal [3].

The prevalence of PAIS has not been clearly determined. Lynch reported an estimated incidence of 71 in 1600 to 5000 births [4]. Laugesaar reported the incidence rate of neonatal stroke in Estonia was 63 per 100 000 live births in 2007 [5]. Lee found that AIS was diagnosed in 20 per 100 000 live births [6]. Estimate incidence rate ranges from 17 to 93 per 100 000 live births [2,7–9]. Possibly due to more widespread use of sophisticated neuro-imaging techniques, recent studies show that the incidence of stroke was significantly higher than before. Meanwhile, a case series of neonates with AIS suggests that newborn boys are at higher risk of ischemic stroke than girls [10,11], with increased frequency in black children [12]. The incidence of neonatal stroke is higher than old children [5,13].

Perinatal arterial ischemic stroke is a main cause of cerebral palsy and other neurologic disabilities, thus making it a clinically relevant type of brain injury, yet the etiology is poorly understood.

The pathogenesis of AIS is complex and multifactorial. Risk factors may be related to both maternal and placental problems as well as fetal and neonatal disorders, such as preeclampsia, chorioamnionitis, congenital heart malformations, hemolytic anemias, thrombophilic abnormalities, heart rate abnormalities, resuscitation at birth, low Apgar score, and abnormal cord ph [6,8,14]. Investigators have implicated hypoxia as a potential cause of AIS [15]. In a series of 250 newborns examined in the 1980s and 1990s, 35% of strokes occurred in the context of perinatal asphyxia [16]. Some term newborns were found with hypoxic-ischemic encephalopathy, particularly in cases of arterial infarction, (stroke). In a prospective cohort study of 124 term newborns with hypoxia-ischemia encephalopathy, 6 neonates had arterial stroke identified by neuroimaging [17]. Although there was an increased incidence of hypoxia factors in the stroke group, some studies reported there was no significant difference between cases and controls in those diagnosed with birth asphyxia or with meconium-stained liquor [9,18]. Although a relatively large number of potential risk factors have been implicated in the etiology of AIS, some of the information published to date is conflicting.

The objective of this meta-analysis was to determine the impact of clinical risk factors or markers for hypoxia in neonates with arterial stroke. Our hypothesis is that clinical risk factors for hypoxia differ between newborns with stroke compared to normal controls.

Methods and Patients

Study Inclusion Criteria and Exclusion Criteria

Studies included should be published, regardless of its design, publication language or date. Neonatal arterial ischemic stroke is generally defined as a cerebrovascular event occurring from birth to 28 days postnatal with radiological evidence of focal arterial infarction [3,5]. Published studies of arterial ischemic stroke in infants less than 28 days of age were evaluated for inclusion. We only included studies comparing risk factors between patients with AIS and control subjects. Studies with titles and abstracts discussing risk factors about AIS were further examined, and those where stroke cases were objectively confirmed by suitable imaging methods were included, the suitable imaging methods referred to ischemic lesions revealed by neuro-imaging (CT and/ or MR scan). In addition, the included studies have reported the country of origin, study design, ethnicity, and numbers of patients/ control subjects. Case reports and case series/studies lacking these controls were excluded, as were cases of cerebral sinovenous thrombosis or hemorrhagic stroke.

Types of Participants

AIS neonates had to be with neurological clinical symptoms during the 28 first days of life, ischemic lesions in an arterial distribution revealed by suitable imaging methods. Neonates with infection of the central nervous system, brain malformations, venous infarction, cystic periventricular Leukomalaeia (PVL), or sinovenous thrombosis were excluded.

The controls were randomly selected and were individually matched to the infants with PAIS for age and gestational age from the birth registry database or the same birth cohort. Those of a contemporaneous dataset from the general population selected as controls were also included.

Search Strategy and Identification of Studies

Two investigators (Lili Luo and Dapeng Chen) searched case-control or cohort studies published electronically and listed in database PubMed, EMBASE, Web of Science and Cochrane Library from initial to July 2013. The search terms were perinatal stroke, perinatal and neonatal ischemic stroke, neonatal arterial ischemic stroke, fetal stroke, and presumed prenatal or perinatal arterial ischemic stroke; prepartum complications, intrapartum complications and risk factor. Search consisted of a combination of one term from each group. Potential related studies about the association between hypoxia factors and AIS were first identified by screening the titles and abstracts of candidate articles, full manuscripts were then obtained. Further criteria for inclusion were then applied manually. Furthermore, a manual search was carried out from references cited in these articles. Otherwise we excluded studies with five or fewer cases, because of unreliability.

Quality Assessment

We used the Newcastle-Ottawa Quality Assessment Scale to assess the quality of both cohort studies and case-control studies [19]. This scale uses an eight-step process that allows for assessment of patient population and selection, study comparability, follow-up, and outcome of interest. Interpretation of the scale is performed by awarding points, (or "stars"), for high-quality elements. Stars are then added up and used to compare study quality in a quantitative manner, as recommended by the Cochrane Non-Randomized Studies Methods Working Group. Studies with 5 or more stars are defined as high quality studies and were included. Quality assessment was independently performed by two investigators (Lili Luo and Dapeng Chen). Data was then independently compiled by two investigators (Lili Luo and Dapeng Chen) after data extraction and assessment. Any areas of discrepancy will be presented in the discussion.

Data Extraction

For data collection, two investigators used a form of data extraction, independently. Any areas of debate will be presented in the discussion. Studies were included in the meta-analysis only if approved by both investigators. First, we scrutinized in detail the literature on neonatal AIS to identify all possible risk factors which might cause hypoxia. We restricted our analysis to those for which an outcome was assessed by at least 5 cases, because of unreliability. During data extraction we recorded characteristics of the studies, including publication time, study design, country, sample size, gestational week, odds ratio, and 95% confidence intervals (CIs). We have included the studies with the largest number of participants if participant overlap between studies occurred. If original odds ratio and its 95% CI was not reported, the original number of participants was determined in order to calculate the odds ratio.

Statistical Analysis

We reviewed the possible hypoxia-related risk factors for AIS, included prepartum complications, intrapartum complications and infant characteristics. Among these factors exclusion criteria were: (1) patients less than 5 cases because of the uncertainty; (2) inconsistency of the diagnostic criteria. The association between risk factors and AIS was expressed as odds ratio (OR).

All statistical analysis was performed using Stata 12.0. The pooled OR and its 95% confidence intervals (CIs) were calculated using either the Mantel–Haenszel formula (fixed-effect model) or the Dersimonian–Laird formula (random-effect model). A fixed-effect model was used when heterogeneity was not detected ($P>0.10$); otherwise, a random-effect model was used. For quantitative evaluation, OR was used to estimate the impact of risk factors on incidence of AIS. OR, variance, 95% CI, log (OR) and se (log (OR)) for each study were extracted or calculated by Stata 12.0 based on the published studies. The weight for each study is the inverse of study variance and variability between studies. A significant two-way P value for comparison was defined as $P<0.05$. Results are described using forest plots, where a single square represents an individual study's OR estimate. The pooled OR is symbolized by a solid diamond at the bottom of the forest plot and the width of the square represents the 95% CI of the OR. The size of the square represents the weight that the corresponding study exerts in the meta-analysis.

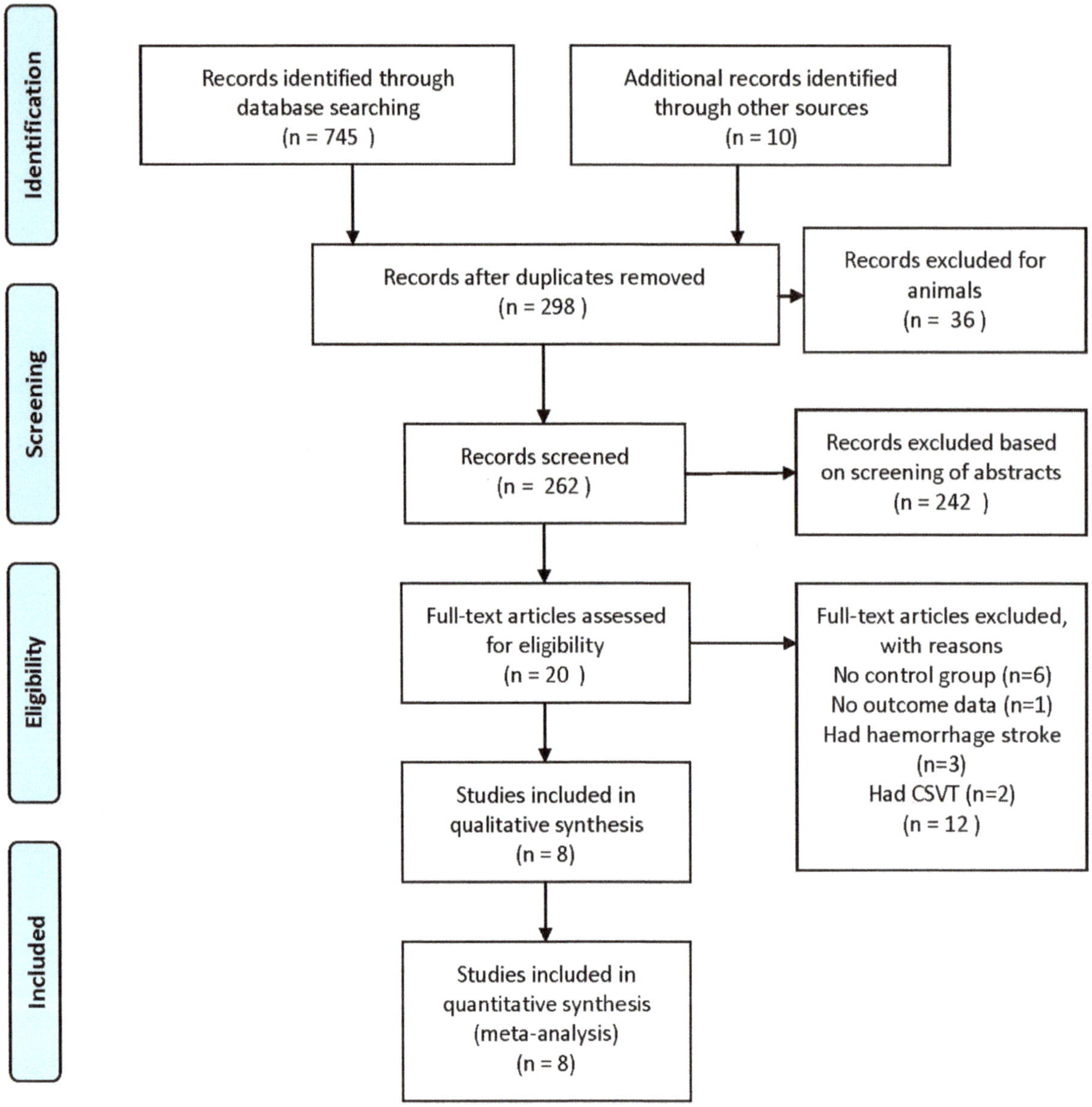

Figure 1. Flow chart showing the results of the search strategy.

Assessment of heterogeneity and publication bias

Statistical heterogeneity between studies was examined using both the Q statistic (significant at $P<0.1$) and the I^2 value. $I^2>50\%$ were considered to represent significant heterogeneity. Assessment of publication bias was performed for each of the pooled study groups using the Beggar's bias indicator test. The analysis of heterogeneity and publication bias was carried out using the statistical software Stata version 12.0.

Results

Search Results and Characteristics of Included Studies

We identified 298 publications by our search strategy, except for the duplicate articles. Initial evaluation of abstracts identified 20 related articles, seven case-control studies and one cohort study with 550 patients were selected for analyses. Figure 1 is the flow diagram depicting the reasons for exclusion of the identified studies. The study dates ranged from 1987 to 2010. Table 1 summarizes the characteristics of the studies included in the meta-analysis.

Selection of Risk factors

After scrutinizing the literature, we yielded 18 possible risk factors (Table 2). Among these factors, forceps delivery, vaginal blood loss, abruption placenta, and infant with congenital heart disease were excluded because of less than 5 cases. We did not include emergency caesarean section, premature rupture of membranes, prolonged second stage of labour and cord abnormality owing to the inconsistency of the diagnostic criteria. Breech delivery was excluded for this factor might or might not lead to hypoxia. Finally, in this meta-analysis, preeclampsia, ventouse delivery, oxytocin induction, fetal heart rate abnormalities, reduced fetal movement, meconium-stained liquor, low Apgar

Table 1. Characteristic of the included studies.

Study	Years	Country	Study type	Study design	Case number	Controls number	Neonate	Birth weight	Imaging confirm	Risk of bias
Benders 2007 [20]	1990–2005	US	retrospective	case-control	31	93	preterm	Cases:1599±633 Controls:1607±720	MRI	different detecting method, only preterm neonates
Chabrier 2010 [21]	2003–2006	France	prospective	cohort study	100	100	both	NR	CT/MRI	different detecting method, no description of those lost to follow up
Darmency-Stamboul 2012 [22]	2000–2007	France	retrospective	case-control	32	96	term	NR	CT/MRI	different detecting method, only term neonates
Estan 1997 [8]	1987–1993	UK	retrospective	case-control	12	24	term	Cases:3496(2541–4460) Controls:3673 (2748–4707)	CT	different detecting method, only term neonates
Harteman 2012 [14]	2000–2010	Utrecht	retrospective	case-control	52	156	term	Cases:3420(2145–5230) Controls:3520(2155–4925)	MRI	different detecting method, only term neonates
Lee 2005 [6]	1997–2002	US	retrospective	nested case-control	37	111	both	Cases:3127±852 Controls:3203±923	CT/MRI	different detecting method
Wu 2004 [9]	1991–1998	US	retrospective	nested case-control	38	218	term	NR	CT/MRI	different detecting method, only term neonates
Kirton 2011 [23]	2003–2007	IPSS	prospective	case-control	248	population	both	NR	CT/MRI	different detecting method

NR: not reported. IPSS: Europe, Canada, US, South America, Asia, Australia; NR: not reported.

score, abnormal arterial umbilical cord ph and resuscitation at birth were included.

Preeclampsia

Four studies (158 cases with AIS) were included in the meta-analysis. No significant heterogeneity was found ($Chi^2 = 3.90$, $P = 0.272$, $I^2 = 23.2\%$) (Figure 2), so fixed-effect model was used. The association between preeclampsia and AIS were seen in all meta-analyses (OR 2.14; 95% CI, 1.25 to 3.66). Visual assessment of a funnel plot and Beggar's test provided no evidence of obviously publication bias ($P = 1.000$) (Figure 3).

Ventouse delivery

Four studies (158 cases with AIS) were included in the meta-analysis. No heterogeneity was found ($Chi^2 = 1.94$, $P = 0.584$, $I^2 = 0\%$) (Figure 4), we used fixed-effect model. The ventouse delivery is associated with AIS based on the data from the meta-analyses, (OR 2.23; 95% CI, 1.26 to 3.97). Visual assessment of a funnel plot and Beggar's test provided no evidence of obviously publication bias ($P = 1.000$) (Figure 3).

Oxytocin induction

Four studies (152 cases with AIS) were included in the meta-analysis. No significant heterogeneity was found ($Chi^2 = 3.74$, $P = 0.291$, $I^2 = 19.7\%$) (Figure 5), so fixed-effect model was used. Analysis of the data showed that oxytocin induction is associated with AIS (OR 1.33; 95% CI, 0.84 to 2.11). Visual assessment of a funnel plot and Beggar's test provided no evidence of obviously publication bias ($P = 1.000$) (Figure 3).

Fetal heart rate abnormalities

Four case-control studies (152 cases with AIS) were included in the meta-analysis. No heterogeneity was found ($Chi^2 = 0.95$, $P = 0.813$, $I^2 = 0\%$) (Figure 6), so fixed-effect model was used. The association between fetal heart rate abnormalities and AIS were seen in all meta-analyses (OR 6.3; 95% CI, 3.84 to 10.34). Visual assessment of a funnel plot and Beggar's test provided no evidence of obviously publication bias ($P = 1.000$) (Figure 3).

Reduced fetal movement

Two studies (68 cases) included in the meta-analysis. There was not heterogeneity among included studies ($Chi^2 = 0.03$, $P = 0.867$, $I^2 = 0\%$) (Figure 7), fixed-effect model was used. Analysis of the findings showed that reduced fetal movement is associated with AIS (OR 5.35; 95% CI, 2.17 to 13.23). We did not carry out the test of publication bias because of only two studies.

Meconium-stained liquor

Estimates were reported from five retrospective case–control studies with 171 cases. No heterogeneity was found ($Chi^2 = 3.04$, $P = 0.551$, $I^2 = 0\%$), we chose fixed-effect model to do the meta-analysis. This meta-analysis showed that meconium-stained liquor is significantly associated with AIS (OR 3.05; 95% CI, 2.02 to 4.60) (Figure 8). Visual assessment of a funnel plot and Beggar's test provided no evidence of obviously publication bias ($P = 1.000$) (Figure 3).

Low Apgar score

Six studies compared Apgar score between groups, however, Apgar score below 7 at 5 minutes is usually considered asphyxia, and we regarded this as the inclusion standard. Four case-control studies (158 cases) contributed to the meta-analysis. There was significant heterogeneity among included studies ($Chi^2 = 8.46$,

Table 2. Potential Hypoxia-related Risk Factors for AIS.

Complications	Numbers of studies	Cases of AIS
Prepartum complications		
Preeclampsia	4	27
Reduced fetal movement	2	16
Intrapartum complications		
Fetal heart rate abnormalities	4	72
Meconium-stained liquor	5	58
Oxytocin induction	4	50
Ventouse delivery	4	27
Breech delivery	4	9
Prolonged second stage of labour	3	13
Emergency caesarean section	7	NR
Premature rupture of membranes	6	35
Vaginal blood loss	1	2
Cord abnormality	4	NR
Forceps delivery	2	3
abruption placenta	1	5
Infant characteristics		
Arterial umbilical cord ph	3	26
Apgar score below 7 at 5 min	4	37
Congenital heart disease	1	3
Resuscitation at birth	4	NR

NR: not reported.

$P = 0.037$, $I^2 = 64.5\%$) (Figure 9), random-effect model was used. Analysis of the findings showed that low Apgar score is associated with AIS (OR 5.77; 95% CI, 1.66 to 20.04). No evidence of obviously publication bias was found according to funnel plot and Beggar's test ($P = 1.000$) (Figure 3).

Arterial umbilical cord ph

Four studies compared arterial umbilical cord ph between groups. Arterial umbilical cord ph below 7.1 is considered mild or moderate academia, we regarded 7.1 as the inclusion standard. Three studies (121 cases) were included in the meta-analysis. There was heterogeneity among included studies ($Chi^2 = 9.66$, $P = 0.008$, $I^2 = 79.3\%$) (Figure 10), random-effect model was used. Based on the data from the studies, the meta-analysis did not show any significant change of the mean risk estimate (OR 4.63; 95% CI 2.14 to 9.98). No evidence of obviously publication bias was found according to funnel plot and Beggar's test ($P = 1.000$) (Figure 3).

Resuscitation at birth

Three retrospective and one prospective case-control studies (423 cases) contributed to the meta-analysis. There was not heterogeneity among included studies ($Chi^2 = 0.21$, $P = 0.976$, $I^2 = 0\%$) (Figure 11), fixed-effect model was used. Analysis of the findings showed that resuscitation at birth is associated with AIS (OR 4.59; 95% CI, 3.23 to 6.52). No evidence of obviously publication bias was found according to funnel plot and Beggar's test ($P = 1.000$) (Figure 3).

Discussion

Our Study included 8 studies and 550 newborns with AIS. The pooled analysis indicates that the associations were found for AIS:

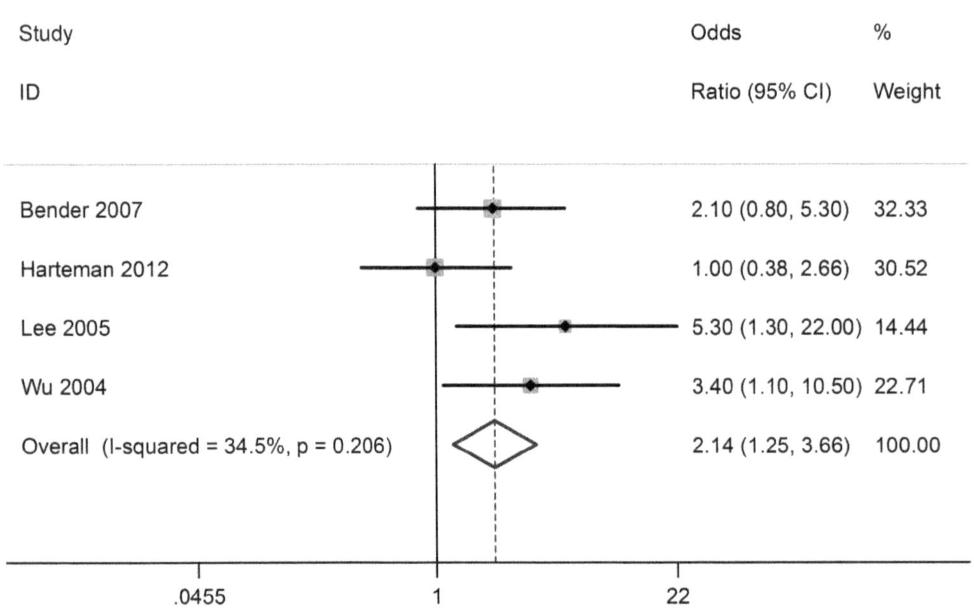

Figure 2. Fixed-effect model forest plot of odds ratio of the association between preeclampsia and AIS. The pooled OR of preeclampsia is symbolized by a solid diamond at the bottom of the forest plot and the width of which represents the 95% CI.

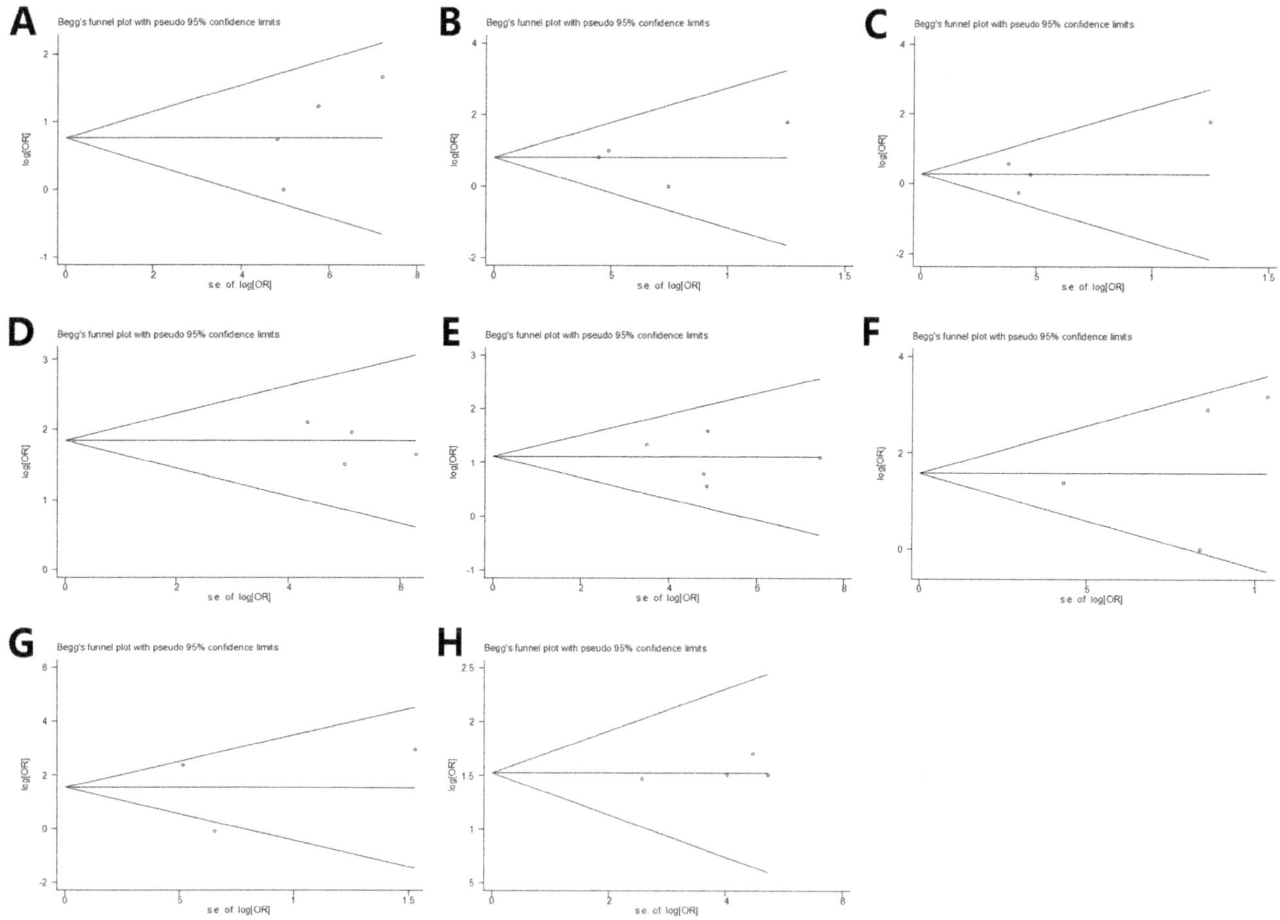

Figure 3. Begg's Funnel plot for publication bias test. The two oblique lines indicate the pseudo 95% confidence limits. a. funnel plot with pseudo 95% CI of preeclampsia b. funnel plot with pseudo 95% CI of ventouse delivery c. funnel plot with pseudo 95% CI of oxytocin induction d. funnel plot with pseudo 95% CI of heart rate abnormalities e. funnel plot with pseudo 95% CI of meconium-stained liquor f. funnel plot with pseudo 95% CI of Apgar scores g. funnel plot with pseudo 95% CI of arterial umbilical cord ph h. funnel plot with pseudo 95% CI of resuscitation at birth.

preeclampsia (OR 2.14; 95% CI, 1.25 to 3.66), ventouse delivery (OR 2.23; 95% CI, 1.26 to 3.97), fetal heart rate abnormalities (OR 6.3; 95% CI, 3.84 to 10.34), reduced fetal movement (OR 5.35; 95% CI, 2.17 to 13.23), meconium-stained liquor (OR 3.05; 95% CI, 2.02 to 4.60), low Apgar score (OR 5.77; 95% CI, 1.66 to 20.04) and resuscitation at birth (OR 4.59; 95% CI, 3.23 to 6.52). Our data did not show any significant change of the mean risk estimate for oxytocin induction (OR 1.33; 95% CI, 0.84 to 2.11) and low arterial umbilical cord ph (OR 4.63; 95% CI 2.14 to 9.98).

Neonatal arterial ischemic stroke is the most common form of cerebral infarction in children, and a leading cause of lifelong neurodevelopmental disabilities. Although the diagnosis is easily confirmed by neuro-imaging [24], about half the children arouse no concern during the neonatal period. However, when neonates are unstable, neuro-imaging can be difficult, particularly MRI and CT. In neonates, cranial ultrasound is a noninvasive and easily accessible intervention for the evaluation of stroke [25]. But it may not accurately diagnose stroke, (the cranial ultrasound is known to miss smaller cortical infarcts), especially since these events do not necessarily lead to neurologic symptoms later in infancy [20]. So identifying newborns at high risk of AIS is important.

The preeclampsia usually is associated with abnormalities in the development of placental vessels. And hypoxia is one of the critical components in the pathogenesis of preeclampsia [26]. Birth asphyxia was more common in the ventouse delivery cohort compared with normal delivery [27]. Our study suggests that preeclampsia and ventouse delivery may be one of the risk factors of AIS. Appropriate use of oxytocin induction generally may not lead to neonatal hypoxia. Our study did not show any association between oxytocin induction and AIS.

Fetal heart rate abnormalities and reduced fetal movement have been routinely considered as predictors of fetal distress. As meconium passage is associated with reduced cerebral artery pulsatility index, some evidence suggests that meconium-stained amniotic fluid may reflect fetal hypoxia [28]. Analysis of our results shows that for studies evaluating AIS, fetal heart rate abnormalities, reduced fetal movement and meconium-stained amniotic fluid may be risk factors.

Apgar score is a sum of values assigned to an infant, with a score of 7 or more indicating that the baby is in good to excellent condition [29]. An Apgar score <7, suggestive of fetal distress, is more commonly associated with AIS than previously reported, according to our meta-analysis. But because of the heterogeneity, further study is needed to confirm this conclusion. We speculate that the reason may be the clinical heterogeneity, one study took the Apgar score <5 at 5 min as the inclusion criteria [20], while the rest studies took the Apgar score <7 at 5 min as the inclusion

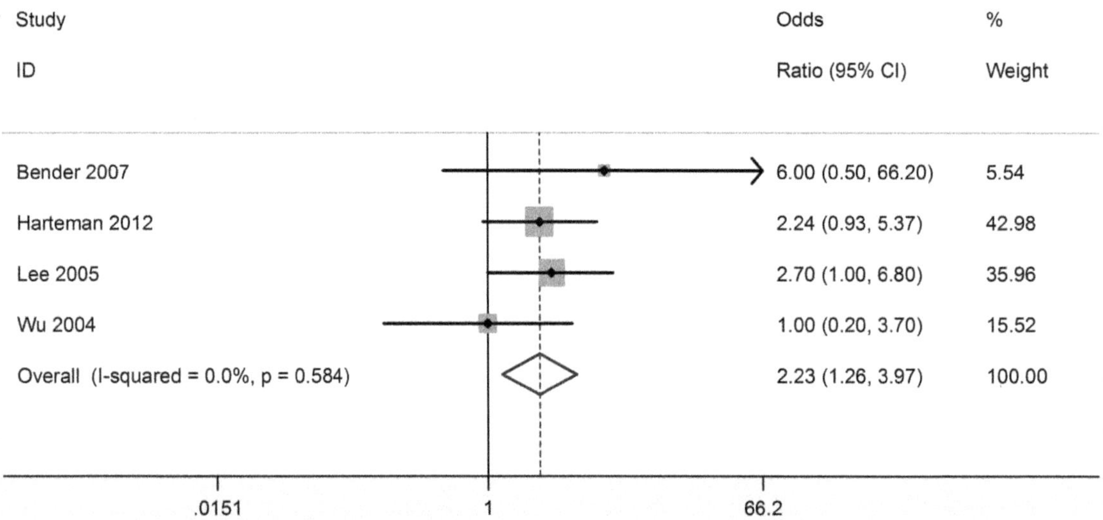

Figure 4. Fixed-effect model forest plot of odds ratio of the association between ventouse delivery and AIS. The pooled OR of ventouse delivery is symbolized by a solid diamond at the bottom of the forest plot and the width of which represents the 95% CI.

criteria. Low Apgar score likely reflects adverse events during delivery and suggests an important role for subsequent hypoxia-ischemia in the pathogenic pathway of AIS [14].

In most centers, an umbilical cord ph of 7 to 7.1 is considered mild or moderate academia, with severe acidemia occurring when the ph is below 7. It has been proposed that neonatal complications are associated with metabolic rather than respiratory acidosis [30]. Respiratory acidosis arises in the early stages of impaired blood supply to the fetus, with a subsequent reduction in the cord ph [31]. Other studies suggest that neurologic injury is more likely to occur in an infant who is distressed but has a normal ph [32]. Hermansen suggested there is an acidosis paradox, or a beneficial effect of a mild to moderate acidosis [33]. We did not find any association between umbilical cord ph and AIS. But as

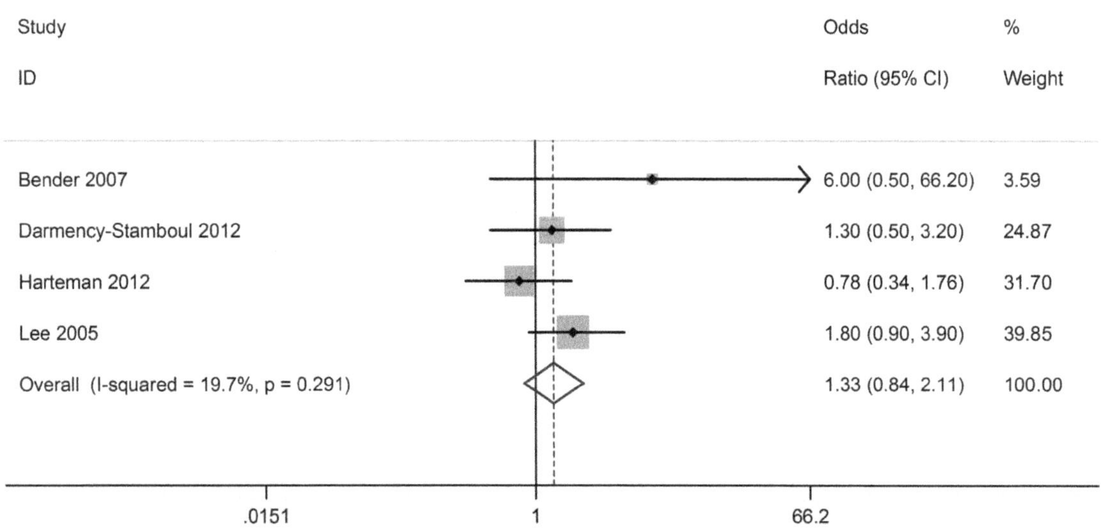

Figure 5. Fixed-effect model forest plot of odds ratio of the association between oxytocin induction and AIS. The pooled OR of oxytocin induction is symbolized by a solid diamond at the bottom of the forest plot and the width of which represents the 95% CI.

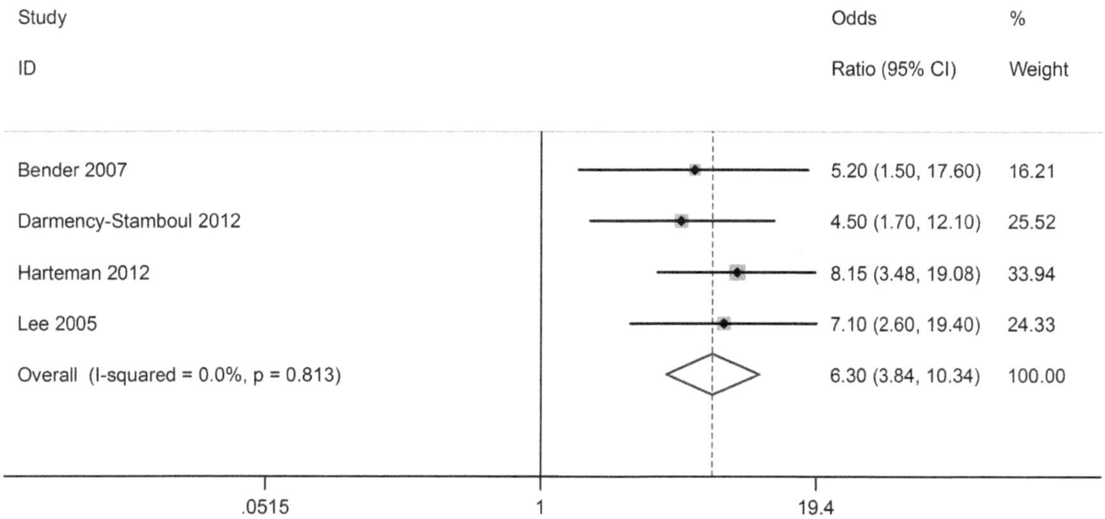

Figure 6. Fixed-effect model forest plot of odds ratio of the association between fetal heart rate abnormalities and AIS. The pooled OR of fetal heart rate abnormalities is symbolized by a solid diamond at the bottom of the forest plot and the width of which represents the 95% CI.

measurement of umbilical cord ph is not part of routine care in some obstetrics facilities, we only had these data in three studies. There was heterogeneity among these studies, the reason may be the clinical and statistical heterogeneity, one study included preterm newborns [20], full term was admitted to another [14]; one used univariable analysis [14], another used multivariable analysis [20]. Thus, more clinical studies are required to assess the relationship between arterial umbilical cord ph and AIS.

Resuscitation at birth usually refers to intubation, assisted ventilation, chest compressions, or cardiac medication. Neonates had transient hypoxia that needed resuscitation at birth. Kirton found that children with arterial presumed perinatal ischemic

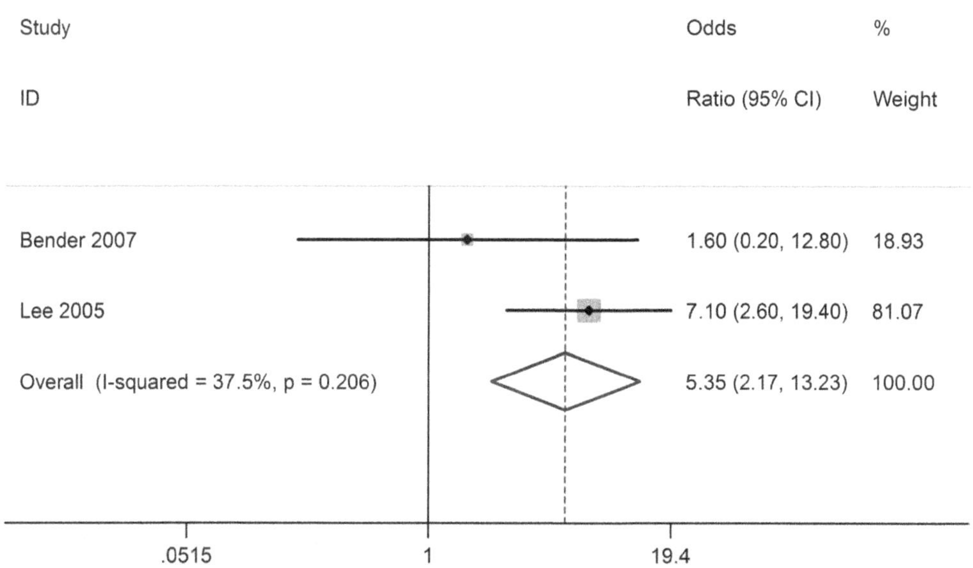

Figure 7. Fixed-effect model forest plot of odds ratio of the association between reduced fetal movement and AIS. The pooled OR of reduced fetal movement is symbolized by a solid diamond at the bottom of the forest plot and the width of which represents the 95% CI.

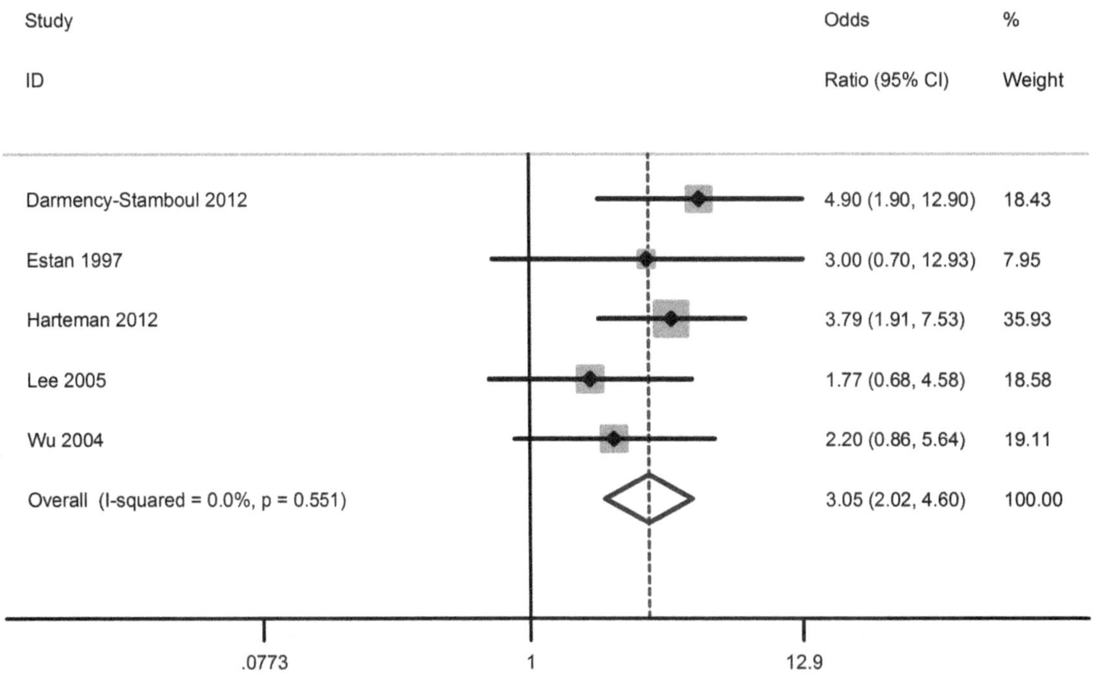

Figure 8. Fixed-effect model forest plot of odds ratio of the association between meconium-stained liquor and AIS. The pooled OR of meconium-stained liquor is symbolized by a solid diamond at the bottom of the forest plot and the width of which represents the 95% CI.

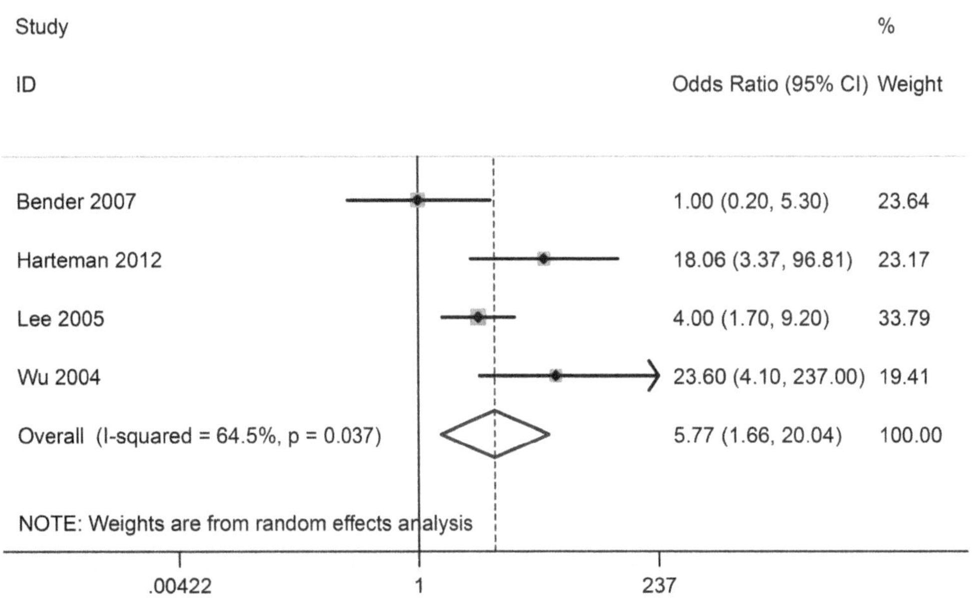

Figure 9. Random-effect model forest plot of odds ratio of the association between low Apgar scores and AIS. The pooled OR of low Appgar scores is symbolized by a solid diamond at the bottom of the forest plot and the width of which represents the 95% CI.

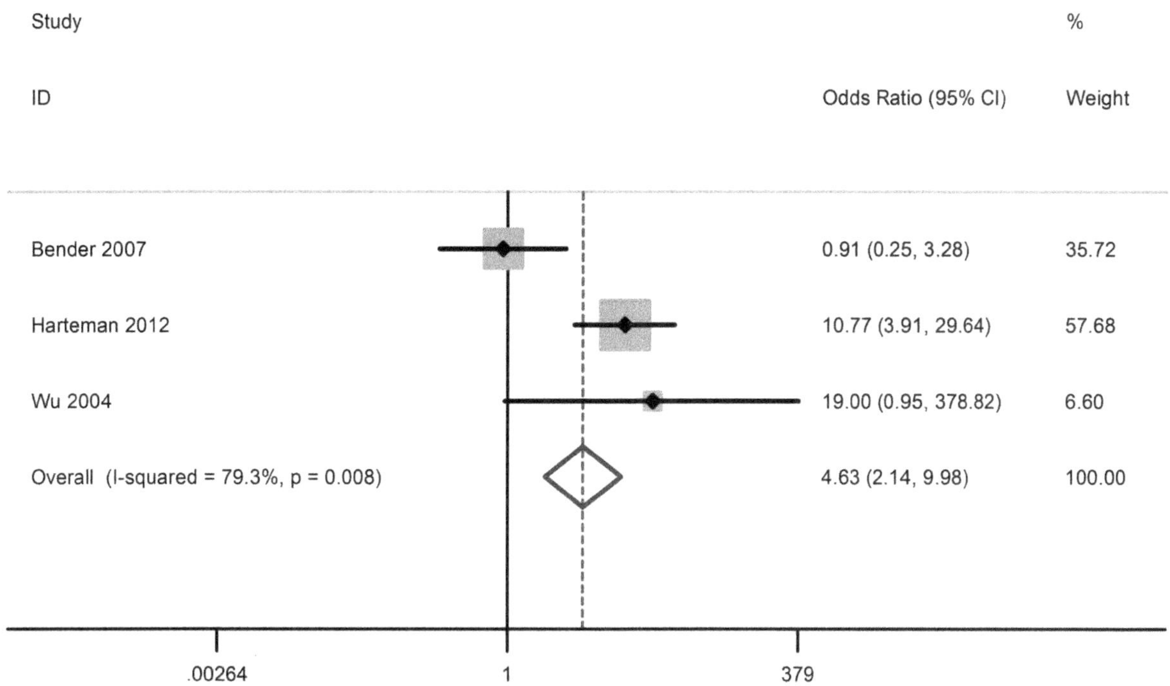

Figure 10. Random-effect model forest plot of odds ratio of the association between arterial umbilical cord ph and AIS. The pooled OR of arterial umbilical cord ph is symbolized by a solid diamond at the bottom of the forest plot and the width of which represents the 95% CI.

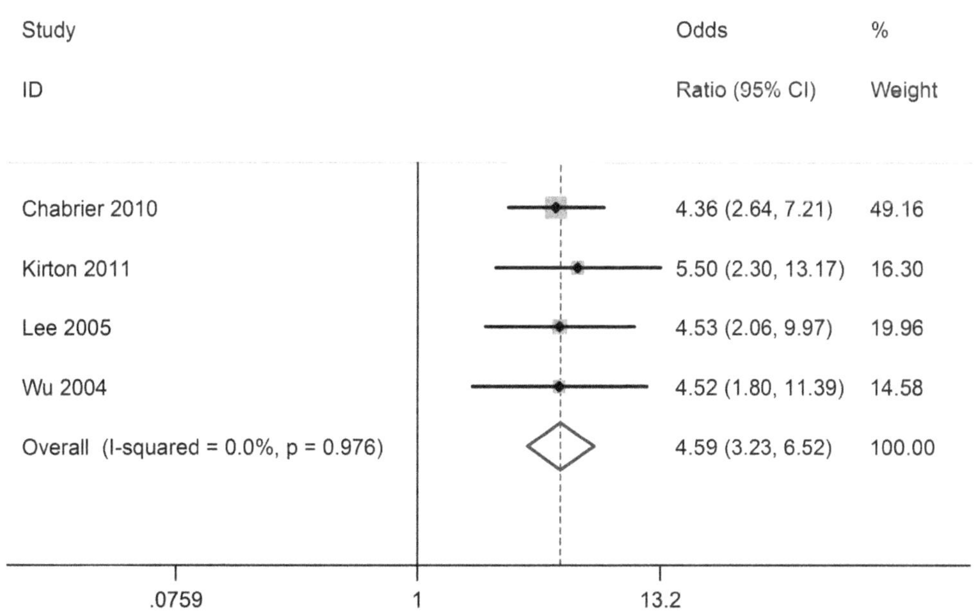

Figure 11. Fixed-effect model forest plot of odds ratio of the association between resuscitation at birth and AIS. The pooled OR of resuscitation at birth is symbolized by a solid diamond at the bottom of the forest plot and the width of which represents the 95% CI.

stroke were more likely to have neonatal resuscitation [34], which was consistent with ours.

Preeclampsia and ventouse delivery are intrapartum complications, both may cause neonatal hypoxia. Fetal heart rate abnormalities reduced fetal movement, meconium-stained amniotic fluid, low Apgar score and resuscitation at birth, all of which are recognized markers of perinatal hypoxia. All of them were more common in AIS cases than in control subjects. Our results suggested a role of perinatal hypoxia in the development of AIS. The same characteristics of neonatal distress suggest that shared pathological mechanisms for perinatal stroke and neonatal encephalopathy may exist, and both pathologies can furthermore coexist in the same baby, as shown by Ramaswamy [17].

AIS and global hypoxic-ischemic encephalopathy likely share risk factors and AIS can occur alongside hypoxic-ischemic encephalopathy. In Wu et al, 17% of infants with AIS had a low Apgar score, but 0.9% from a normal cohort had a low Apgar score [9].

Our findings imply that AIS is more often associated with a complicated gestational course and delivery, resulting in fetal distress or hypoxia. Since the occurrence of stroke in this cohort was more frequent than in population-based data, neuro-imaging should be performed in these infants. And the study comparing neonates with seizures caused by stroke with seizures caused by HIE reported that seizure onset >12 h and clinically observed focal seizures are more often associated with AIS [35]. So our findings suggest the use of MRI as the first-line imaging modality in most cases of neonatal encephalopathy, which facilitates the accurate diagnosis of AIS [23].

Although there is data about the risk factors for AIS, knowledge is still limited. In our meta-analysis, most of the included studies were designed retrospectively. Given the retrospective nature of these studies, it follows that bias towards risk factors may have occurred in the more severe cases [22]. The relatively small number of cases in subgroups resulted in statistical imprecision, and the results should accordingly be interpreted with caution. This study was subject to a number of limitations. However, there is a significant association between perinatal hypoxia factors, likewise preeclampsia, ventouse delivery, fetal heart rate abnormalities, reduced fetal movement, meconium-stained liquor, low Apgar score, resuscitation at birth and AIS. The results indicate that perinatal hypoxia maybe one of causes of AIS. Large scale prospective clinical studies are still warranted.

Author Contributions

Conceived and designed the experiments: LLL DZM. Performed the experiments: LLL DPC DZM. Analyzed the data: LLL DZM YQ. Contributed reagents/materials/analysis tools: LLL DZM YQ XHL. Wrote the paper: LLL DZM JLW.

References

1. Zadro R, Herak DC (2012) Inherited prothrombotic risk factors in children with first ischemic stroke. Biochemia Medica. 22(3):298–310.
2. Raju TN, Nelson KB, Ferriero D, Lynch JK (2007) Ischemic perinatal stroke: summary of aworkshop sponsored by the National Institute of Child Health and Human Development and the National Institute of Neurological Disorders and Stroke. Pediatrics. 120(3):609–616.
3. Chalmers EA (2005) Perinatal stroke—risk factors and management. Br J Haematol. 130(3):333–343.
4. Lynch JK (2009) Epidemiology and classification of perinatal stroke. Semin Fetal Neonatal Med. 14(5):245–9.
5. Laugesaar R, Kolk A, Tomberg T, Metsvaht T, Lintrop M, et al. (2007) Acutely and retrospectively diagnosed perinatal stroke: a population-based study. Stroke. 38(8):2234–2240.
6. Lee J, Croen LA, Backstrand KH, Yoshida CK, Henning LH, et al. (2005) Maternal and infant characteristics associated with perinatal arterial stroke in the infant. JAMA. 293(6):723–729.
7. Andrew ME, Monagle P, deVeber G, Chan AK (2001) Thromboembolic disease and antithrombotic therapy in newborns. Hematology Am Soc Hematol Educ Program. 358–374.
8. Estan J, Hope P (1997) Unilateral neonatal cerebral infarction in full term infants. Arch Dis Child Fetal Neonatal Ed. 76(2):F88–93.
9. Wu YW, March WM, Croen LA, Grether JK, Escobar GJ, et al. (2004) Perinatal stroke in children with motor impairment: a population-based study. Pediatrics. 114(3):612–619.
10. Golomb MR, Dick PT, MacGregor DL, Curtis R, Sofronas M, et al. (2004) Neonatal Arterial Ischemic Stroke and Cerebral Sinovenous Thrombosis Are More Commonly Diagnosed in Boys. J Child Neurol. 19(7):493–7.
11. Günther G, Junker R, Sträter R, Schobess R, Kurnik K, et al. (2000) Symptomatic ischemic stroke in full-term neonates : role of acquired and genetic prothrombotic risk factors. Stroke. 31(10):2437–41.
12. Laugesaar R, Kolk A, Uustalu U, Ilves P, Tomberg T, et al. (2010) Epidemiology of childhood stroke in Estonia. Pediatr Neurol. 42(2):93–100.
13. Tuckuviene R, Christensen AL, Helgested J, Hundborg HH, Kristensen SR, et al. (2012) Infant, obstetrical and maternal characteristics associated with thromboembolism in infancy: a nationwide population-based case-control study. Arch Dis Child Fetal Neonatal Ed. 97(6):F417–22.
14. Harteman JC, Groenendaal F, Kwee A, Welsing PM, Benders MJ, et al. (2012) Risk factors for perinatal arterial ischaemic stroke in full-term infants: a case-control study. Arch Dis Child Fetal Neonatal Ed. 97(6):F411–6.
15. Ment LR, Duncan CC, Ehrenkranz RA (1984) Perinatal cerebral infarction. Ann Neurol. 16(5):559–568.
16. Michoulas A, Basheer SN, Roland EH, Poskitt K, Miller S, et al. (2011) The role of hypoxia-ischemia in term newborns with arterial stroke. Pediatr Neurol. 44(4):254–258.
17. Ramaswamy V, Miller SP, Barkovich AJ, Partridge JC, Ferriero DM (2004). Perinatal stroke in term infants with neonatal encephalopathy. Neurology. 62(11):2088–2091.
18. Mercuri E, Rutherford M, Cowan F, Pennock J, Counsell S, et al. (1999) Early prognostic indicators of outcome in infants with neonatal cerebral infarction: a clinical, electroencephalogram, and magnetic resonance imaging study. Pediatrcs. 103(1):39–46.
19. Wells GA (2012). The Newcastle-Ottawa Scale (NOS) for Assessing the Quality of Nonrandomised Studies in Meta-analyses. Ottawa: Ottawa Hospital Research Institute. Available via DIALOG. http://www.ohri.ca/programs/clinical_epidemiology/oxford.asp. Accessed 2 Apr 2012.
20. Benders MJ, Groenendaal F, Uiterwaal CS, Nikkels PG, Bruinse HW, et al. (2007) Maternal and infant characteristics associated with perinatal arterial stroke in the preterm infant. Stroke. 38(6):1759–1765.
21. Chabrier S, Saliba E, Nguyen The Tich S, Charollais A, Varlet MN, et al. (2010) Obstetrical and neonatal characteristics vary with birth weight in a cohort of 100 term newborns with symptomatic arterial ischemic stroke. Eur J Paediatr Neurol. 14(3):206–13.
22. Darmency-Stamboul V, Chantegret C, Ferdynus C, Mejean N, Durand C, et al. (2012) Antenatal factors associated with perinatal arterial ischemic stroke. Stroke. 43(9):2307–2312.
23. Kirton A, Armstrong-Wells J, Chang T, Deveber G, Rivkin MJ, et al. (2011) Symptomatic neonatal arterial ischemic stroke: the International Pediatric Stroke Study. Pediatrics. 128(6):e1402–1410.
24. Nelson KB (2007) Perinatal ischemic stroke. Stroke. 38(2 Suppl):742–745.
25. Caravale B, Allemand F, Libenson MH (2003) Factors predictive of seizures and neurologic outcome in perinatal depression. Pediatr Neurol. 29(1):18–25.
26. Kim YJ (2013) Pathogenesis and promising non-invasive markers for preeclampsia. Obstet Gynecol Sci.56(1):2–7.
27. Palsdottir K, Dagbjartsson A, Thorkelsson T, Hardardottir H (2007) Birth asphyxia and hypoxic ischemic encephalopathy, incidence and obstetric risk factors. Laeknabladid.93(9):595–601.
28. Xu H, Mas-Calvet M, Wei SQ, Luo ZC, Fraser W (2009) Abnormal fetal heart rate tracing patterns in patients with thick meconium staining of the amniotic fluid: association with perinatal outcomes. Am J Obstet Gynecol. 200(3):283.e1–7
29. Leuthner SR, Das UG (2004) Low Apgar scores and the definition of birth asphyxia. Pediatr Clin North Am. 51(3):737–745.
30. Goldaber KG, Gilstrap LC 3rd, Leveno KJ, Dax JS, McIntire DD (1991) Pathologic fetal acidemia. Obstet Gynecol 78:1103–1107.
31. Fahey J, King TL (2005) Intrauterine asphyxia: clinical implications for providers of intrapartum care. Midwifery Women's Health. 50:498–506.
32. Dennis J, Johnson A, Mutch L, Yudkin P, Johnson P (1989) Acid-base status at birth and neurodevelopmental outcome at four and one-half years. Am J Obstet Gynecol. 161(1):213–220.

33. Hermansen MC (2003) The acidosis paradox: asphyxial brain injury without coincident acidemia. Dev Med Child Neurol. 45(5):353–356.
34. Kirton A, Shroff M, Pontigon AM, deVeber G (2010) Risk factors and presentations of periventricular venous infarction vs arterial presumed perinatal ischemic stroke. Arch Neurol. 67(7):842–848.
35. Rafay MF, Cortez MA, de Veber GA, Tan-Dy C, Al-Futaisi A, et al. (2009) Predictive value of clinical and EEG features in the diagnosis of stroke and hypoxic ischemic encephalopathy in neonates with seizures. Stroke. 40(7):2402–2407.

5

Association between 9p21 Genomic Markers and Ischemic Stroke Risk: Evidence Based on 21 Studies

Xiaoqing Ni[1], Jiawei Zhang[2]*

1 Department of Geriatrics, 107th Hospital of Chinese People's Liberation Army, Binzhou Medical University, Yantai, Shandong, People's Republic of China, **2** Department of Urology, 107th Hospital of Chinese People's Liberation Army, Binzhou Medical University, Yantai, Shandong, People's Republic of China

Abstract

Epidemiological studies indicate a genetic contribution to ischemic stroke risk, but specific genetic variants remain unknown. Recently independent studies reported an association between coronary heart disease and single-nucleotide polymorphisms (SNPs) located at chromosome 9p21 (rs10757278 and proxy SNPs). Given that stroke is a common complication after myocardial infarction, several validation studies have been conducted among various ethnic populations to investigate if the same loci was associated with ischemic stroke (IS), but the results have been inconsistent. To investigate this inconsistency and derive a more precise estimation of the relationship, a meta-analysis of 34,128 cases and 153,428 controls from 21 studies was performed. Potential sources of heterogeneity including ethnicity, sample size, control source and ischemic stroke subtypes were also assessed. Overall, the summary odds ratio of IS was 1.11 (95% CI: 1.07–1.15, $P<10^{-5}$) for rs10757278. In the subgroup analysis by ethnicity, significantly increased risks were found in East Asians (3188 cases and 4503 controls; OR = 1.14, 95% CI: 1.07–1.21, $P<10^{-5}$) and Caucasians (30505 cases and 145153controls; OR = 1.08, 95% CI: 1.04–1.12, $P<10^{-5}$) for the polymorphism; while no significant associations were found among African Americans (435 cases and 3772 controls; OR = 0.97, 95% CI: 0.63–1.51, P = 0.90) in all genetic models. In the subgroup analyses by IS subtypes, significant association was detected only in large vessel stroke group, while no significant associations among small vessel or cardioembolic stroke. When stratified by sample size, and control source, significantly increased risks were found for the polymorphism in all genetic models. This meta-analysis provides accurate and comprehensive estimates of the association of genetic variant at chromosome 9p21 and IS, but these associations vary in different ethnic populations.

Editor: Owen A. Ross, Mayo Clinic, United States of America

Funding: The authors have no support or funding to report.

Competing Interests: The authors have declared that no competing interests exist.

* E-mail: Jiawei_Zhang001@163.com

Introduction

Ischemic stroke (IS) is a leading cause of death and disability worldwide [1]. Traditional risk such as dyslipidemia, hypertension, atrial fibrillation smoking, and diabetes mellitus can only explain a small proportion of the observed clinical events [2]. However, a large proportion of the population attributable risk for ischemic stroke has remained unexplained [3]. Twin and familial aggregation studies suggest that the risk of stroke has a substantial genetic component [4], but the genes underlying this risk in the general population remain undetermined. Since the pathogenesis of ischemic stroke is yet to be elucidated completely, the candidate-gene approach is limited in power to detect novel disease-susceptibility genes.

Recently, significant advance was made in identifying susceptible genes underlying the risk of complex diseases such as type 2 diabetes and coronary disease through genome-wide association strategy (GWAS) [5–7]. The strongest association signal in the genome in GWAS for myocardial infarction (MI) and coronary artery disease (CAD) that has been published thus far comes from a number of SNPs with a high degree of linkage disequilibrium between each other on chromosome 9p21 [7–9]. Given the fact that ischemic stroke shares several common risk factors and pathophysiological mechanism with CAD and MI [10,11], the genomic interval on chromosome 9p21 could be a candidate locus for IS as well. Only recently, several small studies have looked for an association between sequence variants on 9p21 and IS risk [8,12,13].

A number of studies have been conducted to investigate the association between chromosome 9p21 polymorphisms and the risk of IS in humans; however, these studies have yielded inconsistent result. Genetic association studies can be problematic to reproduce due to multiple hypothesis testing, relatively small sample size, population stratification, source of controls, publication bias, and phenotypic heterogeneity. In addition, with the increased studies in recent years among Asian, and other populations, there is a need to reconcile these data. We therefore performed a meta-analysis of the published studies to clarify this inconsistency and to establish a comprehensive picture of the relationship between genetic markers of chromosome 9p21 and IS.

Materials and Methods

Literature Search Strategy and Selection Criteria

Genetic association studies published before the end of August 2013 on ischemic stroke and polymorphisms within chromosome 9p21 gene were identified through a search of PubMed, ISI Web of Science, EMBASE and CNKI (Chinese National Knowledge Infrastructure) without language restrictions. Search term combinations were keywords relating to chromosome 9p21 (e.g., "chromosome 9p21", "CDKN2A/B", or "ANRIL") in combination with words related to IS (e.g., "ischemic stroke", "stroke", "cerebral infarction", "cerebral ischemia", or "cerebrovascular disease") and polymorphism or variation. We replaced one term each time until all possible combination mode were searched to avoid any missing literature. The titles and abstracts of potential articles were screened to determine their relevance, and any clearly irrelevant studies were excluded. The full texts of the remaining articles were read to determine whether they contained information on the topic of interest. All reference lists from the main reports and relevant reviews were hand searched for additional eligible studies.

Eligible studies had to meet all of the following criteria: (a) original papers containing independent data, (b) case–control or cohort studies, (c) identification of IS case was confirmed pathologically and (d) genotype distribution information or odds ratio (OR) with its 95% confidence interval (CI) and P-value. The major reasons for exclusion of studies were (a) overlapping data and (b) case-only studies, (c) family-based studies and review articles.

Data Extraction

Information was carefully extracted from all eligible publications independently by two authors according to the inclusion criteria listed above. For each included study, the following data was extracted from each report according to a fixed protocol: first author, publication year, definition and numbers of cases and controls, diagnostic criterion, frequency of genotypes, source of controls, body mass index (BMI), age, sex, Hardy–Weinberg equilibrium (HWE) status, ethnicity and genotyping method. Discrepancies in data extraction were resolved by discussion between all authors through consensus. Studies with different ethnic groups were considered as individual studies for our analyses. Not all researchers use the same 9p21 SNPs, and most articles reported results for multiple SNPs (uniquely identified by their rs number). We extracted data for all SNPs used by the 21 included articles, but we report herein 1 common SNP (rs10757278) that was widely investigated, as other SNPs (rs2383207, rs2383206, rs10757274, and rs4977574) are in high linkage disequilibrium with rs10757278 (r^2>0.85) [6,8,14,15,16].

Statistical Methods

The strength of association between chromosome 9p21 polymorphisms and IS risk was assessed by OR with corresponding 95% CI. Deviation from Hardy–Weinberg equilibrium was examined by Chi-square test. If controls of studies were found not to be in HWE, sensitivity analyses were performed with and without these studies to test the robustness of the findings. The meta-analysis examined the association between chromosome 9p21 polymorphisms and the risk of IS: (1) allele contrast (effect of each additional risk allele), (2) dominant model (presence vs. absence of the risk allele), and (3) recessive model (presence vs. absence of two copies of the risk allele). Random-effects summary measure was calculated as inverse-variance-weighted average of the log odds ratio [17]. The results of random-effects summary were reported in the text because it takes into account the variation between studies. Heterogeneity was assessed with standard Q-statistic test and I^2 test [18,19].

In addition, sources of heterogeneity were investigated by stratified meta-analyses based on ethnicity, sample size (IS cases ≥ 500 or <500), ischemic stroke subtype and control source (hospital or population based study). Ethnic group was defined as Caucasian (i.e., people of white European origin), East Asian (e.g., Chinese, Japanese, Korean), and African American. BMI, sample size, age, sex and ethnicity were analyzed as covariates in meta-regression. The 95% CIs were constructed using Woolf's method [20]. The significance of the overall OR was determined by the Z-test. Funnel plots and Egger's linear regression test were used to assess evidence for potential publication bias [21]. In order to assess the stability of the result, sensitivity analyses were performed, each study in turn was removed from the total, and the remaining were reanalyzed. All the analyses were carried out with the STATA software version 10.0 (Stata Corporation, College Station, TX, USA). All P values are two-sided at the P = 0.05 level.

Results

Study Characteristics

The combined search yielded 105 references. 84 articles were excluded because they clearly did not meet the criteria or overlapping references (Figure 1). Finally, a total of 21 studies were finally included with 34,128 patients and 153, 428 controls [12–15,22–38]. The detailed characteristics of the studies included in this meta-analysis are shown in Table 1. The polymorphism on chromosome 9p21 was found to occur in frequencies consistent with HWE in the control populations of the vast majority of the published studies. There are 26 data sets with 30505 cases and 145153 controls concerning Caucasians and 5 data sets with 3188 cases and 4503 controls concerning East Asians. For the African American, 4 data sets involved a total of 435 cases and 3772 controls.

Meta-analysis Results

The main results of this meta-analysis were listed in Table 2. In the overall analysis, the risk allele of rs10757278 polymorphism was significantly associated with elevated IS risk. Under a random-effect model, the per-allele OR for IS was 1.11 (95% CI: 1.07–1.15, $P<10^{-5}$; Figure 2) with corresponding results under dominant and receive genetic model of 1.19 (95% CI: 1.11–1.25, $P<10^{-5}$) and 1.23 (95% CI: 1.19–1.29, $P<10^{-5}$), respectively.

When studies were stratified for ethnicity, significant risks were found among East Asians in all genetic model [allele contrast: OR = 1.14, 95% CI: 1.06–1.21; dominant model: OR = 1.19, 95% CI: 1.10–1.31; recessive model: OR = 1.17, 95% CI: 1.05–1.32]. Similar results were also found in Caucasian populations [allele contrast: OR = 1.11, 95% CI: 1.07–1.15; dominant model: OR = 1.18, 95% CI: 1.14–1.27; recessive model: OR = 1.26, 95% CI: 1.19–1.31]. However, no significant association was found for African American populations in all genetic models. Subsidiary analyses of sample size yielded a per-allele OR for small studies of 1.11 (95% CI: 1.05–1.17, P = 0.001) and large studies of 1.10 (95% CI: 1.06–1.15, $P<10^{-5}$). By considering control source subgroups, the OR was 1.10 (95% CI: 1.06–1.14, $P<10^{-5}$) in population-based controls compared to 1.27 (95% CI: 1.10–1.47, P = 0.001) in hospital-based controls. In the subgroup analyses by ischemic stroke subtype, significant associations were found for large vessel stroke in all genetic modes [allele contrast: OR = 1.15, 95% CI: 1.10–1.19; dominant model: OR = 1.19, 95% CI: 1.08–1.30; recessive model: OR = 1.24, 95% CI: 1.07–1.45]. However, we failed to detect any association between small vessel stroke, cardioembolic stroke, or other type of stroke risk and the polymorphism (Figure 3 and Table S1). After adjusting for multiple testing using Bonferroni correction, all significant associations for rs10757278 under the three different genetic models remained.

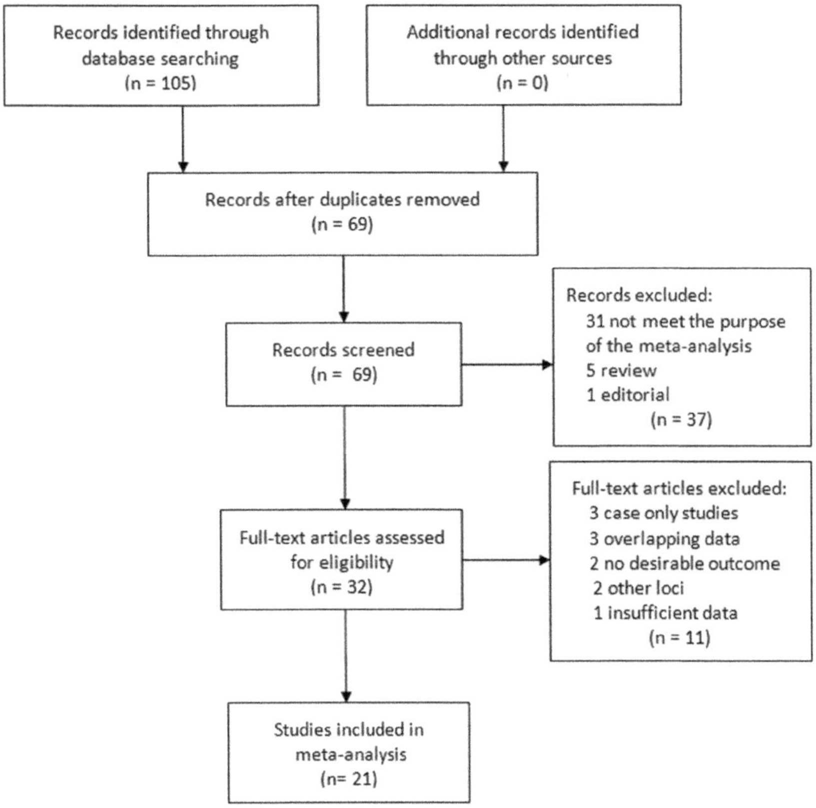

Figure 1. Study selection process.

Although the formal test for heterogeneity was not significant (P>0.05), we conducted meta-regression as there were also grounds for considering the ethnicity, sample size, IS subtype, and clinical characteristics of cases and controls (age, BMI, and sex distribution) as potential sources of heterogeneity. However, the meta-regression showed that none of these covariates significantly contributed to the heterogeneity among the individual study results except for ethnicity (P = 0.01) and IS subtype (P = 0.002).

Sensitivity Analyses and Publication Bias

Sensitivity analysis indicated that no single study influenced the pooled OR qualitatively, suggesting that the results of this meta-analysis are stable (Figure S1). The shape of the funnel plots was symmetrical (Figure S2). The statistical results still did not show publication bias in these studies (Begg test, P = 0.55; Egger test, P = 0.45).

Discussion

Genome-wide association studies have identified a locus for risk of coronary artery disease on chromosome 9p21 [7–9]. Recent studies have also analyzed the association between 9p21 and overall ischemic stroke, with diverse outcomes [22–27]. The present meta-analysis provides the most comprehensive assessment of the risk of IS and 9p21 variant (rs10757278). Its strength was based on the accumulation of published data giving greater information to detect significant differences. In total, the meta-analysis involved 21 studies for IS which provided 34,128 cases and 153, 428 controls.

Our results demonstrated that the rs10757278 polymorphism on chromosome 9p21 is a risk factor for developing ischemic stroke. In the stratified analysis by ethnicity, significant associations were found in East Asian and Caucasian populations for the polymorphism in all genetic models. However, no significant associations were detected among African populations. There are several possible reasons for such differences. In fact, the frequencies of the risk-association alleles in chromosome 9p21 are similar in European and East Asian populations, but substantially lower in African descent [22,27,37,38]. Thus, failing to identify any significant association in African populations could be due to substantially lower statistical power caused by the relatively lower prevalence of the risk allele. In addition, study design or small sample size or some environmental factors may affect the results. Most of these studies did not consider most of the important environmental factors. It is possible that variation at this locus has modest effects on IS, but environmental factors may predominate in the progress of IS, and mask the effects of this variation. Specific environmental factors like lifestyle and diabetes that have been already well studied in recent decades. The unconsidered factors mixed together may cover the role of the polymorphism. Furthermore, different populations usually have different linkage disequilibrium patterns. A polymorphism may be in close linkage with another nearby causal variant in one ethnic population but not in another. The rs10757278 polymorphism may be in close linkage with different nearby causal variants in different populations. Nevertheless, owing to the limited number of relevant studies among African Americans included in this meta-analysis, the observed ethnic difference in this meta-analysis is also likely to be caused by chance because studies with small sample sizes may have insufficient statistical power to detect a slight effect or may have generated a fluctuated risk estimate.

Table 1. Characteristics of the studies included in the meta-analysis.

Reference	Year	Ethnicity	Ethnic groups	Polymorphism	Case	Match criteria for control	No. of cases/ controls	Source of control	Genotyping method
Zee [12]	2007	American	Caucasian	rs10757274	CT or MRI confirmed	Age, ethnicity, smoking status	254/254	Population	NA
Matarin [13]	2008	American	Caucasian	rs2383207	IS per WHO criteria	Age, sex, ethnicity	249/268	Population	Chip
Helgadottir [14]	2008	European	Caucasian	rs10757278	CT or MRI confirmed	Ethnicity	705/14993	Population	Chip
Smith [15]	2009	Swedish	Caucasian	rs2383207	IS per WHO criteria	Age, sex, ethnicity, time of baseline investigation	2725/1840	Population	MassArray
Gschwendtner [22]	2009	European, African American	Caucasian, African American	rs10757278	CT or MRI confirmed	Age, sex, ethnicity, site of enrolment	932/4150	Population	TaqMan
Lemmens [23]	2009	Belgian	Caucasian	rs10757278	IS per WHO criteria	Sex, ethnicity	636/809	Population	Taqman
Karvanen [24]	2009	European	Caucasian	rs1333049	IS per ICD-9 criteria	Age, sex, ethnicity, site of enrolment	209/2064	Population	MassArray
Ikram [25]	2009	European	Caucasian	rs1537378	CT or MRI confirmed	Age, ethnicity	1164/18438	Population	Chip
Luke [26]	2009	Austrian	Caucasian	rs10757274	CT or MRI confirmed	Ethnicity	503/784	Population	Kinetic PCR
Yamagishi [27]	2009	American	Caucasian, African American	rs10757274	IS per ICD-9 criteria	Ethnicity	524/12856	Population	Taqman
Ding [28]	2009	Chinese	East Asian	rs10757278	IS per ICD-9 criteria	Ethnicity, resident area	999/1055	Population	TaqMan
Wahlstrand [29]	2009	Swedish	Caucasian	rs10757278	IS patients	Ethnicity, time of follow-up	163/5099	Hospital	MassArray
Hu [30]	2009	Chinese	East Asian	rs2383206	CT or MRI confirmed	Ethnicity	352/423	Hospital	SNPstream
Plant [31]	2011	American	Caucasian	rs10757278	CT or MRI confirmed	Age, sex, ethnicity	229/229	Population	Taqman
Olsson [32]	2011	Swedish	Caucasian	rs10757278	CT or MRI confirmed	Age, sex, ethnicity	834/665	Population	Golden Gate
Lin [33]	2011	Chinese	East Asian	rs1333049	IS per WHO criteria	Ethnicity	642/1361	Population	Taqman
Bellenguez [34]	2012	European, American	Caucasian	rs2383207	CT or MRI confirmed	Age, sex, ethnicity	1780/12253	Population	Chip
Traylor [35]	2012	European	Caucasian	rs2383207	CT or MRI confirmed	Ethnicity	12389/65004	Population	Chip, Taqman
Cheng [36]	2012	European, American	Caucasian	rs4977574	CT or MRI confirmed	Age, sex, ethnicity	6865/11395	Population	KASPar, Taqman
Zhang [37]	2012	Chinese	East Asian	rs10757278	IS per WHO criteria	Age, sex, resident area	1195/1664	Population	LDR
Heckman [38]	2013	American	Caucasian, African American	rs2383207	IS per WHO criteria	Ethnicity	879/824	Population	MassArray

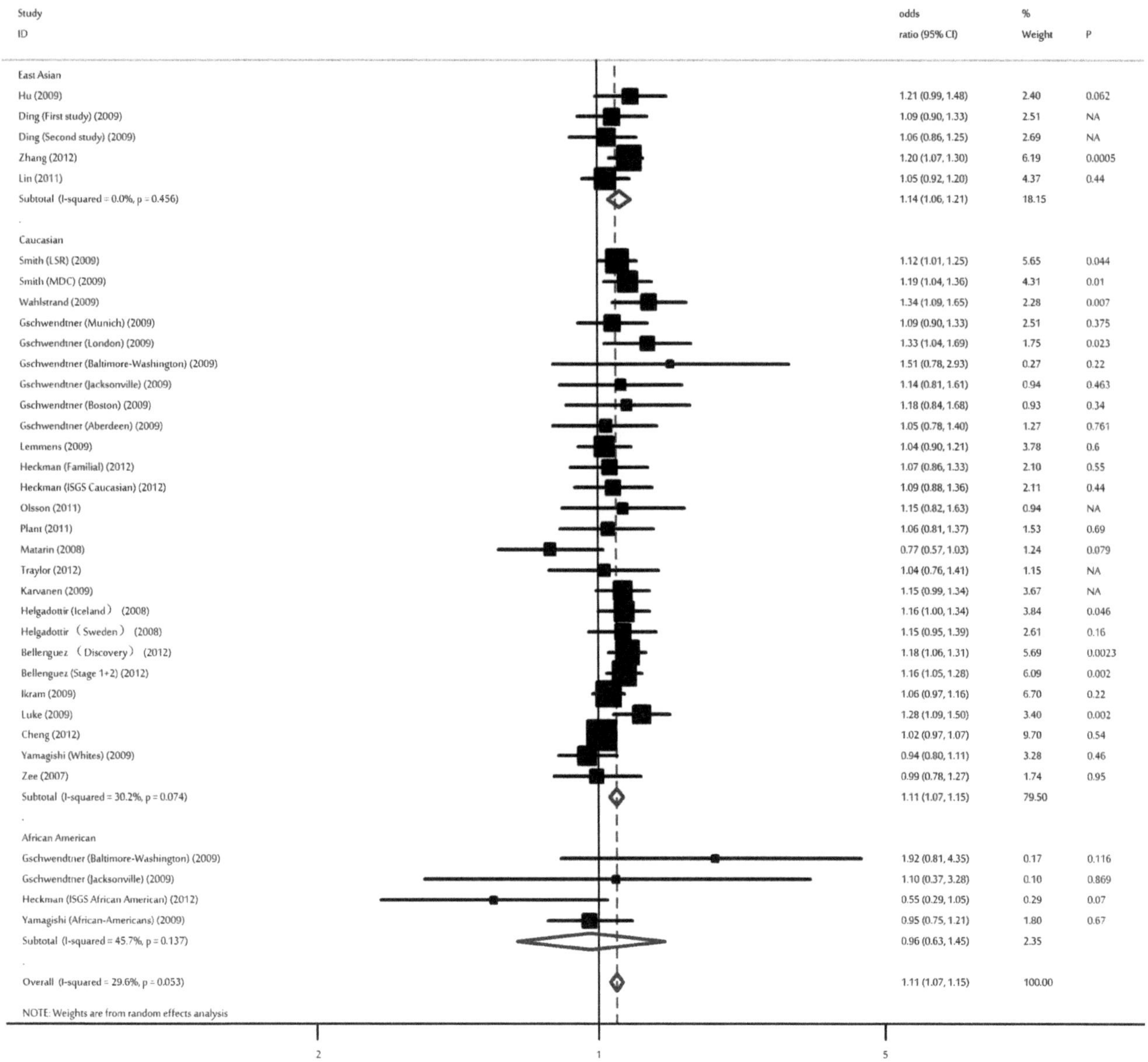

Figure 2. Meta-analysis of studies on the association of rs10757278 on chromosome 9p21 with ischemic stroke.

Thus, further studies including a wider spectrum of subjects to investigate the role of chromosome 9p21 variants in this population will be needed.

Meta-analysis is often dominated by a few large studies, which markedly reduces the evidence from smaller studies. However, in the stratified analysis according to sample size, significantly increased IS susceptibility in risk allele carriers rs10757278 polymorphism was also found both in large and small studies for all genetic models.

Ischemic stroke itself has a number of subtypes with the most common being large-vessel atherosclerotic stroke, small-vessel disease, and cardioembolism. As ischemic stroke subtypes was the main source of heterogeneity in our meta-analysis, we performed subgroup analyses by IS subtypes. We found that the risk allele has an increased risk in large-vessel stroke subgroup but not in small-vessel or cardioembolic stroke subgroup. This finding is in line with previous family history studies on ischemic stroke subtypes, showing a greater risk associated with large vessel stroke than small vessel stroke [39]. Recently, Zhang et al. [37] reported that family history of stroke further increased the stroke risk to 2.37-fold in subjects carrying 4 copies of G-allele of rs10757274 and rs10757278, and also increased the risk of stroke recurrence (2.45-fold). Thus, a combination of the risk variants on 9p21.3 with family stroke history could help to predict an individual's risk of stroke. The reason for the observed stroke-specific difference in the risk conferred by the rs10757278 polymorphism is unknown. It has been suggested that genetic predisposition may differ for these subtypes [40], and of note, most monogenic forms of stroke predispose to individual stroke subtypes [40]. This genetic heterogeneity seems likely to reflect heterogeneity in the underlying pathogenic mechanisms and reinforces the need for the consideration of stroke subtypes separately in research and clinical contexts.

The association between ischemic stroke and SNPs at a locus previously associated with coronary artery disease and diabetes

Table 2. Meta-analysis of the chromosome 9p21 genetic marker on ischemic stroke risk.

Sub-group analysis	No. of data sets	No. of case/ control	Allele contrast					Dominant model					Recessive model				
			OR (95% CI)	P-value	P(Q)[a]	I^2 (%)	P(Q)[b]	OR (95% CI)	P-value	P(Q)[a]	I^2 (%)	P(Q)[b]	OR (95% CI)	P-value	P(Q)[a]	I^2 (%)	P(Q)[b]
Overall	35	34128/153428	1.11 (1.07–1.15)	$<10^{-5}$	0.05	30		1.19 (1.11–1.25)	$<10^{-5}$	0.19	21		1.23 (1.19–1.29)	$<10^{-5}$	0.07	33	
Ethnicity							0.14					0.20					0.11
Caucasian	26	30505/145153	1.11 (1.07–1.15)	$<10^{-5}$	0.07	30		1.18 (1.14–1.27)	$<10^{-5}$	0.24	15		1.26 (1.19–1.31)	$<10^{-5}$	0.19	14	
East Asian	5	3188/4503	1.14 (1.06–1.21)	$<10^{-5}$	0.46	0		1.19 (1.10–1.31)	$<10^{-5}$	0.39	0		1.17 (1.05–1.32)	$<10^{-4}$	0.36	7	
African American	4	435/3772	0.96 (0.63–1.45)	0.83	0.14	46		1.06 (0.90–1.26)	0.58	0.14	10		1.08 (0.98–1.22)	0.13	0.46	0	
Sample size							0.03					0.05					0.18
Small	23	5340/42445	1.11 (1.05–1.17)	0.001	0.12	22		1.16 (1.10–1.24)	$<10^{-5}$	0.20			1.20 (1.05–1.39)	$<10^{-5}$	0.17	12	
large	12	28788/110983	1.10 (1.06–1.15)	$<10^{-5}$	0.09	27		1.21 (1.09–1.24)	$<10^{-5}$	0.31	8		1.25 (1.17–1.29)	$<10^{-5}$	0.48	0	
Control source							0.02					0.13					0.08
Hospital	2	515/5522	1.27 (1.10–1.47)	0.001	0.49	0		1.28 (1.15–1.46)	$<10^{-4}$	0.27	16		1.45 (1.18–1.99)	0.0008	0.10	21	
Population	33	33613/147906	1.10 (1.06–1.14)	$<10^{-5}$	0.08	26		1.18 (1.10–1.25)	$<10^{-5}$	0.12	11		1.22 (1.17–1.31)	$<10^{-5}$	0.03	30	
IS subtypes							$<10^{-5}$					$<10^{-5}$					$<10^{-5}$
Large vessel	9	6226/89235	1.15 (1.10–1.19)	$<10^{-5}$	0.54	0		1.19 (1.08–1.30)	$<10^{-5}$	0.27	19		1.24 (1.07–1.45)	$<10^{-4}$	0.39	0	
Cardioembolic	5	4744/78485	1.03 (0.95–1.13)	0.47	0.09	50		1.17 (0.95–1.46)	0.31	0.05	62		1.22 (0.92–1.68)	0.46	0.13	20	
Small vessel	6	4272/80149	1.02 (0.98–1.07)	0.31	0.87	0		1.01 (0.96–1.06)	0.17	0.58	0		1.07 (0.98–1.19)	0.08	0.46	0	
Other determined causes	2	535/15657	1.01 (0.85–1.19)	0.91	0.33	0		1.09 (0.95–1.25)	0.26	0.12	7		1.52 (0.53–4.35)	0.41	0.27	0	
Undetermined causes	2	3358/15657	1.02 (0.96–1.08)	0.46	0.62	0		1.07 (0.97–1.26)	0.71	0.48	0		1.10 (0.97–1.26)	0.21	0.54	0	

[a]Cochran's chi-square Q statistic test used to assess the heterogeneity in subgroups.
[b]Cochran's chi-square Q statistic test used to assess the heterogeneity between subgroups.
Allele contrast (effect of each additional risk allele).
Dominant model (presence vs. absence of the risk allele).
Recessive model (presence vs. absence of two copies of the risk allele).

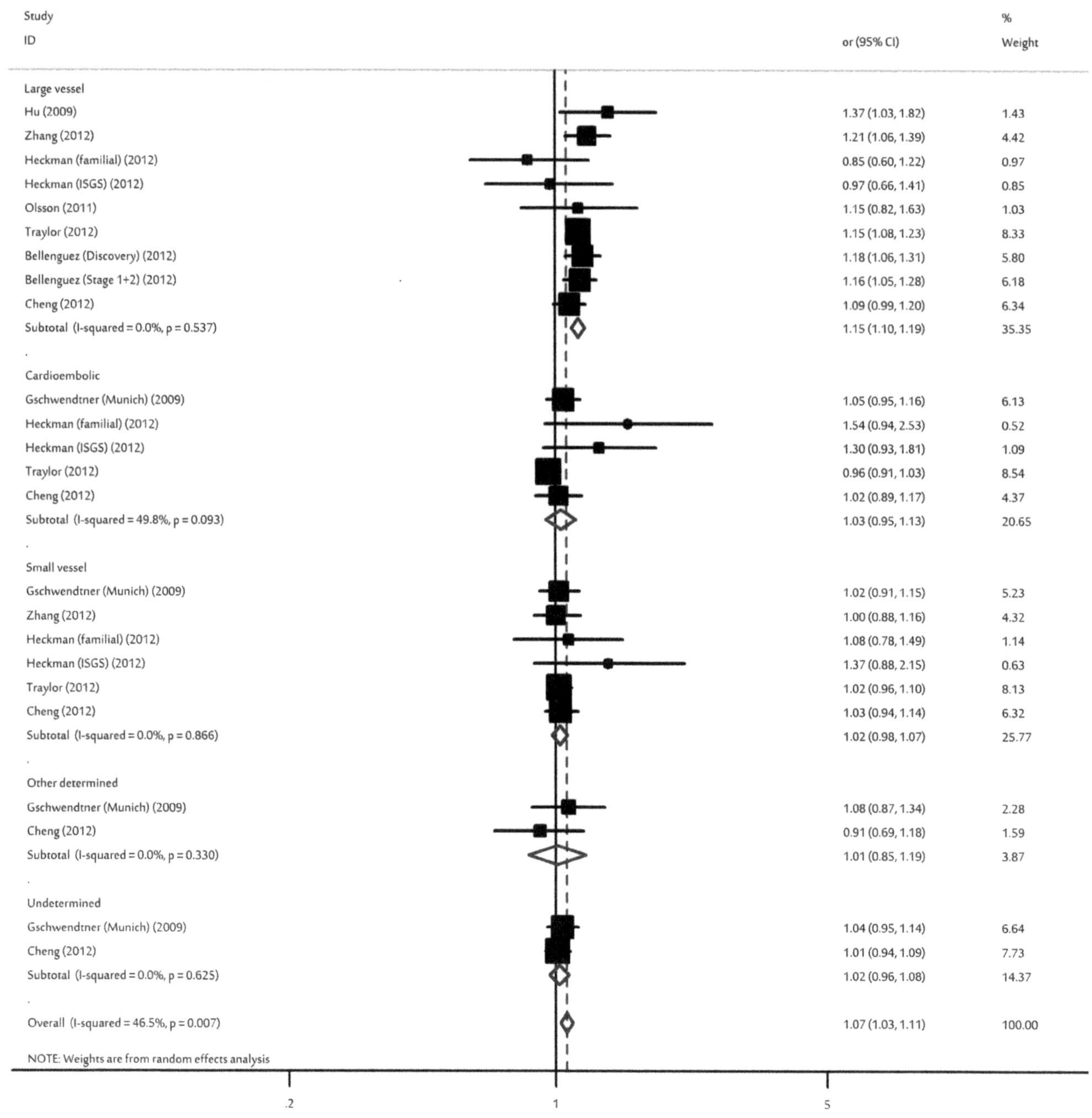

Figure 3. Forest plot for the association between rs10757278 and ischemic stroke risk by stroke subtype status.

suggest that ischemic stroke shares common pathophysiological pathways with these diseases. Recently, a common variant near the CDKN2B gene in the chromosome 9p21 locus is associated with a lower ankle-brachial index which is a simple and reliable method to detect peripheral arterial disease [41]. The cardiovascular disease-associated regions at the chromosome 9p21 locus are adjacent to the last exons of a long noncoding RNA (lncRNA), ANRIL (also known as CDKN2BAS) [42]. Two cyclin-dependent kinases inhibitors, CDKN2A and CDKN2B (encoding p15INK4B, p16INK4A, and p14ARF) lie close to the association spot (~100 kb from the associated SNPs). CDKN2A/B are known to be repressed by Polycomb proteins during cell growth and then activated during senescence [43]. There is strong evidence to support the role of ANRIL in the regulation of the CDKN2A/B locus through histone modification [44,45]. ANRIL has been proposed to regulate senescence at the CDKN2A locus, and it showed a senescence-dependant role in proliferation [44]. These findings emphasize the importance of ANRIL in cell proliferation and regulation of the locus CDKN2A/B in a cell line directly involved in the pathogenesis of atherosclerosis.

In summary, this study provides the most comprehensive evidence that 9p21 is a susceptibility locus in ischemic stroke, particularly in East Asian and Caucasian populations. More important, these variants may have different degrees of influence on various subtypes of ischemic stroke. Larger studies of different ethnic populations, especially strict selection of patients, well-matched controls, are needed to confirm our findings. An improved understanding of the pathogenesis of IS will be beneficial in the diagnosis of prodromal symptoms and in establishing appropriate therapeutic intervention to prevent the onset and the progression of IS.

Supporting Information

Figure S1 Result of sensitivity analyses for rs10757278 polymorphism and ischemic stroke risk.

Figure S2 Funnel plot for rs10757278 polymorphism and ischemic stroke risk.

Table S1 Per-allele OR for rs10757278 variant and risk of IS subtype stratified by ethnic groups.

Checklist S1 CONSORT Checklist.

Author Contributions

Conceived and designed the experiments: XQN JWZ. Performed the experiments: XQN JWZ. Analyzed the data: XQN JWZ. Contributed reagents/materials/analysis tools: XQN JWZ. Wrote the paper: XQN JWZ.

References

1. Rosamond W, Flegal K, Furie K, Go A, Greenlund K, et al. (2008) Heart disease and stroke statistics–2008 update: a report from the American Heart Association Statistics Committee and Stroke Statistics Subcommittee. Circulation 117: e25–e146.
2. Sacco RL, Ellenberg JH, Mohr JP, Tatemichi TK, Hier DB, et al. (1989) Infarcts of undetermined cause: the NINCDS Stroke Data Bank. Ann Neurol 25: 382–390.
3. Conroy RM, Pyörälä K, Fitzgerald AP, Sans S, Menotti A, et al. (2003) Estimation of ten-year risk of fatal cardiovascular disease in Europe: the SCORE project. Eur Heart J 24: 987–1003.
4. Dichgans M (2007) Genetics of ischaemic stroke. Lancet Neurol 6: 149–161.
5. Scott LJ, Mohlke KL, Bonnycastle LL, Willer CJ, Li Y, et al. (2007) A genome-wide association study of type 2 diabetes in Finns detects multiple susceptibility variants. Science 316: 1341–1345.
6. Wellcome Trust Case Control Consortium (2007) Genome-wide association study of 14,000 cases of seven common diseases and 3,000 shared controls. Nature 447: 661–678.
7. McPherson R, Pertsemlidis A, Kavaslar N, Stewart A, Roberts R, et al. (2007) A common allele on chromosome 9 associated with coronary heart disease. Science 316: 1488–1491.
8. Helgadottir A, Thorleifsson G, Manolescu A, Gretarsdottir S, Blondal T, et al. (2007) A common variant on chromosome 9p21 affects the risk of myocardial infarction. Science 316: 1491–1493.
9. Samani NJ, Erdmann J, Hall AS, Hengstenberg C, Mangino M, et al. (2007) Genome wide association analysis of coronary artery disease. N Engl J Med 357: 443–453.
10. Pasternak RC, Criqui MH, Benjamin EJ, Fowkes FG, Isselbacher EM, et al. (2004) Atherosclerotic Vascular Disease Conference: Writing Group I: epidemiology. Circulation 109: 2605–2612.
11. Adams RJ, Chimowitz MI, Alpert JS, Awad IA, Cerqueria MD, et al. (2003) Coronary risk evaluation in patients with transient ischemic attack and ischemic stroke: a scientific statement for healthcare professionals from the Stroke Council and the Council on Clinical Cardiology of the American Heart Association/American Stroke Association. Circulation 108: 1278–1290.
12. Zee RY, Ridker PM (2007) Two common gene variants on chromosome 9 and risk of atherothrombosis. Stroke 38: e111.
13. Matarin M, Brown WM, Singleton A, Hardy JA, Meschia JF, et al. (2008) Whole genome analysis suggests ischemic stroke and heart disease share an association with polymorphisms on chromosome 9p21. Stroke 39: 1586–1589.
14. Helgadottir A, Thorleifsson G, Magnusson KP, Grétarsdottir S, Steinthorsdottir V, et al. (2008) The same sequence variant on 9p21 associates with myocardial infarction, abdominal aortic aneurysm and intracranial aneurysm. Nat Genet 40:217–224.
15. Smith JG, Melander O, Lövkvist H, Hedblad B, Engström G, et al. (2009) Common genetic variants on chromosome 9p21 confers risk of ischemic stroke: a large-scale genetic association study. Circ Cardiovasc Genet 2: 159–164.
16. Palomaki GE, Melillo S, Bradley LA (2010) Association between 9p21 genomic markers and heart disease: a meta-analysis. JAMA 303: 648–56.
17. DerSimonian R, Laird N (1986) Meta-analysis in clinical trials. Control Clin Trials 7: 177–188.
18. Cochran WG (1954) The combination of estimates from different experiments. Biometrics 10: 101–129.
19. Higgins JP, Thompson SG (2002) Quantifying heterogeneity in a meta-analysis. Stat Med 21: 1539–1558.
20. Woolf B (1955) On estimating the relation between blood group and disease. Ann Hum Genet 19: 251–253.
21. Egger M, Davey Smith G, Schneider M, Minder C (1997) Bias in meta-analysis detected by a simple, graphical test. BMJ 315: 629–634.
22. Gschwendtner A, Bevan S, Cole JW, Plourde A, Matarin M, et al. (2009) Sequence variants on chromosome 9p21.3 confer risk for atherosclerotic stroke. Ann Neurol 65: 531–539.
23. Lemmens R, Abboud S, Robberecht W, Vanhees L, Pandolfo M, et al. (2009) Variant on 9p21 strongly associates with coronary heart disease, but lacks association with common stroke. Eur J Hum Genet 17: 1287–1293.
24. Karvanen J, Silander K, Kee F, Tiret L, Salomaa V, et al. (2009) The impact of newly identified loci on coronary heart disease, stroke and total mortality in the MORGAM prospective cohorts. Genet Epidemiol 33: 237–246.
25. Ikram MA, Seshadri S, Bis JC, Fornage M, DeStefano AL, et al. (2009) Genomewide association studies of stroke. N Engl J Med 360: 1718–1728.
26. Luke MM, Lalouschek W, Rowland CM, Catanese JJ, Bolonick JI, et al. (2009) Polymorphisms associated with both noncardioembolic stroke and coronary heart disease: vienna stroke registry. Cerebrovasc Dis 28: 499–504.
27. Yamagishi K, Folsom AR, Rosamond WD, Boerwinkle E; ARIC Investigators (2009) A genetic variant on chromosome 9p21 and incident heart failure in the ARIC study. Eur Heart J 30: 1222–1228.
28. Ding H, Xu Y, Wang X, Wang Q, Zhang L, et al. (2009) 9p21 is a shared susceptibility locus strongly for coronary artery disease and weakly for ischemic stroke in Chinese Han population. Circ Cardiovasc Genet 2: 338–346.
29. Wahlstrand B, Orho-Melander M, Delling L, Kjeldsen S, Narkiewicz K, et al. (2009) The myocardial infarction associated CDKN2A/CDKN2B locus on chromosome 9p21 is associated with stroke independently of coronary events in patients with hypertension. J Hypertens 27: 769–773.
30. Hu WL, Li SJ, Liu DT, Wang Y, Niu SQ, et al. (2009) Genetic variants on chromosome 9p21 and ischemic stroke in Chinese. Brain Res Bull 79: 431–435.
31. Plant SR, Samsa GP, Shah SH, Goldstein LB (2011) Exploration of a hypothesized independent association of a common 9p21.3 gene variant and ischemic stroke in patients with and without angiographic coronary artery disease. Cerebrovasc Dis 31: 117–122.
32. Olsson S, Jood K, Blomstrand C, Jern C (2011) Genetic variation on chromosome 9p21 shows association with the ischaemic stroke subtype large-vessel disease in a Swedish sample aged ≤70. Eur J Neurol 18: 365–367.
33. Lin HF, Tsai PC, Liao YC, Lin TH, Tai CT, et al. (2011) Chromosome 9p21 genetic variants are associated with myocardial infarction but not with ischemic stroke in a Taiwanese population. J Investig Med 59: 926–930.
34. Bellenguez C, Bevan S, Gschwendtner A, Spencer CC, Burgess AI, et al. (2012) Genome-wide association study identifies a variant in HDAC9 associated with large vessel ischemic stroke. Nat Genet 44: 328–333.
35. Traylor M, Farrall M, Holliday EG, Sudlow C, Hopewell JC, et al. (2012) Genetic risk factors for ischaemic stroke and its subtypes (the METASTROKE Collaboration): a meta-analysis of genome-wide association studies. Lancet Neurol 11: 951–962.
36. Cheng YC, Anderson CD, Bione S, Keene K, Maguire JM, et al. (2012) Are myocardial infarction–associated single-nucleotide polymorphisms associated with ischemic stroke? Stroke 43: 980–986.
37. Zhang W, Chen Y, Liu P, Chen J, Song L, et al. (2012) Variants on chromosome 9p21.3 correlated with ANRIL expression contribute to stroke risk and recurrence in a large prospective stroke population. Stroke 43: 14–21.
38. Heckman MG, Soto-Ortolaza AI, Diehl NN, Rayaprolu S, Brott TG, et al. (2013) Genetic variants associated with myocardial infarction in the PSMA6 gene and Chr9p21 are also associated with ischaemic stroke. Eur J Neurol 20: 300–8.
39. Jerrard-Dunne P, Cloud G, Hassan A, Markus HS (2003) Evaluating the genetic component of ischemic stroke subtypes. A family history study. Stroke 34: 1364–1369.
40. Markus HS (2010) Unravelling the genetics of ischaemic stroke. PLoS Med 7: e1000225.
41. Murabito JM, White CC, Kavousi M, Sun YV, Feitosa MF, et al. (2012) Association between chromosome 9p21 variants and the ankle-brachial index identified by a meta-analysis of 21 genome-wide association studies. Circ Cardiovasc Genet 5: 100–12.
42. Pasmant E, Laurendeau I, Héron D, Vidaud M, Vidaud D et al. (2007) Characterization of a germ-line deletion, including the entire INK4/ARF locus, in a melanoma-neural system tumor family: identification of ANRIL, an

antisense noncoding RNA whose expression coclusters with ARF. Cancer Res 67: 3963–3969.
43. Gil J, Peters G (2006) Regulation of the INK4b–ARF–INK4a tumour suppressor locus: all for one or one for all. Nat Rev Mol Cell Biol 7: 667–677.
44. Yap KL, Li S, Muñoz-Cabello AM, Raguz S, Zeng L et al. (2010) Molecular Interplay of the noncoding RNA ANRIL and methylated histone H3 lysine 27 by Polycomb CBX7 in transcriptional silencing of INK4a. Mol Cell 38: 662–674.
45. Kotake Y, Nakagawa T, Kitagawa K, Suzuki S, Liu N, et al. (2011) Long non-coding RNA ANRIL is required for the PRC2 recruitment to and silencing of p15INK4B tumor suppressor gene. Oncogene 30: 1956–1962.

6

Effects of Early Blood Pressure Lowering on Early and Long-Term Outcomes after Acute Stroke

Hongxuan Wang[9], Yamei Tang[9], Xiaoming Rong, Hui Li, Rui Pan, Yidong Wang, Ying Peng*

Department of Neurology, Sun Yat-sen Memorial Hospital, Sun Yat-sen University, Guangzhou, Guangdong Province, China

Abstract

Background: Hypertension is common after acute stroke onset. Previous studies showed controversial effects of early blood pressure (BP) lowering on stroke outcomes. The aim of this study is to assess the effects of early BP lowering on early and long-term outcomes after acute stroke.

Methods: A meta-analysis was conducted with prospective randomized controlled trials assessing the effects of early BP lowering on early and long-term outcomes after acute stroke compared with placebo. Literature searching was performed in the databases from inception to December 2013. New evidence from recent trials were included. Outcomes were analyzed as early (within 30 days) and long-term (from 3 to 12 months) endpoints using summary estimates of relative risks (RR) and their 95% confidence intervals (CI) with the fixed-effect model or random-effect model.

Results: Seventeen trials providing data from 13236 patients were included. Pooled results showed that early BP lowering after acute stroke onset was associated with more death within 30 days compared with placebo (RR: 1.34 and 95% CI: 1.02, 1.74, $p = 0.03$). However the results showed that early BP lowering had no evident effect on early neurological deterioration, early death within 7 days, long-term death, early and long-term dependency, early and long-term combination of death or dependency, long-term stroke recurrence, long-term myocardial infarction and long-term CVE.

Conclusions: The new results lend no support to early BP lowering after acute stroke. Early BP lowering may increase death within 30 days after acute stroke.

Editor: Jean-Claude Baron, INSERM U894, Centre de Psychiatrie et Neurosciences, Hopital Sainte-Anne and Université Paris 5, France

Funding: This work was supported by the sub-program of "12-5" National Science & Technique Support Program of China (2011BAI08B11 to YP), National Natural Science Foundation of China (NSFC 30973479, 31070953 to YP) and Science & Technique Plan fund of Guangdong Province (2009B060700040 to YP), and also supported in part by NSFC (No. 30600164 and No. 81072242 to YT), the Natural Science Foundation of Guangdong Province (No. S2011010004708 to YT), the Fundamental Research Funds for the Central Universities and Funds for Pearl River Science & Technology Star of Guangzhou City to YT. The funders had no role in study design, data collection and analysis, decision to publish, or preparation of the manuscript.

Competing Interests: The authors have declared that no competing interests exist.

* E-mail: 2353352460@qq.com

[9] These authors contributed equally to this work.

Introduction

Elevated blood pressure (BP) is common in acute phase of stroke onset; about more than 75% of patients with acute stroke have elevated blood pressure at presentation[1–3]. It may reflect untreated or uncontrolled hypertension before stroke, or it may relate to stress response, autonomic dysfunction or increased intracranial pressure after stroke onset[2,3]. Observation studies have found that high blood pressure in acute stroke is associated with poor short-term and long-term outcomes[2,4–6]. High blood pressure in acute stroke may be accompanied by higher risk of cerebral edema[7], hemorrhagic transformation of the infarct following thrombolysis in ischemic stroke[8] or expansion of the hematoma in hemorrhagic stroke[9]. In view of the potential risks of hypertension in acute stroke, epidemiologists suggest that high BP should be lowered. However, the high blood pressure usually decreases spontaneously in 4–10 days after stroke onset[10]. Observation studies have reported that low blood pressure in acute ischemic stroke is also associated with a poor prognosis[11,12]. The mechanism may be that BP lowering may result in the reduction of cerebral blood flow because of the impaired autoregulation after ischemic stroke, which leads to further ischemia in penumbra[13]. In consideration of similar mechanism, hypoperfusion in the perihematoma region of intracerebral hemorrhage may also occur after BP lowering. Hence, pathophysiologists argue that lowering BP should be of caution. Therefore, it is a clinical problem whether to lower high BP after acute stroke or not. The benefits of lowering the initial BP remain debated.

Previous studies about the effects of early BP lowering on the outcomes after acute stroke had given conflicting results. Several randomized controlled trials (RCTs) suggested that early BP lowering after acute stroke was safe[14–16]: The CHHIPS study showed early BP lowering in combination group of ischemic stroke and hemorrhagic stroke could improve long-term mortality[16];

the ACCESS study found early BP lowering in ischemic stroke could reduce recurrent vascular events[14]; and the INTERACT study reported early BP lowering in hemorrhagic stroke could reduce hematoma growth[15]. While the other RCTs found no evident benefit of early BP lowering after acute stroke[11,17]. Therefore, previous cochrane meta-analyses had yielded neutral results[18,19]. However, not all the trials included in previous analyses did achieve BP reduction in the intervention group, such as some studies with nimodipine in previous meta-analysis[19]. We argue that they could not lend direct support to the potential association between BP lowering and outcomes after acute stroke, and that they would also confound the association resulting in the obscure effects.

For recent years, some new studies with large sample focusing on the early BP lowering after acute stroke have still noted inconsistent results: the COSSACS study which enrolled patients with either ischemic stroke or hemorrhagic stroke, and the PRoFESS study which enrolled patients with ischemic stroke suggested safe but non-significant benefit of early BP intervention[20,21], while the SCAST study which enrolled patients with either ischemic stroke or hemorrhagic stroke indicated a harmful effect of early BP lowering[22]. The INTERACT2 which enrolled patients with hemorrhagic stroke study indicated the trend to improve functional outcomes after intensive lowering of BP[23], but the CATIS study which enrolled patients with ischemic stroke[24] showed no difference between presence and absence of the antihypertensive medication in acute stroke. Considering these new evidence which was not included in previous meta-analyses[18,19] and the aim to elucidate a new conclusion on the effects of early BP lowering after acute stroke, we update this meta-analysis. Additionally, we also assess the early neurological deterioration after BP lowering in acute stroke, which had not been discussed in previous meta-analyses.

Methods

Search strategy

We conducted the meta-analysis by reviewing published literature. We searched the following data sources: MELINE via Pubmed (from 1966 to December 2013), Science Citation Index (ISI Web of Science, from 1970 to December 2013), Cochrane Database of Systematic Reviews (CDSR) and the Cochrane Central Register of Controlled Trials (CENTRAL) with the search terms, key words or medical subject heading which included "blood pressure lowering", "hypertension", "anti-hypertension", "antihypertensive" and "acute" and "stroke", "cerebrovascular disease", "cerebral infarction", "brain infarction", "cerebral ischemia", "brain ischemia", "cerebral hemorrhage", "intracranial hemorrhage" and "randomized controlled trial". The search was limited to trials in human beings and that published in English. In addition, we also screened the references of identified articles and previous reviews or meta-analyses on blood pressure lowering in acute stroke.

Selection criteria and data extraction

We included the eligible trials which met the following criteria: (1) participants were aged 18 years or older with acute ischemic or hemorrhagic stroke; (2) study design was prospective randomized controlled trial; (3) intervention compared with placebo was initiated within 7 days of stroke onset; (4) intervention aimed to lower blood pressure or intervention achieved BP reduction; (5) one or more functional outcomes were reported, such as death or dependency. We excluded the studies with the patients of subarachnoid hemorrhage, studies without available full-text or relevant data, studies about ongoing trials and those written in languages other than English.

We extracted the data from each trial by reviewing published papers and even requesting detailed information from original authors if needed. Outcomes including early neurological deterioration (END), death, dependency, death or dependency, stroke recurrence, myocardial infarction and combined vascular events (CVE) were collected. We defined END and dependency as the original authors' definition in each study (END was defined as an increase in NIHSS of 4 or more points, or as a decrease in GCS score of 2 or more points in the CHHIPS, INTERACT and INTERACT2 study; dependency was defined as a mRS score of 3 or more points), and we stratified the outcomes to two phases as early outcome (within 30 days) and long-term outcome (3 to 12 months). We also defined CVE as the original authors' definitions (CVE included myocardial infarction, all types of stroke recurrence and peripheral vascular diseases).

Two authors (HW and XR) conducted the literature searches, data extraction and study assessment independently. Any disagreement in study selection or data collection was discussed by HW, XR and YT until agreement was reached. We also discussed the quality of trials such as randomization, blinded method, eligibility criteria and intention-to-treat analysis before they were finally included.

Statistical analysis

Individual study relative risks (RR) and 95% confidence intervals (CI) were calculated from event numbers extracted from each trial before data pooling. In calculation of risk ratios, the total number of patients randomly assigned in each group was used as the denominator. Summary estimates of RR ratios were obtained with fixed-effect models or random-effect models. The percentage of variability across studies attributable to heterogeneity beyond chance was estimated with the I^2 statistic. Potential heterogeneity was explored in estimates of treatment effect with univariate meta-regression and by comparing summary results obtained from the studies. A two-sided p value less than 0.05 was regarded as significant for all analyses. If the value of I^2 was >50% in the analysis, the heterogeneity between studies was defined as significant, and the random-effect model was used for analyses. Otherwise, fixed-effect models was used. Funnel plots were used for analyses of bias. The Cochrane Collaboration's Review Manager software package (RevMan, Edition 5.2) was used for the meta-analyses.

Results

Summaries of included trials

The literature search and the review of previous meta-analyses or reviews finally yielded 17 studies which met the inclusion criteria (Figure 1). The characteristics of the included studies are summarized in Table 1.These studies included a total of 13236 patients from various countries such as UK, USA, Germany, Japan, China, and so on. The process of identifying the included articles is shown in Figure 1. All data included in this analysis were extracted from original papers only because of no additional data available from requested authors.

The trials had a sample size ranging from 18 to 4071 patients, of which eleven were multi-centre randomized controlled trials (RCT) and the others were single centre RCT. Eight trials[11,14,20,24–28] included patients with acute ischemic stroke (IS) only and two trials[15,23] included patients with acute hemorrhagic stroke (HS) only, while seven trials[16,17,21,22,29–31] included patients with either type of stoke except subarachnoid

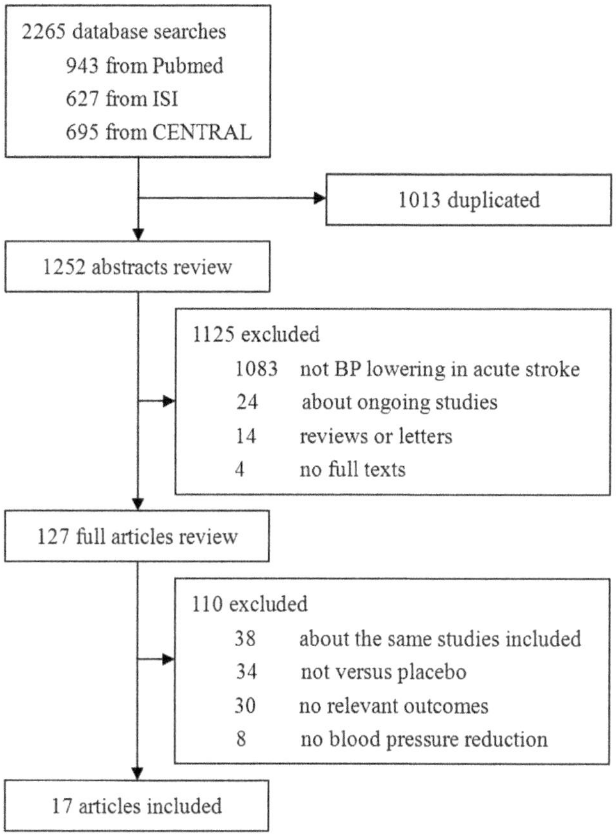

Figure 1. Identification process for included studies. The figure shows detailed information in the process of search, review, exclusion and inclusion of the potential articles.

hemorrhage. Most trials had recruited more male than female. Patients had a mean age ranging from 57 to 76 years old. Patients were recruited into trials within 6 to 120 hours from stroke onset and the mean time to randomize to intervention ranged from 3.6 to 105.6 hours. The trials studied the effect of one or more kinds of antihypertensive agents including the following types: angiotensin converting enzyme inhibitors (ACEI), angiotensin receptor blockers (ARB), beta receptor antagonists (BRA), calcium channel blockers (CCB), glyceryl trinitrate (GTN) and prostacyclin. Intervention period ranged from 3 to 21 days except that the intervention period of the PRoFESS study was 3 months. Follow-up durations ranged from 14 days to 12 months (Table 1).

Early neurological deterioration

Six trials mentioned early neurological deterioration (END) after early BP lowering in acute stroke (Table 1, Figure 2). Of them, three studies reported END within 72 hours after intervention assigned (Figure 2A), which enrolled the patients within 6 to 36 hours after stroke onset. And the other three studies recorded END within 14 days (Figure 2B), which enrolled the patients within 24 to 72 hours after stroke onset. The pooled result showed that early BP lowering after acute stroke yielded no effect on END within 72 hours (RR: 0.97 and 95% CI: 0.82, 1.14) or within 14 days (RR: 2.10 and 95% CI: 0.59, 7.51). And the heterogeneity between studies was not evident (both $I^2 = 0\%$, $p > 0.05$).

Early and long-term death

Three studies recorded early death within 7 days after early BP lowering in acute stroke, which enrolled the patients within 36 to 72 hours after stroke onset (Table 1, Figure 3A). Overall, no significant effect of early death after early BP lowering within 7 days was showed (RR: 0.81 and 95% CI: 0.08, 8.29, Figure 3A). Although the heterogeneity between studies was noted ($I^2 = 72\%$, $p = 0.03$) and it was due to the discrepant data from the BEST trials, however, there was no clinical reason to exclude it from the analysis and no other potential subgroup analysis to eliminate the heterogeneity.

Eleven studies followed up early death for 14 to 30 days after early BP lowering in acute stroke, which enrolled the patients within 24 to 120 hours after stroke onset (Table 1, Figure 3B). Pooled results indicated the significant harmful effect that early BP lowering after acute stroke onset was associated with more death within 30 days (RR: 1.34 and 95% CI: 1.02, 1.74, $p = 0.03$, without significant heterogeneity between studies). Considering the broad span of admission time after stroke onset in the trials included in the analysis, we narrowed the inclusion criteria for the remaining 10 trials which enrolled the patients within 24 to 72 hours after stroke onset (excluding the Willmot's study), and the pooled results were not changed and the adverse effect of early BP lowering on death within 30 days was still evident (data not shown).

Fourteen studies followed up long-term death from 3 to 12 months after acute stroke, which enrolled the patients within 6 to 120 hours after stroke onset (Table 1, Figure 3C). No effect of early BP lowering was shown (RR: 1.05 and 95% CI: 0.93, 1.19). If we re-evaluated the pooled results by narrowing the inclusion criteria for the remaining 12 trials with the admission time within 6 to 72 hours after stroke onset, the result was not changed (data not shown).

Early and long-term dependency, combination of death or dependency

Five studies reported early dependency and early death or dependency, which enrolled the patients within 24 to 72 hours after stroke onset (Table 1, Figure 4A, 4B). Pooled results showed that early BP lowering had no effect on early dependency (RR: 1.02 and 95% CI: 0.95, 1.09; without significant heterogeneity between studies) or early death or dependency (RR: 1.02 and 95% CI: 0.96, 1.09; without significant heterogeneity between studies).

Nine studies reported long-term dependency and long-term death or dependency, which enrolled the patients within 6 to 120 hours after stroke onset (Table 1, Figure 4C, 4D). Pooled results showed that early BP lowering had no effect on long-term dependency (RR: 0.97 and 95% CI: 0.91, 1.02; without significant heterogeneity between studies) and long-term death or dependency (RR: 0.99 and 95% CI: 0.94, 1.04; without significant heterogeneity between studies). Further analysis by narrowing the inclusion criteria for the remaining trials (excluding the Bath's study) with the admission time within 6 to 72 hours after stroke onset did not changed the neutral results (data not shown).

Long-term vascular events

Seven studies considered the long-term effect of early BP lowering on stroke recurrence and combined vascular events (CVE) (Figure 5A, 5C) and six studies reported the long-term effect of early BP lowering on myocardial infarction (MI) (Figure 5B) from 3 to 12 months after acute stroke onset, which enrolled the patients within 6 to 72 hours after stroke onset. Pooled data showed that early BP lowering had no effect on long-term stroke

Table 1. Summary of included studies.

Study	Year	Country of origin	No. of patients	Male (%) (I; C)	Mean age (years) (I; C)	Stroke type	Inclusion of onset (hours)	Mean admission time (hours) (I; C)	Agent class	Intervention period (days)	Duration of follow-up (months)	Study scale	Outcome
ACCESS[14]	2003	Multicentre in Germany	339	51(50;52)	68;68	IS	36	29.9;29.7	ARB	7	12	BI	Death, stroke recurrence, MI
Bath *et al*[30]	2001	Single centre in UK	37	49(38;57)	76;72	IS+HS	120	105.6;93.6	GTN	12	3	RS	Death, dependency
BEST[29]	1988	Single centre in UK	302	54;49	70;69	IS+HS	48	23.4;25.3	BRB	21	6	Ordinal scale	Death, SAE
CATIS[24]	2013	Multicentre in China	4071	64(65;63)	62;62	IS	48	15.3;14.9	All kinds	7	3	NIHSS,mRS	Death, dependency
CHHIPS[16]	2009	Multicentre in UK	179	55(57;53)	74;74	IS+HS	36	19.8;17.4	ACEI/BRB	14	3	NIHSS, mRS	Neurological worsening, death, dependency
COSSACS[21]	2010	Multicentre in UK	763	56(55;56)	74;74	IS+HS	48	23.6;23.4	All kinds	14	6	NIHSS, mRS, BI	Death, dependency, stroke recurrence, MI
Eveson *et al*[26]	2007	Single centre in UK	40	63(44;77)	73;75	IS	24	18.0;20.0	ACEI	14	3	NIHSS, mRS, BI	Death, dependency
Hsu *et al*[28]	1987	Multicentre in USA	80	61(58;65)	63;65	IS	24	15.3;17.4	PGI_2	3	1	Neurologic Grading Scale	Neurological worsening, death
INTERACT[15]	2008	Multicenter from Australia, China and South Korea	404	65(61;69)	63;62	HS	6	3.6;3.7	All kinds	7	3	NIHSS, GCS, mRS	Neurological worsening, death, dependency, stroke recurrence
INTERACT2[23]	2013	Multicentre from Australia, China and South Korea	2839	63(64;62)	63;64	HS	6	3.7;3.7	All kinds	7	3	NIHSS, mRS	Death, dependency, SAE
INWEST[11]	2000	Multicentre from Sweden	295	45	72	IS	24	/	CCB (iv.)	21	6	BI	Death, dependency
Kaste *et al* [27]	1994	Multicentre in Finland	350	67(69;65)	57;58	IS	48	/	CCB (po.)	21	12	Sum score, RS	Death, dependency
Nakamura *et al*[25]	2010	Single centre in Japan	40	83(81;85)	62;81	IS	72	45;41	ARB/ACEI	14	0.5	NIHSS, mRS	Neurological worsening, death, stroke recurrence, MI, SAE
PRoFESS[20]	2009	Multicentre in 35 countries	1360	65(65;65)	67;67	IS	72	57.6;57.6	ARB	90	3	NIHSS, mRS	Death, dependency, stroke recurrence, MI, SAE
Rashid *et al*[17]	2003	Single centre in UK	90	46(47;43)	71;74	IS+HS	72	51.0;49.5	GTN	10	3	SNSS, mRS, BI	Neurological worsening, death, dependency
SCAST[22]	2011	Multicentre in 9 north European countries	2029	58(60;56)	71;71	IS+HS	30	17.6;17.9	ARB	7	6	SSS, mRS, BI	Death, dependency, stroke recurrence, MI
Willmot *et al*[31]	2006	Single centre in UK	18	28(17;50)	69;70	IS+HS	120	79;77	GTN	7	3	SSS, mRS	Death

I: intervention; C: control. ACEI, angiotensin converting enzyme inhibitors; ARB, angiotensin receptor blockers; BRA, beta receptor antagonists; CCB, calcium channel blockers; GTN, glyceryl trinitrate. BI, Barthel Index; GCS, Glasgow Coma Scale; NIHSS, NIH Stroke Scale; RS, Rankin Scale; SSS, Scandinavian Stroke Scale.

A.

Study or Subgroup	Intervention Events	Intervention Total	Control Events	Control Total	Weight	Risk Ratio M-H, Fixed, 95% CI
CHHIPS 2009	7	113	3	59	1.6%	1.22 [0.33, 4.54]
INTERACT 2008	31	203	30	201	12.4%	1.02 [0.64, 1.62]
INTERACT2 2013	198	1369	211	1395	86.0%	0.96 [0.80, 1.14]
Total (95% CI)		**1685**		**1655**	**100.0%**	**0.97 [0.82, 1.14]**
Total events	236		244			

Heterogeneity: Chi² = 0.19, df = 2 (P = 0.91); I² = 0%
Test for overall effect: Z = 0.38 (P = 0.71)

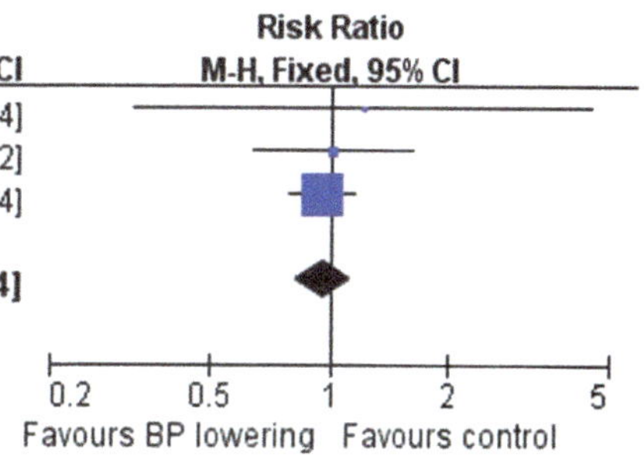

B.

Study or Subgroup	Intervention Events	Intervention Total	Control Events	Control Total	Weight	Risk Ratio M-H, Fixed, 95% CI
Hsu 1987	5	43	2	37	61.8%	2.15 [0.44, 10.44]
Nakamura 2010	2	27	0	13	19.2%	2.50 [0.13, 48.62]
Rashid 2003	1	60	0	30	19.1%	1.52 [0.06, 36.34]
Total (95% CI)		**130**		**80**	**100.0%**	**2.10 [0.59, 7.51]**
Total events	8		2			

Heterogeneity: Chi² = 0.05, df = 2 (P = 0.97); I² = 0%
Test for overall effect: Z = 1.14 (P = 0.25)

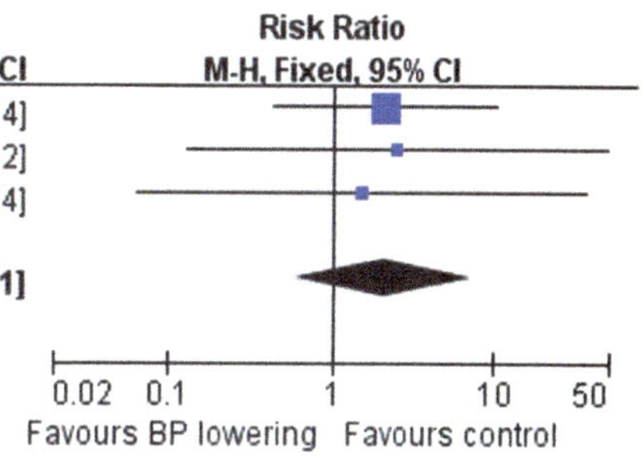

Figure 2. Early neurological deterioration after acute stroke. The figure shows meta-analysis of early BP lowering on early neurological deterioration within 72 hours (A.) or within 14 days (B.) after acute stroke. Risk ratios (RR) and their 95% confidence intervals (CI) were estimated event rates of intervention (BP lowering) compared with control (placebo). Overall effects were tested by Z tests and the heterogeneity of between-studies was tested by χ^2 test and measured as the value of I^2.

recurrence (RR: 0.92 and 95% CI: 0.76, 1.12; with no evidence of heterogeneity between studies), long-term MI (RR: 1.09 and 95% CI: 0.69, 1.71; with no evidence of heterogeneity between studies) and CVE (RR: 0.95 and 95% CI: 0.82, 1.12; with no evidence of heterogeneity between studies).

We used funnel plots to evaluated the publication bias. It showed no evident publication bias in the majority of outcomes such as END within 72 hours, END within 14 days, early death within 30 days, long-term death, early and long-term dependency, early and long-term combination of death or dependency and long-term stroke recurrence (data and plots not shown). Asymmetric funnel plots were shown in few results such as early death within 7 days, long-term MI and long-term CVE, which just only yielded neutral results in our analysis (data not shown).

Discussion

Whether to lower high blood pressure early after acute stroke or not still remains debated. One cochrane meta-analysis failed to analyze the effect of BP lowering on stroke because the author could not obtain enough data[32]. The other two meta-analyses showed no significant effects of early BP lowering on outcomes after acute stroke[18,19]. However, they did not include recent new trials and they did not assess the early neurological deterioration after BP lowering. Furthermore, they included some trials in which the intervention groups did not achieve BP reduction during the study[19]. We doubt that the results were confounded. In this study, we review the evidence from several new trials with large sample such as PRoFESS[20], COSSACS[21], SCAST[22], INTERACT2[23] and CATIS[24] which have not been included in previous meta-analyses[18,19]. We also assess the early neurological deterioration after BP lowering in acute stroke, which has not been discussed in previous meta-analysis. This updated meta-analysis including overall 13236 patients from 17 trials notes the evidence that early BP lowering in acute stroke increases death within 30 days. However there is still no evident effect of early BP lowering after acute stroke on early neurological deterioration, early death within 7 days, long-term death, early and long-term dependency, early and long-term death or dependency, long-term stroke recurrence, long-term myocardial infarction and long-term CVE.

This analysis assesses early neurological deterioration after early BP lowering in acute stroke, which has not been discussed in previous reviews or meta-analyses. How ever, limited trials reported relevant data so that no certain effect can be found. So far, we could not draw any conclusion that early BP lowering after acute stroke is safe enough. More RCTs concerning BP lowering on early neurological deterioration within 72 hours are needed.

Considering potential confounding effect in previous meta-analyses because they included several trials without achieving BP reduction indeed (e.g. the Norris's study[33] and the VENUS study[34] in the Geeganage's analysis[19]). We doubt that probable harmful effects of BP lowering in these trials was attenuated because of no significant BP changes, so we just include the trials aiming to or achieving BP reduction in the intervention groups. The new result yields evident harmful effect of early BP lowering on early death within 30 days.

Because admission time after stroke onset may also be critical in the effect of BP lowering, it is best to make further subgroup analyses according to different admission time to show potential different effects of BP lowering on stroke outcomes. However, nearly no relevant data could be extracted or provided from the origin studies for further subgroup analyses. For it seems non-reasonable to combine the data from the patients enrolled within 6 hours after stroke onset with those from the patients enrolled within 120 hours after stroke onset[18,19], therefore we further evaluated the pooled results by narrowing the inclusion criteria of admission time. In the included trials, only 2 trials (the Bath's study and the Willmot's study) enrolled the patients of wide admission time span up to 5 days (120 hours) after stroke onset, all the other

A.

Study or Subgroup	Intervention Events	Intervention Total	Control Events	Control Total	Weight	Risk Ratio M-H, Random, 95% CI
BEST 1988	26	202	3	100	42.2%	4.29 [1.33 13.83]
CHHIPS 2009	1	113	3	59	32.8%	0.17 [0.02, 1.64]
PRoFESS 2009	0	647	1	713	24.9%	0.37 [0.01, 9.00]
Total (95% CI)		**962**		**872**	**100.0%**	**0.81 [0.08, 8.29]**
Total events	27		7			

Heterogeneity: Tau^2 = 2.98; Chi^2 = 7.26, df = 2 (P = 0.03); I^2 = 72%
Test for overall effect: Z = 0.18 (P = 0.86)

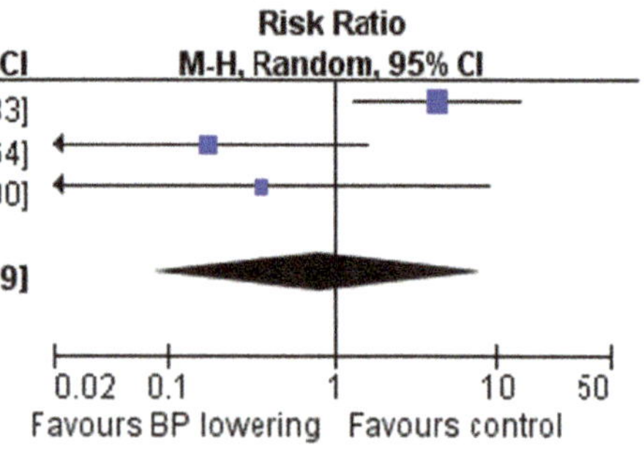

B.

Study or Subgroup	Intervention Events	Intervention Total	Control Events	Control Total	Weight	Risk Ratio M-H, Fixed, 95% CI
BEST 1988	52	202	14	100	21.1%	1.84 [1.07, 3.15]
CATIS 2013	25	2038	25	2033	28.2%	1.00 [0.57, 1.73]
CHHIPS 2009	6	113	6	59	8.9%	0.52 [0.18, 1.55]
COSSACS 2010	4	379	7	384	7.8%	0.58 [0.17, 1.96]
Eveson 2007	1	18	1	22	1.0%	1.22 [0.08, 18.20]
Hsu 1987	1	43	2	37	2.4%	0.43 [0.04, 4.56]
INWEST 2000	36	173	14	92	20.6%	1.37 [0.78, 2.40]
Kaste 1994	20	176	7	174	7.9%	2.82 [1.23, 6.51]
Nakamura 2010	0	27	0	13		Not estimable
PRoFESS 2009	4	647	2	713	2.1%	2.20 [0.41, 11.99]
Willmot 2006	0	12	0	6		Not estimable
Total (95% CI)		**3828**		**3633**	**100.0%**	**1.34 [1.02, 1.74]**
Total events	149		78			

Heterogeneity: Chi^2 = 11.42, df = 8 (P = 0.18); I^2 = 30%
Test for overall effect: Z = 2.14 (P = 0.03)

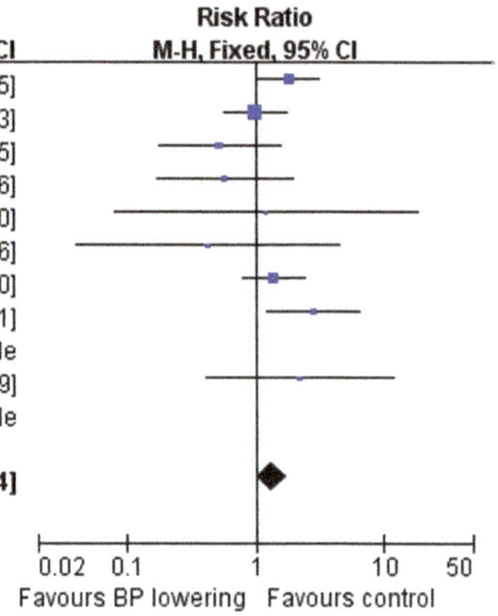

C.

Study or Subgroup	Intervention Events	Intervention Total	Control Events	Control Total	Weight	Risk Ratio M-H, Fixed, 95% CI
ACCESS 2003	5	173	12	166	2.7%	0.40 [0.14, 1.11]
Bath 2001	3	16	1	21	0.2%	3.94 [0.45, 34.41]
BEST 1988	67	202	23	100	6.9%	1.44 [0.96, 2.17]
CATIS 2013	68	1988	54	1987	12.1%	1.26 [0.89, 1.79]
CHHIPS 2009	11	113	12	59	3.5%	0.48 [0.22, 1.02]
COSSACS 2010	32	379	29	384	6.4%	1.12 [0.69, 1.81]
Eveson 2007	2	18	1	22	0.2%	2.44 [0.24, 24.83]
INTERACT 2008	21	203	25	201	5.6%	0.83 [0.48, 1.44]
INTERACT2 2013	166	1382	170	1412	37.6%	1.00 [0.82, 1.22]
Kaste 1994	29	176	22	174	5.0%	1.30 [0.78, 2.18]
PRoFESS 2009	5	647	6	713	1.3%	0.92 [0.28, 2.99]
Rashid 2003	3	60	3	30	0.9%	0.50 [0.11, 2.33]
SCAST 2011	84	1017	78	1012	17.5%	1.07 [0.80, 1.44]
Willmot 2006	0	12	0	6		Not estimable
Total (95% CI)		**6386**		**6287**	**100.0%**	**1.05 [0.93, 1.19]**
Total events	496		436			

Heterogeneity: Chi^2 = 15.51, df = 12 (P = 0.21); I^2 = 23%
Test for overall effect: Z = 0.85 (P = 0.39)

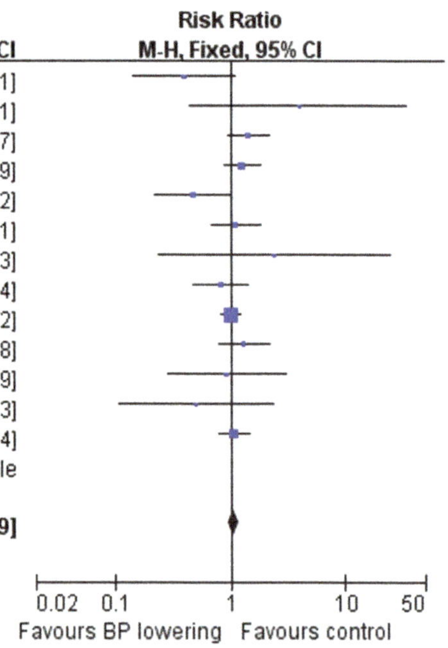

Figure 3. Early and long-term death after acute stroke. The figure shows meta-analysis of early BP lowering on early death within 7 days (A.) or within 30 days (B.) and long-term death from 3 to 12 months (C.) after acute stroke. Risk ratios (RR) and their 95% confidence intervals (CI) were estimated event rates of intervention (BP lowering) compared with control (placebo). Overall effects were tested by Z tests and the heterogeneity of between-studies was tested by χ^2 test and measured as the value of I^2.

A.

Study or Subgroup	Intervention Events	Intervention Total	Control Events	Control Total	Weight	Risk Ratio M-H, Fixed, 95% CI
CATIS 2013	658	2038	656	2033	60.8%	1.00 [0.92, 1.09]
CHHIPS 2009	63	113	29	59	3.5%	1.13 [0.83, 1.54]
COSSACS 2010	68	379	75	384	6.9%	0.92 [0.68, 1.23]
INWEST 2000	107	173	48	92	5.8%	1.19 [0.94, 1.49]
PRoFESS 2009	246	647	261	713	23.0%	1.04 [0.90, 1.19]
Total (95% CI)		**3350**		**3281**	**100.0%**	**1.02 [0.95, 1.09]**
Total events	1142		1069			

Heterogeneity: Chi² = 2.87, df = 4 (P = 0.58); I² = 0%
Test for overall effect: Z = 0.55 (P = 0.58)

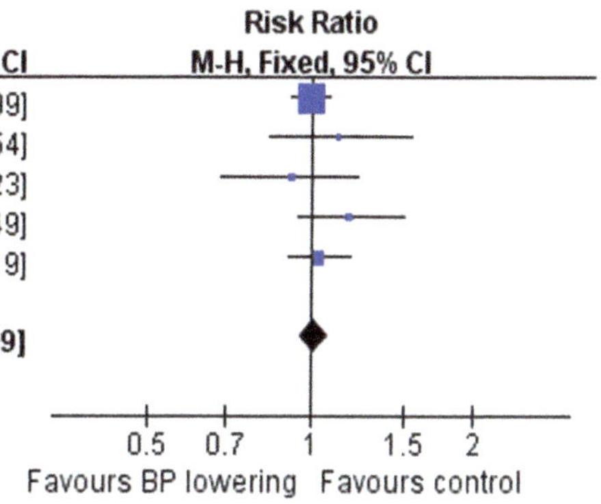

B.

Study or Subgroup	Intervention Events	Intervention Total	Control Events	Control Total	Weight	Risk Ratio M-H, Fixed, 95% CI
CATIS 2013	683	2038	681	2033	59.8%	1.00 [0.92, 1.09]
CHHIPS 2009	69	113	35	59	4.0%	1.03 [0.80, 1.33]
COSSACS 2010	72	379	82	384	7.1%	0.89 [0.67, 1.18]
INWEST 2000	143	173	62	92	7.1%	1.23 [1.05, 1.44]
PRoFESS 2009	250	647	263	713	21.9%	1.05 [0.91, 1.20]
Total (95% CI)		**3350**		**3281**	**100.0%**	**1.02 [0.96, 1.09]**
Total events	1217		1123			

Heterogeneity: Chi² = 6.49, df = 4 (P = 0.17); I² = 38%
Test for overall effect: Z = 0.60 (P = 0.55)

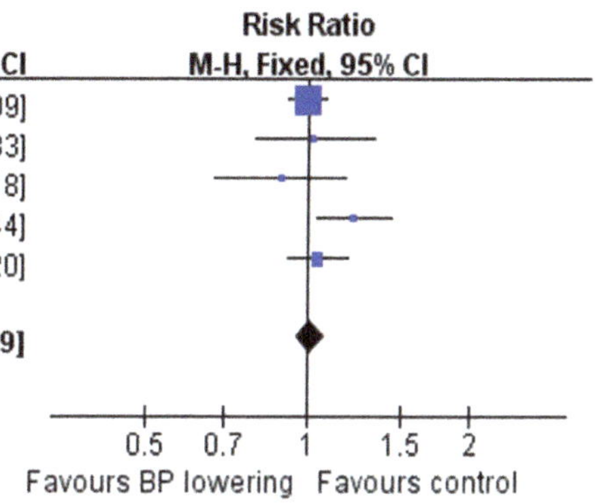

C.

Study or Subgroup	Intervention Events	Intervention Total	Control Events	Control Total	Weight	Risk Ratio M-H, Fixed, 95% CI
Bath 2001	7	16	7	21	0.4%	1.31 [0.58, 2.98]
CATIS 2013	432	1988	448	1987	28.4%	0.96 [0.86, 1.08]
COSSACS 2010	110	379	112	384	7.0%	1.00 [0.80, 1.24]
Eveson 2007	5	18	7	22	0.4%	0.87 [0.33, 2.29]
INTERACT 2008	74	203	70	201	4.5%	1.05 [0.81, 1.36]
INTERACT2 2013	553	1382	615	1412	38.5%	0.92 [0.84, 1.00]
Kaste 1994	50	176	54	174	3.4%	0.92 [0.66, 1.26]
Rashid 2003	34	60	16	30	1.4%	1.06 [0.71, 1.59]
SCAST 2011	264	1000	253	1004	16.0%	1.05 [0.90, 1.22]
Total (95% CI)		**5222**		**5235**	**100.0%**	**0.97 [0.91, 1.02]**
Total events	1529		1582			

Heterogeneity: Chi² = 3.74, df = 8 (P = 0.88); I² = 0%
Test for overall effect: Z = 1.16 (P = 0.25)

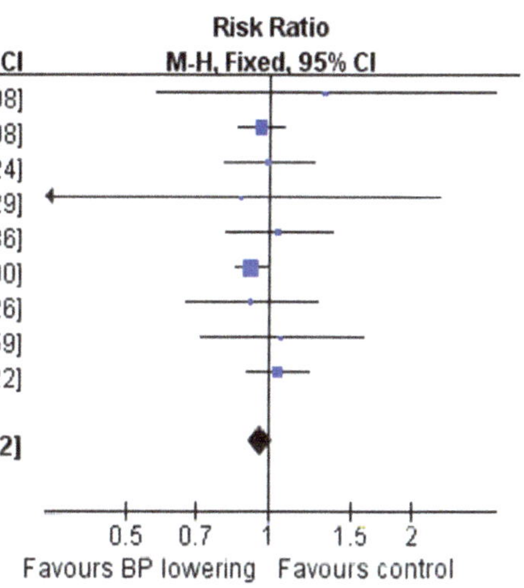

D.

Study or Subgroup	Intervention Events	Intervention Total	Control Events	Control Total	Weight	Risk Ratio M-H, Fixed, 95% CI
Bath 2001	10	16	8	21	0.4%	1.64 [0.84, 3.19]
CATIS 2013	500	1988	502	1987	25.6%	1.00 [0.89, 1.11]
COSSACS 2010	142	379	141	384	7.1%	1.02 [0.85, 1.23]
Eveson 2007	7	18	8	22	0.4%	1.07 [0.48, 2.38]
INTERACT 2008	95	203	95	201	4.9%	0.99 [0.81, 1.22]
INTERACT2 2013	719	1382	785	1412	39.6%	0.94 [0.87, 1.00]
Kaste 1994	79	176	76	174	3.9%	1.03 [0.81, 1.30]
Rashid 2003	37	60	19	30	1.3%	0.97 [0.69, 1.36]
SCAST 2011	348	1000	331	1004	16.9%	1.06 [0.93, 1.19]
Total (95% CI)		**5222**		**5235**	**100.0%**	**0.99 [0.94, 1.04]**
Total events	1937		1965			

Heterogeneity: Chi² = 6.01, df = 8 (P = 0.65); I² = 0%
Test for overall effect: Z = 0.53 (P = 0.60)

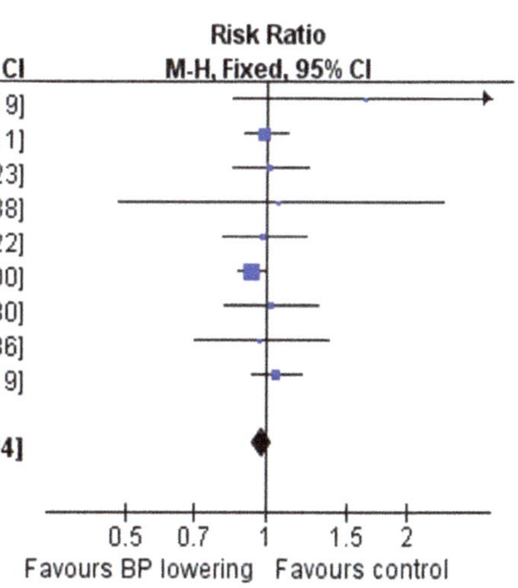

Figure 4. Early and long-term dependency, the combination of death or dependency after acute stroke. The figure shows meta-analysis of early BP lowering on early dependency (A.), early death or dependency (B.), long-term dependency from 3 to 12 months (C.) and long-term death or dependency from 3 to 12 months (D.) after acute stroke. Risk ratios (RR) and their 95% confidence intervals (CI) were estimated event rates of intervention (BP lowering) compared with control (placebo). Overall effects were tested by Z tests and the heterogeneity of between-studies was tested by χ^2 test and measured as the value of I^2.

studies enrolled the patients within 6 to 72 hours after stroke onset. If the 2 trials were excluded for a stricter inclusion criteria of admission time, similarly, the adverse effects on death within 30 days was still significant and the other neutral results would not be changed (data not shown). However, more studies concerning the timing of the intervention and different effects on outcomes after stroke onset are extremely required in future. In addition, we also included the studies of which admission time was within 72 hours (such as the PRoFESS study), because the studies did include part of patients who were enrolled within 48 hours after stroke onset. If we restricted a more stricter inclusion criteria of admission time which was from 6 hours to 48 hours, three more studies (the Nakamura's study, Rashid's study and the PRoFESS study) would be excluded but the pooled results of adverse effects on death

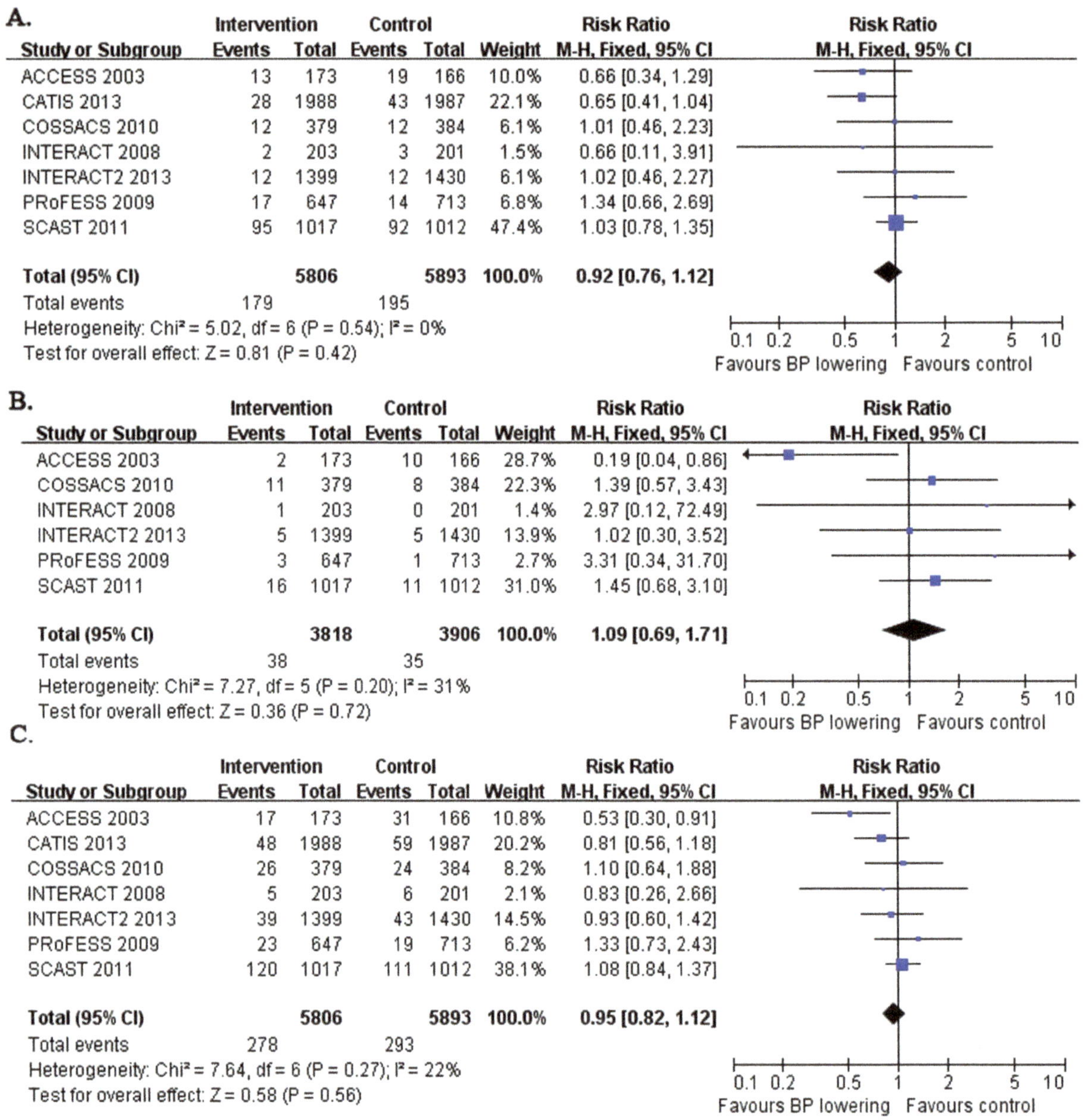

Figure 5. Long-term vascular events. The figure shows meta-analysis of early BP lowering on long-term stroke recurrence (A.), long-term myocardial infarction (B.) and long-term combined vascular events (CVE) from 3 to 12 months (C.) after acute stroke. Risk ratios (RR) and their 95% confidence intervals (CI) were estimated event rates of intervention (BP lowering) compared with control (placebo). Overall effects were tested by Z tests and the heterogeneity of between-studies was tested by χ^2 test and measured as the value of I^2.

within 30 days was still significant and the other neutral results would not be changed (data not shown).

Although the PRoFESS study was designed to focus on the effects of BP-lowering and antiplatelet strategies on secondary stroke prevention which enrolled totally 20332 patients, however, about 7% (1360) of the patients were enrolled within 72 hours after stroke onset and the intervention or placebo was assigned in the acute phase of stroke. Further more, the PRoFESS study was a 2×2 factorial design trial, which also had sufficient statistical power to detect the independent effect of BP lowering on outcomes after stroke. Therefore, the PRoFESS subgroup analysis can reasonably represent a single trial to test the effects of BP lowering on outcomes after acute stroke. On the other hand, the period of intervention in the PRoFESS study was longer (90 days) than other studies because of its initial aim for the secondary stroke prevention. We can not exclude the confounding effects due to mixed effects of short-term and long-term BP lowering. In our analysis, we found that the data from PRoFESS study showed different trends of effects of BP lowering on early death within 30 days after acute stroke (Figure 3B) and long-term death after 3 months after acute stroke (Figure 3C). On the basis of this results, we assumed that the PRoFESS study did show some effect of BP lowering after acute stroke and we could not exclude this trial from our analysis.

This updated meta-analysis differentiate from previous studies[19] with two more important aspects other than adding new data from recent trials or analyzing new outcome. Firstly, we just include the trials aiming to or achieving BP reduction in the intervention groups. In addition, we further evaluate the results by narrowing admission time span with a stricter inclusion criteria of the trials, and still find similar pooled results.

However,there are still several limitations in this analysis. Firstly, we could not obtain enough the data from the original authors, so several pooled outcomes could not be evaluated with sufficient studies and data, and it may affect our results more or less. Secondly, we could not make further subgroup analysis between ischemic stroke and hemorrhagic stroke because of the unavailable data of individual patients in each trial. But we did a crude subgroup analysis by different types of stroke with insufficient data and found that early BP lowering had a trend to increase early death within 30 days in ischemic stroke, which was similar to the combined result, however, no trend could be found in hemorrhagic stroke (data and figure not shown). Thirdly, we also could not make further subgroup analysis of the effects between different timing of intervention for the above reason. Finally, we could not assess the effects of different types of antihypertensive agents because of limited data available for detailed subgroup analyses. Therefore, more studies concerning the above problems are required in future and they will help to clarify the specific question more clearly on BP lowering after acute stroke, such as whether or when to intervene and which agent to use.

In conclusion, this updated meta-analysis with new evidence lend no support to early blood pressure lowering after acute stroke. It indicates that early BP lowering significantly increases death within 30 days after acute stroke.

Author Contributions

Conceived and designed the experiments: HW YT XR YP. Performed the experiments: HW XR. Analyzed the data: HW YT XR YP. Contributed reagents/materials/analysis tools: HW XR. Wrote the paper: HW HL. Discussed and revised the manuscript: HW XR RP YW YP.

References

1. Robinson TG, Potter JF (2004) Blood pressure in acute stroke. Age Ageing 33: 6–12.
2. Willmot M, Leonardi-Bee J, Bath PM (2004) High blood pressure in acute stroke and subsequent outcome: a systematic review. Hypertension 43: 18–24.
3. Qureshi AI (2008) Acute hypertensive response in patients with stroke: pathophysiology and management. Circulation 118: 176–87.
4. Ahmed N, Wahlgren G (2001) High initial blood pressure after acute stroke is associated with poor functional outcome. J Intern Med 249: 467–73.
5. Robinson TG, Dawson SL, Ahmed U, Manktelow B, Fotherby MD, et al. (2001) Twenty-four hour systolic blood pressure predicts long-term mortality following acute stroke. J Hypertens 19: 2127–34.
6. Leonardi-Bee J, Bath PM, Phillips SJ, Sandercock PA (2002) Blood pressure and clinical outcomes in the International Stroke Trial. Stroke 33: 1315–20.
7. Sare GM, Geeganage C, Bath PM (2009) High blood pressure in acute ischaemic stroke—broadening therapeutic horizons. Cerebrovasc Dis 27 Suppl 1: 156–61.
8. Ko Y, Park JH, Yang MH, Ko SB, Han MK, et al. (2010) The significance of blood pressure variability for the development of hemorrhagic transformation in acute ischemic stroke. Stroke 41: 2512–8.
9. Ohwaki K, Yano E, Nagashima H, Hirata M, Nakagomi T, et al. (2004) Blood pressure management in acute intracerebral hemorrhage: relationship between elevated blood pressure and hematoma enlargement. Stroke 35: 1364–7.
10. Britton M, Carlsson A, de Faire U (1986) Blood pressure course in patients with acute stroke and matched controls. Stroke 17: 861–4.
11. Ahmed N, Nasman P, Wahlgren NG (2000) Effect of intravenous nimodipine on blood pressure and outcome after acute stroke. Stroke 31: 1250–5.
12. Mistri AK, Robinson TG, Potter JF (2006) Pressor therapy in acute ischemic stroke: systematic review. Stroke 37: 1565–71.
13. Eames PJ, Blake MJ, Dawson SL, Panerai RB, Potter JF (2002) Dynamic cerebral autoregulation and beat to beat blood pressure control are impaired in acute ischaemic stroke. J Neurol Neurosurg Psychiatry 72: 467–72.
14. Schrader J, Luders S, Kulschewski A, Berger J, Zidek W, et al. (2003) The ACCESS Study: evaluation of Acute Candesartan Cilexetil Therapy in Stroke Survivors. Stroke 34: 1699–703.
15. Anderson CS, Huang Y, Wang JG, Arima H, Neal B, et al. (2008) Intensive blood pressure reduction in acute cerebral haemorrhage trial (INTERACT): a randomised pilot trial. Lancet Neurol 7: 391–9.
16. Potter JF, Robinson TG, Ford GA, Mistri A, James M, et al. (2009) Controlling hypertension and hypotension immediately post-stroke (CHHIPS): a randomised, placebo-controlled, double-blind pilot trial. Lancet Neurol 8: 48–56.
17. Rashid P, Weaver C, Leonardi-Bee J, Bath F, Fletcher S, et al. (2003) The effects of transdermal glyceryl trinitrate, a nitric oxide donor, on blood pressure, cerebral and cardiac hemodynamics, and plasma nitric oxide levels in acute stroke. J Stroke Cerebrovasc Dis 12: 143–51.
18. Geeganage C, Bath PM (2008) Interventions for deliberately altering blood pressure in acute stroke. Cochrane Database Syst Rev CD000039.
19. Geeganage C, Bath PM (2010) Vasoactive drugs for acute stroke. Cochrane Database Syst Rev CD002839.
20. Bath PM, Martin RH, Palesch Y, Cotton D, Yusuf S, et al. (2009) Effect of telmisartan on functional outcome, recurrence, and blood pressure in patients with acute mild ischemic stroke: a PRoFESS subgroup analysis. Stroke 40: 3541–6.
21. Robinson TG, Potter JF, Ford GA, Bulpitt CJ, Chernova J, et al. (2010) Effects of antihypertensive treatment after acute stroke in the Continue or Stop Post-Stroke Antihypertensives Collaborative Study (COSSACS): a prospective, randomised, open, blinded-endpoint trial. Lancet Neurol 9: 767–75.
22. Sandset EC, Bath PM, Boysen G, Jatuzis D, Korv J, et al. (2011) The angiotensin-receptor blocker candesartan for treatment of acute stroke (SCAST): a randomised, placebo-controlled, double-blind trial. Lancet 377: 741–50.
23. Anderson CS, Heeley E, Huang Y, Wang J, Stapf C, et al. (2013) Rapid blood-pressure lowering in patients with acute intracerebral hemorrhage. N Engl J Med 368: 2355–65.
24. He J, Zhang Y, Xu T, Zhao Q, Wang D, et al. (2013) Effects of Immediate Blood Pressure Reduction on Death and Major Disability in Patients With Acute Ischemic Stroke: The CATIS Randomized Clinical Trial. JAMA
25. Nakamura T, Tsutsumi Y, Shimizu Y, Uchiyama S (2010) Renin-angiotensin system blockade safely reduces blood pressure in patients with minor ischemic stroke during the acute phase. J Stroke Cerebrovasc Dis 19: 435–40.

26. Eveson DJ, Robinson TG, Potter JF (2007) Lisinopril for the treatment of hypertension within the first 24 hours of acute ischemic stroke and follow-up. Am J Hypertens 20: 270–7.
27. Kaste M, Fogelholm R, Erila T, Palomaki H, Murros K, et al. (1994) A randomized, double-blind, placebo-controlled trial of nimodipine in acute ischemic hemispheric stroke. Stroke 25: 1348–53.
28. Hsu CY, Faught RJ, Furlan AJ, Coull BM, Huang DC, et al. (1987) Intravenous prostacyclin in acute nonhemorrhagic stroke: a placebo-controlled double-blind trial. Stroke 18: 352–8.
29. Barer DH, Cruickshank JM, Ebrahim SB, Mitchell JR (1988) Low dose beta blockade in acute stroke ("BEST" trial): an evaluation. Br Med J (Clin Res Ed) 296: 737–41.
30. Bath PM, Pathansali R, Iddenden R, Bath FJ (2001) The effect of transdermal glyceryl trinitrate, a nitric oxide donor, on blood pressure and platelet function in acute stroke. Cerebrovasc Dis 11: 265–72.
31. Willmot M, Ghadami A, Whysall B, Clarke W, Wardlaw J, et al. (2006) Transdermal glyceryl trinitrate lowers blood pressure and maintains cerebral blood flow in recent stroke. Hypertension 47: 1209–15.
32. Perez MI, Musini VM, Wright JM (2009) Effect of early treatment with anti-hypertensive drugs on short and long-term mortality in patients with an acute cardiovascular event. Cochrane Database Syst Rev CD006743.
33. Norris JW LLAB (1994) Intravenous Nimodipine in Acute Ischaemic Stroke. Cerebrovasc Dis 4: 194–196.
34. Horn J, de Haan RJ, Vermeulen M, Limburg M (2001) Very Early Nimodipine Use in Stroke (VENUS): a randomized, double-blind, placebo-controlled trial. Stroke 32: 461–5.

7

Efficacy and Dose-Dependent Safety of Intra-Arterial Delivery of Mesenchymal Stem Cells in a Rodent Stroke Model

Dileep R. Yavagal[1,2,3]*, Baowan Lin[1], Ami P. Raval[1,2], Philip S. Garza[1], Chuanhui Dong[2], Weizhao Zhao[2], Erika B. Rangel[3], Ian McNiece[3], Tatjana Rundek[2], Ralph L. Sacco[2], Miguel Perez-Pinzon[1,2], Joshua M. Hare[3,4]

1 Cerebral Vascular Disease Research Laboratories, Leonard M. Miller School of Medicine, University of Miami, Miami, Florida, United States of America, **2** Department of Neurology, Leonard M. Miller School of Medicine, University of Miami, Miami, Florida, United States of America, **3** Interdisciplinary Stem Cell Institute, Leonard M. Miller School of Medicine, University of Miami, Miami, Florida, United States of America, **4** The Department of Medicine, Leonard M. Miller School of Medicine, University of Miami, Miami, Florida, United States of America

Abstract

Intra-arterial (IA) delivery of mesenchymal stem cells (MSCs) for acute ischemic stroke is attractive for clinical translation. However, studies using rat model of stroke have demonstrated that IA MSCs delivery can decrease middle cerebral artery (MCA) flow, which may limit its clinical translation. The goal of this study is to identify a dose of IA MSCs (maximum tolerated dose; MTD) that does not compromise MCA flow and evaluate its efficacy and optimal timing in a rat model of reversible middle cerebral artery occlusion (rMCAo). We sought to determine if there is a difference in efficacy of acute (1 h) versus sub-acute (24 h) IA MSCs treatment after rMCAo. Adult female Sprague-Dawley rats underwent rMCAo (90 min) and an hour later a single dose of MSCs (at de-escalating doses 1×10^6, 5×10^5, 2×10^5, 1×10^5 and 5×10^4) was given using IA route. MSCs were suspended in phosphate buffered saline (PBS) and PBS alone was used for control experiments. We measured the percent change in mean laser Doppler flow signal over the ipsilateral MCA in de-escalating doses groups to determine MTD. The results demonstrated that the lowering of IA MSC dose to 1×10^5 and below did not compromise MCA flow and hence an IA MSC dose of 1×10^5 considered as MTD. Subsequently, 1 h and 24 h after rMCAo, rats were treated with IA MSCs or PBS. The 24 h delivery of IA MSCs significantly improved neurodeficit score and reduced the mean infarct volume at one month as compared to control, but not the 1 h delivery. Overall, this study suggests that the IA delivery of MSCs can be performed safely and efficaciously at the MTD of 1×10^5 delivered at 24 hours in rodent model of stroke.

Editor: Toru Hosoda, Tokai University, Japan

Funding: This study was supported by Department of Neurology, University of Miami (DRY); James and Esther King Biomedical Research Program, Florida Department of Health Grant # 2KN09 (DRY); University of Miami intramural grant: Interdepartmental Research Development Initiative grant 2009–2010 (DRY) and the Anderson Family Gift 2010–2011, 2012–2014 (DRY). The funders had no role in study design, data collection and analysis, decision to publish, or preparation of the manuscript.

Competing Interests: The authors have declared that no competing interests exist.

* E-mail: dyavagal@med.miami.edu

Introduction

Stroke is the main cause of long-term disability and the third leading cause of death in the United States. The public health burden of stroke continues to be staggering with an estimated cost of 73.3 billion in 2010 [1]. Despite the approval of intravenous recombinant tissue plasminogen activator (rtPA) 18 years ago, and rapid growth in number of endovascular recanalization therapies for acute ischemic stroke (AIS), their impact on reducing stroke-related long-term disability is limited [2,3]. Hence, there continues to be a critical need for novel therapies for AIS. In this regard, over the last decade, various types of stem cell have been tested in several pre-clinical studies suggesting improved functional neurological outcomes after AIS [4–7]. The leading type of stem cell for clinical translation in stroke is the mesenchymal stem cell, which is an adult, non-hematopoietic progenitor cell with capacity to differentiate into a variety of cell lineages including osteoblasts, chondrocytes and neuron-like cells [8–11].

Mesenchymal stem cells (MSCs) are multipotent non-hematopoietic stem cells found mainly in the stromal fraction of the bone marrow as well as in the connective tissue of most organs [9–11]. MSCs can be easily isolated from adipose tissue, amniotic fluid, placenta and umbilical cord, though they are most commonly and efficiently derived from adult bone marrow. MSCs are an attractive cell source because they are relatively easy to obtain, expand and manipulate *in vitro* [12]. Moreover, adult MSCs do not confer the risk of tumorgenicity that pluripotent cells carry [13]. Importantly, MSCs are also immunoprivileged, with low MHC I and no MHC II antigen expression [12,13]. Their immunoprivileged nature obviates the need for immunosuppression in allogeneic administration of MSCs. Thus allogeneic MSCs, already produced from a healthy donor, can be given as an off-the-shelf product without delay if needed without the need of immunosuppression. This feature is especially attractive for future translation of MSCs into a treatment for ischemic stroke, which is presents most often without warning and may benefit from early administration of cell therapy [14–16].

There are multiple routes of stem cell delivery to the brain in AIS. Among these, the intra-arterial (IA) route of stem cell delivery has a high potential for clinical translation, in view of the increasing clinical application of endovascular therapy in the treatment of AIS [6,17–20]. Furthermore, IA delivery of stem cells after AIS is minimally invasive and results in a larger number and more diffuse distribution of stem cells in and around the infarcted area when compared to intra-parenchymal, intra-cerebroventricular and intravenous stem cell delivery [21]. IA delivery avoids the first pass trapping of stem cells in the lungs and liver seen with intravenous delivery [22]. Also, a recent study has shown superior functional and histological outcomes with IA delivery of stem cells as compared to intravenous administration [23]. However MSCs range in size from 5–50 microns and a major limitation to IA delivery of MSCs is the possibility of compromise of regional cerebral blood flow (rCBF) owing to those MSCs in the larger size range of 20–50 microns; thus a potentially novel therapeutic strategy can paradoxically worsen of cerebral ischemia outcome [10].

In the current study, first we hypothesized that compromise of MCA blood flow during IA delivery of MSCs was dose-dependent and therefore, lowering the dose of IA MSCs would mitigate rCBF compromise. The efficacy of IA MSC in focal cerebral ischemia, with doses lower than 1×10^6 has not been studied. Hence, we also hypothesized that the lower safe dose we identify, based on our first hypothesis, would be efficacious in focal cerebral ischemia. Furthermore, the efficacy of IA MSCs given immediately after reperfusion (within 60 minutes) as compared to the efficacy when given at 24-hours is unknown. Hence, we additionally hypothesized that the efficacy of the MTD of IA MSCs delivered at 24 hours (sub-acute) and 60 minutes (acute) in a rodent cerebral ischemia model would be the same.

Materials and Methods

All animal procedures were carried out in accordance with the Guide for the Care and Use of Laboratory Animals published by the U.S. National Institutes of Health and approved by the Animal Care and Use Committee of the University of Miami.

Female Sprague-Dawley rats (Charles River Laboratories, Inc., Wilmington, MA) weighing 260–310 g were used. The animals in the experimental groups were allocated in a randomized fashion. Investigators were blinded to dose and treatment group allocation during surgery and during outcome evaluations.

Surgery

The animals underwent Reversible Middle cerebral artery occlusion (rMCAo) following an overnight fast. Anesthesia was induced with 3% isofluorane and 70% nitrous oxide. Rats were intubated endotracheally and ventilated mechanically on a mixture of 1–0.5% isofluorane, 70% nitrous oxide and a balance of oxygen. The right femoral artery and vein were catheterized to permit to monitor blood pressure and to take arterial samples for blood gas and glucose assessments. Arterial PCO_2 and PO_2 were maintained in the normal range by ventilator adjustment. For immobilization, rats received pancuromium bromide 0.75 mg/kg i.v. Rectal temperature was measured continuously and maintained at 37–37.5°C by a heating pat under the rat's body. Cranial temperature was separately monitored by a 29-gauge thermocouple implanted into the right temporalis muscle and was maintained at 36–36.5°C by a warming lamp placed above the rat's head throughout the experiment. Our previous studies have shown that the cranial temperature 36–36.5°C corresponds to a brain temperature of 36.5–37°C [24]. Physiological variables (plasma glucose concentration, pH, PCO_2, PO_2 and mean arterial blood pressure (MABP)) were maintained normal before and after ischemia (Table S1 and S2; presented as supplementary data).

CBF monitoring

The left scalp was opened and the skull was exposed. A 2-mm bur hole was drilled on the left *sphenoid*, 3 mm below the up edge, 0.5 mm anterior and 6 mm lateral to the bregma, leaving the dura intact. A short Laser Doppler Flowmetry (LDF, Perimed Inc.) probe was placed above the dura and fixed on to the skull with glue and dental cement. From this point, the CBF inside the trunk of the ascending vessel from cortical branch of MCA was monitored. The LDF signal reading was recorded, starting at 30 min before the suture insertion and continuously throughout the experiment and 60 min after the cell infusion, using a specific designed monitoring system.

Reversible Middle cerebral artery occlusion (rMCAo)

The previously well-described suture technique for MCAo was utilized in this study [25–28]. The common carotid artery (CCA) was exposed through a midline incision on the ventral neck and carefully separated from the surrounding tissue including the adjacent vagus nerve by blunt dissection using microsurgery. Under an operation microscope, the branches of external carotid artery (ECA), superior thyroid and ascending pharyngeal arteries and further the terminal lingual and maxillary artery branches, were dissected and coagulated. Two long 5–0 silk sutures tied the ECA as distal to carotid bifurcation as possible. Two short (3 cm) 5–0 silk sutures were tied loosely around the segment of ECA closed to the bifurcation. The ICA was exposed, and the origin of the pterygopalatine artery (PPA) was visualized. An intraluminal 3.0 nylon suture, having a spherical and enlarged tip produced by heating near flame, introduced into the distal segment of ECA via a small incision on the vessel and advanced into the ECA lumen to reach the bifurcation. The 2 short silk sutures subsequently were tied to prevent bleeding. The ECA was cut at the distal segment between the 2 long-suture notes. The stump of the ECA was held toward the surgeon; thus the stump and the ICA were on a straight line. The suture was then turned into ICA with a special care not enter the PPA. The suture went advance in ICA until the sharp drop of regional cerebral blood flow confirmed by the LDF. The length of inserted suture inside the ICA from the bifurcation was 19–25 mm. A sudden and sharp decrease in the LDF signal was interpreted to indicate a successful MCA occlusion. The suture was gently withdrawn after the 90-min occlusion period. During the procedure and the 2-h recirculation, blood pressure and the blood gas were maintained in the normal ranges, cranial and rectal temperature were maintained at normal levels.

Inclusion and Exclusion Criteria

Rats that had less than 50% drop in LDF signal on suture insertion and premature mortality during rMCAo were excluded from the study prior to randomization and allocation to treatment groups.

Experimental Design

(1) Safety Study

Forty-three female rats underwent rMCAo. The suture was gently withdrawn after a 90-minute occlusion period (Figure 1A, B). At 60 minutes after recirculation, a 1 ml syringe was filled with the MSCs suspended in phosphate buffered saline (PBS) or PBS alone. The cell suspension in 0.5 mL PBS or PBS alone (0.5 mL) was delivered into the ipsilateral IA over 3 minutes. The different groups of animals received 1×10^6, 5×10^5, 2×10^5, 1×10^5 & 5×10^4 MSCs in PBS or only PBS. Following MSCs or PBS delivery, the catheter was carefully withdrawn and the ECA was tied. During the surgical procedure of rMCAo and IA MSCs deliver, we measure blood flow over ipsilateral MCA using laser Doppler flow signal (LDFS).

(2) Efficacy Study

In another cohort, 34 female rats underwent 90 minutes of rMCAo. Twenty-four hours after induction of rMCAo, rats were assigned to receive IA MSCs (1×10^5) or IA PBS or intravenous (IV) MSCs 1×10^6. In the IV MSCs group, the cells were given into the femoral vein at a 10-fold of the IA MSC dose in order to potentially increase the number of MSCs reaching the injured brain. In an additional experimental group, IA MSCs at 1×10^5 were given at 60 minutes after rMCAo to study the effect of acute timing on efficacy. The primary outcome measure was neurodeficit score and the secondary outcome was infarct volume at 4 weeks.

Donor rodent MSCs

MSCs used in this study were derived from green fluorescence protein (GFP) transgenic male Sprague-Dawley rats. At the Cell Manufacturing Program at the University of Miami, the bone marrow was harvested from rats and the mononuclear cells isolated by density gradient centrifugation. The cells were then cultured at 1 to 5×10^6 cells per ml in 25 ml of alpha MEM plus 20%FCS in T162 cm^2 culture flasks at 5%CO_2 and 37°C. MSCs exhibited spindle-shaped morphology and were characterized by (i) adherence to plastic, (ii) negativity for hematopoietic cell surface markers CD34 and CD45 (0.1±0.1% and 0.2±.0.1%, respectively) and positivity for CD73, CD90.2, and CD105 (88±5.4%, 99.2±0.7% and 95±3.7%, respectively). The cells were expanded to passage 6 and then the MSCs were suspended in 10% of cryopreservant dimethylsulfoxide (DMSO) and frozen in liquid nitrogen. Prior to injection, the cells were thawed rapidly and washed to remove (DMSO), and then re-suspended in PBS to the required cell dose. We evaluated cell viability prior to infusion using trypan blue technique. Only cell doses at and above 70% viability were administered in the study.

The presence of hematopoietic cell surface markers was investigated using fluorescence-activated cell sorting (FACS). Briefly, a total of $0.5-1\times10^6$ MSCs was used for FACS characterization. GFP positivity was detected in 79±5% of MSCs in culture. For surface markers, cells were incubated for 1 hour with FACS buffer (1% bovine serum albumin and 5% FBS diluted in distilled water) on ice, and subsequently 1 hour with the primary and secondary antibodies (washed 3 times for 5 minutes during centrifugation between the primary and secondary and after the secondary). Each analysis included at least 10,000 events and was performed on at least three separate cell preparations (BD FACSAria, University of Miami). All experiments for MSCs characterization were performed between passages 8 to 11 after isolation. Cells were incubated with anti-mouse PE-fluorochrome-conjugated antibodies against CD45, CD73, and CD90.2 (BD Biosciences, San Jose, CA), PE-fluorochrome-conjugated against CD34 (Santa Cruz Biotechnology, Santa Cruz, CA), PE/Cy7-fluorochrome-conjugated against CD105 (BioLegend, San Diego, CA), and their respective isotype controls (BD Biosciences, San Jose, CA).

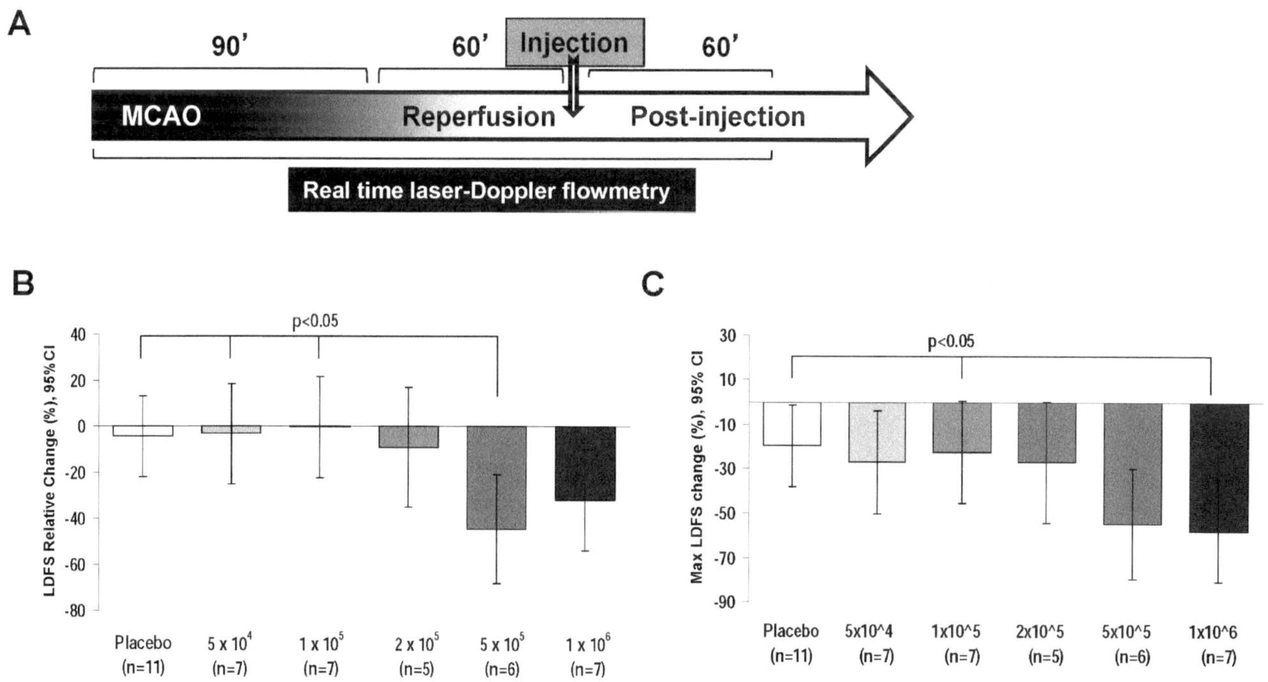

Figure 1. Lower doses of IA MSCs mitigate adverse effect IA injection on MCA blood flow. (A) Experimental timeline showing rMCAo for 90 minutes followed by withdrawal of the suture to allow reperfusion. At 60 minutes of reperfusion, IA MSC or vehicle only injection was given, followed by LDF monitoring for 60 min. (B) Comparison of relative LDFS worsening from baseline to final recording, among de-escalating dose groups (C) The 1×10^5 dose and placebo has significantly less maximum LDFS worsening as compared to the 1×10^6 dose. The comparisons in B and C were done using general linear modeling (GLM) to compare mean differences among groups. LDFS= Laser Doppler Flow Signal.

Intra-arterial MCA infusion

A PE-10 polyethylene catheter connected to a 30G needle and a 1-ml syringe was inserted into the stump of left ECA through an incision on the vessel under the operation microscope and was tightened to ECA by a 5–0 silk suture. The catheter went forward into ICA and avoided PPA, the extracranial branch of ICA, to approach the skull base [29]. The catheter was filled with heparinized physiological saline to prevent air bubble and coagulation. The syringe was filled with MSCs in PBS or PBS only. Using slow hand injection over 3 minutes, 0.5 ml volume of the cells in PBS or PBS only were then delivered into the ICA via the PE-10 catheter.

Histology and detection of MSCs in the brain

Under anesthesia rats were perfused via ascending aorta with FAM (a mixture of 40% formaldehyde, glacial acetic acid, and methanol, 1:1:8 by volume) for 20 min following a 2-min initial perfusion with physical saline. The rat heads were immersed in FAM for 1 day before the brains were removed. The brains were placed in FAM at 4°C for at least 1 additional day, and then coronal brain blocks were embedded in paraffin. All brains were cut into 10- μm thick sections from 5.5 mm to −7.5 mm from bregma at 9 standard levels to cover the whole infracted areas. Sections of the 9 levels were stained with hematoxylin and eosin to display the infracted areas and to obtain infarct volumes.

In a parallel study, adjacent sections were subjected to immunohistochemistry (IHC) studies with Vectastain ABC peroxidase method (Vector Labs, Burlingame, CA). Sections from levels 2–8 in the dose group 1×10^5 & 5×10^5 were tested by GFP-IHC to reveal the MSCs immigration inside the brain via injection through IA. To detect GFP positive MSCs, sections were incubated in the working dilution of 1:100 of anti-GFP (SC-101525, Santa Cruz Biotech, CA.) for 90 min at room temperature, and 3, 3″-diaminobenzidine (DAB) was used for visualization of the primary antibody binding. The dark-brown appearance was considered the specific labeling to indicate the MSCs. Hematoxylin counterstain was conducted to identify cells and brain regions. Blocked vessels were defined as: complete filling of the microvessel caliber with MSCs in axial section or segment of vessel in sagittal section of a vessel. The absolute total number of blocked microvessels per section was reported.

Both positive control, to confirm the negative labeling being truly negative, and negative control, to confirm the positive staining not false positive, were applied in the present study. The two negative controls including 1) mouse IgG 1 (X0931, Dako, Carpenteria, CA) replaced anti-GFP in the female brains of the present study and 2) anti-GFP applied to male rat brains having infarction from previous study were performed. Negative labeling represented in the 2 negative controls supported that the positive staining were true positive. Anti-glial fibrillary acidic protein (GFAP, Dako, Carpenteria) was employed in the IHC study as the positive control to ensure that the reduced sensitivity of reaction not due to improper technique because positive control slide, i.e. the known histological slide containing the specific antigen unavailable [26].

Neurodeficit Scoring

A standardized neurobehavioral test battery was conducted as described previously [27], which includes tests for postural reflex, sensorimotor integration and proprioception. Total neurological score ranged from a normal score of 0 to a maximal possible score of 12.

Statistical analyses

Descriptive statistics for physiological continuous variables were presented as means with standard deviations. For safety analysis, the primary outcome was the relative change in MCA blood flow from pre-injection to the final assessment after injection of MSCs or saline, whereas the secondary outcome was the maximum relative reduction in blood flow within the 60 minutes after injection. General linear model (GLM) was used to compare mean differences among groups in the relative change at the final LDFS measurement and in the maximum relative reduction in blood flow. Mixed model was used for analyzing for comparing LDFS over time between two groups. For efficacy analysis, mixed-effects model was used to assess differences among groups in neurodeficit scores based on the repeated measures. Due to skewed distribution, log transformation was first performed for infarct volume and ANOVA was used to compare the differences among groups at week 4 after treatment. All analyses were performed with SAS 9.3 (SAS Institute Inc., Cary, NC) or SPSS 16.0 (SPSS Inc., Chicago, IL).

Results

Lower IA MSC doses mitigate adverse impact on MCA blood flow

We first determined the impact of lowering the dose of IA MSC on MCA blood flow, starting with a dose of 1 million cells, which was previously shown to severely decrease MCA flow in one-thirds of animals [10]. In the animals receiving $1\times10^6$and 5×10^5 MSCs, there was a considerable decrease in the final post-injection MCA flow by 32% and 45% respectively, compared to the pre-IA MSC injection MCA flow (Figure 1B). Lowering the dose below 5×10^5 resulted in mitigation of the adverse effect of IA MSC injection on MCA flow. At the dose of 2×10^5, the MCA flow compromise was less as compared to the 5×10^5 dose group, but this was non-significant (LDFS decreased by 9% vs 45%, $p=0.06$). At the next lowered dose level of 1×10^5 MSCs, the MCA flow compromise was significantly less as compared to 5×10^5 dose group (LDFS decreased by 0.2% vs 45%, $p=0.01$). When we analyzed the maximum reduction in LDFS among the dose groups, the rats receiving $1\times10^6$and 5×10^5 MSCs had a maximum reduction of LDFS over 50%, whereas those receiving a dose at 1×10^5 MSCs had a maximum reduction in LDFS of 23%, similar to 20% in placebo group (Figure 1C). Furthermore, we found that as compared to the 5×10^5 dose, the 1×10^5 IA MSC dose injection led to less worsening in LDFS post injection over the course of 60 minutes post injection, becoming significantly improved at 45 minutes and 60 minutes post-injection (Figure 2A). Based on these results the 1×10^5 IA MSCs dose was utilized for subsequent studies and defined as maximum tolerated dose (MTD).

Mortality with MCAo and IA MSCs

The mortality rate of the MCAo procedure (premature mortality) in this study was 13.46%. In the part of the study evaluating safety of de-escalating doses, the mortality rate after IA MSC dose administration was: 8.3%, 28.6%, 12.5%, 42.9%, 42.9% and 42.9% in the placebo, 5×10^4, 1×10^5, 2×10^5, 5×10^5 and 1×10^6 IA MSC dose groups respectively.

Impact of MSC Dose on Microvascular Occlusion and MSC Distribution

Consistent with the effect on MCA flow, at 3–5 days post injection, we found a significantly higher number of brain microvessels showing complete occlusion with MSCs in rats

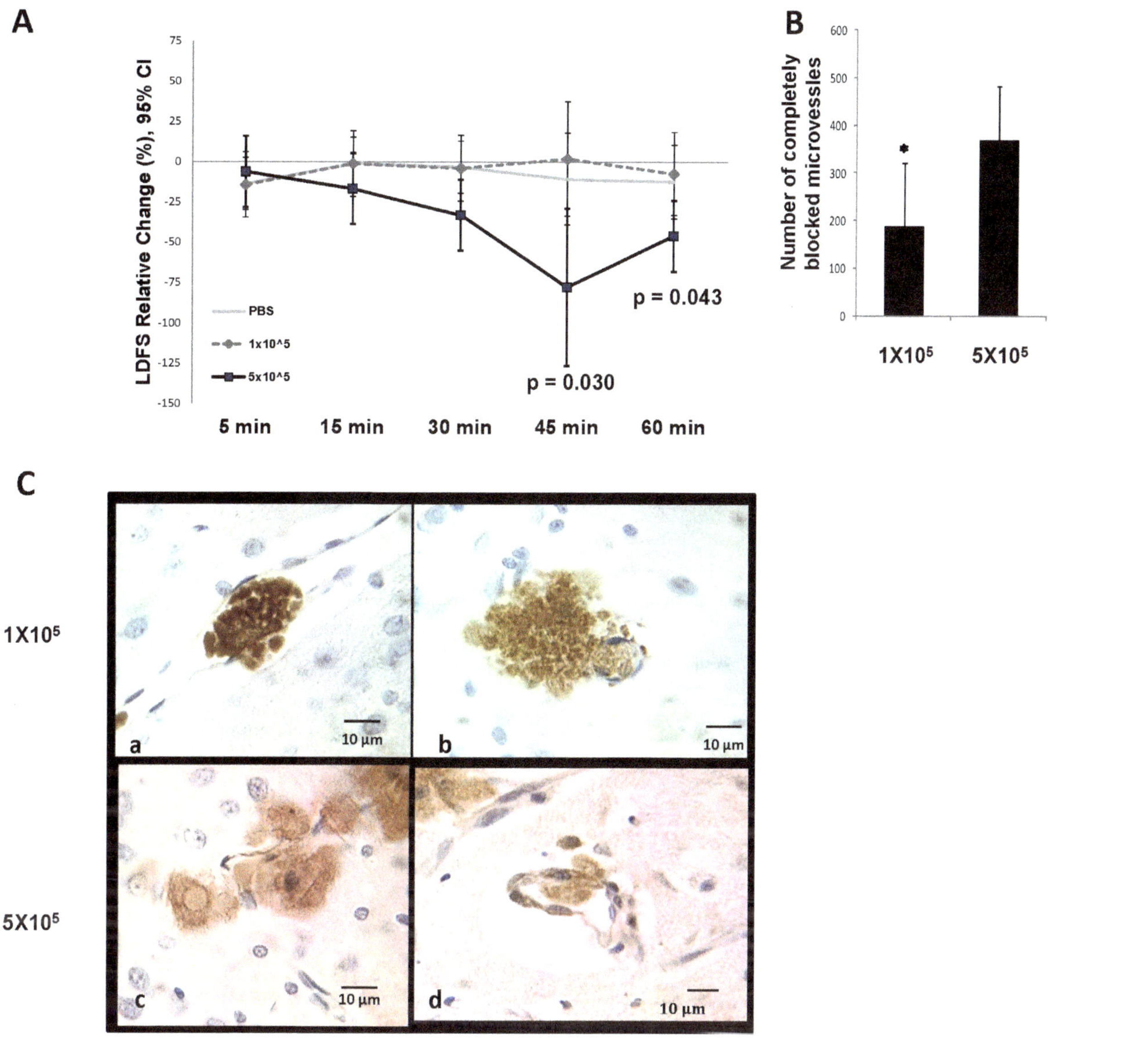

Figure 2. Comparison of LDFS changes over time and microvascular occlusion between dose-groups. (A) IA MSC dose of 1×10^5 and IA placebo have a transient and less MCA LDF worsening during 60 minutes post injection as compared to 5×10^5 dose using mixed model. LDFS = Laser Doppler Flow Signal. (B) On comparing the total number of microvessels with complete occlusion among the two dose groups, there were a significantly lower number of complete occlusions in the lower dose group. Mean ±SD, * P<0.05, ANOVA. (C) Representative brain sections from IA MSC 1×10^5 dose group showing GFP+ MSCs identified by 3, 3″-diaminobenzidine (DAB), showing localized complete filling of microvessels at 3–5 days post-injection, as well as MSCs just outside the vessel wall in brain parenchyma and (D) high power field of representative brain sections from IA 5×10^5 dose group showing single MSC partly inside and partly outside microvessel wall.

receiving IA MSCs at the higher dose of 5×10^5 as compared to the MTD of 1×10^5(366.5 vs. 185.75, $p = 0.047$) (Figure 2B). However, in rats in both dose groups, MSCs were also seen in the brain parenchyma just outside the microvessels at the level of the blockage. (Fig. 2C) We noted two sections in one rat from the larger dose group in which individual MSCs were located across the vessel wall partly inside the vessel and rest in the adjacent brain parenchyma, consistent with them being in the process of diapedesis.

Efficacy Study of MTD of IA MSCs

We chose the 1×10^5 MSCs as the dose to use for our efficacy study of IA MSCs in rMCAo based on the above results showing that this was the highest dose group that had minimal adverse effect on MCA LDF post-injection. We compared the efficacy of IA MSCs given at 24 hours (IA MSC_24 h), at one hour (IA MSC_1 h), IV MSCs at a ten-fold dose given at 24 hours (IV MSC_24 h) and IC PBS given at 24 hours (IA PBS_24 h) post rMCAo. On mixed model analysis we found a significant interaction between treatment group and time point ($p = 0.02$), with no significant difference among the groups at day 1 ($p = 0.49$) and most significant difference at 28 days ($p<0.0001$) after treatment (Figure 3B). The IA MSC_24 h group had a significantly lower neurodeficit score (5.8, 95% CI: 4.4 to 7.2) at 28 days after treatment as compared to IA PBS_24 h (10.4, 8.5 to 12.3, $p<0.0001$), as well as to IV MSC_24 h at dose of 1×10^6 (10.3, 8.8 to 11.7, $p = 0.0002$), and IA MSC_1 h (9.2, 7.3 to 11.1,

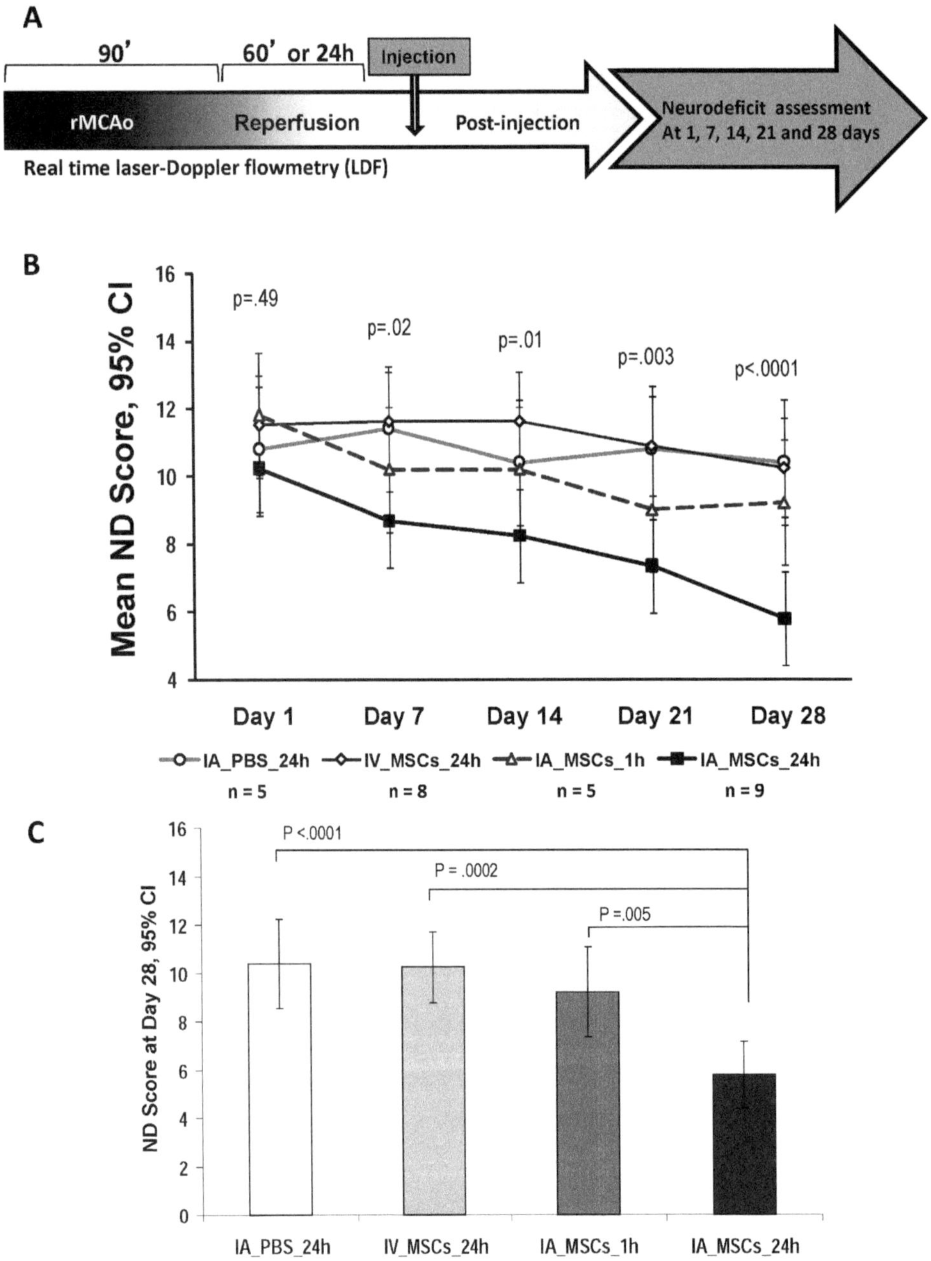

Figure 3. Functional neurologic outcomes are superior in the IA MSC_24 h group. (A) Experimental timeline of the efficacy study showing 90 min rMCAo followed by 24 hour reperfusion except in group receiving IA MSCs at 1 hour reperfusion followed by ND score assessment at 1,7,14,21 & 28 days. (B) On day 1 post rMCAo, the ND scores were not significantly different among groups. The ND score of the 1×10^5 group progressively decreased over time and at 28 days was significantly lower than the other groups. C, The day 28 ND score was significantly lower in the IA MSC_24 h group as compared to all the remaining groups. ND = Neurodeficit

p = 0.005) groups. The IA MSC_1 h group showed no significant difference in functional outcome compared to the IA PBS_24 h (p = 0.37) and IV MSC_24 h (p = 0.38) groups (Figure 3C).

Also, the mean infarct volume of the group treated with IA MSC_24 h group (4.6 mm3, 1.2 to 12.72) was significantly lower as compared to IA PBS_24 h (39.5, 11 to 136.1, p = 0.01) The groups treated with IV_24 h MSCs and IA MSC_24 h did not show a significant reduction in their infarct volume as compared to IA PBS_24 h (Fig. 4A). In order to compare the location of infarcted brain, we used an infarct topography frequency map, which showed a significantly decreased volume of infarction in the penumbral region in the IA MSC_24 h group as compared to the IA PBS_24 h group (Fig 4B).

Discussion

The major challenge to the IA method of delivery of MSCs is the possibility of vascular occlusion in small arterioles and capillaries owing to the large size of the cells ranging from 15–50 microns [10]. We report a major new finding of a dose response relationship in safety of IA delivery of allogeneic IA MSCs and

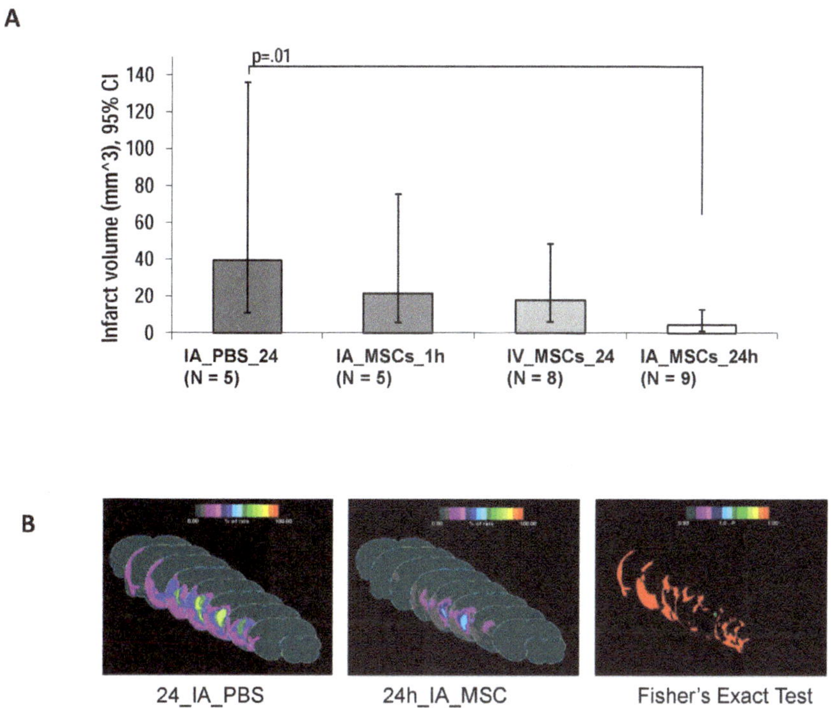

Figure 4. Comparison of infarct volume among treatment groups. (A) Geometric mean infarct volumes are compared among groups after log transformation to achieve normal distribution. Only the IA MSC_24 h group shows significantly reduced infarct volume as compared to the IA PBS_24 h. B, Frequency infarct map statistically comparing the location of the mean infarct volume in the IA MSC_24 h and IA PBS_24 h groups using color- coded representation of the percent of rats showing infarction in each brain region using "Fisher's exact test" with a color-coded representation of the "p-value", the color bar in "1-p" format. Displays are in "Coronal presentation"; middle sections are selected. The IA MSC_24 h group shows a much reduced infarction frequency, particularly surrounding the core as quantized by the Fisher test.

that lowering of the IA dose overcomes the decrease in blood flow in the middle cerebral artery after IA MSC injection in a rat model of acute ischemic stroke. Furthermore, the lower safe dose of 1×10^5 MSCs, when given IA at 24 hours results therapeutic effect to reduce infarct volume and improve functional status. Together these findings support further translational investigation to develop intra-arterial allogeneic MSCs as a novel therapy for AIS in the first 24 hours after stroke onset.

With the increasing number of catheter-based endovascular treatments for patients with AIS, intra-arterial delivery of stem cells has tremendous potential for clinical translation. Intra-arterial delivery of bone marrow mononuclear cells into the affected MCA was found to be safe within 3–7 days in a 20 patients trial of patients with MCA strokes [30]. The strategy of endovascular intra-arterial delivery of MSCs has been successfully implemented in early clinical studies of intra-coronary-delivered MSCs after acute myocardial infarction [31,32]. Given this tremendous promise for clinical application, pre-clinical studies addressing crucial translational hurdles in intra-arterial delivery of stem cells, including MSCs in stroke, are crucial in the efforts to bring this therapy to the bedside.

A previous study of IA MSC delivery reported severely reduced ipsilateral MCA blood flow (80–90%) in 35%, and moderately reduced (10–30%) in 47%, of animals after intra-carotid delivery of 1×10^6 MSCs given 30 minutes after rMCAo [10]. On dose de-escalation, starting at the dose of 1×10^6, we found a similar reduction in CBF signal on IA MSC delivery at the doses of 1×10^6 and 5×10^5. This adverse effect was somewhat ameliorated at the 2×10^5dose and resolved with further lowering of the dose to 1×10^5 consistent with a dose-response relationship in the safety of IA delivery of MSCs in rMCAo. In another recent study the safety of MSC delivery was tested using non-MCAo rats [33]. Lowering of MSCs dose from 2×10^6 to 1×10^6 dose decreased stroke lesions on MRI the rodent rMCAo model. Stroke lesions occurred frequently (12 out of 15 animals) when injecting 2×10^6 MSCs, but not after lowering the dose to 1×10^6 cells. While the decrease in dose of MCSs led to better safety, similar to our study, the safety of the 1×10^6 dose is likely due to the use of non-MCAo rats in that study. The twice bigger dose 2×10^6 produced frequent micro-strokes – mostly in the area of corpus callosum. With regards to mortality post cell injection, the groups receiving 2×10^5 and higher doses of MSCs had a mortality rate of 42.9% similar to that seen in other studies [10]. The 1×10^5 dose group and the PBS group had a numerically a lower mortality rate (12.5% and 8.3% respectively) as compared to the higher dose groups although not statistically significant. Similarly, mortality in 5×10^4 group is numerically higher than 1×10^5 however, there is no statistically significant difference between two groups. The surgical procedure of MCAo is highly invasive and observed mortality could be confounded by the mortality related to the MCAo in the safety phase of our study.

Despite approximately three times slower speed of injection as compared to a previous study we did not see mitigation of the adverse effect on blood flow in the MCA at the dose of 1×10^6 MSCs, the only dose tested in that study [10]. The speed of cell injection from our rodent study and others cannot be directly translated in humans. Apart from the large difference in scale, the size of microcatheters available for clinical use allow for excellent blood flow around the microcatheters in the ICA whereas, the PE 10 has a very snug fit in the rodent ICA. Testing of the IA injection speed into ICA in larger animal species may hence be needed.

The reduction of CBF signal over the MCA at the dose of 5×10^5 is seen shortly after intra-carotid delivery of MSCs at the higher doses and progressively worsens over 60 minutes (Figure 2A), suggesting a mechanical obstruction in the MCA, likely caused by microvascular "sludging" owing to stacking of cells in the microvasculature at higher doses. This is supported by our histology results that showed significantly increased microvascular occlusion at 3–5 days at the higher dose as compared to the lower dose and no evidence for other possible mechanisms for microvascular occlusion such as thrombosis or spasm. The occlusion of microvessels might be due to the higher ratio of the size of some MSCs (some being 15–50 microns in size) to the microvessels size. Along with intravascular MSCs, we found the vast majority of extravascular MSCs to be in the peri-vascular regions at this early time point. We found two separate instances in two separate animal brains of MSCs positioned across the endothelial lining partly inside a capillary and partly in the parenchyma, suggestive of transendothelial migration as the mechanism of transport of these cells into the brain, (Figure 2C, D) as seen in previous studies of intra-carotid stem cell infusion [34].

In the current study we observed the maximum reduction in LDFS was 20% following PBS delivery. Most importantly, the observed reduction in LDFS after PBS delivery occurred shortly after injection and was transient, lasting for short duration (~5 min) and reverted back to the baseline. In contrast, at the higher doses of 5×10^5 and 1×10^6 of IA MSCs, the reduction in LDFS lasted throughout the period of recording (60 min). Hence, the observed transient initial reduction with PBS injection is very unlikely to lead to worsening of ischemic injury

In our study, the animals receiving IA MSCs at the safe dose of 1×10^5 at 24 hours post rMCAo had a clearly superior functional neurologic outcome at one month as compared to controls receiving IA saline as well as compared to IV MSCs at the same time point. In parallel with the superior functional outcome, we also found the infarct volume to be significantly smaller only in the IA MSC_24 h group as compared to IA PBS_24 h. This decrease in infarct volume was found to be in the penumbral area (Figure 4B) in this group as compared to control suggesting that MSC-mediated neuroprotection as the likely mechanism of benefit. This mechanism has been confirmed in other studies that showed increased concentration of anti-apoptotic factors in the peri-infarct area in animals treated with MSCs.

While previous studies have shown efficacy of IA autologous bone marrow mononuclear cells (BMMCs) and fetal-derived neural stem cells [34,35], we found that allogeneic MSCs given via the IA route are efficacious in ameliorating neurological deficits in rodent cerebral ischemia without a need for immunosuppression. The application of allogeneic MSCs can facilitate rapid "off-the-shelf" therapy in patients with acute ischemic stroke. We found that not only of 1×10^5 IA MSCs lead to superior functional neurological recovery as compared to the control group given IA PBS, but also as compared to the group given IV MSCs at a 10-fold higher dose, indicating a robust relative efficacy of the IA route of delivery and its superiority to the IV route when MSCs are administered at 24 hours post rMCAo. Our results are consistent with the functional neurological benefit previously reported [15] with intra-arterial allogeneic MSCs administered at 24 hours post rMCAo. However, the dose of IA MSCs in our study was 10-fold lower as compared to the previous study. Our finding of efficacy at the MTD being safer as compared to higher doses, is novel and supports careful dose escalation studies in clinical translation of IA MSC therapy. In a previous study comparing the IA and IV routes of delivery of autologous BMMCs, efficacy was seen in the IA group but not the IV group [23]. Our results confirm a similar superiority of the IA route but add to this previous finding, as we also found a clear superiority of IA over the IV route on direct comparison of the effect of the two routes of delivery on functional recovery. Of note, in order to compensate for this systemic trapping of IV delivered MSCs, we chose an IV MSC dose that is 10 fold higher than the IA MSC dose so as to serve as an adequate control to IA MSCs that do not undergo systemic trapping. The choice of the IV dose was based on studies showing that IA administration of cells leads to a 7 to 12 times higher number of cells reaching the brain as compared to IV cell administration [34,36,37].

The optimal timing of IA stem cell delivery after AIS is unknown. We found that allogeneic IA MSCs given at 24 hours results in efficacy but not when given at 60 minutes after cerebral ischemia. The fact that there was no reduction in the infarct volume in the IA MSC_1 h group indicates that neuroprotection was not significant when MSCs are given at this hyperacute timing after rMCAo. This important finding may be a result of higher concentration of chemoattractant factors for transendothelial transport of MSCs at the more delayed time point, but we did not test this hypothesis. Another study has shown results consistent with the need to delay the administration of IA stem cells after stroke for efficacy [38]. In the prior study of IA neural stem cells in a mouse model of hypoxia-ischemia, authors found that increased phagocytosis of the cells in the post-ischemic brain when transplanted within 24 hours whereas transplantation at 3 days led to lower co-localization of MSCs with pan-monocytic marker Iba-1. These findings suggest that in the hyperacute phase the environment in the post-ischemic brain tissue may be detrimental to the administered IA cells and waiting for this inflammatory response to wane in the first few days is advantageous [38]. Therefore, while administration of IA stem cells via intra-carotid catheters immediately after endovascular reperfusion therapy for ischemic stroke in patients would avoid a second endovascular procedure to administer the cells a few days later, our data suggest that this hyperacute phase may not be an optimal treatment time point for IA cell therapy. Thus early clinical trial designs of IA allogeneic MSCs in ischemic stroke should consider administration of the cells in the first few days after stroke and not in conjunction or immediately following IA thrombolytic therapy.

One of the major limitations of the current study is that we did not test the possibility of slower IA injection to decrease cell sludging. However, the finding of efficacy at the MTD in our study offsets the concern that the higher doses than MTD may be necessary for benefit. Also, we did not comprehensively study the mechanism of action of MSCs, as our primary goal was safety and efficacy of the IA route of MSC delivery. We did not test for time points beyond 24 hours for IA allogeneic MSC injection. Although there is evidence for lack of efficacy of IA BMMC, as beyond 24 hours after rMCAo [39], the outer limit of the treatment time window remains to be established for allogeneic IA MSCs. Additionally, in the present study we monitored the LDF in the MCA for 60 minutes after IA MSCs delivery. However, effect of IA MSCs on LDF beyond 60 minutes is not known and remains to be investigated. Apart from LDF, the information such as presence of MSCs at perivascular locations and overall MSCs survival following IA MSCs needs investigation.

The present study used an experimental model of ischemic stroke in female rats to investigate efficacy of IA MSCs. The MSCs used for IA delivery were generated from male rats. Our approach of delivering MSCs derived from male rats in to the female experimental animals offer an added advantage of localizing MSCs in the brain by cytogenetic approach after IA or IV delivery in future. On the other hand, our use of female rats remains a limitation because it is well known that the circulating ovarian hormones influence ischemic pathology [40]. Future studies employing ovarian hormones-deprived (ovariectomized) female rats are needed to confirm the findings of current study.

In conclusion IA delivery of MSCs at low dose (1×10^5 cells) did not compromise MCA blood flow in a rat model of MCAo. Importantly, sub-acute delivery of MSCs at lowered dose protected brain from ischemic damage. Our study findings outline the core principles of MSC therapy for ischemic stroke using IA delivery. A clinical translational impact of these results needs to be determined in the future.

Supporting Information

Table S1 Physiological variables of protocol I. Values are mean ± SD (MABP, mean arterial blood pressure).

Table S2 Physiological variables of protocol II. Values are mean ± SD (MABP, mean arterial blood pressure).

Acknowledgments

We thank Drs. Myron Ginsburg, MD and Brant Watson, PhD for their critical review of the manuscript.

Author Contributions

Conceived and designed the experiments: DRY JH. Performed the experiments: BL. Analyzed the data: PSG AR CD WZ. Contributed reagents/materials/analysis tools: JH IM ER. Wrote the paper: DRY AR. Critically read manuscript: TR MAPP RLS JH.

References

1. Lloyd-Jones D, Adams RJ, Brown TM, Carnethon M, Dai S, et al. (2010) Executive summary: heart disease and stroke statistics—2010 update: a report from the American Heart Association. Circulation 121: 948–954.
2. Del Zoppo GJ, Saver JL, Jauch EC, Adams HP, Jr., American Heart Association Stroke C (2009) Expansion of the time window for treatment of acute ischemic stroke with intravenous tissue plasminogen activator: a science advisory from the American Heart Association/American Stroke Association. Stroke 40: 2945–2948.
3. Del Zoppo GJ, Moskowitz MA (2009) Translating interventions from ischemic stroke models to patients: the view in 2009. Front Neurol Neurosci 25: 34–38.
4. STEPS (2009) Stem Cell Therapies as an Emerging Paradigm in Stroke (STEPS): bridging basic and clinical science for cellular and neurogenic factor therapy in treating stroke. Stroke 40: 510–515.
5. Chen J, Li Y, Wang L, Zhang Z, Lu D, et al. (2001) Therapeutic benefit of intravenous administration of bone marrow stromal cells after cerebral ischemia in rats. Stroke 32: 1005–1011.
6. Mimura T, Dezawa M, Kanno H, Yamamoto I (2005) Behavioral and histological evaluation of a focal cerebral infarction rat model transplanted with neurons induced from bone marrow stromal cells. J Neuropathol Exp Neurol 64: 1108–1117.
7. Bliss T, Guzman R, Daadi M, Steinberg GK (2007) Cell transplantation therapy for stroke. Stroke 38: 817–826.
8. Williams BA, Keating A (2008) Cell therapy for age-related disorders: myocardial infarction and stroke—a mini-review. Gerontology 54: 300–311.
9. Pittenger MF, Martin BJ (2004) Mesenchymal stem cells and their potential as cardiac therapeutics. Circ Res 95: 9–20.
10. Walczak P, Zhang J, Gilad AA, Kedziorek DA, Ruiz-Cabello J, et al. (2008) Dual-modality monitoring of targeted intraarterial delivery of mesenchymal stem cells after transient ischemia. Stroke 39: 1569–1574.
11. Uccelli A, Moretta L, Pistoia V (2006) Immunoregulatory function of mesenchymal stem cells. Eur J Immunol 36: 2566–2573.
12. Bhatia R, Hare JM (2005) Mesenchymal stem cells: future source for reparative medicine. Congest Heart Fail 11: 87–91; quiz 92–83.
13. Williams AR, Hare JM (2011) Mesenchymal stem cells: biology, pathophysiology, translational findings, and therapeutic implications for cardiac disease. Circ Res 109: 923–940.
14. Liu X, Ye R, Yan T, Yu SP, Wei L, et al. (2013) Cell based therapies for ischemic stroke: From basic science to bedside. Prog Neurobiol pii: S03010082(13)00131–7.
15. Chen J, Li Y, Wang L, Lu M, Zhang X, et al. (2001) Therapeutic benefit of intracerebral transplantation of bone marrow stromal cells after cerebral ischemia in rats. J Neurol Sci 189: 49–57.
16. Blum A, Balkan W, Hare JM (2012) Advances in cell-based therapy for peripheral vascular disease. Atherosclerosis 223: 269–277.
17. Ikeda N, Nonoguchi N, Zhao MZ, Watanabe T, Kajimoto Y, et al. (2005) Bone marrow stromal cells that enhanced fibroblast growth factor-2 secretion by herpes simplex virus vector improve neurological outcome after transient focal cerebral ischemia in rats. Stroke 36: 2725–2730.
18. Li Y, Chen J, Wang L, Lu M, Chopp M (2001) Treatment of stroke in rat with intracarotid administration of marrow stromal cells. Neurology 56: 1666–1672.
19. Zhang L, Li Y, Romanko M, Kramer BC, Gosiewska A, et al. (2012) Different routes of administration of human umbilical tissue-derived cells improve functional recovery in the rat after focal cerebral ischemia. Brain Res 1489: 104–112.
20. Cloft HJ, Rabinstein A, Lanzino G, Kallmes DF (2009) Intra-arterial stroke therapy: an assessment of demand and available work force. AJNR Am J Neuroradiol 30: 453–458.
21. Li L, Jiang Q, Ding G, Zhang L, Zhang ZG, et al. (2010) Effects of administration route on migration and distribution of neural progenitor cells transplanted into rats with focal cerebral ischemia, an MRI study. J Cereb Blood Flow Metab 30: 653–662.
22. Fischer UM, Harting MT, Jimenez F, Monzon-Posadas WO, Xue H, et al. (2009) Pulmonary passage is a major obstacle for intravenous stem cell delivery: the pulmonary first-pass effect. Stem Cells Dev 18: 683–692.
23. Kamiya N, Ueda M, Igarashi H, Nishiyama Y, Suda S, et al. (2008) Intra-arterial transplantation of bone marrow mononuclear cells immediately after reperfusion decreases brain injury after focal ischemia in rats. Life Sci 83: 433–437.
24. Busto R, Dietrich WD, Globus MY, Valdes I, Scheinberg P, et al. (1987) Small differences in intraischemic brain temperature critically determine the extent of ischemic neuronal injury. J Cereb Blood Flow Metab 7: 729–738.
25. Longa EZ, Weinstein PR, Carlson S, Cummins R (1989) Reversible middle cerebral artery occlusion without craniectomy in rats. Stroke 20: 84–91.
26. Lin B, Ginsberg MD (2000) Quantitative assessment of the normal cerebral microvasculature by endothelial barrier antigen (EBA) immunohistochemistry: application to focal cerebral ischemia. Brain Res 865: 237–244.
27. Ley JJ, Vigdorchik A, Belayev L, Zhao W, Busto R, et al. (2005) Stilbazulenyl nitrone, a second-generation azulenyl nitrone antioxidant, confers enduring neuroprotection in experimental focal cerebral ischemia in the rat: neurobehavior, histopathology, and pharmacokinetics. J Pharmacol Exp Ther 313: 1090–1100.
28. Belayev L, Busto R, Zhao W, Fernandez G, Ginsberg MD (1999) Middle cerebral artery occlusion in the mouse by intraluminal suture coated with poly-L-lysine: neurological and histological validation. Brain Res 833: 181–190.
29. Woitzik J, Schilling L (2007) A new method for superselective middle cerebral artery infusion in the rat. J Neurosurg 106: 872–878.
30. Friedrich MA, Martins MP, Araujo MD, Klamt C, Vedolin L, et al. (2011) Intra-Arterial Infusion of Autologous Bone-Marrow Mononuclear Cells in Patients with Moderate to Severe Middle-Cerebral-Artery Acute Ischemic Stroke. Cell Transplant 21 Suppl 1:S13–21.
31. Strauer BE, Brehm M, Zeus T, Kostering M, Hernandez A, et al. (2002) Repair of infarcted myocardium by autologous intracoronary mononuclear bone marrow cell transplantation in humans. Circulation 106: 1913–1918.
32. Assmus B, Schachinger V, Teupe C, Britten M, Lehmann R, et al. (2002) Transplantation of Progenitor Cells and Regeneration Enhancement in Acute Myocardial Infarction (TOPCARE-AMI). Circulation 106: 3009–3017.
33. Janowski M, Lyczek A, Engels C, Xu J, Lukomska B, et al. (2013) Cell size and velocity of injection are major determinants of the safety of intracarotid stem cell transplantation. J Cereb Blood Flow Metab 33: 921–927.
34. Guzman R, De Los Angeles A, Cheshier S, Choi R, Hoang S, et al. (2008) Intracarotid injection of fluorescence activated cell-sorted CD49d-positive neural stem cells improves targeted cell delivery and behavior after stroke in a mouse stroke model. Stroke 39: 1300–1306.
35. Brenneman M, Sharma S, Harting M, Strong R, Cox CS, Jr., et al. (2010) Autologous bone marrow mononuclear cells enhance recovery after acute ischemic stroke in young and middle-aged rats. J Cereb Blood Flow Metab 30: 140–149.
36. Pendharkar AV, Chua JY, Andres RH, Wang N, Gaeta X, et al. (2010) Biodistribution of neural stem cells after intravascular therapy for hypoxic-ischemia. Stroke 41: 2064–2070.

37. Pluchino S, Zanotti L, Rossi B, Brambilla E, Ottoboni L, et al. (2005) Neurosphere-derived multipotent precursors promote neuroprotection by an immunomodulatory mechanism. Nature 436: 266–271.
38. Rosenblum S, Wang N, Smith TN, Pendharkar AV, Chua JY, et al. (2012) Timing of intra-arterial neural stem cell transplantation after hypoxia-ischemia influences cell engraftment, survival, and differentiation. Stroke 43: 1624–1631.
39. Minnerup J, Seeger FH, Kuhnert K, Diederich K, Schilling M, et al. (2010) Intracarotid administration of human bone marrow mononuclear cells in rat photothrombotic ischemia. Exp Transl Stroke Med 2: 3.
40. Raval AP, Saul I, Dave KR, DeFazio RA, Perez-Pinzon MA, et al. (2009) Pretreatment with a single estradiol-17beta bolus activates cyclic-AMP response element binding protein and protects CA1 neurons against global cerebral ischemia. Neuroscience 160: 307–318.

8

Targeted Delivery of Erythropoietin by Transcranial Focused Ultrasound for Neuroprotection against Ischemia/Reperfusion-Induced Neuronal Injury: A Long-Term and Short-Term Study

Sheng-Kai Wu[1], Ming-Tao Yang[2,4], Kai-Hsiang Kang[2], Houng-Chi Liou[2], Dai-Hua Lu[2], Wen-Mei Fu[2]*, Win-Li Lin[1,3]*

1 Institute of Biomedical Engineering, College of Medicine and College of Engineering, National Taiwan University, Taipei, Taiwan, **2** Institute of Pharmacology, College of Medicine, National Taiwan University, Taipei, Taiwan, **3** Division of Medical Engineering Research, National Health Research Institutes, Miaoli, Taiwan, **4** Department of Pediatrics, Far Eastern Memorial Hospital, New Taipei City, Taiwan

Abstract

Erythropoietin (EPO) is a neuroprotective agent against cerebral ischemia/reperfusion (I/R)-induced brain injury. However, its crossing of blood-brain barrier is limited. Focused ultrasound (FUS) sonication with microbubbles (MBs) can effectively open blood-brain barrier to boost the vascular permeability. In this study, we investigated the effects of MBs/FUS on extending the therapeutic time window of EPO and its neuroprotective effects in both acute and chronic phases. Male Wistar rats were firstly subjected to two common carotid arteries and right middle cerebral artery occlusion (three vessels occlusion, 3VO) for 50 min, and then the rats were treated with hEPO (human recombinant EPO, 5000 IU/kg) with or without MBs/FUS at 5 h after occlusion/reperfusion. Acute phase investigation (I/R, I/R+MBs/FUS, I/R+hEPO, and I/R+hEPO+MBs/FUS) was performed 24 h after I/R; chronic tests including cylinder test and gait analysis were performed one month after I/R. The experimental results showed that MBs/FUS significantly increased the cerebral content of EPO by bettering vascular permeability. In acute phase, both significant improvement of neurological score and reduction of infarct volume were found in the I/R+hEPO+MBs/FUS group, as compared with I/R and I/R+hEPO groups. In chronic phase, long-term behavioral recovery and neuronal loss in brain cortex after I/R injury was significantly improved in the I/R+hEPO+MBs/FUS group. This study indicates that hEPO administration with MBs/FUS sonication even at 5 h after occlusion/reperfusion can produce a significant neuroprotection.

Editor: Vardan Karamyan, School of Pharmacy, Texas Tech University HSC, United States of America

Funding: This work was supported by research grants from the National Science Council of Taiwan (NSC 99-2221-E-002-005-MY3) and National Health Research Institutes of Taiwan (NHRI ME-100-PP-13). The funders had no role in study design, data collection and analysis, decision to publish, or preparation of the manuscript.

Competing Interests: The authors have declared that no competing interests exist.

* E-mail: winli@ntu.edu.tw (WL); wenmei@ntu.edu.tw (WF)

Introduction

The American Stroke Association [1] estimates that stroke accounts for 1 out of every 18 deaths and occurs every 40 seconds in the United States. In the 2012 update, the majority of strokes were ischemic (87%); 10% were intracerebral hemorrhage; 3% were due to subarachnoid hemorrhage. Ischemic stroke results from the occlusion of a cerebral artery, leading to a blocked cerebral blood flow to certain part of the brain. Two emergent clinical therapies for acute ischemic stroke are: reperfusion of the blood flow and neuroprotection of the injured brain cells. Early reperfusion within 3 h is beneficial to improve the outcome of acute human ischemic stroke. However, late recovery of circulation might cause reperfusion injury, resulting in blood-brain barrier (BBB) breakdown, or brain edema [2].

Although many animal stroke models have been developed, no single model can fully mimic clinical human stroke because of its heterogeneity. The transient three vessels occlusion (3VO, two common carotid arteries and middle cerebral artery) method provides a model for the study of ischemia-reperfusion injury [3]. This method can build a stable focal infarction in the brain. In addition, reperfusion is performed easily by untying the suture without plasminogen activator (t-PA) injection, and the effect of neuroprotection can be directly reflected in this animal model.

It has been recently reported that focused ultrasound (FUS) with microbubbles (MBs), which are ultrasound contrast agents in clinical use, can disrupt the local BBB for providing trans-vascular delivery of macromolecules [4,5]. The mechanism of MBs/FUS-induced vascular permeability change may be caused by the opening of tight junction [6]. This disruption of BBB is transient and reversible within several hours [5,7]. In recent study, MBs/FUS has been used to facilitate the delivery of liposomal doxorubicin into normal animal brains by opening the BBB[8]. The benefits of this delivery method have been demonstrated in animal models with brain tumors [9–11] and Alzheimer's disease [12,13]. Although MBs/FUS may damage the brain parenchyma,

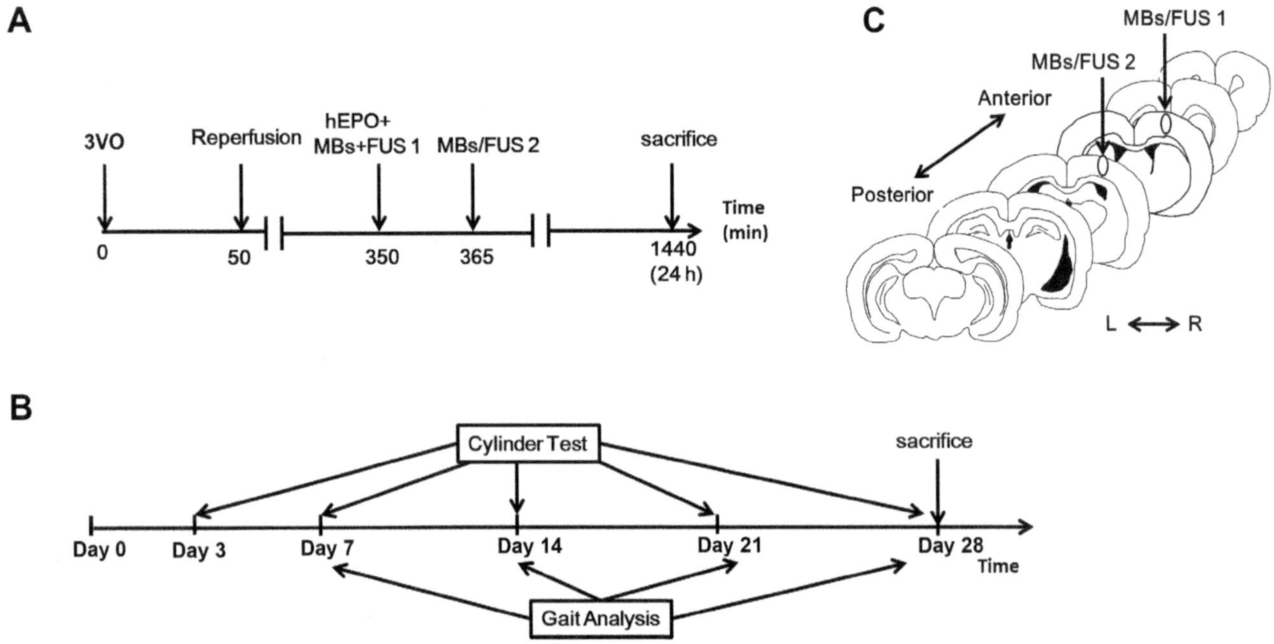

Figure 1. Experimental procedures. (A) For the hEPO+MBs/FUS group in the acute phase study, hEPO (i.v. injection) and first MBs/FUS were applied approximately 5 h after a 50-min 3VO. A second MBs/FUS was given 15 min later. Animals were sacrificed 24 h after 3VO. (B) In the chronic study, experimental groups were tested for motor deficits with gait analysis and cylinder test at indicated time points. Animals were sacrificed on Day 28. (C) Coronal brain section showed the cortex locations with a 2-mm interval for the two MBs/FUS application.

a safe sonication can be achieved by regulating ultrasound sonication and the dosage of MBs [4,14].

Erythropoietin (EPO) is a secreted glycoprotein produced primarily by the kidney and is used clinically to treat anemia [15,16]. EPO is induced by hypoxia within the central nervous system. It has been reported that EPO is a promising acute therapeutic agent for cerebral ischemia in animal studies [17]. The protective mechanisms may include the activation of endogenous survival pathways that inhibit apoptosis and further reduce inflammatory responses [18,19]. Systemic administration of EPO after induction of focal cerebral ischemia has been demonstrated to exert a potential neuroprotective effect on the outcome of stroke; however, there is a limited therapeutic time window. The best application time is up to 3 h after ischemia with a leaky BBB [20].

The aim of this study is to investigate the feasibility of utilizing FUS with MBs to deliver hEPO to ischemia/reperfusion injured rat brains beyond the conventional therapeutic time window and to examine the efficacy of this treatment in both acute and chronic phases.

Materials and Methods

All the experimental protocols were approved by Institutional Animal Care and Use Committees of Medical College, National Taiwan University.

Three Vessels Occlusion (3VO) Model

Male Wistar rats (230 to 250 g) were used in this study. The available data suggest that the 3VO model provides more consistent cortical injury compared to the MCAO model [21]. In this study, we employed the 3VO model to form a focal cortical infarction, and this kind of infarction is more suitable for the evaluation of the BBB opening with microbubbles/focused ultrasound (MBs/FUS). Temporary focal ischemia were based on the model described by Chen et al [22]. The rats were anesthetized by exposure to 1 to 3% isoflurane, and two common carotid arteries (CCAs) were occluded by artery clips. A burr hole was drilled at the anterior junction of the zygoma and the squamosal bone, and the exposed middle cerebral artery (MCA) was tied with a 10-0 suture. The above procedures were conducted within 10 to 15 minutes. Rectal temperature was maintained at $37\pm0.5°C$. After an occlusion of 50 min, the suture was untied and the reflow of the right MCA and two CCAs was confirmed under a microscope.

Experimental Grouping

The experiments in this study include three parts: hEPO quantification in brain tissues, acute response and chronic response following ischemia/reperfusion (I/R). First, to quantify the amount of hEPO entering the sonicated brain, normal rats were divided into two groups: received hEPO (CBC #329871, Merck KGaA, Darmstadt, Germany) (5000 IU/kg, i.v. injection) only or hEPO plus MBs/FUS. The procedure was shown in Fig. 1A. Second, to examine the neuroprotective effect of the execution of hEPO and MBs/FUS on I/R, rats were randomly divided into four groups. Group A (denoted as I/R (Control)): rats received a 50-min 3VO. Group B (I/R+MBs/FUS): a 50-min 3VO, and then received twice MBs/FUS at 5 h after reperfusion. Group C (I/R+hEPO): a 50-min 3VO, and then received hEPO alone at 5 h after reperfusion. Group D (I/R+hEPO+MBs/FUS): a 50-min 3VO, and then received hEPO plus MBs/FUS at 5 h after reperfusion. The flowchart was displayed in Fig. 1B. Third, to evaluate the chronic response, rats were randomly divided into four groups: Group A (denoted as sham control), Group B (I/R), Group C (I/R+hEPO), and Group D (I/R+hEPO+MBs/FUS). The investigation of long-term response included: cylinder test and automated gait analysis. The time courses were shown in Fig. 1C.

Focused Ultrasound (FUS) Sonication

A 480 KHz FUS transducer with a diameter of 10 cm, 10 cm radius of curvature was used. The acoustic beam was transmitted to the brain directly by a removable cone replete with degassed water. The FUS was precisely targeted using a stereotaxic apparatus (Stoelting, Wood Dale, IL) and the center of the focal spot was about 1 mm below the cone tip. The FUS transducer was driven by a power amplifier (500-012, Advanced Surgical Systems, Tucson, AZ) connected to a function generator (33220A, Agilent, Palo Alto, CA). The rats were laid prone beneath the cone tip, and ultrasound transmission gel (Pharmaceutical Innovations, Newark, NJ) was used to maximize the transmission of ultrasound to the brain. The focal zone is 3 mm and 13 mm in diameter and length, respectively. Pulsed sonication was applied with a peak negative pressure of 0.57 MPa, a burst length of 10 ms, a duty cycle of 1%, and a repetition frequency of 1 Hz. The duration of each sonication was 20 s. MBs (microbubbles) (SonoVue, Bracco, Amsterdam, The Netherlands) was injected as a bolus (10 μl/kg) about 15 s before each sonication. The FUS was delivered at two locations with 2 mm apart in the right hemisphere cortex: 4 mm lateral to the bregma and 1 mm or 3 mm posterior to the bregma, respectively, and both 1 mm below the skull surface (Fig. 1C).

Quantification of hEPO Entering the Brain Tissue

CSF sample was obtained at 3 h after the execution of hEPO+MBs/FUS or hEPO alone. The rats were then perfused with saline and decapitated, and the brain was removed and sliced into six coronal sections. The sonicated region of each section was dissected and the quantity of hEPO in the sonicated brain tissue was measured by ELISA method using Quantikine human erythropoietin kit (R&D Systems, Minneapolis, MN), which did not cross-react with rat EPO

Infarct Volume and Residual Brain Volume Evaluation

The infarct volume was analyzed 24 h after ischemia. Six consecutive coronal sections with 2 mm thick each were sliced from the frontal tip with the aid of a rat brain matrix and immersed in a 2% solution of 2,3,5-triphenyltetrazolium chloride (TTC). The stained brain sections were then fixed by immersion in phosphate-buffer containing 4% paraformaldehyde. Section images were analyzed with ImageJ (National Institutes of Health, Bethesda, MD) to calculate the infarct volume. The residual brain volume was analyzed one month after I/R. The brains were removed and sliced into six consecutive coronal sections with 2 mm thick. Section images were analyzed with ImageJ to calculate the residual brain volume.

Behavioral Evaluation

The neurological status of the rats was evaluated 24 h after ischemia. Neurological score was based on Menzies behavioral function [23]. Score from 0 to 4 represents the extent of damage from normality to severity. Score 0: rats can extend both forelimbs; score 1: the contralateral forelimb is consistently flexed during suspension; score 2: decreased grip of the contralateral forelimb when pulled by the tail; score 3: rats show a mono-directional circling at a slight jerk of the tail; and score 4: a consistent circling occurs. One author (H.-C. Liou) blind to the treatment condition performed the neurological evaluation. To quantify the asymmetric forelimb use for the stroke animals, the cylinder test was performed on Day-3, Day-7, Day-14, Day-21, and Day-28 after I/R. The animals were placed in a 20-cm-diameter cylinder with transparent glass and at least 25 contacts of the forelimbs on the wall of the cylinder were recorded for each rat[24]. The contact percentage of impaired forelimb was expressed as contacts of impaired forelimb divided by total contacts. The theoretical value was 50% for the sham group. Animals were subjected to gait measurement every week for one month after I/R utilizing CatWalk-automated gait analysis system (Noldus Information Technology, Wageningen, The Netherlands)[25,26]. For gait assessment, the animals were subjected to three consecutive runs. After identifying each footprint, the images were converted into digital signals and stroke-related gait data were generated including intensity of paws (pressure) and angle of the paw axis relative to the body axis (inward angles expressed as minus; outward angles as plus).

Immunohistochemistry

Immunohistochemical staining was obtained both 24 h and 28 days after 3VO. The rats were perfused with saline and then fixed with phosphate buffer containing 4% paraformaldehyde. The brain was removed, post-fixed with 4% paraformaldehyde at 4°C overnight, and then stored in a 30% sucrose solution at 4°C for two days. Brain tissue slices (30 μm thick) were pretreated with 3% hydrogen peroxide to block endogenous peroxidase activity before incubation of primary antibody. After blocking in 4% non-fat milk containing 1% Triton X-100 for 1 h, brain tissue slices were incubated overnight at 4°C with the following primary antibody: NeuN (1:500; Millipore, Billerica, MA), CD-11b (1:500; AbD Serotec, Oxford, UK), and GFAP (1:500; Millipore, Billerica, MA) in PBS. After a brief wash, brain tissue slices were then incubated with horse anti-mouse biotinylated secondary antibodies, and processed with avidin-biotin complex system (ABC kit; Vector Laboratories, Burlingame, CA), which was visualized by incubating with 0.5% diaminobenzidine and 0.01% hydrogen peroxide in PBS. Finally, the brain tissue slices were washed in PBS and mounted on slides. Usually microglia activation reaches the peak at ~72 h after ischemia, and some reports demonstrated that microglia activation may appear as early as 24 h after ischemia [27,28]. In this study, we like to display the delivery of hEPO into the sonicated brain tissue and to see its resulting effect as early as possible, and hence we performed the difference between I/R and I/R+hEPO+MBs/FUS groups at 24 hr after ischemia. For detecting Nissl body in the cytoplasm of neurons, the brain was fixed with 4% paraformaldehyde, embedded in paraffin, and then was sectioned. The brain sections were sequentially conducted with the following steps: deparaffinized in xylene for 10 min, hydrated in 100% ethanol for 10 min, in 95% ethanol for 5 min, in 70% ethanol for 5 min, rinsed in water for 2 min, stained in a 0.1% cresyl violet solution for 20 min, and then rinsed in water. After dehydration with ethanol, sections were mounted with xylene-based mounting solution.

Statistical Analysis

Values are expressed as mean ± S.E.M. The results were analyzed with one-way ANOVA with post hoc test. Statistical significance was defined as $p<0.05$.

Results

Amount of hEPO Delivered into Brain and CSF by MBs/FUS

To study the quantity of hEPO delivered into brain, hEPO was intravenously injected first and then MBs/FUS were applied twice at a 15 min interval on the right cortex (Fig. 1D). The hEPO levels in the brain sections were measured at 3 h after hEPO injection. It was found that hEPO levels in sections 3 and 4 of the cortex were significantly higher in the hEPO+MBs/FUS group ($n = 3$) than in

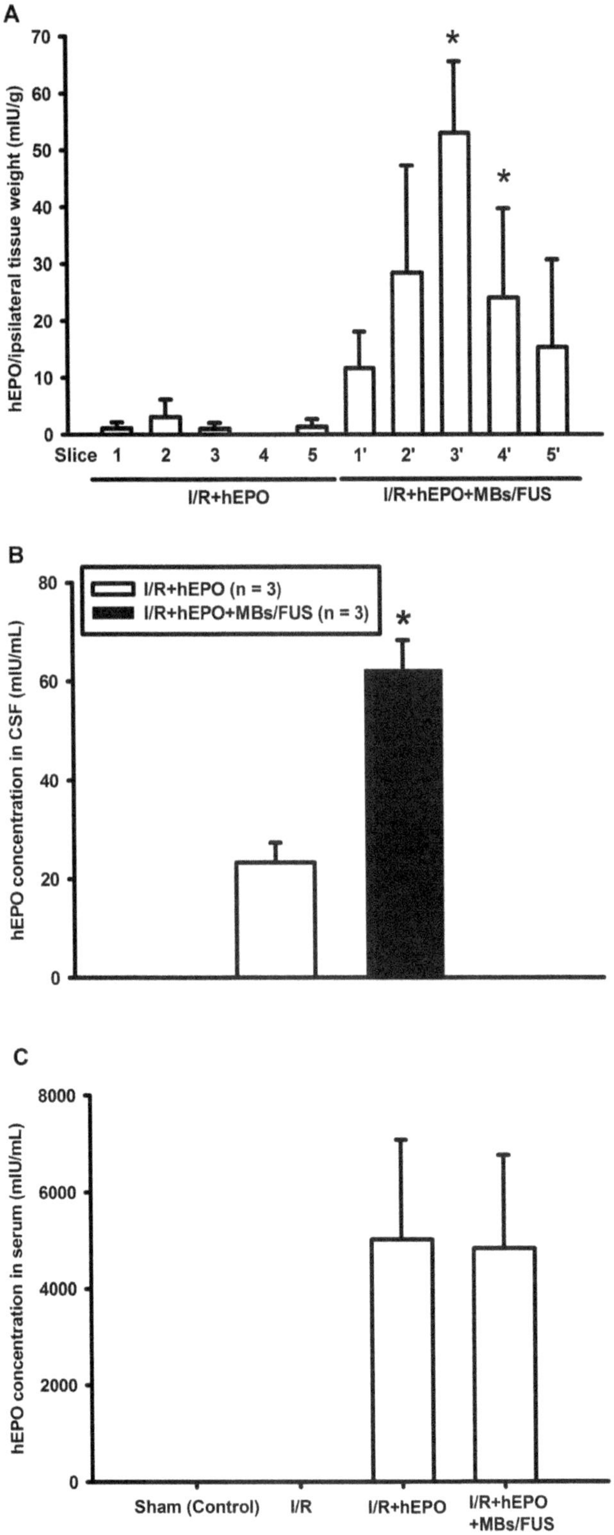

Figure 2. Enhancement of hEPO delivery into the brain tissues by MBs/FUS. hEPO and MBs were intravenously administered and FUS was transcranially applied. (A) Rat brains were perfused and sliced into sections at 3 h after hEPO injection. Sonicated region of the brain was dissected and quantified. The hEPO levels in sections 3 and 4 were significantly higher in the I/R+hEPO+MBs/FUS group compared to the I/R+hEPO group (n = 3 for each). Data were given as means ± S.E.M., * $p<0.05$, as compared with the I/R+hEPO group. (B) CSF was sampled at 3 h after hEPO injection. The hEPO concentration of CSF in the I/R+hEPO+MBs/FUS group showed significant enhancement compared with the I/R+hEPO group. (C) The serum hEPO was also sampled at 3 h after hEPO injection. No hEPO was found in the sham and I/R groups without hEPO injection.

the hEPO group (n = 3) (Fig. 2A). These results indicate that sonication with microbubbles increased the entry of hEPO through the BBB. The hEPO concentration of CSF in the I/R+hEPO+MBs/FUS group showed a significant enhancement compared with the I/R+hEPO group (Fig. 2B). The serum hEPO was also sampled at 3 h after hEPO injection, and the results showed that both groups had quite high levels of hEPO. No hEPO was found in both the sham and I/R groups indicated that hEPO ELISA kit did not cross-react with rat EPO.

Reduction of Infarct Volume by hEPO+MBs/FUS

Rats were induced cerebral infarct by 3VO for 50 min, followed by reperfusion. The infarction was demonstrated by TTC staining with white color in infarct area and red color in non-infarct area (Fig. 3A). The ratio of infarct volume was presented as percentage of contralateral side of cortex. The infarct region was 59.5±6.62% (n = 7), 66.16±7.05% (n = 6), 58.62±2.93% (n = 5), and 26.87±4.92% (n = 5) in the I/R, I/R+MBs/FUS, I/R+hEPO, and I/R+hEPO+MBs/FUS groups, respectively. The I/R+hEPO+MBs/FUS group displayed a significant reduction of infarct volume, as compared with the I/R and I/R+hEPO groups ($p<0.05$, Fig. 3B). No significant difference was observed among the I/R, I/R+MBs/FUS, and I/R+hEPO groups. These results indicate that the enhancement of hEPO entry into ischemic area by MBs/FUS exerted neuroprotection against I/R-induced neuronal injury.

Improvement of Neurological Behavior

The neurological scores were evaluated at 24 h after brain I/R. It was found that treatment with hEPO+MBs/FUS significantly improved neurological function ($p<0.05$, Fig. 3C), while treatment with hEPO or MBs/FUS individually did not show any significant difference as compared with the I/R group.

Neuroprotective Effect of hEPO+MBs/FUS

All the brain slice samples for immunohistochemical staining were obtained 24 h after 3VO and the representative slices were shown in Fig. 4. The neuronal nuclear (NeuN) staining was used to recognize neuronal nuclei in the brain. Fig. 4E showed the marked reduction of neuronal nuclei in the I/R group. On the contrary, the sham and the I/R+hEPO+MBs/FUS group displayed an intact presence of neuronal nuclei (Fig. 4, B and H). It has been reported that microglia activation occurs following neuronal death. Neuroinflammation was thus evaluated by immunohistochemical staining for CD-11b. CD-11b positive cells with large cell bodies were observed throughout the I/R group (Fig. 4F). In contrast, the I/R+hEPO+MBs/FUS group showed more homogenous distribution of cells with long fine processes extending from small cell bodies (Fig. 4I). Glial fibrillary acidic protein (GFAP) recognized astrocytes which were also activated in stroke. Fig. 3G showed that the expression of GFAP was increased in the I/R group, whereas the astroglia activation was less in the I/R+hEPO+MBs/FUS group (Fig. 4J).

Increase of Residual Brain Volume by hEPO+MBs/FUS in Chronic Phase

To further study the effect of hEPO+MBs/FUS against the I/R-induced brain injury, we examined whether this treatment exerted a long-term protection. After I/R operation, the cortex volume of rat brain may gradually shrink as time goes by. Representative Nissl staining showed a drastic loss of cortex tissue in the I/R, I/R+hEPO, and I/R+MBs/FUS groups, whereas the group treated with hEPO+MBs/FUS displayed a rather intact cortex (Fig. 5A). The residual brain volume was presented as the percentage of contralateral side of cortex, and the value was 99.67±0.18% (n = 5), 60.62±5.53% (n = 5), 59.01±9.03% (n = 5), 64.41±4.29% (n = 5) and 85.97±5.85% (n = 5) for the sham, I/R, I/R+hEPO, I/R+MBs/FUS, and I/R+hEPO+MBs/FUS groups, respectively. The I/R+hEPO+MBs/FUS group displayed a significant increase of residual brain volume as compared with the I/R, I/R+hEPO, and I/R+MBs/FUS groups ($p<0.05$, Fig. 5B).

Improvement of Asymmetric Limb-Use and Recovery of Gait Deficits by hEPO+MBs/FUS in Chronic Phase

One month after 3VO, the behavioral tests were performed to examine the deficit of limb and there were no animals dead due to the 3VO surgery. A general linear model (GLM) with repeated measure procedure and Greenhouse-Geisser correction was used and the results showed that usage of the contralateral forepaw differed significantly among the treatment groups (F(3, 16)

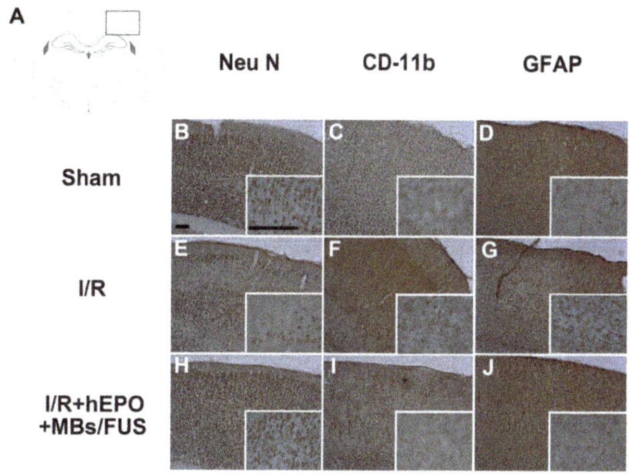

Figure 4. hEPO+MBs/FUS inhibits the ischemia/reperfusion-induced neuronal death and inflammation in rat experiments. Immunohistochemical staining of NeuN, CD-11b, and GFAP was performed 24 h after I/R. (A) illustrated the position of FUS sonication. In NeuN staining (B, E, and H), the I/R group showed a marked loss of neurons, whereas, neurons were intact in the sham and I/R+hEPO+MBs/FUS groups. In CD-11b staining (C, F, and I), the I/R group showed microglia activation (condensed nuclei), whereas the sham and I/R+hEPO+MBs/FUS groups showed ramified microglia. In GFAP staining (D, G, and J), there was an increase of GFAP in the I/R group but not in the sham and I/R+hEPO+MBs/FUS groups. (Scale bar = 200 μm).

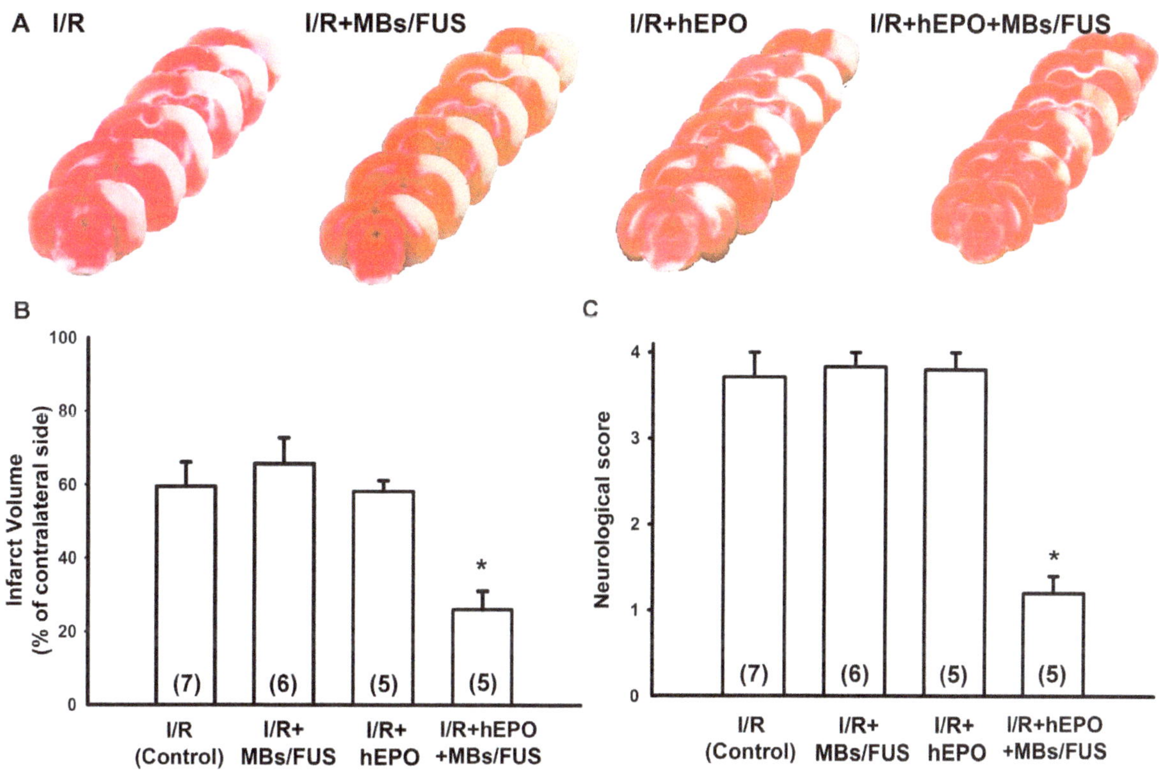

Figure 3. Reduction of brain infarct volume and neurological score by hEPO+MBs/FUS in rat experiments. (A) All rats were induced ischemia by 3VO for 50 min. The brain was removed and stained with TTC 24 h after 3VO. Representative sections of TTC-stained coronal brain showed the infarct area 24 h after 3VO for the I/R (control), I/R+MBs/FUS, I/R+hEPO, and I/R+hEPO+MBs/FUS groups. (B) Infarct volume was presented as the percentage of contralateral cortex. Note that the infarct volume was significantly reduced in the hEPO+MBs/FUS group. (C) Neurological score was performed 24 h after I/R. Note that hEPO combined with MBs/FUS significantly reduced the neurological scores. Data were presented as mean ± SEM, * $p<0.05$ as compared with the control group.

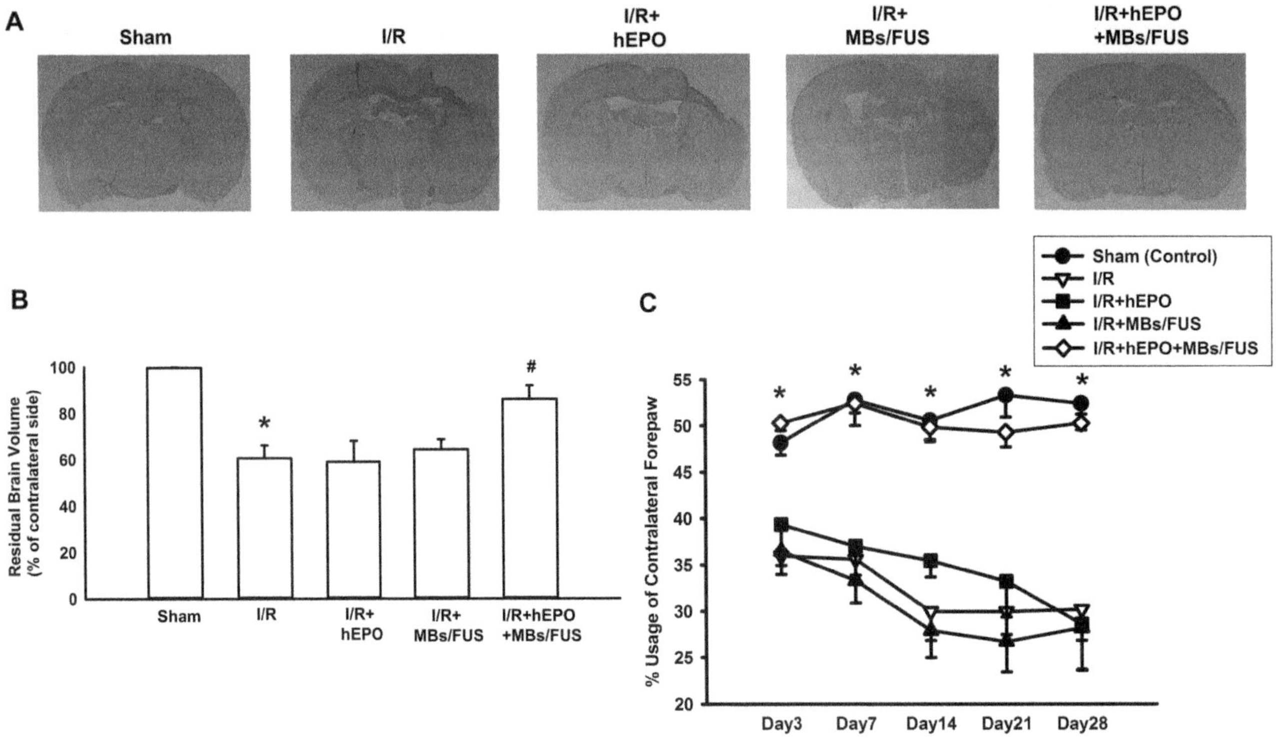

Figure 5. Increase of residual brain volume and improvement of limb-use in chronic phase of 3VO by hEPO+MBs/FUS. (A) Representative Nissl staining showed the residual neurons 28 days after I/R. (Scale bar = 5 mm) (B) Residual brain volume was presented as the percentage of contralateral cortex. 28 days after I/R, residual brain volume was reduced markedly, while it was antagonized by I/R+hEPO+MBs/FUS. (C) The cylinder test was used to evaluate the rat behavior after brain injury. The I/R group showed a deficit in the usage of the left forepaw from Day-3 to Day-28, while it was reversed by hEPO+MBs/FUS. The average percentage of paw usage in normal rats was 50%. Data were presented as mean ± SEM (n = 5 for each group), * $p<0.05$ as compared with sham control group, # $p<0.05$ as compared with the I/R group.

= 23.602, $p<0.001$). Post hoc tests using the Tukey's HSD precedure revealed that the usage of the contralateral forepaws in the IR+hEPO+MBs/FUS group was significantly reduced when compared with the I/R group (Fig. 5C, $p<0.05$). The differences between the I/R+hEPO+MBs/FUS group and the I/R group during all the examining days were statistically significant (Dunnet's test, $p<0.05$ for all). Dynamic gait information was also assessed via an automated gait analysis system. In the paw-intensity measurement, the intensity of the left forepaw in the I/R group was significantly decreased from Day-7 to Day-28 as compared with the sham group (Fig. 6A), while in the I/R+hEPO+MBs/FUS group, the paw intensity significantly recovered from Day-14 to Day-28 ($p<0.05$). The measurement of the left-paw angle indicated that the left-paw axis was more inward in the I/R group than in the sham group ($p<0.05$, Fig. 6B). Treatment with hEPO+MBs/FUS had a significant recovery in the long-term response.

Discussion

Drug treatment for brain diseases is usually hampered by the BBB, which prevents the therapeutic agents from entering the target brain tissues. Cerebral ischemia can induce BBB disruption and permit macromolecular drug to transport into the infarcted brain tissues. However, the therapeutic time window is short, and beyond this window, the efficacy of treatment is limited due to inability to achieve a sufficiently high dose of drug in the infarcted region[29]. In this study, we employed MBs/FUS to transiently open the BBB to extend the hEPO treatment for the I/R brain injury beyond the conventional therapeutic time window. We investigated the amount of hEPO delivered into the sonicated brain tissues and the effectiveness in neuroprotection.

Focused ultrasound sonication with microbubbles could effectively boost the vascular permeability and then extend the therapeutic time window of EPO as well as its neuroprotective effects in both acute and chronic phases after I/R injury. In the acute phase, the total sonication volume was smaller than the size of infarction and hence the enhancement of hEPO delivery was only beneficial to part of the infarcted brain. As shown in Fig. 2A, the concentrations of hEPO in sections 3 and 4 (the sonicated region) were significantly higher, and the TTC staining showed that the infarct volume was reduced over 50% as compared with the control or I/R+hEPO groups (Fig. 3B). Furthermore, in the chronic phase, both limb-use asymmetry and dynamic gait test for the evaluation of the chronic behavioral recovery showed that there was a significant improvement for the hEPO+MBs/FUS treatment. The chronic loss of brain cortex was reduced by the hEPO+MBs/FUS treatment (Fig. 5A). These results indicated that MBs/FUS enhanced the hEPO entry even 5 h after I/R, which resulted in neuron protection in both acute and chronic phases. Although stroke itself might alter hEPO delivery, the amount of hEPO entering the infarction area did not produce significant therapeutic effect. As hEPO combined with MBs/FUS, it can result in a significant neuroprotection on both acute and chronic phases.

It has been demonstrated that intracerebraventricular administration of hEPO inhibits the I/R-induced brain injury [30–32]. However, direct injection of hEPO into the brain is not a practical

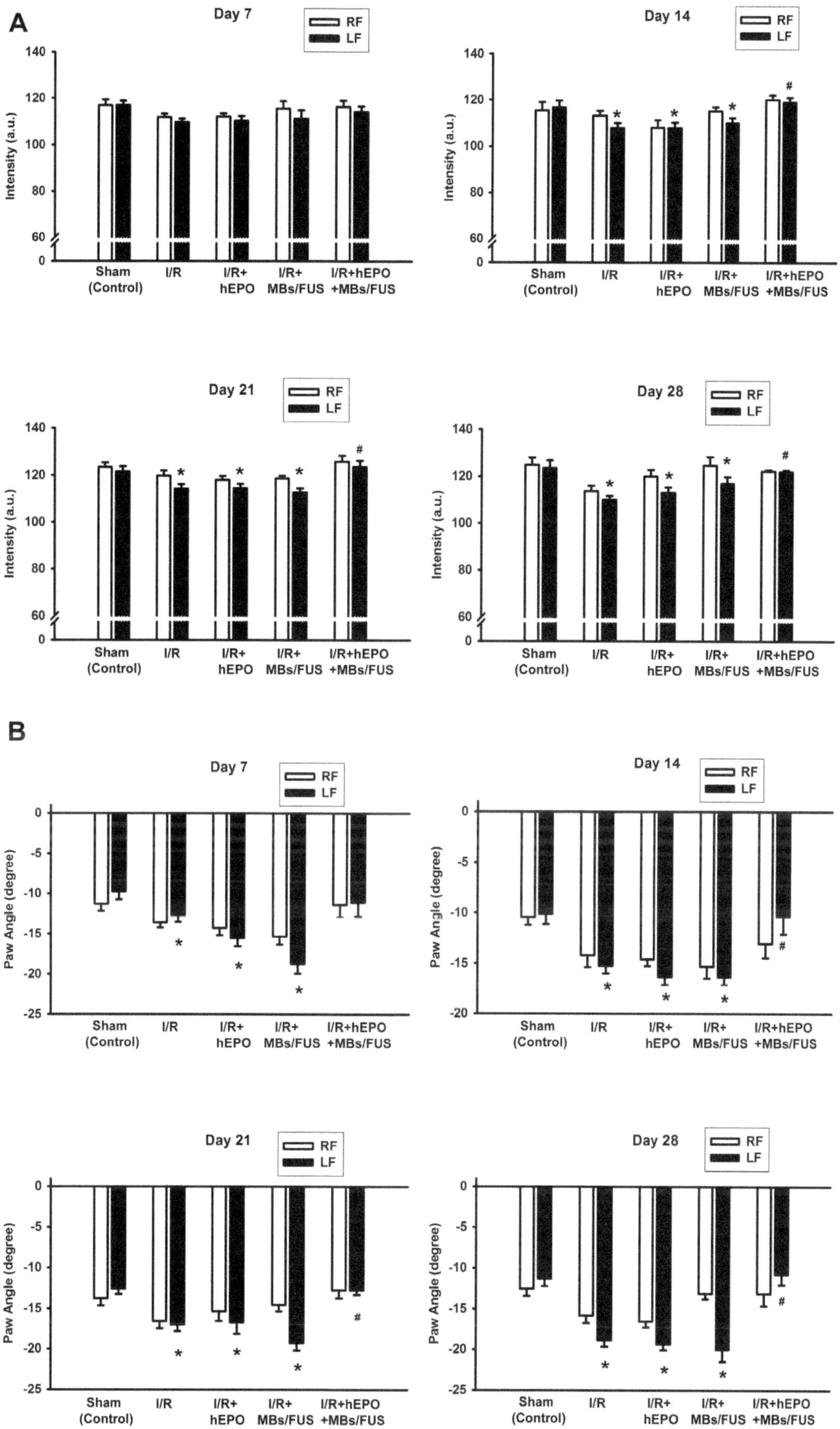
A
Day 7
RF
LF
Intensity (a.u.)
Sham (Control)
I/R
I/R+ hEPO
I/R+ MBs/FUS
I/R+hEPO +MBs/FUS
Day 14
Day 21
Day 28
B
Paw Angle (degree)

Figure 6. Improvement in catwalk automated gait analysis test by hEPO plus MBs/FUS in chronic phase of 3VO. Two gait analysis parameters, paw intensity (A) and paw angle (B), were assessed from Day-7 to Day-28 after I/R. In both paw intensity and paw angle, treatment with hEPO+MBs/FUS significantly improved the performance of impaired limb. Data were shown as mean ± SEM (n = 5 for each group), * $p<0.05$ as compared with the sham (control group), # $p<0.05$ as compared with the I/R group.

approach to have an appropriate hEPO distribution in the entire infarcted region. In the meanwhile, this kind of interstitial method can result in severe hemorrhages and brain trauma. On the contrary, systemic delivery of hEPO can have a much more uniform distribution of hEPO in the infarcted volume but may be limited by the therapeutic time window. In this study, transcranial, noninvasive FUS technology was demonstrated to be a useful modality to transiently open the localized BBB for the targeted delivery of neuroprotectant to treat the ischemic stroke-induced brain injury beyond the conventional therapeutic time window.

Brines et al. reported that animals receiving hEPO ~3 h after occlusion (equal to 2 h after reperfusion) showed significant reduction of necrosis volume compared with controls [33]. Animals receiving hEPO 6 h after occlusion (equal to 5 h after reperfusion) exhibited a significant decrease in injury volume, but the effect was substantially smaller compared with animals receiving hEPO earlier. Gan et al. reported that EPO exerted significantly neuroprotective effects when administered up to 4 h after I/R in MCAO model, but the effects were significantly diminished and lost when administered 6 h after I/R [34]. In our study, we employed 3VO for 50 min and injected EPO at 5 h after reperfusion and the result showed that there was no significant neuroprotection. These might be due to different stroke models with various occlusion and ischemic duration would produce different levels of impact on the brain.

EPO-TAT administered at the onset of post-stroke reperfusion [35] showed the ability across the BBB for neuroprotection. Derivatives of EPO such as CEPO had the neuroprotection ability only within 4 h after occlusion, which is equal to 3 h after reperfusion, in a rat model of focal ischemia [36]. BBB is more permeable for these EPO derivatives within 3 h after reperfusion due to leaky vascularity. Mutant EPO exerted neuroprotective effects up to 4 h after reperfusion but gradually lose its efficacy as time went by [34]. However, the neuroprotective effects were diminished and lost when the mutant EPO was administered 6 h after reperfusion. Ischemia is an acute pathological process and cells die rapidly within first several hours after ischemia. Therefore, neuroprotective drugs must be delivered within their therapeutic window. In this study, we demonstrated that MBs/FUS had the ability to enhance EPO into the brain at 5 h after reperfusion (~6 h after the onset of occlusion). MBs/FUS can open the intact BBB and extend the therapeutic time window of EPO.

The parameters used in this study are based on our previous work [14], which is able to minimize the brain tissue damage. Ultrasound pressure would have caused the microbubbles in the acoustic beam oscillation and even cavitation during sonication [37,38]. These oscillation and cavitation may open vascular walls to enhance hEPO transport into brain tissues. However, the above phenomena may produce some small hemorrhages for the brain tissue in the focal zone, which might cause some damage. To achieve effective drug delivery and minimize this side-effect, we can control acoustic pressure, duty cycle, sonication time, MB dose, etc.

For clinical patient treatments, FUS transducers should be combined with magnetic resonance imaging (MRI) system and thus the MR imaging can be used to guide the FUS transducer to have a precision sonication and to monitor the treatment response. Recently, it has been shown the feasibility of using MRI-guided FUS with MBs to noninvasively open the localized BBB on non-human primates [39,40]. In this preliminary study, the neuroprotective agent was used only one dose and one time. It requires further scrutiny and examination for the combination of FUS sonication with multiple treatments of neuroprotectants.

MBs/FUS can transcranially and transiently open the localized BBB for the transport of macromolecular drug into the desired brain region. In this study, we utilized this modality for the localized delivery of neuroprotective agent into the infarcted brain of rats beyond the conventional therapeutic time window. The results of acute and chronic investigation show that this modality can provide an alternative treatment option to deliver neuroprotectants or drugs to the injured brain.

Author Contributions

Conceived and designed the experiments: SW WF WL. Performed the experiments: SW MY KK HL DL. Analyzed the data: SW. Contributed reagents/materials/analysis tools: SW. Wrote the paper: SW.

References

1. Roger VL, Go AS, Lloyd-Jones DM, Benjamin EJ, Berry JD, et al. (2012) Heart disease and stroke statistics—2012 update: a report from the American Heart Association. Circulation 125: e2–e220.
2. Aronowski J, Strong R, Grotta JC (1997) Reperfusion injury: demonstration of brain damage produced by reperfusion after transient focal ischemia in rats. J Cereb Blood Flow Metab 17: 1048–1056.
3. Nagasawa H, Kogure K (1989) Correlation between cerebral blood flow and histologic changes in a new rat model of middle cerebral artery occlusion. Stroke 20: 1037–1043.
4. Hynynen K, McDannold N, Sheikov NA, Jolesz FA, Vykhodtseva N (2005) Local and reversible blood-brain barrier disruption by noninvasive focused ultrasound at frequencies suitable for trans-skull sonications. Neuroimage 24: 12–20.
5. Hynynen K, McDannold N, Vykhodtseva N, Jolesz FA (2001) Noninvasive MR imaging-guided focal opening of the blood-brain barrier in rabbits. Radiology 220: 640–646.
6. Sheikov N, McDannold N, Vykhodtseva N, Jolesz F, Hynynen K (2004) Cellular mechanisms of the blood-brain barrier opening induced by ultrasound in presence of microbubbles. Ultrasound Med Biol 30: 979–989.
7. Hynynen K, McDannold N, Vykhodtseva N, Raymond S, Weissleder R, et al. (2006) Focal disruption of the blood-brain barrier due to 260-kHz ultrasound bursts: a method for molecular imaging and targeted drug delivery. J Neurosurg 105: 445–454.
8. Treat LH, McDannold N, Vykhodtseva N, Zhang Y, Tam K, et al. (2007) Targeted delivery of doxorubicin to the rat brain at therapeutic levels using MRI-guided focused ultrasound. Int J Cancer 121: 901–907.
9. Liu HL, Hua MY, Chen PY, Chu PC, Pan CH, et al. (2010) Blood-brain barrier disruption with focused ultrasound enhances delivery of chemotherapeutic drugs for glioblastoma treatment. Radiology 255: 415–425.
10. Park EJ, Zhang YZ, Vykhodtseva N, McDannold N (2012) Ultrasound-mediated blood-brain/blood-tumor barrier disruption improves outcomes with trastuzumab in a breast cancer brain metastasis model. J Control Release 163: 277–284.
11. Yang FY, Wong TT, Teng MC, Liu RS, Lu M, et al. (2012) Focused ultrasound and interleukin-4 receptor-targeted liposomal doxorubicin for enhanced targeted drug delivery and antitumor effect in glioblastoma multiforme. J Control Release 160: 652–658.
12. Raymond SB, Treat LH, Dewey JD, McDannold NJ, Hynynen K, et al. (2008) Ultrasound enhanced delivery of molecular imaging and therapeutic agents in Alzheimer's disease mouse models. PLoS One 3: e2175.
13. Jordao JF, Ayala-Grosso CA, Markham K, Huang Y, Chopra R, et al. (2010) Antibodies targeted to the brain with image-guided focused ultrasound reduces

amyloid-beta plaque load in the TgCRND8 mouse model of Alzheimer's disease. PLoS One 5: e10549.

14. Weng JC, Wu SK, Lin WL, Tseng WY (2011) Detecting blood-brain barrier disruption within minimal hemorrhage following transcranial focused ultrasound: a correlation study with contrast-enhanced MRI. Magn Reson Med 65: 802–811.
15. Nagao M, Suga H, Okano M, Masuda S, Narita H, et al. (1992) Nucleotide sequence of rat erythropoietin. Biochim Biophys Acta 1171: 99–102.
16. Wen D, Boissel JP, Tracy TE, Gruninger RH, Mulcahy LS, et al. (1993) Erythropoietin structure-function relationships: high degree of sequence homology among mammals. Blood 82: 1507–1516.
17. Siren AL, Fratelli M, Brines M, Goemans C, Casagrande S, et al. (2001) Erythropoietin prevents neuronal apoptosis after cerebral ischemia and metabolic stress. Proc Natl Acad Sci U S A 98: 4044–4049.
18. Villa P, Bigini P, Mennini T, Agnello D, Laragione T, et al. (2003) Erythropoietin selectively attenuates cytokine production and inflammation in cerebral ischemia by targeting neuronal apoptosis. J Exp Med 198: 971–975.
19. Villa P, van Beek J, Larsen AK, Gerwien J, Christensen S, et al. (2007) Reduced functional deficits, neuroinflammation, and secondary tissue damage after treatment of stroke by nonerythropoietic erythropoietin derivatives. J Cereb Blood Flow Metab 27: 552–563.
20. Ishii T, Asai T, Urakami T, Oku N (2010) Accumulation of macromolecules in brain parenchyma in acute phase of cerebral infarction/reperfusion. Brain Res 1321: 164–168.
21. Yanamoto H, Nagata I, Niitsu Y, Xue JH, Zhang Z, et al. (2003) Evaluation of MCAO stroke models in normotensive rats: standardized neocortical infarction by the 3VO technique. Exp Neurol 182: 261–274.
22. Chen ST, Hsu CY, Hogan EL, Maricq H, Balentine JD (1986) A model of focal ischemic stroke in the rat: reproducible extensive cortical infarction. Stroke 17: 738–743.
23. Menzies SA, Hoff JT, Betz AL (1992) Middle cerebral artery occlusion in rats: a neurological and pathological evaluation of a reproducible model. Neurosurgery 31: 100–106; discussion 106–107.
24. Schallert T, Fleming SM, Leasure JL, Tillerson JL, Bland ST (2000) CNS plasticity and assessment of forelimb sensorimotor outcome in unilateral rat models of stroke, cortical ablation, parkinsonism and spinal cord injury. Neuropharmacology 39: 777–787.
25. Wang Y, Bontempi B, Hong SM, Mehta K, Weinstein PR, et al. (2008) A comprehensive analysis of gait impairment after experimental stroke and the therapeutic effect of environmental enrichment in rats. J Cereb Blood Flow Metab 28: 1936–1950.
26. Vandeputte C, Taymans JM, Casteels C, Coun F, Ni Y, et al. (2010) Automated quantitative gait analysis in animal models of movement disorders. BMC Neurosci 11: 92.
27. Hamby AM, Suh SW, Kauppinen TM, Swanson RA (2007) Use of a poly(ADP-ribose) polymerase inhibitor to suppress inflammation and neuronal death after cerebral ischemia-reperfusion. Stroke 38: 632–636.
28. Morioka T, Kalehua AN, Streit WJ (1991) The microglial reaction in the rat dorsal hippocampus following transient forebrain ischemia. J Cereb Blood Flow Metab 11: 966–973.
29. Menzies SA, Betz AL, Hoff JT (1993) Contributions of ions and albumin to the formation and resolution of ischemic brain edema. J Neurosurg 78: 257–266.
30. Sadamoto Y, Igase K, Sakanaka M, Sato K, Otsuka H, et al. (1998) Erythropoietin prevents place navigation disability and cortical infarction in rats with permanent occlusion of the middle cerebral artery. Biochem Biophys Res Commun 253: 26–32.
31. Sakanaka M, Wen TC, Matsuda S, Masuda S, Morishita E, et al. (1998) In vivo evidence that erythropoietin protects neurons from ischemic damage. Proc Natl Acad Sci U S A 95: 4635–4640.
32. Bernaudin M, Marti HH, Roussel S, Divoux D, Nouvelot A, et al. (1999) A potential role for erythropoietin in focal permanent cerebral ischemia in mice. J Cereb Blood Flow Metab 19: 643–651.
33. Brines ML, Ghezzi P, Keenan S, Agnello D, de Lanerolle NC, et al. (2000) Erythropoietin crosses the blood-brain barrier to protect against experimental brain injury. Proc Natl Acad Sci U S A 97: 10526–10531.
34. Gan Y, Xing J, Jing Z, Stetler RA, Zhang F, et al. (2012) Mutant erythropoietin without erythropoietic activity is neuroprotective against ischemic brain injury. Stroke 43: 3071–3077.
35. Zhang F, Xing J, Liou AK, Wang S, Gan Y, et al. (2010) Enhanced Delivery of Erythropoietin Across the Blood-Brain Barrier for Neuroprotection against Ischemic Neuronal Injury. Transl Stroke Res 1: 113–121.
36. Leist M, Ghezzi P, Grasso G, Bianchi R, Villa P, et al. (2004) Derivatives of erythropoietin that are tissue protective but not erythropoietic. Science 305: 239–242.
37. Vykhodtseva N, McDannold N, Hynynen K (2008) Progress and problems in the application of focused ultrasound for blood-brain barrier disruption. Ultrasonics 48: 279–296.
38. McDannold N, Vykhodtseva N, Hynynen K (2006) Targeted disruption of the blood-brain barrier with focused ultrasound: association with cavitation activity. Phys Med Biol 51: 793–807.
39. Hynynen K, McDannold N, Clement G, Jolesz FA, Zadicario E, et al. (2006) Pre-clinical testing of a phased array ultrasound system for MRI-guided noninvasive surgery of the brain—a primate study. Eur J Radiol 59: 149–156.
40. Marquet F, Tung YS, Teichert T, Ferrera VP, Konofagou EE (2011) Noninvasive, transient and selective blood-brain barrier opening in non-human primates in vivo. PLoS One 6: e22598.

9

Increased Risk of Ischemic Stroke in Young Patients with Ankylosing Spondylitis: A Population-Based Longitudinal Follow-Up Study

Chia-Wei Lin[1], Ya-Ping Huang[2], Yueh-Hsia Chiu[3], Yu-Tsun Ho[1], Shin-Liang Pan[1,4]*

1 Department of Physical Medicine and Rehabilitation, National Taiwan University Hospital, Taipei, Taiwan, **2** Department of Physical Medicine and Rehabilitation, National Taiwan University Hospital Yu-Lin Branch, Yunlin, Taiwan, **3** Department and Graduate Institute of Health Care Management, Chang Gung University, Tao-Yuan, Taiwan, **4** Department of Physical Medicine and Rehabilitation, National Taiwan University College of Medicine, Taipei, Taiwan

Abstract

Background: Prospective data on the association between ischemic stroke and ankylosing spondylitis (AS) in the young are sparse. The purpose of this population-based, age- and sex-matched longitudinal follow-up study was to investigate the risk of developing ischemic stroke in young patients with AS.

Methods: A total of 4562 patients aged 18- to 45-year-old with at least two ambulatory visits in 2001 with a principal diagnosis of AS were enrolled in the AS group. The non-AS group consisted of 22810 age- and sex-matched, randomly sampled subjects without AS. The two-year ischemic stroke-free survival rate for each group were calculated using the Kaplan-Meier method. Cox proportional hazards regression analysis was used to estimate the hazard ratio of ischemic stroke after adjusting for demographic and clinical covariates.

Results: During follow-up, 21 patients in the AS group and 53 in the non-AS group developed ischemic stroke. The ischemic stroke-free survival rate over the 2 year follow-up was lower in the AS group than the non-AS group (p = 0.0021). The crude hazard ratio of ischemic stroke for the AS group was 1.98 (95% CI, 1.20–3.29; p = 0.0079) and the adjusted hazard ratio after controlling for demographic and comorbid medical disorders was 1.93 (95% CI, 1.16–3.20; p = 0.0110).

Conclusion: Our study showed an increased risk of developing ischemic stroke in young patients with AS.

Editor: James T. Rosenbaum, Oregon Health & Science University, United States of America

Funding: This work was supported by grants DOH93-TD-M-113-030, DOH94-TD-M-113-004, and DOH95-TD-M-113-002 from the Department of Health (DOH), Executive Yuan, Republic of China and grant NSC101-2314-B-002-088 from the National Science Council, Executive Yuan, Republic of China. This study used the complete National Health Insurance Research Database provided by the Bureau of National Health Insurance, Department of Health. The conclusions in our study are not necessarily those of the Department of Health, Executive Yuan, Republic of China. The funders had no role in study design, data collection and analysis, decision to publish, or preparation of the manuscript.

Competing Interests: The authors have declared that no competing interests exist.

* E-mail: panslcb@gmail.com

Introduction

Ankylosing spondylitis (AS), an autoimmune disease with systemic inflammation, predominantly involves the axial skeleton [1]. AS has been associated with an increased risk of ischemic heart disease [2–8], but whether AS patients are at a higher risk of ischemic stroke remains controversial. Two observational studies have reported an increased risk of cerebrovascular disease in AS patients [9,10], whereas another study found that AS patients had no increased prevalence of stroke compared to non-AS patients [11]. In addition, two of these studies were based on a cross-sectional survey [9,11] and prospective data on the relationship between AS and cerebrovascular diseases are sparse. Moreover, these studies were carried out mainly on middle-aged or older AS patients, and little is known about cerebrovascular risk in young AS patients. Thus, the aim of this population-based, age- and sex-matched longitudinal follow-up study was to evaluate the risk of developing ischemic stroke in young patients with AS.

Materials and Methods

Data source

The data used in this study were obtained from the complete National Health Insurance (NHI) claim database in Taiwan for the period 2000 to 2003. The NHI program, a single-payer compulsory social insurance program, has been implemented in Taiwan since 1995, and the coverage rate was 96% of the whole population in 2000 and 97% at the end of 2003, at which time more than 21.9 million inhabitants were enrolled. It should be noted that the rationale for using the NHI database after 2000 is that, from Jan 1st, 2000, according to the rules of the Bureau of NHI, NHI claim data have been encoded using the standardized International Classification of Disease, 9th Revision, Clinical Modification (ICD-9-CM).

Ethics Statement

To keep individual information confidential so as to satisfy regulations on personal privacy in Taiwan, all personal identification numbers in the data were encrypted by converting them into scrambled numbers before data processing. This study was exempt from full review by the National Taiwan University Hospital Research Ethics Committee, and the need for informed consent was waived because the data used consisted of de-identified secondary data released for research purposes and were analyzed anonymously, thus complying with the regulations of the Department of Health, Executive Yuan, Republic of China.

Study Design and Subjects

We used an age- and sex-matched cohort study design to investigate the risk of ischemic stroke in young patients with AS. The study population included an AS group and a non-AS group. The AS group consisted of subjects aged between 18 to 45 years who had received a principal diagnosis of AS (ICD-9-CM code 720.0) in ambulatory medical care visits between January 1, 2001 and December 31, 2001. The index visit was defined as the first ambulatory visit during which the principal diagnosis of AS was made. In order to maximize case ascertainment, only patients with at least two ambulatory visits (including the index visit) with a principal diagnosis of AS in this period were considered for inclusion in the AS group (n = 11428). The exclusion criteria for the recruitment of subjects into the AS group were: (1) a previous diagnosis of AS during year 2000 (n = 6473) to increase the likelihood of identifying AS cases newly diagnosed in 2001; (2) a previous diagnosis of any type of stroke (ICD-9-CM codes 430-438) (n = 91) before the index visit; and (3) a diagnosis of diffuse diseases of connective tissue (ICD-9-CM code 710, n = 252) or rheumatoid arthritis (ICD-9-CM code 714, n = 765) before the index visit; 6866 subjects were excluded because of one or more of these criteria, leaving 4562 subjects in the final AS group.

The non-AS group was constructed by sampling the subjects without a diagnosis of AS in the same 2001 NHI claim database. We assigned the first ambulatory visit during 2001 as the index visit. The exclusion criteria for recruiting subjects into the non-AS group were: (1) a previous diagnosis of AS before the index visit; (2) a previous diagnosis of stroke before the index visit; and (3) a diagnosis of diffuse diseases of connective tissue or rheumatoid arthritis before the index visit. We randomly sampled 5 age- and sex-matched subjects for each subject in the AS group. A total of 22810 subjects was included in the non-AS group.

Outcome

All ambulatory medical care and inpatient records for each subject in the two groups for the 2 year follow-up period were retrieved and the mortality data for those subjects who died during follow-up were obtained from the mortality registry. These medical records and mortality data were linked through a unique encrypted identification number for each subject. We identified the date of the first principal diagnosis of ischemic stroke (ICD-9-CM codes 433–437) during follow-up as the primary endpoint. All subjects were followed from the index visit to the first occurrence of ischemic stroke, death, or end of follow-up (whichever occurred first). We evaluated the effect of AS on the ischemic stroke-free survival, adjusting for the demographic features of age and sex and for the cardiovascular comorbidities of hypertension (ICD-9-CM code 401–405), diabetes (ICD-9-CM code 250), dyslipidemia (ICD-9-CM code 272), coronary heart disease (ICD-9-CM codes 410–414, and 429.2), and other types of heart disease (ICD-9-CM code 393-398, 420–429). Information on these preexisting comorbid medical disorders was obtained by retrieving all the ambulatory medical care and inpatients records in the NHI database for the year before the index visit.

Statistical analysis

The Chi-square test and Student's t test were used to compare differences in demographic characteristics and comorbid medical disorders between the AS and non-AS groups. The ischemic stroke-free survival probabilities for the two groups were estimated using the Kaplan-Meier method and differences in ischemic stroke-free survival between the two groups were tested using the log rank test. Cox proportional hazards regression analysis was used to estimate the effect of AS on the subsequent occurrence of ischemic stroke after adjusting for medical comorbidities. Univariate analysis was initially performed for each variable, then the best subset selection method was used to obtain the final multiple regression model. An alpha level of 0.05 was considered statistically significant. The analyses were performed using SAS 9.2 software (SAS Institute, Cary, NC).

Results

Table 1 shows the distribution of demographic characteristics and medical comorbidities in the AS and non-AS groups. Men made up 73.8% of the AS group, which had a mean age of 31.3 years (SD = 7.6). The AS group had a higher prevalence of dyslipidemia ($p = 0.0157$), coronary heart disease ($p<0.0001$), and other types of heart disease ($p<0.0001$). There was no significant difference between the two groups in the prevalence of diabetes mellitus ($p = 0.3755$) or hypertension ($p = 0.7527$).

Of the 4562 subjects with AS, 21 (0.46%) developed ischemic stroke during the 2-year follow-up compared to 53 (0.23%) of the 22810 subjects in the non-AS group. Comparison of the ischemic stroke-free survival curves showed that the stroke-free survival rate for the AS group was significantly lower than that for the non-AS group ($p = 0.0021$, Figure 1).

The results of the Cox proportional hazards regression analysis are shown in Table 2. The left column shows the crude hazard ratio (HR) for each variable based on the univariate analysis. The covariates with a p value less than 0.05 were age, AS, hypertension, coronary heart disease, and other heart diseases. Compared to the non-AS group, the crude HR of ischemic stroke for the AS group was 1.98 (95% CI, 1.20 to 3.29; $p = 0.0079$). The middle column shows the results using the full multivariate model; age and sex were not included in the multiple regression analysis, since the AS and non-AS groups were matched for these variables. The right column shows the result of the final best subset selected model; the variables included in the final model were AS, hypertension, and coronary heart disease. The adjusted HR of developing ischemic stroke during the 2-year follow-up was 1.93 (95% CI, 1.16 to 3.20; $p = 0.0110$) for the AS group compared to the non-AS group. It should also be noted that hypertension and coronary heart disease were also associated with a higher risk of ischemic stroke.

Of the 21 AS patients who developed stroke, 15 (71.4%) were male. The mean age of these 21 AS patients was 38.0 years (SD = 6.9), elder than that (31.3 years, SD = 7.6) of the remaining 4541 AS patients who did not develop stroke ($p<0.0001$). The prevalence of diabetes mellitus, hypertension, dyslipidemia, coronary heart disease, and other heart disease of these 21 AS patients at baseline were 0%, 4.8%, 9.5%, 4.8%, and 4.8%, respectively. There was lack of significant difference in the prevalence of the above medical co-morbidities between the AS patients who developed stroke or not.

Table 1. Demographic and clinical characteristics of the AS and non-AS groups.

Variable	AS group	Non-AS group	p value
	N=4562	N=22810	
Men	3365 (73.8)	16825 (73.8)	1.0000
Age (years)	31.3±7.6	31.2±7.6	0.2866
Diabetes	72 (1.6)	321 (1.4)	0.3755
Hypertension	102 (2.2)	493 (2.2)	0.7527
Dyslipidemia	122 (2.7)	479 (2.1)	0.0157
Coronary heart disease	61 (1.3)	171 (0.8)	<0.0001
Other heart diseases	122 (2.7)	285 (1.2)	<0.0001

Values are expressed as the mean ± SD or n (%).

Sensitivity analysis

In order to assess the robustness of our results, we carried out the following sensitivity analyses. First, in the present study, the diagnosis of AS was entirely determined by ICD codes from the insurance database, and may be less accurate than those obtained through a standardized procedure. Moreover, the radiographic data are not available in the NHI database. Therefore, we performed additional analysis, using a more rigorous definition that included only AS patients who received two principal diagnosis of AS with at least one being made by a rheumatologist, orthopedist, or physiatrist. The results showed that 3719 (82%) out of the original 4562 patients in the AS group fit this more rigorous case definition. The estimated adjusted HR obtained from this analysis was 1.79 (95% CI, 1.01 to 3.18), consistent with the estimates from the original analysis (Table 2, right column, adjusted HR 1.93, 95% CI, 1.16 to 3.20). Second, while AS patients who had at least 2 ambulatory visits in 2001 were considered for inclusion, the non-AS group consisted of age and gender matched patients who had at least one ambulatory visit in 2001. It may raise a concern that the non-AS group would consist of a potentially healthier population requiring fewer ambulatory visits, which may have had an influence on the risk of stroke. Therefore, we performed additional analysis restricting the non-AS group inclusion criteria to only subjects with at least 2 ambulatory visits in 2001. The majority of the subjects in the non-AS group (21649 out of 22810, 94.9%) had two or more ambulatory visits in 2001. The adjusted HR of ischemic stroke for AS was 1.89 (95% CI, 1.14 to 3.14), which is almost unchanged compared to the original estimates (adjusted HR 1.93, 95% CI, 1.16 to 3.20). Third, as shown in Table 1, the AS group had a higher prevalence of dyslipidemia, coronary heart disease, and other types of heart disease compared to the non-AS group. As these co-morbidities may also contribute to the risk of ischemic stroke, we conducted an analysis excluding all patients (in both the AS and non-AS groups) with any one of the co-morbidities listed in Table 1 (i.e. diabetes mellitus, hypertension, dyslipidemia,

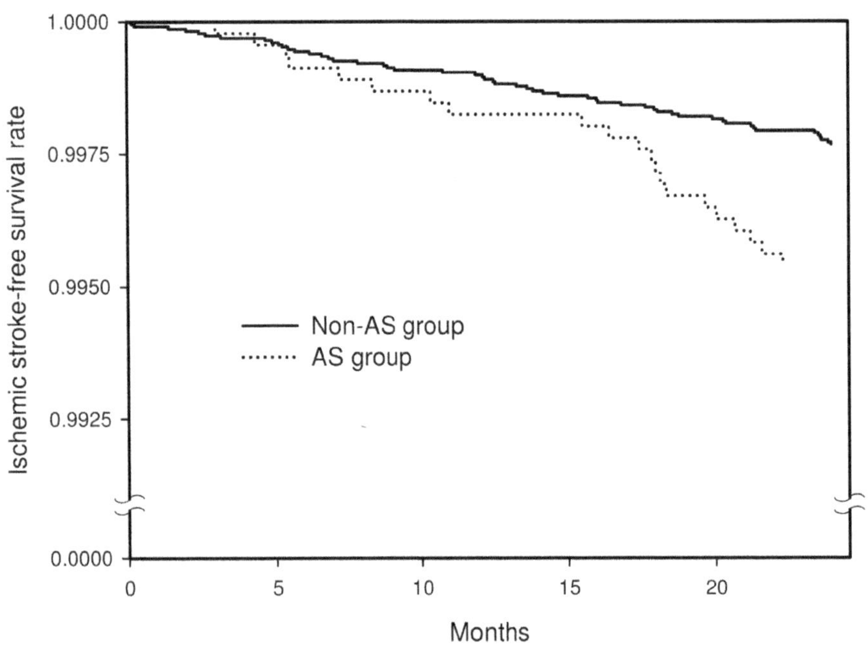

Figure 1. Two-year ischemic stroke-free survival rates for the ankylosing spondylitis (AS) group (dotted line) and non-AS group (solid line).

Table 2. Crude and adjusted hazard ratio (HR) for the occurrence of ischemic stroke during the two-year follow-up period in the AS and non-AS groups.

	Occurrence of ischemic stroke					
	Univariate analysis		**Full multivariate model**		**Best subset selected model**	
Variable	Crude HR (95% CI)	p value	Adjusted HR (95% CI)	p value	Adjusted HR (95% CI)	p value
Age (years)	1.12 (1.08 to 1.16)	<0.0001	NA	NA	NA	NA
Sex (female vs. male)	0.97 (0.58 to 1.63)	0.9060	NA	NA	NA	NA
AS (AS vs. non-AS)	1.98 (1.20 to 3.29)	0.0079	1.92 (1.16 to 3.19)	0.0116	1.93 (1.16 to 3.20)	0.0110
Hypertension (yes vs. no)	6.32 (3.18 to 12.69)	<0.0001	4.55 (2.02 to 10.23)	0.0002	4.66 (2.15 to 10.09)	<0.0001
Diabetes mellitus (yes vs. no)	0.96 (0.13 to 6.86)	0.9633	0.42 (0.06 to 3.19)	0.4031	NA	NA
Dyslipidemia (yes vs. no)	2.56 (0.93 to 7.01)	0.0677	1.39 (0.47 to 4.13)	0.5490	NA	NA
Coronary heart disease (yes vs. no)	8.55 (3.45 to 21.19)	<0.0001	3.78 (1.27 to 11.24)	0.0170	4.18 (1.53 to 11.46)	0.0053
Other heart diseases (yes vs. no)	3.80 (1.39 to 10.40)	0.0095	1.42 (0.45 to 4.48)	0.5467	NA	NA

Abbreviations: AS, ankylosing spondylitis; CI, confidence interval; NA, not applicable.

coronary heart disease, and other heart disease). The adjusted HR of ischemic stroke for AS was 2.20 (95% CI, 1.25 to 3.90, p = 0.0065), still supporting that AS is associated with a higher risk of developing ischemic stroke. Fourth, we performed a competing risk analysis accounting for death due to causes other than stroke as a competing risk. The adjusted HR of ischemic stroke for AS is 1.84 (95% CI, 1.10 to 3.08), which is very close to the original estimates (adjusted HR 1.93, 95% CI, 1.16 to 3.20).

Discussion

The major finding in our study was that, in young patients with AS, AS was associated with a 1.9-fold increased risk of ischemic stroke. This association was still seen after controlling for common vascular risk factors. The 2-year ischemic stroke-free survival rate for the AS subjects was lower than that for the non-AS group. Our findings are consistent with two previous observational studies carried out in the US (prevalence ratio: 1.7, 95% CI, 1.3 to 2.3) [9] and in Quebec (prevalence ratio: 1.25, 95% CI, 1.15 to 1.35) [10]. The mechanism responsible for the association between AS and ischemic stroke is unclear; however, we propose the following explanations.

Inflammation plays an important role in the pathogenesis and progression of atherosclerosis [3,12–15]. Previous studies have shown that, compared to patients without AS, AS patients have higher levels of inflammatory markers, such as interleukin 6, tumor necrosis factor alpha, and C-reactive protein [3,16,17]. In addition, AS patients have been reported to show early features of atherosclerosis, such as an increase in intima media thickness in the carotid arteries [18–22] and impaired flow-mediated dilatation in the brachial arteries [19,23]. Thus, the increased risk of ischemic stroke in the AS group may result from accelerated atherosclerosis caused by systemic inflammation.

Heart disorders, such as aortic insufficiency, mitral valve disease, and cardiomyopathy, are part of the extraskeletal manifestations of AS [24,25]. These heart disorders may also contribute to a higher risk of ischemic stroke [26,27]. However, in our study, although the AS group had a higher prevalence of coronary heart disease and other heart diseases, AS remained an independent risk factor of ischemic stroke after controlling for vascular risk factors and heart diseases in the multivariate analysis. The adjusted hazard ratio of ischemic stroke for the AS group (adjusted HR: 1.93, 95% CI: 1.16 to 3.20) in the multivariate analysis is very close to the crude HR (1.98, 95% CI: 1.20 to 3.29) in the univariate analysis (Table 2). These findings suggest that the increased risk of ischemic stroke in the AS group is independent of the heart involvement in AS.

Non-steroidal anti-inflammatory drugs (NSAIDs) are widely used for treating AS [28,29]. However, the use of NSAID was not evaluated in our study because observational studies on the effects of NSAID exposure on vascular risks are potentially confounded by indication, as patients with more severe rheumatic diseases are likely to receive higher NSAID doses and also to be at higher disease-related vascular risk. In addition, since NSAIDs are widely available as over the counter medications, their use is not readily assessable in the insurance database. It is therefore difficult to separate the effects of NSAIDs from the biological impacts resulting from AS. Moreover, it remains controversial whether NSAIDs is associated with an increased risk of stroke. A recent large-scale meta-analysis of 280 trials of NSAIDs versus placebo and 474 trials of one NSAID versus another NSAID showed there was no evidence that any NSAID, including selective COX-2 inhibitors and traditional NSAIDs, significantly increased the risk of stroke [30]. Therefore, the use of NSAID was not included in our analysis.

In the present population-based study, the estimated prevalence of AS was 0.12% using case definition that requires at least two ambulatory visits with a principal diagnosis of AS in 2001. This prevalence estimate is relatively lower than that obtained from a community-based survey on the prevalence of rheumatic diseases in Taiwan [31] which used a 2-stage screening process in 1992. In that study, the estimated prevalence of AS in the adult Taiwanese population ranged from 0.19 to 0.54% [31]. Since some AS patients with mild symptoms who did not seek medical service would not be recorded in the NHI database, our study may tend to recruit patients with more severe or active AS, and it can be expected that the estimated prevalence of AS in our study would be lower than that reported from the previous community-based survey.

The strength of the present study was the use of a longitudinal population-based NHI database. The NHI program is a single-payer compulsory social insurance program with considerably high coverage rate in Taiwan. The barrier to medical access is negligible because the NHI system allows patients to visit any clinic or hospital freely without referral by a general practitioner, and patients pay only about $5–$15 USD at each visit.

Considering the neurological deficit and functional disability related to stroke, and the minimal barrier to medical access in Taiwan, it can be expected that most patients who developed stroke would seek medical help and would be captured in the NHI database, which enabled us to identify all incident cases of stroke and establish a temporal relationship between AS and ischemic stroke. Nevertheless, several limitations should be acknowledged. First, the diagnoses of AS, ischemic stroke, and medical comorbidities were determined using the ICD codes from the NHI claim database, and there may be concern about the diagnostic accuracy of the database. However, the Bureau of NHI has formed different audit committees that make it a rule to randomly sample the claims data from every hospital and to review charts on a regular basis to verify the diagnostic validity and quality of care. In addition, one validation study that evaluated the validity of the NHI database for patients with a principal diagnosis of ischemic stroke showed that the NHI database appears to be a valid resource for population-based research in ischemic stroke [32]. Accordingly, the NHI claim database is an established research database and independent studies have demonstrated the validity of the data [33]. Furthermore, we performed sensitivity analyses using various case definitions, and found that AS was consistently linked to an increased risk of developing ischemic stroke, suggesting that our results are robust to different case definitions. Second, although we excluded subjects with a previous diagnosis of AS during year 2000 to increase the likelihood of identifying AS patients newly diagnosed in 2001, it was possible that some prevalent AS cases with more longstanding AS who had not sought medical care in 2000 but coded for the first time in 2001 based on our database, were included in the AS group. Third, due to the inherent limitation of the NHI database, information was lacking regarding lifestyle factors, such as smoking, alcohol consumption, and obesity. Moreover, since traditional vascular risk factors, such as diabetes, hypertension and dyslipidemia, are disorders with an insidious onset, some asymptomatic vascular risk factors may not be captured in the NHI database. Therefore, the prevalence of vascular risk factors may be underestimated in both the AS and non-AS groups. These potential confounders may lead to residual confounding and may affect the interpretation of our findings. Fourth, the follow-up time was only 2 years and the long-term effects of AS on the development of ischemic stroke cannot therefore be evaluated. Finally, since Taiwanese are mainly of Chinese ethnicity, it is uncertain whether our findings can be generalized to other ethnic groups.

In conclusion, the present population-based longitudinal follow-up study demonstrates there is an increased risk of ischemic stroke in young patients with AS and highlights the importance of early risk assessment for ischemic stroke in such patients. Further long-term follow-up study would be required to validate our findings and to investigate the underlying pathophysiological mechanism.

Author Contributions

Conceived and designed the experiments: CWL YPH YHC YTH SLP. Performed the experiments: CWL YPH YHC YTH SLP. Analyzed the data: CWL YPH YHC SLP. Contributed reagents/materials/analysis tools: CWL YPH YHC SLP. Wrote the paper: CWL YPH YHC YTH SLP.

References

1. Braun J, Sieper J (2007) Ankylosing spondylitis. Lancet 369: 1379–1390.
2. El Maghraoui A (2011) Extra-articular manifestations of ankylosing spondylitis: prevalence, characteristics and therapeutic implications. Eur J Intern Med 22: 554–560.
3. Divecha H, Sattar N, Rumley A, Cherry L, Lowe GD, et al. (2005) Cardiovascular risk parameters in men with ankylosing spondylitis in comparison with non-inflammatory control subjects: relevance of systemic inflammation. Clin Sci (Lond) 109: 171–176.
4. Peters MJ, van der Horst-Bruinsma IE, Dijkmans BA, Nurmohamed MT (2004) Cardiovascular risk profile of patients with spondylarthropathies, particularly ankylosing spondylitis and psoriatic arthritis. Semin Arthritis Rheum 34: 585–592.
5. Roman MJ, Salmon JE (2007) Cardiovascular manifestations of rheumatologic diseases. Circulation 116: 2346–2355.
6. Mathieu S, Gossec L, Dougados M, Soubrier M (2011) Cardiovascular profile in ankylosing spondylitis: a systematic review and meta-analysis. Arthritis Care Res (Hoboken) 63: 557–563.
7. Bremander A, Petersson IF, Bergman S, Englund M (2011) Population-based estimates of common comorbidities and cardiovascular disease in ankylosing spondylitis. Arthritis Care Res (Hoboken) 63: 550–556.
8. Huang YP, Wang YH, Pan SL (2013) Increased risk of ischemic heart disease in young patients with newly diagnosed ankylosing spondylitis—a population-based longitudinal follow-up study. PLoS One 8: e64155.
9. Han C, Robinson DW Jr, Hackett MV, Paramore LC, Fraeman KH, et al. (2006) Cardiovascular disease and risk factors in patients with rheumatoid arthritis, psoriatic arthritis, and ankylosing spondylitis. J Rheumatol 33: 2167–2172.
10. Szabo SM, Levy AR, Rao SR, Kirbach SE, Lacaille D, et al. (2011) Increased risk of cardiovascular and cerebrovascular diseases in individuals with ankylosing spondylitis: A population-based study. Arthritis Rheum 63: 3294–3304.
11. Kang JH, Chen YH, Lin HC (2010) Comorbidity profiles among patients with ankylosing spondylitis: a nationwide population-based study. Ann Rheum Dis 69: 1165–1168.
12. Ross R (1999) Atherosclerosis—an inflammatory disease. N Engl J Med 340: 115–126.
13. Pearson TA, Mensah GA, Alexander RW, Anderson JL, Cannon RO 3rd, et al. (2003) Markers of inflammation and cardiovascular disease: application to clinical and public health practice: A statement for healthcare professionals from the Centers for Disease Control and Prevention and the American Heart Association. Circulation 107: 499–511.
14. Verma S, Anderson TJ (2002) Fundamentals of endothelial function for the clinical cardiologist. Circulation 105: 546–549.
15. Stoll G, Bendszus M (2006) Inflammation and atherosclerosis: novel insights into plaque formation and destabilization. Stroke 37: 1923–1932.
16. Gratacos J, Collado A, Filella X, Sanmarti R, Canete J, et al. (1994) Serum cytokines (IL-6, TNF-alpha, IL-1 beta and IFN-gamma) in ankylosing spondylitis: a close correlation between serum IL-6 and disease activity and severity. Br J Rheumatol 33: 927–931.
17. Lange U, Teichmann J, Stracke H (2000) Correlation between plasma TNF-alpha, IGF-1, biochemical markers of bone metabolism, markers of inflammation/disease activity, and clinical manifestations in ankylosing spondylitis. Eur J Med Res 5: 507–511.
18. Hamdi W, Chelli Bouaziz M, Zouch I, Ghannouchi MM, Haouel M, et al. (2012) Assessment of preclinical atherosclerosis in patients with ankylosing spondylitis. J Rheumatol 39: 322–326.
19. Bodnar N, Kerekes G, Seres I, Paragh G, Kappelmayer J, et al. (2011) Assessment of subclinical vascular disease associated with ankylosing spondylitis. J Rheumatol 38: 723–729.
20. Cece H, Yazgan P, Karakas E, Karakas O, Demirkol A, et al. (2011) Carotid intima-media thickness and paraoxonase activity in patients with ankylosing spondylitis. Clin Invest Med 34: E225.
21. Peters MJ, van Eijk IC, Smulders YM, Serne E, Dijkmans BA, et al. (2010) Signs of accelerated preclinical atherosclerosis in patients with ankylosing spondylitis. J Rheumatol 37: 161–166.
22. Gonzalez-Juanatey C, Vazquez-Rodriguez TR, Miranda-Filloy JA, Dierssen T, Vaqueiro I, et al. (2009) The High Prevalence of Subclinical Atherosclerosis in Patients With Ankylosing Spondylitis Without Clinically Evident Cardiovascular Disease. Medicine 88: 358–365.
23. Sari I, Okan T, Akar S, Cece H, Altay C, et al. (2006) Impaired endothelial function in patients with ankylosing spondylitis. Rheumatology (Oxford) 45: 283–286.
24. O'Neill TW, Bresnihan B (1992) The heart in ankylosing spondylitis. Ann Rheum Dis 51: 705–706.
25. Ribeiro P, Morley KD, Shapiro LM, Garnett RA, Hughes GR, et al. (1984) Left ventricular function in patients with ankylosing spondylitis and Reiter's disease. Eur Heart J 5: 419–422.
26. Avierinos JF, Brown RD, Foley DA, Nkomo V, Petty GW, et al. (2003) Cerebral ischemic events after diagnosis of mitral valve prolapse: a community-based study of incidence and predictive factors. Stroke 34: 1339–1344.
27. Cohen A, Tzourio C, Chauvel C, Bertrand B, Crassard I, et al. (1997) Mitral valve strands and the risk of ischemic stroke in elderly patients. The French Study of Aortic Plaques in Stroke (FAPS) Investigators. Stroke 28: 1574–1578.

28. Braun J, van den Berg R, Baraliakos X, Boehm H, Burgos-Vargas R, et al. (2011) 2010 update of the ASAS/EULAR recommendations for the management of ankylosing spondylitis. Ann Rheum Dis 70: 896–904.
29. van den Berg R, Baraliakos X, Braun J, van der Heijde D (2012) First update of the current evidence for the management of ankylosing spondylitis with non-pharmacological treatment and non-biologic drugs: a systematic literature review for the ASAS/EULAR management recommendations in ankylosing spondylitis. Rheumatology (Oxford) 51: 1388–1396.
30. Bhala N, Emberson J, Merhi A, Abramson S, Arber N, et al. (2013) Vascular and upper gastrointestinal effects of non-steroidal anti-inflammatory drugs: meta-analyses of individual participant data from randomised trials. Lancet 382: 769–779.
31. Chou CT, Pei L, Chang DM, Lee CF, Schumacher HR, et al. (1994) Prevalence of rheumatic diseases in Taiwan: a population study of urban, suburban, rural differences. J Rheumatol 21: 302–306.
32. Cheng CL, Kao YH, Lin SJ, Lee CH, Lai ML (2011) Validation of the National Health Insurance Research Database with ischemic stroke cases in Taiwan. Pharmacoepidemiol Drug Saf 20: 236–242.
33. Wu CH, Wang YH, Huang YP, Pan SL (2012) Does adhesive capsulitis of the shoulder increase the risk of stroke? A population-based propensity score-matched follow-up study. PLoS One 7: e49343.

10

Plasma D-Dimer Predicts Short-Term Poor Outcome after Acute Ischemic Stroke

Xiao-ying Yang[1], Shan Gao[2]*, Jie Ding[3], Yan Chen[2], Xing-sheng Zhou[2], Jing-E Wang[2]

1 Department of Clinical Laboratory, Shanghai Jiao Tong University, Affiliated the Sixth People Hospital Fengxian Branch, Shanghai, P. R. China, **2** Department of Neurology, Shanghai Jiao Tong University, Affiliated the Sixth People Hospital Fengxian Branch, Shanghai, P. R. China, **3** Department of Neurology, Tianjin Union Medicine Center, Tianjin, P. R. China

Abstract

Objective: Haemostatic biomarkers associated with poor outcome in acute ischemic stroke (AIS). The objective of the study was to evaluate the predictive value of plasma D-dimer (D-D) on functional outcome at 90-day follow-up from stroke onset.

Methods: We conducted a prospective, observational cohort study in the emergency department and enrolled 220 patients with AIS. Plasma D-D concentrations, determined by a particle-enhanced, immunoturbidimetric assay, were measured. Each patient's medical record was reviewed, and demographic, clinical, laboratory and neuroimaging information was abstracted.

Results: There was a positive correlation between levels of D-D and the NIHSS ($r = 0.361$, $p < 0.001$), and the infarct volume ($r = 0.449$, $p < 0.001$). In the 69 patients with an unfavorable functional outcome, D-D levels were higher compared with those in patients with a favorable outcome [3.24(IQR, 2.18–4.60)mg/L vs 0.88(IQR, 0.35–1.77) mg/L; $p < 0.001$]. After adjusting for all other significant outcome predictors, D-D level remained an independent predictor for unfavorable functional outcome and mortality with an odds ratio of 2.18 (95% CI, 1.55–2.83), 3.22 (95% CI, 2.05–6.43); respectively.

Conclusions: D-D levels are a useful tool to predict outcome and mortality 90-day after acute ischemic stroke and have a potential to assist clinicians.

Editor: Jorge I F Salluh, D'or Institute of Research and Education, Brazil

Funding: This study was supported by Shanghai health bureau scientific research plan fund (2011350). The funders had no role in study design, data collection and analysis, decision to publish, or preparation of the manuscript.

Competing Interests: The authors have declared that no competing interests exist.

* E-mail: cams024@163.com

Introduction

Ischemic stroke is one of the major causes of death worldwide. China has 2.5 million new stroke cases each year and 7.5 million stroke survivors [1]. It places a tremendous burden on health resources in China. Timely intervention can dramatically improve outcome and reduce disability.

D-dimer(D-D), the final product of plasmin-mediated degradation of fibrin-rich thrombi, has emerged as a simple blood test that can be used in diagnostic algorithms for the exclusion of venous thromboembolism [2]. D-D levels have certain advantages over other measures of thrombin generation, because it is resistant to ex vivo activation, relatively stable, and has a long half-life [3].

It has been suggested that modestly elevated circulating D-D values reflect minor increases in bloodcoagulation, thrombin formation, and turnover of cross linked intravascular fibrin (which is partly intra-arterialin origin) and that these increases may be associated with coronary heart disease [4]. Mahé et al [5] reported that patients with higher D-D levels are at higher risk of cardiovascular events, even if they are receiving oral anticoagulants.

Goldenberg et al [6] reported that elevated D-D concentrations are prognostic of long-term neurologic outcomes in Childhood-Onset Arterial Ischemic Stroke. Elevated D-D level has also been shown to relate to early clinical progression [7], stroke subtypes [8], infarction volume [9], unfavorable outcome [10] in ischemic stroke patients and poor functional outcome after acute spontaneous intracerebral hemorrhage [11] and subarachnoid hemorrhage [12]. On the contrary, Haapaniemi et al [3] supposed that D-D levels per se are not an independent predictor for poor outcome but reflect stroke etiology. Thus, the purpose of this study was to investigate the association between plasma D-D level at admission and short-term functional outcome in Chinese patients with acute ischemic stroke (AIS).

Subjects and Methods

Patients and Study Design

From February 2011 to December 2012, all consecutive patients with first-ever AIS admission to the emergency department of our hospital were recruited to participate in the study. All patients were admitted within 24 hours of experiencing a new focal or global neurological event. An acute ischemic stroke was defined according to the World Health Organization criteria [13]. Brain MRI was performed routinely within 24 hours after admission. Patients were excluded if any of the following criteria were met: a delay of 24 hours from symptom recognition to admission, age younger than 18 years, coma or epileptic seizure activity, MRI could not be performed, intracranial hemorrhage, malignancy, febrile disorders, acute or chronic inflammatory disease at study enrollment. Patients who were anticoagulated before admission were also excluded.

One hundred and twenty healthy people matched for age and gender were assigned to the normal control group. Those normal cases in our study were from our hospital staff who took part in the health examination. Records of potential controls were reviewed by a neurologist (not an author) to exclude the presence of stroke, other types of diseases. The Institutional Review Committee on Human Research of Shanghai Jiao Tong University Affiliated the Sixth People Hospital Fengxian Branch approved the study protocol. All patients received oral and written information concerning the background and procedures of the study, and the patients or their relatives gave written informed consent prior to entering the study.

Clinical Variables

At baseline, demographic data (age and sex) and history of risk factors (hypertension, diabetes mellitus, atrial fibrillation, hyperlipidemia, smoking habit and alcohol abuse) were obtained. The time from symptom recognition to admission were also recorded. At admission, the neurological deficit was quantified using the National Institutes of Health Stroke Scale (NIHSS) [14] and stroke subtype was classified according to TOAST (Trial of Org 10172 in Acute Stroke Treatment) criteria [15]. The clinical stroke syndrome was determined by applying the criteria of the Oxfordshire Community Stroke Project: total anterior circulation syndrome (TACS); partial anterior circulation syndrome (PACS); lacunar syndrome (LACS); and posterior circulation syndrome (POCS) [16]. All patients received treatment according to current guidelines. The routine treatment of patients with AIS in our institution was thrombolytic therapy, and 62 patients (28.2%) timely receive thrombolytic therapy.

Neuroimaging

MRI with diffusion-weighted imaging (DWI) was available in all stroke patients. In patients, DWI lesion volumes were determined by one experienced neurologist unaware of the clinical and laboratory results. The infarct volume was calculated by using the formula $0.5 \times a \times b \times c$ (where *a* is the maximal longitudinal diameter, *b* is the maximal transverse diameter perpendicular to *a*, and *c* is the number of 10-mm slices containing infarct) [17].

End Points and Follow-up

We considered the following endpoints: (1) the primary endpoint was functional outcome on day 90. Functional outcome was assessed by the modified Rankin Scale (mRS, a favourable functional outcome was defined as a mRS of 0–2 points, whereas an unfavourable outcome was defined as a mRS of 3–6 points) [18]; (2) secondary end-points were all-cause mortality within 90 days. Outcome assessment was performed by one trained medical staff blinded to D-D levels with a structured interview, if discharged, with telephone interview.

Blood Collection and Test

Blood samples of patients and controls were obtained at 7:00 AM in the next morning of the day of admission. Blood samples were collected in 5-ml vacuum tubes containing 0.5 ml buffered sodium citrate. Plasma aliquots were collected and centrifuged at 3000 g for 10 min at ambient room temperature. Plasma was then frozen at −80 C until assayed.

D-D concentration was measured with a particle-enhanced, immunoturbidimetric assay in a calibrated SYSMEX1500 analyzer (Sysmex Corporation, Hyogo, Japan). The median level of D-D in our normal control is 0.33 mg/L, which is slightly higher than other laboratory (0.25 mg/L) [19]. The detection limit was 0.05 mg/L, and the dynamic range was from 0.05 to 30.0 mg/L. The intra-assay coefficient of variation [CV] and inter-assay CV were 1.8–37%, 2.5%–4.6%, respectively. For all measurements, levels that were not detectable were considered to have a value equal to the lower limit of detection of the assay.

Statistical Analysis

Results are expressed as percentages for categorical variables and as medians (interquartile ranges,IQRs) for the continuous variables. Proportions were compared using the $\chi 2$ test, and the Mann–Whitney test to compare continuous variables between groups. Correlations were determined using Spearman critical value rankings. Multivariate analysis was performed by binary logistic regression analysis, which allows adjustment for confounding factors (age, the NIHSS score, infarct volume, stroke syndrome, vascular risk factors, thrombolytic therapy and other laboratory biomarkers). Results were expressed as adjusted odds ratios (OR) with the corresponding 95% confidence intervals (CIs). Receiver operating characteristic (ROC) curves were utilized to evaluate the accuracy of D-D to predict outcomes. All statistical analysis was performed with SPSS for Windows, version 19.0 (SPSS Inc., Chicago, IL, USA). Statistical significance was defined as $p<0.05$.

Results

From 302 screened patients, acute ischemic stroke was diagnosed in 242 patients, and 220 completed 3- month follow-up and were included in the analysis. The median age of patients with ischemic stroke included in this study was 68 (IQR, 54–76) years and 42.3% were women. The median NIHSS score on admission was 8 points (IQR, 5–11). The median time from stroke onset to inclusion in the study was 6.2 (IQR, 3.4–13.7) hours. An unfavorable functional outcome was found in 69 patients (31.4%) with a median mRS score of 4 (IQR, 3–6). 27 patients died, thus the mortality rate was 12.3%. Basal characteristics of patients with acute ischemic stroke are provided in table 1.

Plasma D-D levels were significantly ($p<0.001$) higher in AIS patients as compared to normal controls [1.36 (IQR, 0.55–3.11)mg/L and 0.33 (IQR, 0.18–0.80)mg/L, respectively; Figure 1.). Interestingly, plasma D-D levels were also significantly higher in AIS patients who received thrombolytic therapy as compared to others [1.12 (IQR, 0.47–2.77)mg/L and 0.52 (IQR; 0.35–0.89)mg/L, respectively; $p<0.001$]. There was a positive correlation between levels of D-D and the NIHSS ($r=0.361$, $p<0.001$; Figure 2a.) There was a modest correlation between D-D levels and age($r=0.321$, $p<0.001$). There was no correlation between levels of serum cortisol levels and sex ($p=0.212$). In patients for whom MRI data were available ($n=220$), there was a positive correlation between levels of D-D and the infarct volume ($r=0.449$, $p<0.001$; Figure 2b.).

In the 69 patients with an unfavorable functional outcome, D-D levels were higher compared with those in patients with a favorable outcome [3.24(IQR, 2.18–4.60)mg/L vs 0.88(IQR, 0.35–1.77) mg/L; $p<0.001$). See the figure 3. With an unadjusted OR of 3.56 (95% CI, 1.99–6.34), D-D had a strong association with functional outcome. See the table 2. After adjusting for all other significant outcome predictors, D-D remained can be seen as

Table 1. Basal characteristic of patients with acute ischemic stroke.

Characteristics	All	Good outcomes	Poor outcomes	p[a]
	(n = 220)	(n = 151)	(n = 69)	
Female sex (%)	42.3	41.1	44.9	NS
Age (years), median(IQR)	68(54–76)	60(51–65)	74(63–79)	<0.001
Stroke severity, median NIHSS score (IQR)	8(5–11)	3(2–6)	11(7–16)	<0.001
Infarct volume(mL, IQR)	11(7–22)	6(3–13)	18(12–59)	<0.001
Vascular risk factors no. (%)				
Diabetes mellitus	61(27.7)	30(19.9)	31(44.9)	<0.01
Hypertension	155(70.4)	95(62.9)	60(87.0)	<0.01
Hypercholesterolemia	55(25.0)	39(25.8)	16(23.2)	NS
Coronary heart disease	62(28.2)	40(26.5)	22(31.9)	NS
Atrial fibrillation	48(21.8)	32(21.2)	16(23.2)	NS
Alcohol abuse	44(20.0)	31(20.5)	13(18.8)	NS
Smoking habit	48(21.8)	32(21.2)	14(20.3)	NS
Laboratory findings (median, IQR)				
Total cholesterol (mmol L^{-1})	4.04(3.33–4.90)	4.01(3.30–4.85)	4.07(3.37–4.94)	NS
HDL (mmol L^{-1})	1.40(1.05–1.87)	1.38(1.06–1.73)	1.49(1.05–2.15)	NS
LDL (mmol L^{-1})	2.11(1.37–2.72)	2.10(1.38–2.71)	2.12(1.36–2.72)	NS
Triglycerides(mmol L^{-1})	1.30(1.05–1.63)	1.29(1.05–1.62)	1.31(1.07–1.67)	NS
Glucose(mmol L^{-1})	5.75(4.90–7.03)	5.45(4.75–6.35)	6.32(5.33–7.76)	<0.01
C-reactive protein (mgL^{-1})	4.9(3.3–8.8)	3.9 (3.0–8.1)	5.9(4.3–9.8)	<0.001
FBG(g L^{-1})	3.66(3.25–4.04)	3.17(2.87–3.69)	4.04(3.45–4.54)	<0.01
D-dimer(mg L^{-1})	1.36(0.55–3.11)	0.88(0.35–1.77)	3.24(2.18–4.62)	<0.001
Stroke syndrome no. (%)				
TACS	25(11.4)	9(6.0)	16(23.2)	<0.01
PACS	86(39.1)	59(39.1)	27(39.1)	NS
LACS	43(19.5)	28(18.5)	15(21.7)	NS
POCS	66(30.0)	55(36.4)	11(16.0)	<0.01
Stroke etiology no. (%)				
Small-vessel occlusive	37(16.8)	24(15.9)	13(18.8)	NS
Large-vessel occlusive	43(19.5)	30(19.9)	13(18.8)	NS
Cardioembolic	87(39.5)	59(39.1)	28(40.6)	NS
Other	15(6.8)	9(6.0)	6(8.7)	NS
Unknown	38(17.4)	29(19.1)	9(13.1)	NS

IQR, interquartile range; TACS, total anterior circulation syndrome; LACS, lacunar syndrome; PACS, partial anterior circulation syndrome; POCS, posterior circulation syndrome; NIHSS, National Institutes of Health Stroke Scale; HDL, High-density lipoproteins; LDL, Low-density lipoproteins;FBG, Fibrinogen.
[a]*p* value was assessed using Mann-Whitney *U* test or $\chi 2$ test.

an independent outcome predictor with an adjusted OR of 2.18 (95% CI, 1.55–2.83). See the table 2.

Based on the ROC curve, the optimal cut-off value of plasma D-D levels as an indicator for diagnosis of unfavorable functional outcome was projected to be 1.99 mg/L, which yielded a sensitivity of 81.2% and a specificity of 79.7%, the area under the curve was 0.84(95%CI, 0.79–0.90). See the figure 4. D-D was in the range of the NIHSS with an AUC of 0.83 (0.77–0.89) and had a higher prognostic accuracy as compared to infarct volume (AUC 0.75 (0.58–0.84), p<0.01) and C-reactive protein (AUC 0.71 (0.60–0.79), p = 0.01).

D-D levels in 27 patients who died were more than 4 times greater as compared with patients who survived [3.98 (IQR, 2.25–5.69)mg/L vs 0.75(IQR, 0.32–1.48)mg/L; p<0.001). After adjustment for possible parameters, D-D level remained an independent predictor for mortality with an OR of 3.22 (95% CI, 2.05–6.43). See the table 2.

Discussion

In this study, we firstly assessed plasma D-D levels with regard to their accuracy to predict short-term functional outcome in patients with AIS within 90 days in Chinese population. Our main finding was that elevated levels of D-D is an independent short-term prognostic marker of functional outcome and death in Chinese patients with AIS even after correcting for possible confounding factors. We also found that that plasma D-D levels increased with infarct volume and neurological deficit (assessed by the NIHSS).

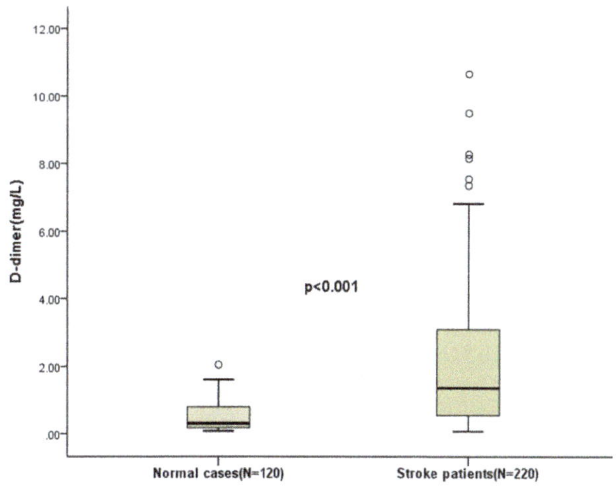

Figure 1. Plasma D-dimer levels in acute ischemic stroke patients and control group. Mann–Whitney U-test. All data are medians and in-terquartile ranges (IQR). Significantly higher in stroke patients as compared to normal cases ($p<0.001$).

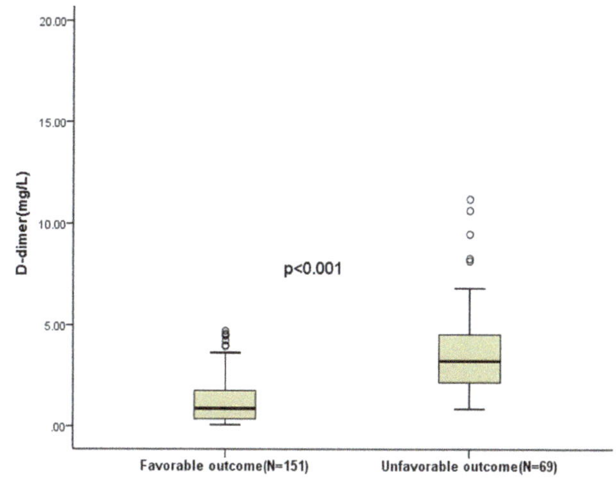

Figure 3

Figure 3. Plasma D-dimer levels in patients with favorable outcomes and unfavorable outcomes. Significantly higher in unfavorable patients as compared to favorable ($p<0.001$).

These results are in accordance with the results from other studies showing that elevated levels of D-D was associated with older age, greater severity of neurological deficit, larger ischemic lesions, stroke subtypes and worse prognoses in stroke patients [8–9,20–21]. In addition, the routine thrombolytic therapy of patients with AIS could alter D-D levels. After adjusted this condition, plasma D-D levels still can be seen as an independent prognostic marker of functional outcome and death.

Over the last two decades numerous studies have explored whether D-D measurements would help stroke clinicians. One study reported that D-D is independently related to acute stroke severity and short-term outcome [10]. Similarly,Yuan et al [7] found that D-D of acute period strongly indicates an unfavorable clinical outcome in a cohort of Chinese patients with AIS. Otherwise,Haapaniemi et al [3] suggested that regarding prediction of patient outcome, good clinical evaluation is clearly superior to D-D testing. From our results, we could confirm that plasma D-D was a valuable and independent short-term prognostic marker of functional outcome and death after stroke, and the prognostic value was in the range of clinical evaluation (assessed by the NIHSS).

Several blood biomarkers had been reported to relevant to functional outcome in AIS patients: inflammation markers [22], neuroendocrine markers [23–24], Vitamin D [25] and haemostatic biomarkers [20,26]. Kang et al [26] reported that elevated levels of D-D in the 24-hour window after acute ischemic stroke are associated with early recurrence of silent brain infarcts independent of other clinical, imaging, and laboratory variables. D-D and CRP are independently associated with poor outcome in acute ischemic stroke [20]. We found that after adjusted with CRP, D-D was still associated with stroke outcome, which was in accordance with another study [27]. In addition, there was a body

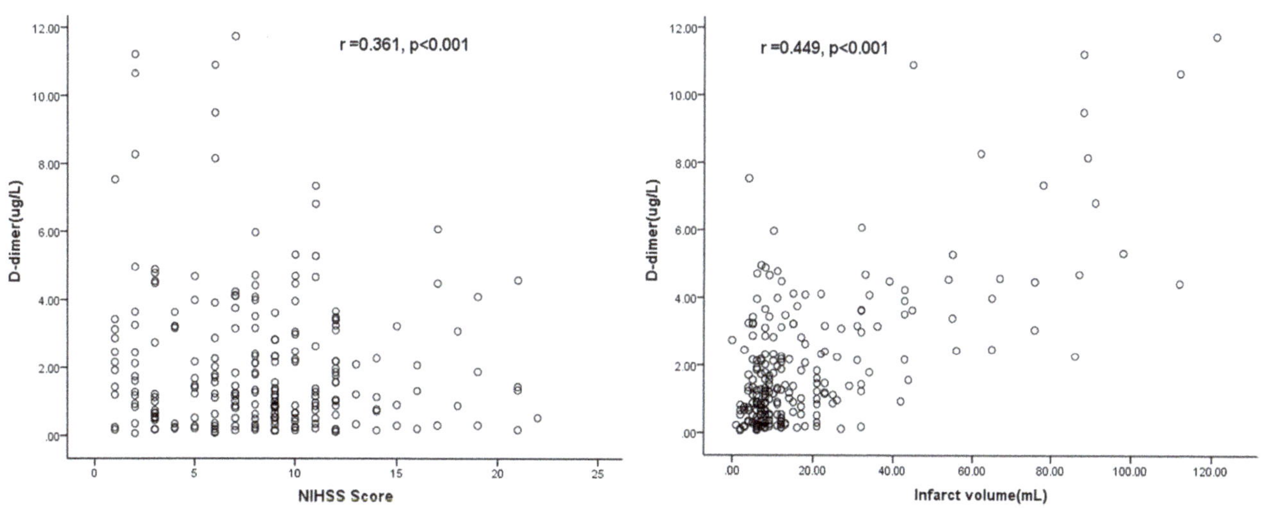

Figure 2(a) Figure 2(b)

Figure 2. Correlation between plasma D-dimer levels and others predictors. (a) Correlation between plasma D-dimer levels and the National Institutes of Health Stroke Scale (NIHSS) score; (b) Correlation between plasma D-dimer levels and infarct volume.

Table 2. Univariate and multivariate logistic regression analysis for outcome and mortality.

Parameter	Univariate Analysis			Multivariate Analysis		
	OR [a]	95% CI [a]	P	OR [a]	95% CI [a]	P
Predictor: functional outcome						
D-dimer (increase per unit)	3.56	1.99–6.34	<0.001	2.18	1.55–2.83	0.005
Age (increase per unit)	1.21	1.05–1.88	0.004	1.06	1.01–1.22	0.001
Hypertension	1.55	1.12–2.45	0.011	1.33	0.82–1.77	0.590
Diabetes mellitus	1.17	1.01–1.44	0.043	1.20	0.70–1.69	0.527
Glucose (increase per unit)	1.08	0.89–1.27	0.027	1.06	0.93–1.31	0.021
FBG(increase per unit)	1.31	1.02–1.65	0.046	1.22	0.97 –1.98	0.053
CRP (increase per unit)	1.08	0.97–1.13	0.012	1.06	1.00–1.24	0.004
Infarct volume(increase per unit)	1.16	1.10–1.22	0.003	1.11	1.01–1.29	0.006
NIHSS (increase per unit)	1.34	1.15–1.54	<0.001	1.31	1.10–1.48	<0.001
TACS	4.01	2.54–8.32	0.024	2.11	1.02–4.35	0.236
Not thrombolytic therapy	1.98	1.16–2.94	0.007	1.65	1.34–2.45	0.006
Predictor: death						
D-dimer (increase per unit)	4.25	1.93–9.28	<0.001	3.22	2.05–6.43	0.002
Age (increase per unit)	1.18	1.04–1.85	<0.001	1.06	1.03–1.09	<0.001
Hypertension	1.16	0.96–1.40	0.090	1.21	0.78–1.54	0.124
Diabetes mellitus	1.24	0.98–1.55	0.027	1.17	0.99–1.77	0.033
Glucose (increase per unit)	1.10	0.93–1.33	0.011	1.08	0.95–1.55	0.036
FBG(increase per unit)	1.40	1.05–1.78	0.033	1.42	0.95–2.07	0.027
CRP (increase per unit)	1.11	1.01–1.28	0.006	1.09	0.99–1.32	0.013
Infarct volume(increase per unit)	1.18	1.11–1.31	0.005	1.17	1.04–1.44	0.009
NIHSS (increase per unit)	1.30	1.12–1.47	<0.001	1.16	1.08–1.24	<0.001
TACS	4.87	2.14–9.02	0.036	1.55	0.56–4.63	0.423
Not thrombolytic therapy	1.96	1.20–2.86	0.005	1.62	1.11–2.87	0.006

[a]Note that the odds ratio corresponds to a unit increase in the explanatory variable.
OR, odds ratio; CI, confidence interval; CRP, C-reactive protein; NIHSS, National Institutes of Health Stroke Scale; TACS, total anterior circulation syndrome.

of evidence from other studies suggested that D-D is associated with poor outcome in acute stroke [28–29].

The mechanism of the hemostatic system activation and the association between D-D concentration and functional outcome in patients with AIS remains unclear. The elevation of D-D concentration thus reflects hypercoagulation and this is considered a poor prognostic factor. First, increased D-Dr levels may reflect ongoing thrombus formation within cerebral vessels or may be a marker of systemic hypercoagulability [7]. Second, D-D may stimulate the inflammatory process. Activated inflammation and activated coagulation, in concert with each other, may contribute to the development of unfavorable outcome [30]. Furthermore, high D-D levels may be resistant to the endogenous fibrinolytic system [31]. In a word, D-D is both an acute phase reactant and a marker of turnover of cross-linked fibrin, generated by activation of coagulation and fibrinolysis; hence, it may represent the biological activation of both the inflammatory, haemostatic and fibrinolytic systems. However, we cannot be certain of the biological mechanisms behind elevated D-D levels predicting acute stroke outcome, and it is necessary to exercise caution in implying causality from epidemiological studies.

There are some limitations to our study. First, our study sample was restricted to individuals with acute ischemic stroke in the first 24 hours of symptom onset and thus is not representative of stroke patients in general. In addition, a single researcher assessed consecutive admissions to the hospital using relatively few exclusion criteria, other than those to establish the diagnosis of acute ischemic stroke also should be considered. Second, we cannot exclude the possibility that D-D levels increased after stroke onset as acute phase reactants. Third, we cannot exclude the possibility that plasma D-D increased under immobile state such as aspiration pneumonia and venous thrombosis. D-D level is very rarely elevated in healthy individuals, however, may increase in many illnesses and physiological conditions associated with thrombosis and thrombolysis [3]. These patients may have had widespread vascular disease before stroke onset and are, therefore, likely to have increased pre-event levels when compared with population controls. Forth, without serial measurement of the circulating D-D levels, this study yielded no data regarding when and how long D-D is elevated in these patients. Haapaniemi et al [3] reported that following AIS, D-D levels gradually increase peaking around 2 weeks, remain high for several weeks, and then gradually decrease. Fifth, long-term MRI and clinical follow-up data were not included in the study protocol, so these relationships were not examined beyond the 90-day clinical outcome. Lastly, all patients in our study were submitted to MRI in order to obtain the MRI results. In this process, the inclusion criterion may have introduced a selection bias, where only the least severe patients (who could stand a MRI) were studied.

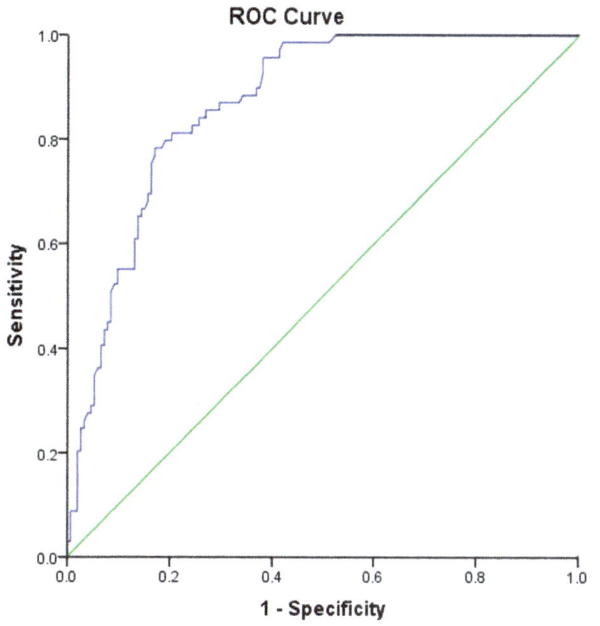

Figure 4. Receiver operating characteristic (ROC) curves were utilized to evaluate the accuracy of D-dimer levels to predict short-term outcomes.

Conclusions

Our study suggests that D-D levels are a useful tool to predict outcome and mortality 90-day after acute ischemic stroke in Chinese population and have a potential to assist clinicians.

Acknowledgments

We are grateful to the Department of emergency; the nurses, physicians, and patients who participated in our study; and the staff of the central laboratory of the Hospital.

Author Contributions

Conceived and designed the experiments: X-YY X-SZ J-EW. Performed the experiments: X-YY X-SZ J-EW. Analyzed the data: X-YY SG J-EW. Contributed reagents/materials/analysis tools: X-YY SG JD YC J-EW. Wrote the paper: X-YY SG.

References

1. Liu L, Wang D, Wong KSL, Wang Y (2011) Stroke and Stroke Care in China Huge Burden, Significant Workload, and a National Priority. Stroke 42: 3651–3654.
2. Meng R, Wang X, Hussain M, Dornbos D 3rd, Meng L, et al (2013) Evaluation of plasma d-dimer plus fibrinogen in predicting acute CVST. International Journal of Stroke, doi: 10.1111/ijs.12034. [Epub ahead of print].
3. Haapaniemi E, Tatlisumak T (2009) Is D-dimer helpful in evaluating stroke patients? A systematic review. Acta Neurologica Scandinavica 119: 141–150.
4. Lowe GD, Rumley A (1999) Use of fibrinogen and fibrin D-dimer in prediction of arterial thrombotic events. Thromb Haemost 82: 667–672.
5. Mahé I, Bergmann JF, Chassany O, dit-Sollier CB, Simoneau G, et al (2012) A multicentric prospective study in usual care: D-dimer and cardiovascular events in patients with atrial fibrillation. Thromb Res 129: 693–699.
6. Goldenberg NA, Jenkins S, Jack J, Armstrong-Wells J, Fenton LZ, et al (2013) Arteriopathy, D-Dimer, and Risk of Poor Neurologic Outcome in Childhood-Onset Arterial Ischemic Stroke. J Pediatr 162: 1041–1046.
7. Yuan W, Shi ZH (2013) The relationship between plasma D-dimer levels and outcome of Chinese acute ischemic stroke patients in different stroke subtypes. J Neural Transm, Doi: 10.1007/s00702-013-1113-y [Epub ahead of print].
8. Koch H J, Horn M, Bogdahn U, Ickenstein GW (2005) The relationship between plasma D-dimer concentrations and acute ischemic stroke subtypes. J Stroke Cerebrovasc Dis 14: 75–79.
9. Park YW, Koh EJ, Choi HY (2011) Correlation between serum D-dimer level and volume in acute ischemic stroke. J Korean Neurosurg Soc 50: 89–94.
10. Berge E, Friis P, Sandset P (2001) Hemostatic activation in acute ischemic stroke. Thromb Res 101: 13–21.
11. Delgado P, Alvarez-Sabin J, Abilleira S, Santamarina E, Purroy F, et al (2006) Plasma D-dimer predicts poor outcome after acute intracerebral hemorrhage. Neurology 67: 94–98.
12. Juvela S, Siironen J (2006) D-dimer as an independent predictor for poor outcome afteraneurysmal subarachnoid hemorrhage. Stroke 37: 1451–1456.
13. Hatano S (1976) Experience from a multicentre stroke register: a preliminary report. Bull World Health Organ 54: 541–553.
14. Brott T, Adams HP Jr, Olinger CP, Marler JR, Barsan WG, et al (1989) Measurements of acute cerebral infarction: A clinical examination scale. Stroke 20: 864–70.
15. Adams HP, Bendixen BH, Kappelle LJ, Biller J, Love BB, et al (1993) Classification of subtype of acute ischemic stroke. Definitions for use in a multicenter clinical trial. TOAST. Trial of Org 10172 in Acute Stroke Treatment. Stroke 24: 35–41.
16. Bamford J, Sandercock P, Dennis M, Burn J, Warlow C (1991)Classification and natural history of clinically identifiable subtypes of cerebral infarction. Lancet 337: 1521–1526.
17. Sims JR, Gharai LR, Schaefer PW, Vangel M, Rosenthal ES (2009) ABC/2 for rapid clinical estimate of infarct, perfusion, and mismatch volumes. Neurology 72: 2104–2110.
18. Bonita R, Beaglehole R (1988) Recovery of motor function after stroke. Stroke 19: 1497–1500.
19. Chiu CC, Li YN, Lin LJ, Hsiao CT, Hsiao KY, et al (2012) Serum D-dimer as a predictor of mortality in patients with acute spontaneous intracerebral hemorrhage. J Clin Neurosci 19: 810–813.
20. Welsh P, Barber M, Langhorne P, Rumley A, Lowe GD,et al (2009) Associations of inflammatory and haemostatic biomarkers with poor outcome in acute ischaemic stroke. Cerebrovascular Dis 27: 247–253.
21. Barber M, Langhorne P, Rumley A, Lowe GD, Stott DJ (2006) D-dimer predictsearly clinical progression in ischemic stroke: confirmation using routineclinical assays. Stroke 37: 1113–1115.
22. Whiteley W, Jackson C, Lewis S, Lowe G, Rumley A, et al (2009) Inflammatory markers and poor outcome after stroke: a prospective cohort study and systematic review of interleukin-6. PLoS medicine 6: e1000145.

23. Tu WJ, Dong X, Zhao SJ, Yang DG, Chen H (2013) Prognostic value of plasma neuroendocrine biomarkers in patients with acute ischemic stroke. J Neuroendocrinol 25: 771–778.
24. Katan M, Fluri F, Morgenthaler NG, Schuetz P, Zweifel C, et al (2009) Copeptin: a novel, independent prognostic marker in patients with ischemic stroke. Ann Neurol 66: 799–808.
25. Tu WJ, Zhao SJ, Xu DJ, Chen H (2014) Serum 25-hydroxyvitamin D predicts the short-term outcomes of Chinese patients with acute ischaemic stroke. Clinical Science 126: 339–346.
26. Kang DW, Yoo SH, Chun S, Kwon KY, Kwon SU, et al (2009) Inflammatory and hemostatic biomarkers associated with early recurrent ischemic lesions in acute ischemic stroke. Stroke 40: 1653–1658.
27. Barber M, Langhorne P, Rumley A, Lowe GD, Stott DJ (2004) Hemostatic-function and progressing ischemic stroke: D-dimer predicts early clinical progression. Stroke 35: 1421–1425.
28. Di Napoli M, Papa F, Villa Pini (2002) Stroke DataBank Investigators: Inflammation, hemostaticmarkers, and antithrombotic agents inrelation to long-term risk of new cardiovascularevents in first ever ischemic stroke patients. Stroke 33: 1763–1771.
29. Ageno W, Finazzi S, Steidl L, Biotti MG, Mera V, et al (2002) Plasmameasurement of D -dimer levels for the earlydiagnosis of ischemic stroke subtypes. Arch Intern Med 162: 2589–2593.
30. Csala M, Lerant I, Banhegyi G, Kardon T, Puskas F, et al (1998) Prostaglandin-independent stimulation ofinterleukin-6 production by fibrinogen degradation product D in perfusedmurine liver. Scand J Immunol 48: 269–271.
31. Urbach H, Hartmann A, Pohl C, Omran H, Wilhelm K, et al (2002) Local intra-arterial thrombolysis in the carotid territory: does recanalization depend on the thromboembolus type? Neuroradiology 44: 695–699.

11

Pre-Existing Hypertension Dominates γδT Cell Reduction in Human Ischemic Stroke

Mateusz G. Adamski[1,2], Yan Li[1], Erin Wagner[1], Hua Yu[1], Chloe Seales-Bailey[1], Helen Durkin[3], Qing Hao[1], Steven A. Soper[4], Michael Murphy[5], Alison E. Baird[1]*

1 Department of Neurology, SUNY Downstate Medical Center, Brooklyn, New York, United States of America, **2** Department of Neurology, Jagiellonian University Medical College, Krakow, Poland, **3** Department of Pathology, SUNY Downstate Medical Center, Brooklyn, New York, United States of America, **4** University of North Carolina, Chapel Hill, North Carolina, United States of America, **5** Louisiana State University, Baton Rouge, Louisiana, United States of America

Abstract

T lymphocytes may play an important role in the evolution of ischemic stroke. Depletion of γδT cells has been found to abrogate ischemia reperfusion injury in murine stroke. However, the role of γδT cells in human ischemic stroke is unknown. We aimed to determine γδT cell counts and γδT cell interleukin 17A (IL-17A) production in the clinical setting of ischemic stroke. We also aimed to determine the associations of γδT cell counts with ischemic lesion volume, measures of clinical severity and with major stroke risk factors. Peripheral blood samples from 43 acute ischemic stroke patients and 26 control subjects matched on race and gender were used for flow cytometry and complete blood count analyses. Subsequently, cytokine levels and gene expression were measured in γδT cells. The number of circulating γδT cells was decreased by almost 50% ($p = 0.005$) in the stroke patients. γδT cell counts did not correlate with lesion volume on magnetic resonance diffusion-weighted imaging or with clinical severity in the stroke patients, but γδT cells showed elevated levels of IL-17A ($p = 0.048$). Decreased γδT cell counts were also associated with older age ($p = 0.004$), pre-existing hypertension ($p = 0.0005$) and prevalent coronary artery disease ($p = 0.03$), with pre-existing hypertension being the most significant predictor of γδT cell counts in a multivariable analysis. γδT cells in human ischemic stroke are reduced in number and show elevated levels of IL-17A. A major reduction in γδT lymphocytes also occurs in hypertension and may contribute to the development of hypertension-mediated stroke and vascular disease.

Editor: Jason R. Lees, Uniform Services University of the Health Sciences, United States of America

Funding: This work was supported by the National Institute of Biomedical Imaging and Bioengineering/NIH (R01-EB010087) to A.E.B., M.M., and S.A.S. The funders had no role in study design, data collection and analysis, decision to publish, or preparation of the manuscript.

Competing Interests: The authors have declared that no competing interests exist.

* E-mail: alison.baird@downstate.edu

Introduction

Stroke is a leading cause of death and disability in the United States [1]. The immune system is recognized as playing a major role in the evolution and pathophysiology of stroke and microvascular dysfunction, with a growing number of reports on the role of T lymphocytes [2–7].

γδT cells are a population of T lymphocytes that comprise between 0 and 7% of circulating $CD3^+$ cells [8]. These cells express γδ T cell receptors (TCR), whereas the majority of T lymphocytes express αβTCR. γδT cells secrete interleukin-17 (IL-17) when stimulated by interleukin-23 (IL-23) and interferon gamma (INF-γ) when stimulated by interleukin-12 (IL-12) [9,10]. As a bridge cell population γδT cells break the classical immune system paradigm by having features of both the adaptive (e.g., the antigen experienced response) and innate (i.e., the rapid response) immune responses. γδT cells that secrete IL-17 have been characterized as ligand-naive and γδT cells that secrete INF-γ have been characterized as ligand-experienced [9].

In a prior study depletion of γδT cells in mice ameliorated ischemia-reperfusion injury in the brain [11]. When analyzing the mechanistic basis of γδT cells in this model, Shichita et al. [11] identified important roles and interactions of IL-23 and IL-17 but not INF-γ. After ischemia reperfusion injury, increased macrophage IL-23 secretion commenced after day 1 and increased γδT cell IL-17 secretion commenced after day 3. In this same model, infarct size was reduced on day 1 in IL-23 knockout (KO) mice and on day 4 in IL-17 KO mice but was not altered in INF-γ KO mice. Intracellular cytokine staining confirmed that γδT cells were the main source of IL-17, $CD4^+$ and γδTCR- T cells were the main sources of INF-γ.

To date there is little data on the role of γδT cells in human stroke [12]. The mice in Shichita et al's study [11] were young and apparently free of vascular risk factors, while older age, a major risk factor for stroke, has been associated with reduced γδT cell counts [13,14]. Furthermore, hypertension and coronary artery disease, other major stroke risk factors, have been associated with alterations in IL-17 and IFN-γ [15–18]. Therefore, our objectives were to determine γδT cell counts and function in the clinical setting of ischemic stroke and the associations of γδT cell counts with lesion volume, measures of clinical severity and with major stroke risk factors. We have investigated whether circulating γδT cell counts are 1) altered in patients presenting with acute ischemic human stroke, and 2) correlate with: lesion volume on diffusion-weighted magnetic resonance imaging (DW MRI), and with clinical severity and demographic and risk factors. Next we

Table 1. Clinical and laboratory characteristics of patients and controls.

Factor	All (n = 69)	Stroke (n = 43)	Control (n = 26)	p
Age	63.0 (52.0, 71.0)	70.0 (60.0, 73.0)	55.5 (50.2,61.0)	0.0002
Gender– male	28 (40)	18 (42)	10 (38)	0.9
Race– black	63 (91)	43 (93)	23 (88)	0.8
Risk factors				
Hypertension	54 (78)	41 (95)	13 (50)	<0.0001
Diabetes	24 (35)	16 (37)	8 (31)	0.8
Coronary artery disease	17 (25)	13 (30)	4 (15)	0.3
Smoking history	33 (48)	11 (25)	22 (85)	<0.0001
Atrial fibrillation	6 (9)	6 (14)	0 (0)	0.12
Hyperlipidemia	29 (42)	19 (44)	10 (38)	0.8
Medications				
Diuretics	13 (20)	11 (27)	2 (8)	0.10
ACEIs/ARBs	20 (30)	18 (45)	2 (8)	0.003
Beta blockers	29 (44)	22 (55)	7 (27)	0.046
Calcium channel blockers	18 (27)	14 (35)	4 (15)	0.14
Antithrombotics	28 (42)	20 (50)	8 (31)	0.2
Statins	24 (36)	16 (40)	8 (31)	0.6
Stroke-Related				
Infarct volume (mm^3)	N/A	2,367.3 (1,028.4, 14,491.5)	N/A	N/A
NIHSS score	N/A	5.0 (3.0, 9.0)	N/A	N/A
Barthel score at 3–6 months	N/A	95.0 (87.5, 100)	N/A	N/A

Results are median (interquartile range) for continuous factors and numbers (%) for categorical factors. ACEI – angiotensin converting enzyme inhibitor, ARB - angiotensin receptor blocker, N/A – not applicable, NIHSS – National Institutes of Health Stroke Scale, Wilcoxon rank sum tests were used to compare the ages between the stroke patients and the control subjects. Chi-square and Fishers' exact tests were used to compare the remaining demographic, risk factors and medications between the stroke patients and the control subjects.

examined γδT cell levels of IL-17A and INF-γ and the cellular gene expression of interleukin-23 receptor (*IL-23R*) and interleukin-23 subunit alpha (*IL-23A*).

Methods

Approval was obtained from the SUNY Downstate Medical Center Institutional Review Board for this prospective observational study. All patients and/or authorized representatives gave full and signed informed consent.

Study Subjects

The peripheral blood samples of 69 subjects were used: 43 acute stroke patients admitted to the University Hospital of Brooklyn at SUNY Downstate Medical Center and at Long Island College Hospital, and 26 gender and race matched healthy control subjects recruited from the local community. The clinical and laboratory characteristics of patients and controls are shown in Table 1. The age range of the subjects was 30–95 years. The median time of blood draw was 36±29 hours post stroke. Stroke was diagnosed according to World Health Organization stroke criteria.

The study inclusion criteria were: over 18 years of age and acute ischemic stroke. The exclusion criteria were: current immunological diseases, taking steroid or immunosuppressive therapies, severe allergies, acute infection and severe anemia. The following clinical data were recorded: age, gender, race, self-reported risk factors, medications at the time of stroke onset (based on 40 subjects) or, in the control subjects, medications at the time of blood draw, National Institutes of Health Stroke Scale (NIHSS) score in the stroke subjects and complete blood counts (CBC), including total white blood cell count and white cell differential counts. Hypertension was defined as a prior (at any time in the

Table 2. Monoclonal antibodies.

Target	Antibody clone	Fluorophore	Volume used	Catalogue number	Manufacturer
CD3	S4.1	PE–Texas Red	0.5 µl	MHCD0317	Invitrogen
CD4	RPA-T4	FITC	2 µl	555346	BD Biosciences
γδTCR	11F2	PE	2 µl	340887	Becton Dickinson
CD8	HIT8a	PE–Cy5	2 µl	555636	BD Pharmingen

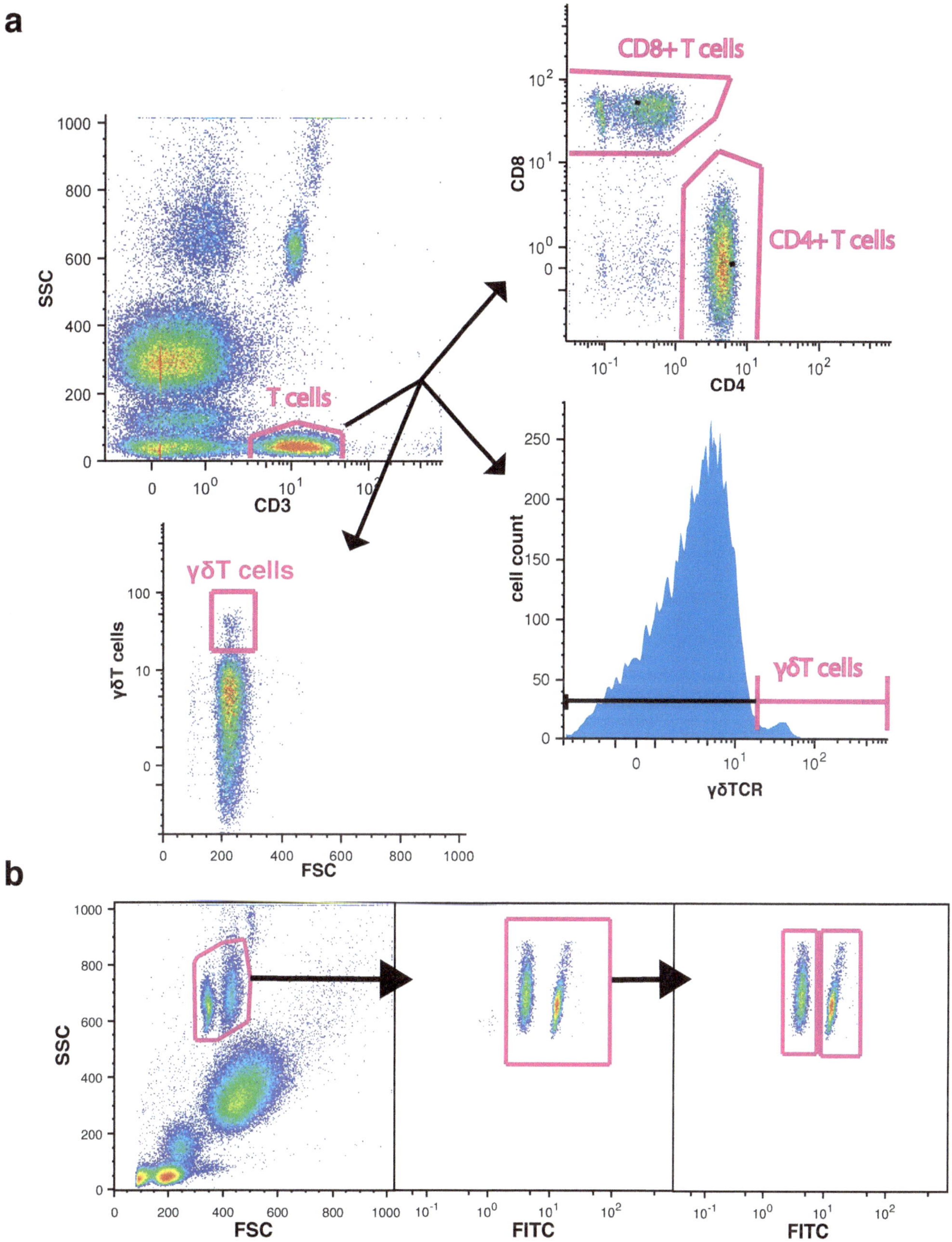

Figure 1. Gating strategy to identify T cell subsets (CD4+, CD8+ and γδTCR+) and counting beads based on a representative sample. (a) Gating strategy to identify T cell subsets. T lymphocytes were selected based on CD3 expression and side scatter (SSC) characteristics. The CD3+ population was further divided into CD4+/CD8+ T lymphocytes (based on CD4 and CD8 expression) and γδT positive and negative CD3 cells (based

on γδTCR expression). (b) Gating strategy to identify counting beads. First, two populations of counting beads were selected based on the forward and side scatter characteristics. Second, FITC positive beads were counted for the cell count analyses. Third, the frequency of each bead population was assessed to compare with bead lot characteristics.

past) diagnosis of hypertension by the subject's physician or currently receiving treatment for hypertension. Diabetes was defined as a past medical history of known diabetes mellitus. Coronary artery disease was defined as a physician-diagnosed past history of ischemic heart disease or angina. Hyperlipidemia was defined as a past history of documented elevation in total cholesterol (>200 mg/dl). Smoking was defined as current or prior smoking. Atrial fibrillation was defined as a past or current history of physician-diagnosed atrial fibrillation.

In the stroke patients lesion volumes were independently measured by two observers with neuroimaging expertise who were blinded to the clinical and laboratory data. Ischemic lesion volumes were measured on magnetic resonance imaging diffusion weighted images using Medical Image Processing Analysis and Visualization software. Neurological severity was based on the admission National Institutes of Health Stroke Scale (NIHSS) score. Follow-up assessment used the Barthel scores at 3 to 6 months (based on 33 patients) that provides a measure of the amount of stroke recovery and disability.

Flow Cytometry

Peripheral blood from the study participants was drawn to BD Vacutainer tubes containing ethylenediaminetetraacetate (EDTA). Within an hour from blood collection 100 μl of blood was stained in the dark for 30 minutes in room temperature with four monoclonal antibodies (Ab) to CD3, CD4, CD8 and γδTCR (Table 2). Following staining, erythrocytes were lysed and leukocytes were fixed according to manufacturer No-Wash Lysis Procedure (Cal-Lyse solution Invitrogen). Counting beads (AccuCheck Counting Beads Invitrogen) were added, following manufacturer protocol, to obtain absolute cell counts (gating strategy presented in the Figure 1). Data were collected on the Epics XL flow cytometer (Beckman Coulter). Three populations of T lymphocytes were analyzed: CD8+, CD4+ and γδTCR+. T lymphocytes were defined as CD3+ cells within the lymphocyte gate. The lymphocyte gate was set based on side scatter characteristics. Gating strategy was set to include CD3+ cells regardless of size, not to exclude activated (larger) and apoptotic (smaller) lymphocytes (Figure 1). Based on forward scatter (FSC) values, size of CD3+ lymphocytes was not different from the size of γδT cells (mean ±standard deviation, respectively: 182±14 and 187±16; $p>0.05$) as presented on FCS vs. γδTCR+ plot (Figure 1). γδT cells size did not differ between stroke and control (mean ±standard deviation, respectively: 188±17 and 184±14; $p>0.05$). 200,000 events were acquired for each sample. Raw data were compensated, analyzed and presented using FlowJo software version 9.2 for Mac (Tree Star, San Carlos, California). Ab were titrated to achieve optimal resolution and gates for CD8+, CD4+ and γδTCR+ T lymphocytes were set using fluorescence minus one (FMO) method [19].

Cytokine Levels and Gene Expression in γδT cells

γδT cells were extracted from 35 study subjects (17 stroke, 18 control). A detailed protocol for γδT cell sorting has been published previously [20]. Briefly, γδT cells were extracted from whole blood using magnetic bead separation (Miltenyi Biotec) – γδT cell purity was over 80%. RNA and proteins were extracted using column separation (Norgen). Quality and concentration of RNA and protein was measured using Qubit 1.0 Fluorometer (Invitrogen). Protein concentration was measured in 28 study subjects (10 stroke, 18 controls). The concentration of IL-17A and INF-γ in proteins extracted from γδT cell was determined by flow cytometry using BD cytometric bead array. Samples processing was performed according to the manufacturers instructions (BD Bioscience) using Human IL-17A Flex Set and Human IFN-γ Flex Set. Results were analyzed using FCAP Array version 3 software (BD Bioscience). Gene expression was measured in 29 study subjects (17 stroke, 12 control). RNA reverse transcription PCR was based on random hexamers (Life Technologies). The primers were designed using NCBI/Primer-Blast (Primer3 and BLAST), and wet tested. High throughput real time PCR run on BioMark HD system (Fluidigm) was used to measure gene expression of IL-23R and IL-23A genes. To compare gene expression between samples relative analytic approach was used. The relative analysis was based on the cell count input for each sample and was normalized to commercial cDNA (Universal cDNA Reverse Transcribed by Random Hexamer: Human Normal Tissues; Biochain, Newark, CA). Subjects selected for cytokine expression and gene expression were representative for the entire group used for cell phenotyping.

Table 3. Leukocyte subset cellular counts in stroke and control subjects.

	All (n = 69)	Stroke (n = 43)	Control (n = 26)	p
$\gamma\delta^{+}$T (cells/μl)	98.6 (52.8, 197.0)	79.4 (45.7, 163.0)	137.0 (85.4, 254.5)	0.005
$CD4^{+}$T (cells/μl)	3972.0 (2471.0, 5252.0	3903.0 (2641.0, 4835.0)	4346.5 (2430.5, 6862.0)	0.14
$CD8^{+}$T (cells/μl)	1463.0 (950.0, 2094.0)	1343.0 (876.5, 1799.0)	1737.5 (993.7, 2487.7)	0.08
Neutrophils (10^{9}/ml)	3.6 (2.8, 4.3)	3.7 (3.1, 4.8)	2.9 (2.4, 4.0)	0.045
Monocytes (10^{9}/ml)	0.4 (0.3, 0.5)	0.4 (0.3, 0.5)	0.4 (0.3, 0.5)	0.99
Lymphocytes (10^{9}/ml)	1.7 (1.3, 2.0)	1.6 (1.0, 1.9)	1.9 (1.5, 2.2)	0.026
Total WBC (10^{9}/ml)	5.8 (4.8,7.3)	5.8 (5.2, 7.4)	5.5 (4.3, 6.8)	0.3

Values are median (interquartile range). $\gamma\delta^{+}$T, $CD4^{+}$T and $CD8^{+}$T count was measured with flow cytometry; Neutrophil, Monocyte, Lymphocyte and Total WBC was measured with complete blood count; WBC – white blood cell. Wilcoxon rank sum tests were used to compare leukocyte cellular counts between the stroke patients and the control subjects.

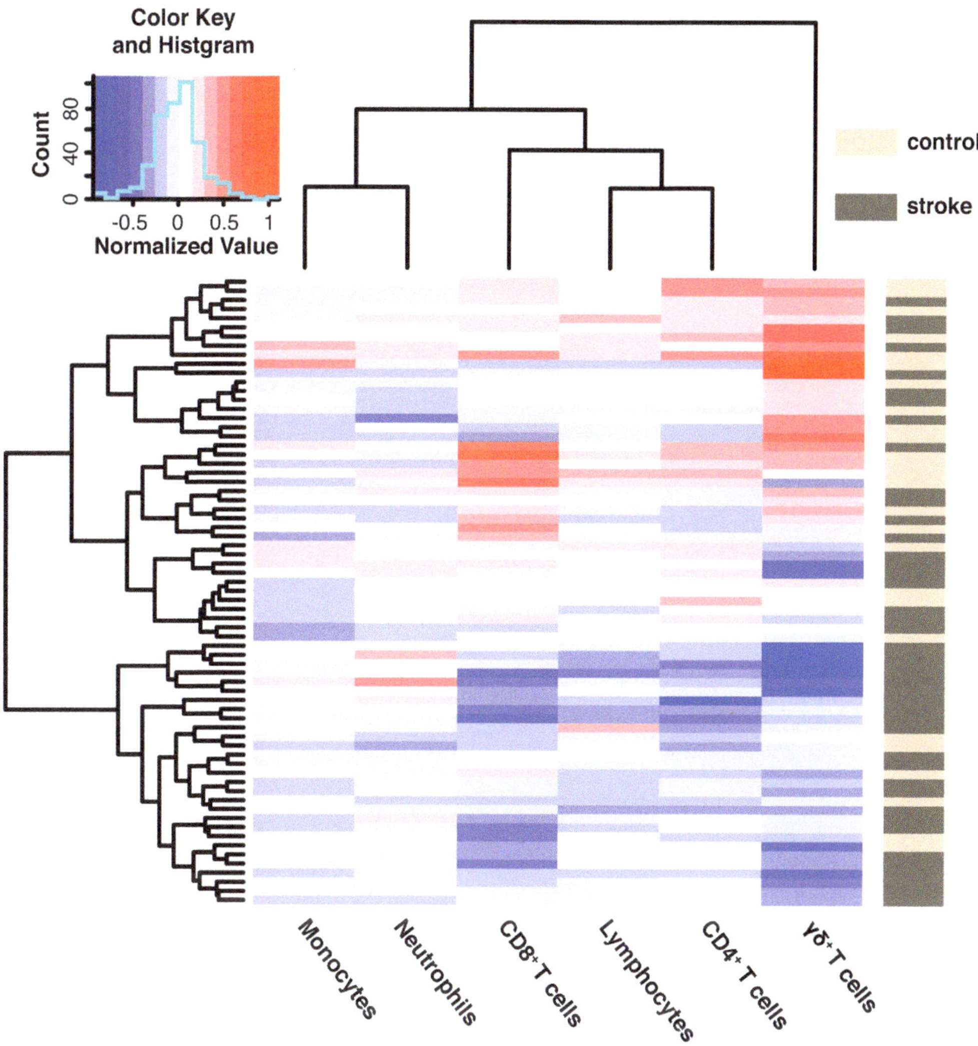

Figure 2. γδT cells were differentially altered in this clinical cohort relative to 5 other leukocyte subsets. This heatmap illustrates the normalized cell counts for 6 leukocyte cell subsets (columns) in the study subjects (rows). Cell numbers for neutrophils, monocytes and total lymphocytes were determined from the complete blood count, and cell numbers for $CD4^+$, $CD8^+$ and $\gamma\delta^+$ T lymphocytes were measured using flow cytometry. The column dendrogram reveals clustering by leukocyte subset, demonstrating that the γδT cell subset formed a separate and dominant cluster from the other five leukocyte subsets. The γδT cell cluster separates into decreased and increased cellular counts, with decreased cellular counts predominating in the stroke subjects. This hierarchical cluster analysis used Ward's method and log-transformed and normalized cell count data.

Statistical Analyses

The data were analyzed using R version 2.15.2 [21]. Non-parametric and parametric tests, as appropriate, were used to compare demographic and laboratory values between the stroke and control subjects (Wilcoxon rank sum and Student's *t*, tests).Spearman correlation coefficients were used for correlational analyses. Chi-square and Fishers' exact tests were used to compare grouped data. The hierarchical cluster analysis used Ward's method and log transformed and normalized cell count data.

A factorial analysis of variance (section 4 of the Results) was used to evaluate for potential interactions in the associations of stroke and hypertension on γδT cell subset counts. Levene's tests confirmed homogeneity of the variances of the independent factors. A linear regression analysis was performed to adjust for baseline differences between patients and controls and to control for major potential confounders in the associations of hypertension and stroke with γδT cell counts. Measurements of the global validation statistic, skewness, kurtosis, link function and heteroscedasticity confirmed that all model assumptions were met. The γδT cell count data were log transformed for this analysis. P values <0.05 were considered statistically significant.

Results

1. Reduction of γδT cell numbers in human ischemic stroke

The absolute number of circulating γδT cells was reduced in the stroke subjects relative to the controls, by almost 50% ($p = 0.005$, **Table 3**). In the stroke patients the median γδT cell count was 79.4 cells/µl while in the control subjects the median number of γδT cells was 137.0 cells/µl. γδT cells accounted for a median of 1.92% (range 0.28–22.9%) of $CD3^+$ lymphocytes.

Table 4. Associations of γδT cell counts with demographic and risk factors for all study subjects (n = 69).

γδT Cell Counts (cells/μl)	Factor Present	Factor Absent	p
Demographic Factors			
Age≥60 years	72.5 (29.8, 171.7)	130.0 (94.1, 238.0)	0.004
Gender - male	96.0 (59.0, 159.7)	102.0 (50.3, 199.0)	0.8
Race - black	102.0 (52.8, 193.5)	77.9 (53.4, 171.7)	0.8
Risk Factors			
Hypertension	80.6 (49.8, 148.5)	217.0 (126.5, 293.0)	0.0005
Diabetes	90.7 (55.6, 195.2)	98.6 (58.2, 197.0)	0.97
Coronary artery disease	59.9 (27.6, 141.0)	109.5 (64.8, 211.0)	0.03
Smoking history	120 (69.2, 209.0)	87.5 (42.2, 171.7)	0.08
Atrial fibrillation	90.2 (55.1, 172.4)	102.0 (52.8, 193.5)	0.7
Hyperlipidemia	102.0 (56.5, 171.0)	97.3 (50.1, 222.2)	0.9
Medications			
Diuretics	102.0 (69.2, 182.0)	96.1 (50.7, 199.0)	0.73
ACEIs/ARBs	87.5 (49.8, 169.2)	109.5 (55.8, 217.2)	0.34
Beta blockers	72.7 (29.3, 157.5)	130.0 (73.5, 228.0)	0.02
Calcium channel blockers	72.5 (51.5, 176.2)	105.0 (52.4, 211.2)	0.32
Antithrombotics	72.5 (46.0, 141.0)	125.0 (70.1, 233.0)	0.03
Statins	97.6 (65.0, 176.0)	102.0 (47.0, 215.0)	0.81

Values are median (interquartile range). Wilcoxon rank sum tests were used to compare γδT cellular counts with demographics, risk factors and medication usage.

γδT cells were disproportionately altered relative to the five other leukocyte subsets studied (**Figure 2**). Mild increases in neutrophils ($p = 0.045$) and decreases in the total number of lymphocytes ($p = 0.03$) were present in the ischemic stroke patients, while $CD4^+$ and $CD8^+$ T cells were non-significantly reduced (**Table 3**) and monocyte counts were unaltered ($p = 0.99$, **Table 3**).

2. γδT cell numbers did not correlate with lesion volume or clinical severity

There was no association of γδT cell count with ischemic lesion volume on DW MRI (coefficient $= -0.03$, $p = 0.9$). There was also no association of γδT cell number with stroke severity as measured by the NIHSS (coefficient $= -012$, $p = 0.4$) or with outcome (coefficient $= 0.02$, $p = 0.9$).

Table 5. T cell numbers in subjects with and without pre-existing hypertension.

Subjects	γδT (cells/μl)	CD4 (cells/μl)	CD8 (cells/μl)
All Subjects			
Normotension (n = 15)	217.0 (126.5, 293.0)	4394.0 (2495.0, 7399.0)	2168.0 (1503.0, 3564.5)
Hypertension (n = 54)	80.6 (49.8, 148.5)	3885.5 (2458.7, 4865.7)	1238.5 (868.2, 1765.2)
p	0.0005	0.14	0.008
Control Subjects			
Normotension (n = 13)	238.0 (199.0, 316.0)	5427.0 (2471.0, 7682.0)	2168.0 (1657.0, 4064.0)
Hypertension (n = 13)	81.8 (59.9, 111.0)	3778.0 (2417.0, 5524.0)	1230.0 (950.0, 1754.0)
p	0.0006	0.5	0.1
Stroke Subjects			
Normotension (n = 2)	73.1 (61.7, 84.6)	3680.5 (3534.8, 3826.2)	2207.0 (1778.0, 2636.0)
Hypertension (n = 41)	79.4 (45.3, 171.0)	3903.0 (2588.0, 4856.0)	1247.0 (860.0, 1769.0)
p	0.8	0.9	0.27

Values are median (interquartile range). Wilcoxon rank sum test were used for the comparisons in T cell numbers between the subject groups.

Table 6. Linear regression model for γδT cell count.

Factor	Estimate	95% CI	T value	p
Age	−0.005	−0.04, 0.03	−0.02	0.80
Gender- male	0.12	−0.34, 0.58	0.53	0.60
Race- white	−0.04	−0.86, 0.77	−0.11	0.91
No hypertension	1.03	0.28, 1.78	2.73	0.008
Stroke	1.44	−1.08, 3.97	1.14	0.26
Hypertension:stroke interaction	−1.28	−2.87, 0.29	−1.62	0.11
Stroke:age interaction	−0.02	−0.06, 0.02	−1.13	0.26

Linear regression modeling was used to determine the relative impacts of hypertension and stroke on γδT cell counts and to adjust for clinical and demographic factors and potential interactions (for age, race and gender). This revealed that pre–existing hypertension was the significant predictor in the model accounting for γδT cell counts. Coronary artery disease had no effect when entered into the model, nor did smoking history, beta-blocker treatment, or antithrombotic treatment. CI– confidence intervals.

3. Correlation of γδT cell numbers with demographic and risk factors

γδT cell numbers were decreased in individuals over age 60 years ($p = 0.004$) and in individuals with a prior history of coronary artery disease ($p = 0.03$). There was no association of γδT cell count with race or gender (**Table 4**). There was a substantial decrease in γδT cell counts in individuals with pre-existing hypertension. γδT cell counts were reduced by over 60% in hypertensive subjects (80.6 cells/μl) relative to normotensive subjects (217.0 cells/μl, $p = 0.0005$, **Table 4**). γδT cell counts were reduced in patients taking antithrombotics ($p = 0.03$) or β-blockers ($p = 0.02$) but not altered in patients taking angiotensin converting enzyme (ACE) inhibitors, angiotensin II receptor blockers (ARB), diuretics or calcium channel blockers.

To further explore this finding, the cellular counts of the other T cell subsets were compared between subjects with and without hypertension. The $CD8^+$ subset ($p = 0.01$) was moderately reduced in individuals with hypertension while there was no significant difference in $CD4^+$ subset numbers in the subjects with hypertension (**Table 5**). γδT cell numbers were compared between the hypertensive and normotensive controls where substantial reductions were found- 81.8 cells/μl in hypertensive control subjects compared to 238.0 cells/μl in the normotensive control subjects ($p = 0.0006$, **Table 5**). This was not explained by age differences, as the median age was not significantly different between the control subjects with and without hypertension (58.0 vs. 52.0 years, respectively). $CD8^+$ T cells were non–significantly decreased in hypertensive control subjects relative to normotensive controls (**Table 5**).

4. Relative contributions of hypertension and stroke on γδT cell counts

In a factorial analysis of variance hypertension was the major determinant of γδT cellular counts (F value = 12.8; $p = 0.0006$). Stroke and hypertension:stroke interaction were not significant (respectively, F value = 1.54; $p = 0.22$ and F value = 2.1; $p = 0.15$). In linear regression analysis, adjusting for age, race and gender, pre–existing hypertension was also the most significant predictor of γδT cell counts ($p = 0.008$, **Table 6**). The estimated effect size of hypertension from the model was 2.77, indicating that hypertension is associated with a 64% reduction in γδT cell counts (**Table 6**). Coronary artery disease had no effect when entered into the model, nor did smoking history or beta-blocker or antithrombotic therapy.

5. Cytokine levels and gene expression in γδT cells

In γδT cells there were increased levels of IL-17A in the stroke patients relative to the controls ($p = 0.048$) with a similar trend in IL-17A/IFN-γ ratio ($p = 0.1$) and with no alterations in IFN γ levels (**Table 7**). There was a 3.3 fold non significant increase in *IL-23R* gene expression in γδT cells in the stroke patients ($p > 0.05$) with a 1.1 fold non significant decrease in *IL-23A* gene expression ($p > 0.05$). γδT cellular cytokine levels and gene expression were not significantly different between individuals with and without hypertension, with and without CAD and those over age 60 years relative to those less than age 60 years.

Table 7. γδT cellular cytokine levels (n = 28).

	Stroke	Control	p
IL-17A (ng/μl)*	7.01±2.3	4.78±3.1	0.048
IFN-γ (ng/μl)	2.4 (0.72, 3.58)	3.31 (1.43, 4.07)	0.4
IL-17A/IFN-γ ratio	3.3 (1.7, 6.2)	1.5 (0.9, 2.4)	0.1

Results are median (IQR) or mean* ± SD, as appropriate. Wilcoxon rank sum and Student's t tests, as appropriate, were used for the between group comparisons.

Discussion

In this study we found that γδT cell numbers were reduced in human ischemic stroke and that γδT cells showed elevated IL-17A secretion. Reductions in γδT lymphocytes were also associated with hypertension, older age and, to a lesser degree, with prevalent coronary artery disease. Hypertension was associated with γδT cell count reductions of almost 65%. To the best of our knowledge this is the first clinical study showing the potential roles of γδT lymphocytes in stroke, hypertension and hypertension-mediated stroke.

In this study, the increase in IL-17A but not in INF-γ levels in the γδT cells of the stroke patients suggests activation of the IL-23 and IL-17 cytokine expression pathway. This is in line with previous reports by Shichita et al. from a murine stroke model and by Li et al. from human ischemic brain tissues [11,22]. This increase in IL-17 expression from antigen-naive γδT cells may reflect a non-specific/antigen naive immune response to stroke [9,10,23]. Contrary to this murine study of Shichita et al. where γδT cell depletion ameliorated ischemia-reperfusion injury [11] we did not find associations of γδT cell counts with lesion volume, stroke severity and outcome. However, associations with lesion size and outcome and severity might be found in a larger patient sample.

Changes in leukocyte numbers, as reflected by elevated neutrophil counts and reductions in lymphocyte counts are common in acute stroke and reflect the phenomenon of adrenergic mediated stroke-induced immunodepression [24]. In stroke, activation of the sympathetic nervous system causes shrinkage of the spleen due to the release of residual cells [25–27] and is essential to the release of hepatic invariant NKT cells [6]. Blockade of the sympathetic nervous system has been shown to modulate circulating regulatory T cell numbers [28] and to change the activity of $CD8^+$ and $CD4^+$ T cells [29]. Stimulation of the sympathetic nervous system by acute stress has also been associated with increased numbers of circulating T cells expressing receptors for chemokines secreted by activated endothelial cells [30]. The reductions in γδT cells seen in this study may indicate that this is one of the populations of T lymphocytes that are regulated by the stress induced sympathetic response [6,30]. Although, we did not specifically study the role of sympathetic activation in this study, we note that patients treated with β-blockers had significantly decreased numbers of circulating γδT cells.

The reductions of γδT cellular numbers in the stroke patients were disproportionately larger than reductions in the other lymphocyte subsets. Our results show that older age, hypertension and coronary artery disease were also associated with γδT cellular counts, with hypertension dominating γδT cell reductions. Older age has previously been reported to be associated with altered γδT cell counts [13,14]. In CAD, no alterations in γδT cell counts have been reported to date, but decreases in $CD3^+$ lymphocytes and increases of IFN–γ secreting $CD8^+CD56^+$ T lymphocytes and of $CD28^-CD4^+$ T lymphocytes - also a significant source of IFN–γ - have been reported [15–17]. Coronary artery infiltrating T lymphocytes producing IL–17 and IFN–γ [18] have been described. Given that γδT cells are a major source of both IL-17 and IFN–γ, our finding of decreased numbers of γδT cells in CAD is deserving of further study.

Hence, while the stroke patients and control subjects were matched on race and gender the subjects were not matched on age and hypertension status, which were associated with γδT cell counts. Given this finding, and given that most stroke patients are hypertensive, in order to fully and further explore the decrease in the gamma delta T cell counts in stroke patients stroke patients should be matched with controls based on their hypertension score.

Hypertension was overall the strongest determinant of γδT cell counts. Hypertension was the factor that was most strongly associated with γδT cell counts and was the most significant predictor in factorial and linear regression analyses. Markedly reduced cellular counts were also seen in the hypertensive control subjects, relative to the normotensive control subjects.

Hypertension is by far the most significant, modifiable risk factor for both ischemic and hemorrhagic stroke [31–33]. The high prevalence of hypertension in our non–Hispanic Black Caribbean stroke population is typical of many stroke cohorts. Hypertension has classically been considered a disorder of the renin angiotensin system or of the brain. Recently in rodent studies it has been demonstrated that T lymphocytes are required for the full development of angiotensin II induced hypertension [34]. T lymphocytes were found to infiltrate the adventitia and peri-adventitial fat of vessels [34] and T cells secreting IL–17 have been found in the vessel walls of hypertensive animals [34–36], potentially due to induction of hypertension-induced expression of homing receptors [35]. Furthermore, plasma and tissue levels of IL–17 and IFN–γ have been independently related with the development of hypertension, but the cellular sources were not identified [36]. As γδT cells secrete and are key sources of IL–17 and IFN–γ in the blood and IL–17 in the brain [4,8,37], the decrease in the number of circulating γδT cells in our study may be due to their active role in the evolution of hypertension and possible mobilization into vascular walls or their removal from the circulation. As the number of γδT cells distinguished the already diagnosed hypertensive subjects from non–hypertensive subjects, regardless of the medications being taken, as yet unrecognized pathophysiological mechanisms may be involved- other than targeted by current antihypertensive agents [38].

The implications of our results are that we have recognized two T lymphocyte subsets – the γδT and the CD8 subsets - that may be involved in human hypertension [39], with γδT cells possibly linking hypertension to stroke. γδT cells were identified for the first time as a potential marker of stroke risk in hypertensive individuals or of vascular disease burden. Alterations in $CD8^+$ T lymphocytes support a recent finding where subsets of these cells were found to contribute to human hypertension [40]. The importance of these findings are highlighted by the fact that hypertension is the most common vascular disease worldwide with 5–30% of individuals remaining resistant to available treatments [31]. Hypertension–related morbidity comes largely from its downstream vascular consequences that include atherosclerotic vascular disease, heart disease and stroke, with stroke being the preeminent complication. Elucidating as yet unrecognized mechanisms of both hypertension and stroke could give new perspectives to the understanding of these diseases and possibly lead to novel treatments. Furthermore, this study demonstrates the importance of incorporating vascular risk factors in stroke translational research studies.

Author Contributions

Conceived and designed the experiments: MGA AEB. Performed the experiments: MGA YL. Analyzed the data: AEB MGA QH HY. Contributed reagents/materials/analysis tools: AEB HD EW CS-B SAS MM. Wrote the paper: MGA AEB HD.

References

1. Go AS, Mozaffarian D, Roger VL, Benjamin EJ, Berry JD, et al. (2013) Heart disease and stroke statistics—2013 update: a report from the American Heart Association. Circulation 127: e6–e245. doi:10.1161/CIR.0b013e31828124ad.
2. Iadecola C, Anrather J (2011) The immunology of stroke: from mechanisms to translation. Nat Med 17: 796–808. doi:10.1038/nm.2399.
3. Macrez R, Ali C, Toutirais O, Le Mauff B, Defer G, et al. (2011) Stroke and the immune system: from pathophysiology to new therapeutic strategies. Lancet Neurol 10: 471–480. doi:10.1016/S1474-4422(11)70066-7.
4. Gelderblom M, Weymar A, Bernreuther C, Velden J, Arunachalam P, et al. (2012) Neutralization of the IL-17 axis diminishes neutrophil invasion and protects from ischemic stroke. Blood 120: 3793–3802. doi:10.1182/blood-2012-02-412726.
5. Yilmaz G, Arumugam TV, Stokes KY, Granger DN (2006) Role of T lymphocytes and interferon-gamma in ischemic stroke. Circulation 113: 2105–2112. doi:10.1161/CIRCULATIONAHA.105.593046.
6. Wong CHY, Jenne CN, Lee W-Y, Léger C, Kubes P (2011) Functional Innervation of Hepatic iNKT Cells Is Immunosuppressive Following Stroke. Science 334: 101–105. doi:10.1126/science.1210301.
7. Liesz A, Suri-Payer E, Veltkamp C, Doerr H, Sommer C, et al. (2009) Regulatory T cells are key cerebroprotective immunomodulators in acute experimental stroke. Nat Med 15: 192–199. doi:10.1038/nm.1927.
8. Roark CL, Simonian PL, Fontenot AP, Born WK, O'Brien RL (2008) gammadelta T cells: an important source of IL-17. Curr Opin Immunol 20: 353–357. doi:10.1016/j.coi.2008.03.006.
9. Jensen KDC, Su X, Shin S, Li L, Youssef S, et al. (2008) Thymic selection determines gammadelta T cell effector fate: antigen-naive cells make interleukin-17 and antigen-experienced cells make interferon gamma. Immunity 29: 90–100. doi:10.1016/j.immuni.2008.04.022.
10. Nakamura R, Shibata K, Yamada H, Shimoda K, Nakayama K, et al. (2008) Tyk2-signaling plays an important role in host defense against Escherichia coli through IL-23-induced IL-17 production by gammadelta T cells. J Immunol 181: 2071–2075.
11. Shichita T, Sugiyama Y, Ooboshi H, Sugimori H, Nakagawa R, et al. (2009) Pivotal role of cerebral interleukin-17-producing gammadeltaT cells in the delayed phase of ischemic brain injury. Nat Med 15: 946–950. doi:10.1038/nm.1999.
12. Peterfalvi A, Molnar T, Banati M, Pusch G, Miko E, et al. (2009) Impaired function of innate T lymphocytes and NK cells in the acute phase of ischemic stroke. Cerebrovasc Dis 28: 490–498. doi:10.1159/000236527.
13. Roux A, Mourin G, Larsen M, Fastenackels S, Urrutia A, et al. (2013) Differential impact of age and cytomegalovirus infection on the γδ T cell compartment. J Immunol 191: 1300–1306. doi:10.4049/jimmunol.1202940.
14. Andreu-Ballester JC, García-Ballesteros C, Benet-Campos C, Amigó V, Almela-Quilis A, et al. (2012) Values for αβ and γδ T-lymphocytes and CD4+, CD8+, and CD56+ subsets in healthy adult subjects: assessment by age and gender. Cytometry B Clin Cytom 82: 238–244. doi:10.1002/cyto.b.21020.
15. Brunetti ND, D'Antuono C, Rana M, D'Arienzo G, De Gennaro L, et al. (2012) Lymphocyte subset characterization in patients with early clinical presentation of coronary heart disease. J Thromb Thrombolysis 34: 475–482. doi:10.1007/s11239-012-0761-3.
16. Kolbus D, Ljungcrantz I, Andersson L, Hedblad B, Fredrikson GN, et al. (2013) Association between CD8+ T-cell subsets and cardiovascular disease. J Intern Med 274: 41–51. doi:10.1111/joim.12038.
17. Dumitriu IE, Baruah P, Finlayson CJ, Loftus IM, Antunes RF, et al. (2012) High levels of costimulatory receptors OX40 and 4-1BB characterize CD4+CD28null T cells in patients with acute coronary syndrome. Circ Res 110: 857–869. doi:10.1161/CIRCRESAHA.111.261933.
18. Eid RE, Rao DA, Zhou J, Lo SL, Ranjbaran H, et al. (2009) Interleukin-17 and interferon-gamma are produced concomitantly by human coronary artery-infiltrating T cells and act synergistically on vascular smooth muscle cells. Circulation 119: 1424–1432. doi:10.1161/CIRCULATIONAHA.108.827618.
19. Herzenberg L a, Tung J, Moore W a, Herzenberg L a, Parks DR (2006) Interpreting flow cytometry data: a guide for the perplexed. Nat Immunol 7: 681–685. doi:10.1038/ni0706-681.
20. Adamski MG, Li Y, Wagner E, Yu H, Seales-Bailey C, et al. (2013) Next-Generation qPCR for the High-Throughput Measurement of Gene Expression in Multiple Leukocyte Subsets. J Biomol Screen 18: 1008–1017. doi:10.1177/1087057113489882.
21. RDevelopment C (2012) TEAM (2008): R: A language and environment for statistical computing. Vienna, Austria. Internet http//www R-project org.
22. Li G-Z, Zhong D, Yang L-M, Sun B, Zhong Z-H, et al. (2005) Expression of interleukin-17 in ischemic brain tissue. Scand J Immunol 62: 481–486. doi:10.1111/j.1365-3083.2005.01683.x.
23. Shibata K, Yamada H, Hara H, Kishihara K, Yoshikai Y (2007) Resident Vdelta1+ gammadelta T cells control early infiltration of neutrophils after Escherichia coli infection via IL-17 production. J Immunol 178: 4466–4472.
24. Dirnagl U, Klehmet J, Braun JS, Harms H, Meisel C, et al. (2007) Stroke-induced immunodepression: experimental evidence and clinical relevance. Stroke 38: 770–773. doi:10.1161/01.STR.0000251441.89665.bc.
25. Sahota P, Vahidy F, Nguyen C, Bui T-T, Yang B, et al. (2013) Changes in spleen size in patients with acute ischemic stroke: a pilot observational study. Int J Stroke 8: 60–67. doi:10.1111/ijs.12022.
26. Offner H, Vandenbark AA, Hurn PD (2009) Effect of experimental stroke on peripheral immunity: CNS ischemia induces profound immunosuppression. Neuroscience 158: 1098–1111. doi:10.1016/j.neuroscience.2008.05.033.
27. Yu H, Adamski MG, Wagner E, Seales-Bailey C, Baird AE (2013) Splenic measurements in ischemic stroke: assessment of baseline size. Int J Stroke 8: E57. doi:10.1111/ijs.12175.
28. Bhowmick S, Singh A, Flavell RA, Clark RB, O'Rourke J, et al. (2009) The sympathetic nervous system modulates CD4(+)FoxP3(+) regulatory T cells via a TGF-beta-dependent mechanism. J Leukoc Biol 86: 1275–1283. doi:10.1189/jlb.0209107.
29. Grebe KM, Hickman HD, Irvine KR, Takeda K, Bennink JR, et al. (2009) Sympathetic nervous system control of anti-influenza CD8+ T cell responses. Proc Natl Acad Sci U S A 106: 5300–5305. doi:10.1073/pnas.0808851106.
30. Bosch JA, Berntson GG, Cacioppo JT, Dhabhar FS, Marucha PT (2003) Acute stress evokes selective mobilization of T cells that differ in chemokine receptor expression: a potential pathway linking immunologic reactivity to cardiovascular disease. Brain Behav Immun 17: 251–259.
31. O'Donnell MJ, Xavier D, Liu L, Zhang H, Chin SL, et al. (2010) Risk factors for ischaemic and intracerebral haemorrhagic stroke in 22 countries (the INTERSTROKE study): a case-control study. Lancet 376: 112–123. doi:10.1016/S0140-6736(10)60834-3.
32. Kengne AP, Patel A, Barzi F, Jamrozik K, Lam TH, et al. (2007) Systolic blood pressure, diabetes and the risk of cardiovascular diseases in the Asia-Pacific region. J Hypertens 25: 1205–1213. doi:10.1097/HJH.0b013e3280dce59e.
33. Lewington S, Clarke R, Qizilbash N, Peto R, Collins R (2002) Age-specific relevance of usual blood pressure to vascular mortality: a meta-analysis of individual data for one million adults in 61 prospective studies. Lancet 360: 1903–1913.
34. Guzik TJ, Hoch NE, Brown KA, McCann LA, Rahman A, et al. (2007) Role of the T cell in the genesis of angiotensin II induced hypertension and vascular dysfunction. J Exp Med 204: 2449–2460. doi:10.1084/jem.20070657.
35. Kim CH, Vaziri ND (2005) Hypertension promotes integrin expression and reactive oxygen species generation by circulating leukocytes. Kidney Int 67: 1462–1470. doi:10.1111/j.1523-1755.2005.00223.x.
36. Von Victinghoff S, Ley K (2010) Interleukin 17 in vascular inflammation. Cytokine Growth Factor Rev 21: 463–469. doi:10.1016/j.cytogfr.2010.10.003.
37. Ribot JC, DeBarros A, Pang DJ, Neves JF, Peperzak V, et al. (2009) CD27 is a thymic determinant of the balance between interferon-gamma- and interleukin 17-producing gammadelta T cell subsets. Nat Immunol 10: 427–436. doi:10.1038/ni.1717.
38. Chon H, Gaillard CAJM, van der Meijden BB, Dijstelbloem HM, Kraaijenhagen RJ, et al. (2004) Broadly altered gene expression in blood leukocytes in essential hypertension is absent during treatment. Hypertension 43: 947–951. doi:10.1161/01.HYP.0000123071.35142.72.
39. Touyz RM (2012) New insights into mechanisms of hypertension. Curr Opin Nephrol Hypertens 21: 119–121. doi:10.1097/MNH.0b013e328350a50f.
40. Youn J-C, Yu HT, Lim BJ, Koh MJ, Lee J, et al. (2013) Immunosenescent CD8+ T cells and C-X-C chemokine receptor type 3 chemokines are increased in human hypertension. Hypertension 62: 126–133. doi:10.1161/HYPERTENSIONAHA.113.00689.

Increased Risk of Ischemic Stroke after Hyperosmolar Hyperglycemic State: A Population-Based Follow-Up Study

Jen-Yu Wang[1]☯, Cheng-Yi Wang[1]☯, Yung-Sung Huang[2], Pin-Fan Chen[3], Kuang-Yung Huang[4,5], Pesus Chou[6], Wei-Cheng Lian[3,4]*, Ching-Chih Lee[4,6,7,8,9]*

1 Department of Internal Medicine, Cardinal Tien Hospital, School of Medicine, Fu-Jen Catholic University, New Taipei City, Taiwan, **2** Division of Neurology, Department of Internal Medicine, Buddhist Dalin Tzu Chi General Hospital, Chiayi, Taiwan, **3** Division of Metabolism and Endocrinology, Department of Internal Medicine, Buddhist Dalin Tzu Chi General Hospital, Chiayi, Taiwan, **4** School of Medicine, Tzu Chi University, Hualian, Taiwan, **5** Division of Allergy, Immunology, and Rheumatology, Department of Internal Medicine, Buddhist Dalin Tzu Chi General Hospital, Chiayi, Taiwan, **6** Community Medicine Research Center and Institute of Public Health, National Yang-Ming University, Taipei, Taiwan, **7** Department of Otolaryngology, Buddhist Dalin Tzu Chi General Hospital, Chiayi, Taiwan, **8** Department of Education, Buddhist Dalin Tzu Chi General Hospital, Chiayi, Taiwan, **9** Center for Clinical Epidemiology and Biostatistics, Buddhist Dalin Tzu Chi General Hospital, Chiayi, Taiwan

Abstract

Background: Although much attention has been focused on the association between chronic hyperglycemia and cerebrovascular diseases in type 2 diabetes mellitus (DM) patients, there is no data regarding the risk of ischemic stroke after a hyperosmolar hyperglycemic state (HHS) attack. The objective of this study was to investigate the risk of ischemic stroke in type 2 DM patients after an HHS attack.

Methods: From 2004 to 2008, this retrospective observational study was conducted on a large cohort of Taiwanese using Taiwan's National Health Insurance Research Database (NHIRD). We identified 19,031 type 2 DM patients who were discharged with a diagnosis of HHS and 521,229 type 2 DM patients without an HHS diagnosis. Using the propensity score generated from logistic regression models, conditional on baseline covariates, we matched 19,031 type 2 DM patients with an HHS diagnosis with the same number from the comparison cohort. The one-year cumulative rate for ischemic stroke was estimated using the Kaplan-Meier method. After adjusting covariates, Cox proportional hazard regression was used to compute the adjusted one-year rate of ischemic stroke.

Results: Of the patients sampled, 1,810 (9.5%) of the type 2 DM patients with HHS and 996 (5.2%) of the comparison cohort developed ischemic stroke during the one-year follow-up period. After adjusting for covariates, the adjusted HR for developing ischemic stroke during the one-year follow-up period was 1.8 (95% C.I., 1.67 to 1.95, $P<0.001$) for type 2 DM patients with HHS compared with those without HHS.

Conclusion: Although DM is a well-recognized risk factor for atherosclerosis, type 2 DM patients that have suffered a HHS attacks are at an increased risk of developing ischemic stroke compared with those without HHS.

Editor: Xiaoying Wang, Massachusetts General Hospital, United States of America

Funding: The authors have no support or funding to report.

Competing Interests: The authors have declared that no competing interests exist.

* E-mail: hematcd2@hotmail.com (WCL); hematcd@hotmail.com (CCL)

☯ These authors contributed equally to this work.

Introduction

Atherosclerosis, with its complications of ischemic stroke and coronary artery diseases, is responsible for the highest morbidity and mortality in patients with type 2 diabetes mellitus (DM) [1]. The metabolic abnormalities that accompany type 2 DM, (particularly chronic hyperglycemia, dyslipidemia, and insulin resistance) impair normal functioning of endothelial cells, vascular smooth muscle cells, and platelets which render arteries in type 2 DM patients susceptible to atherosclerosis [2] and increase the likelihood of ischemic stroke.

In particular, acute hyperglycemia has been shown to worsen the size of the infarct in ischemic stroke [3,4] and retrospective studies in humans have shown that hyperglycemia on admission may worsen the clinical outcome in ischemic stroke [5,6]. Hyperglycemic crisis may also be associated with an increased risk of stroke. The hyperosmolar hyperglycemic state (HHS) is typically characterized by hyperglycemia and dehydration caused by osmotic diuresis, which leads to hyperviscosity and a hypercoagulable state [7,8]. Besides ischemic stroke, complications include myocardial infarction, pulmonary embolism and mesenteric vessel thrombosis [9,10].

Although most studies have demonstrated that hyperglycemia on admission is associated with increased risk of ischemic stroke [11], there is no data regarding the post-discharge risk of ischemic stroke after an HHS attack in type 2 DM patients. The objective of this study was to investigate the risk of ischemic stroke after an HHS attack in type 2 DM patients using Taiwan's National Health Insurance Research Database (NHIRD).

Materials and Methods

Ethics Statement

This study was approved by the Institutional Review Board of Buddhist Dalin Tzu Chi General Hospital, Taiwan. Since all identifying personal information was removed from the secondary files prior to analysis, the review board waived the requirement for written informed consent from the patients involved.

Database

From 2004 to 2008, this retrospective observational study was conducted on a large cohort of Taiwanese using Taiwan's NHIRD. The National Health Insurance program, which provides compulsory universal health insurance, was implemented in Taiwan in 1995. It enrolls up to 99% of the Taiwanese population and contracts with 97% of all medical providers. The database contains comprehensive information on insured subjects, including dates of clinical visits, diagnostic codes, details of prescriptions, and expenditure amounts.

Our study cohort consisted of all type 2 DM patients in Taiwan with International Classification of Diseases, Ninth Revision, Clinical Modification (ICD-9-CM) codes, 250.X0 or 250.X2, who had been hospitalized for HHS (ICD-9-CM, 250.20 or 250.22) between 2004 and 2008, compared to hospitalized type 2 DM patients without HHS. We excluded those patients with any type of stroke (ICD-9-CM, 430–438) diagnosed before or during the index hospitalization.

Each patient was tracked for a one-year after his or her first discharge to identify outcomes, including ischemic stroke diagnosis codes (ICD-9-CM, 430, 431, 433.x1, 434.x1, or 436.x). The NHIRD has an accuracy of up to 95% in recording diagnoses of ischemic stroke [12]. To maximize case ascertainment, only patients hospitalized for cerebrovascular events were included. These patients were then linked to the administrative data for the period from 2004–2008 to calculate cerebrovascular disease-free survival time, with cases censored for patients who drew back guarantees from the National Health Insurance Program or were still robust without defined events at the end of follow-up.

Variables

Patient characteristics included age, gender, co-morbidities, geographic location, level of urbanization, and socioeconomic status (SES), as previous studies have shown that the incidence of ischemic stroke was associated with geographic location, level of urbanization, and SES [13–15]. Co-morbid conditions, such as coronary artery disease, atrial fibrillation, dyslipidemia, and

Table 1. Characteristics in type 2 DM patients,2004–2008.

Characteristics	Before matched			Propensity score-matched		
	Patients without HHS	Patients with HHS	*p* value	Patients without HHS	Patients with HHS	*p* value
Patient no.	521229	19031		19031	19031	
Mean age (s.d.), year	64.5±13.6	66.0±14.7	<0.001	66.1±13.3	66.1±14.7	0.80
Male gender	269273(51.7)	10444(54.9)	<0.001	10476(55.0)	10444(54.9)	0.74
Comorbidity						
Hypertension	293150(56.2)	10976(57.7)	<0.001	10889(57.2)	10976(57.7)	0.37
Coronary artery disease	120287(23.1)	5732(30.1)	<0.001	5750(30.2)	5732(30.1)	0.84
Atrial fibrillation	22137(4.2)	1090(5.7)	<0.001	1089(5.7)	1090(5.7)	0.98
Hyperlipidemia	67296(12.9)	3300(17.3)	<0.001	3255(17.1)	3300(17.3)	0.54
Chronic renal failure	37583(7.2)	2565(13.5)	<0.001	2397(12.6)	2565(13.5)	0.01
Socioeconomic status			<0.001			
High	159115(30.5)	4949(26.0)		4934(25.9)	4949(26.0)	0.88
Moderate	234088(44.9)	9005(47.3)		8976(47.2)	9005(47.3)	
Low	128026(24.6)	5077(26.7)		5121(26.9)	5077(26.7)	
Geographic region			<0.001			0.98
Northern	260703(50.0)	8547(44.9)		8575(45.1)	8547(44.9)	
Central	93495(17.9)	3784(19.9)		3771(19.8)	3784(19.9)	
Southern	149458(28.7)	6146(32.3)		6121(32.2)	6146(32.3)	
Eastern	17573(3.4)	554(2.9)		564(3.0)	554(2.9)	
Urbanization level			<0.001			0.40
Urban	167143(32.1)	7164(37.7)		7159(37.6)	7164(37.7)	
Suburban	223195(42.8)	7811(41.0)		7913(41.6)	7811(41.0)	
Rural	130891(25.1)	4056(21.3)		3959(20.8)	4056(21.3)	

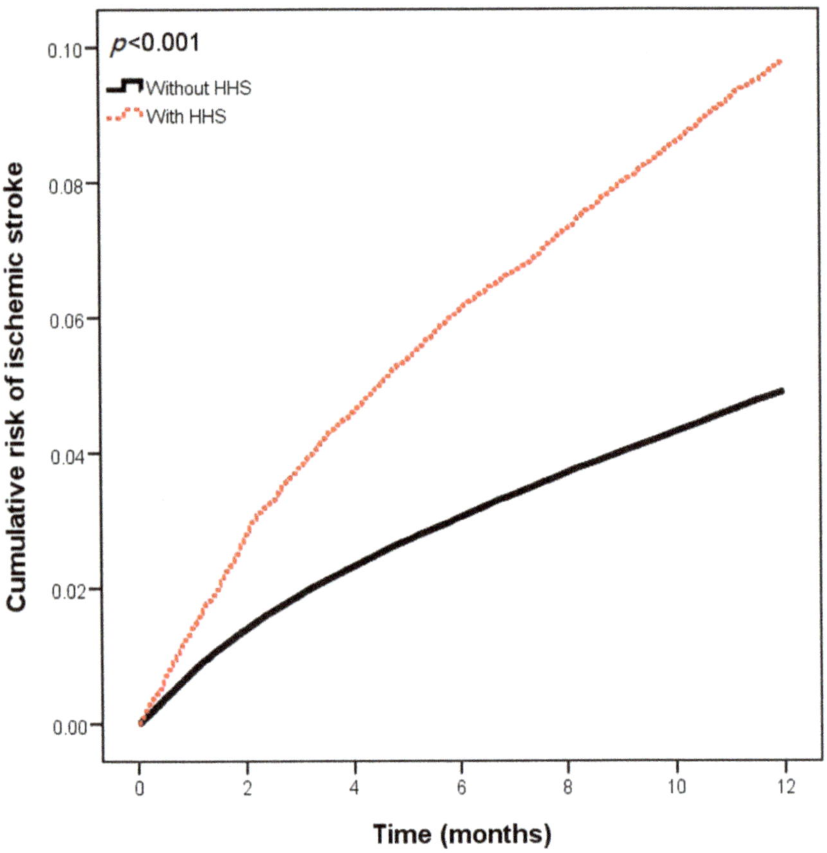

Figure 1. Cumulative risk of ischemic stroke for the DM patients with HHS and those without HHS.

chronic renal failure, were identified according to the ICD-9-CM system.

Patients were classified into two sub-groups: (1) high individual SES (civil servants, regular or full-time paid personnel with a government affiliation, employees of privately owned institutions), and (2) low individual SES (self-employed individuals, members of the farmers' or fishermen's associations, other employees, military veterans, substitute service draftees, and members of low-income families) [16]. The urbanization level of residences were classified in seven levels based on five indices in Taiwan: (1) population density, (2) percentage of residents with college level or higher education, (3) percentage of residents above 65 years old, (4) percentage of residents who were agriculture workers, and (5) the number of physicians per 100,000 people [17]. We recorded the urbanization level of residences as urban (urbanization level 1), sub-urban (urbanization levels 2–3), or rural (urbanization levels 4–7). The geographic regions where the DM patients resided were subdivided into northern, central, southern and eastern Taiwan.

Statistical Analyses

The SPSS (version 15, SPSS Inc., Chicago, IL, USA) was used for data analysis. Propensity score stratification was applied to replace the wide host of confounding factors that may be present in an observational study with such variable factors. Pearson's chi-

Table 2. The cumulative rate of ischemic stroke in type 2 DM patients with and without HHS.

Characteristics	**6 months**			**1-year**		
	n	**Events (%)**	***p* value**	*n*	**Events (%)**	***p* value**
Ischemic stroke						
Before matched			<0.001			<0.001
Without HHS	521229	15391 (3.0)		521229	24042(4.6)	
With HHS	19031	1143 (6.0)		19031	1810(9.5)	
Propensity score-matched			<0.001			<0.001
Without HHS	19031	631(3.3)		19031	996(5.2)	
With HHS	19031	1143(6.0)		19031	1810(9.5)	

Table 3. Hazard ratios for the ischemic stroke in DM patients with and without HHS.

Characteristics	Before matched		Propensity score-matched	
	Hazard ratio (95%CI)	***p* value**	**Hazard ratio (95%CI)**	***p* value**
Univariate model				
Without HHS	1		1	
With HHS	2.05(1.96–2.15)	<0.001	1.81(1.68–1.96)	<0.001
*Multivariable regression model**				
Without HHS	1		1	
With HHS	1.75(1.67–1.84)	<0.001	1.80(1.67–1.95)	<0.001
Age	1.04(1.03–1.04)	<0.001	1.03(1.02–1.03)	<0.001
Gender				
Male	1		1	
Female	0.90(0.88–0.92)	<0.001	0.96(0.89–1.04)	0.32
Comorbidity				
Hypertension	2.55(2.47–2.64)	<0.001	2.40(2.18–2.64)	<0.001
Coronary artery disease	1.49(1.45–1.52)	<0.001	1.42(1.31–1.53)	<0.001
Atrial fibrillation	1.55(1.48–1.61)	<0.001	1.29(1.14–1.46)	<0.001
Hyperlipidemia	1.38(1.34–1.43)	<0.001	1.15(1.05–1.27)	0.004
Chronic renal failure	1.50(1.45–1.56)	<0.001	1.25(1.14–1.38)	<0.001
Socioeconomic status				
High	1		1	
Moderate	1.06(1.02–1.09)	0.001	1.12(1.01–1.24)	0.03
Low	1.08(1.04–1.12)	<0.001	1.06(0.95–1.18)	0.29
Geographic region				
Northern	1		1	
Central	1.20(1.16–1.25)	<0.001	1.20(1.09–1.33)	<0.001
Southern	1.08(1.05–1.12)	<0.001	1.02(0.93–1.13)	0.69
Eastern	0.95(0.88–1.02)	0.16	0.91(0.72–1.16)	0.45
Urbanization level				
Urban	1		1	
Suburban	0.94(0.91–0.98)	<0.001	0.99(0.91–1.09)	0.89
Rural	0.87(0.84–0.91)	<0.001	0.97(0.86–1.09)	0.61

*Adjusted for patient age, gender, Charlson Comorbidity Index Score, geographic region, urbanization level, hospital ownership, and comorbidity.

square test was used for categorical variables such as gender, comorbidities, level of urbanization, geographic regions of residence, and SES. Continuous variables were analyzed with a one way ANOVA test. The Cox proportional hazards regression model, adjusting for patients' characteristics (age, gender, Charlson Comorbidity Index Score, urbanization, area of residence and SES) was used to compare outcomes between the two cohorts. The one-year cumulative rate of ischemic stroke was estimated using the log rank test to examine the differences in the risk of developing ischemic stroke between type 2 DM patients with and without HHS. We calculated hazard ratios (HR) along with 95% confidence intervals (C.I.) using a significance level of 0.05. A two-sided p-value ($P<0.05$) was used to determine statistical significance.

Results

We identified 19,031 type 2 DM patients who were discharged with a diagnosis of HHS and 521,229 type 2 DM patients without a HHS diagnosis. Using the propensity score generated from logistic regression models, conditional on baseline covariates, we matched 19,031 type 2 DM patients with an HHS diagnosis with the same number from the comparison cohort. The demographic characteristics and selected morbidities for the two cohorts are shown in Table 1.

During the one-year follow-up period, 1,810 (9.5%) type 2 DM patients with HHS and 996 (5.2%) patients from the comparison cohort developed ischemic stroke (Table 2). The HRs and 95% C.I.s of the various risk factors for ischemic stroke are presented in Table 3. Age, hypertension, coronary artery disease, atrial fibrillation, hyperlipidemia, chronic kidney disease, and moderate SES were associated with an increased risk of ischemic stroke. After adjusting for the covariates, the adjusted HR for developing ischemic stroke during the one-year follow-up period was 1.8 (95% C.I., 1.67 to 1.95, $P<0.001$) for type 2 DM patients with HHS compared with those without HHS. Figure 1 shows the Kaplan-Meier failure curve of developing ischemic stroke in type 2 DM patients with and without HHS. The type 2 DM patients with HHS had a significantly higher one-year cumulative rate of

Table 4. Hazard ratios for the ischemic stroke in HHS patients.

Characteristics	Univariate model			Multivariable regression model*		
	HR	95% CI	*p* value	HR	95% CI	*p* value
Age	1.03	1.02–1.03	<0.001	1.03	1.02–1.03	<0.001
Gender						
Male	1			1		
Female	1.29	1.18–1.42	0.03	1.01	0.92–1.11	0.84
Comorbidity						
Hypertension	2.94	2.62–3.29	<0.001	2.36	2.10–2.66	<0.001
Coronary artery disease	1.85	1.69–2.03	<0.001	1.39	1.26–1.52	<0.001
Atrial fibrillation	1.82	1.56–2.13	<0.001	1.24	1.06–1.46	0.007
Hyperlipidemia	1.04	0.92–1.17	0.51	1.11	0.98–1.25	0.11
Chronic renal failure	1.46	1.30–1.64	<0.001	1.22	1.08–1.38	0.001
Socioeconomic status						
High	1			1		
Moderate	1.31	1.16–1.47	<0.001	1.20	1.05–1.36	0.007
Low	1.20	1.05–1.37	0.007	1.08	0.94–1.23	0.29
Geographic region						
Northern	1			1		
Central	1.29	1.14–1.45	<0.001	1.24	1.10–1.41	0.001
Southern	1.00	0.90–1.12	0.94	0.99	0.87–1.12	0.99
Eastern	0.99	0.74–1.32	0.95	0.93	0.70–1.25	0.93
Urbanization level						
Urban	1			1		
Suburban	0.90	0.81–1.00	0.05	1.03	0.92–1.15	0.67
Rural	0.88	0.77–0.99	0.04	1.05	0.91–1.22	0.50

*Adjusted for patient age, gender, Charlson Comorbidity Index Score, geographic region, urbanization level, hospital ownership, and accreditation level.

ischemic stroke than patients in the comparison cohort ($P<0.001$), after adjusting for the covariates.

Among the type 2 DM patients with HHS, predictors of ischemic stroke were analyzed using the Cox regression model. In univariate analysis, age, hypertension, coronary artery disease, atrial fibrillation, chronic kidney disease, moderate SES and residence in central Taiwan were associated with increased risk for ischemic stroke. Increased age (HR = 1.03; 95% C.I., 1.02 to 1.03), hypertension (HR = 2.36; 95% C.I., 2.10 to 2.66), coronary artery disease (HR = 1.39, 95% C.I., 1.26 to 1.52), atrial fibrillation (HR = 1.24; 95% C.I., 1.10 to 1.41), chronic renal failure (HR = 1.22; 95% C.I., 1.08–1.38), moderate SES (HR = 1.20; 95% C.I., 1.05 to 1.36), and residence in central Taiwan (HR = 1.24; 95% C.I., 1.10 to 1.41) remained independent risk factors for ischemic stroke using the multivariable model (Table 4).

Discussion

Compared with type 2 DM patients without HHS, we found that type 2 DM patients that had suffered an HHS attack were at an increased risk of developing subsequent ischemic stroke (HR, 1.8; 95% C.I., 1.67 to 1.95, $P<0.001$). Using a multivariable model, we also found that increased age, hypertension, coronary artery disease, atrial fibrillation, chronic renal failure, moderate SES, and residence in central Taiwan were independent risk factors for ischemic stroke.

DM has been shown to be an important risk factor for ischemic stroke. In the Multiple Risk Factor Intervention Trial (MRFIT) [18], the risk of stroke was three times higher in DM subjects. However, data regarding the risk of ischemic stroke after stabilization following an HHS attack are lacking. According to the one-year follow-up data, the risk of developing ischemic stroke after an HHS attack increased by 80% after adjusting for other cerebrovascular risks.

Several possible pathophysiological processes may explain the unexpectedly high risk of ischemic stroke observed after treatment for HHS. First, we hypothesize that a worse metabolic profile among the HHS group (compared to the non-HHS group) may partially explain the increased incidence of stroke observed during the one year follow-up in our study. In a study of HHS patients in Taiwan, poor compliance with medication (21.0%) and undiagnosed DM (10.9%) were the second and third most common precipitating factors in HHS [19]. A second theory links attacks of HHS in DM patients with marked fluctuations in glucose levels. Intermittent hyperglycemia may induce endothelial cell dysfunction and is associated with high oxidative stress [20]. Other studies have shown that fluctuations in glucose levels can enhance cell proliferation, induce the release of cytokines, and impair endothelial function, all of which contribute to the mechanisms underlying cerebrovascular events [21,22]. Finally, among the HHS precipitating factors (such as infections, alcohol abuse, gastrointestinal bleeding, acute pancreatitis, silent myocardial infarction, mesenteric ischemia, use of certain medications, and noncompliance with diabetic treatment [23]), infection, in particular, is associated with an increased risk of ischemic stroke. Such infections include respiratory tract infections [24], tuberculosis [25], herpes zoster attacks [26], chronic Helicobacter pylori infections [27], and chronic hepatitis C infections [28]. Despite adjusting for several well-known cerebrovascular risk factors, the general health condition of our patients could not be inferred from the database. Therefore, the possibility that development of ischemic stroke was associated with an underlying infection or other stressful condition cannot be excluded.

Our study had several additional limitations related to the NHIRD database. The diagnoses of HHS, DM, ischemic stroke, and any other comorbid conditions were dependent on ICD codes from the NHIRD database. The National Health Insurance Bureau of Taiwan, however, has made every effort to verify the accuracy of diagnosis based upon random chart review and patient interview [29]. In fact, since inclusion criteria involved hospitalized type 2 DM patients, the dataset used in our study was the most accurate available. An additional limitation of the NHIRD database was its lack of information on tobacco use, dietary habits, physical activity, metabolic profiles, and body mass index, or the status of DM control, which also may be risk factors for ischemic stroke among DM patients. Nonetheless, given the magnitude and statistical significance of the observed effects in this study, these limitations were unlikely to have compromised our results. In fact, the strength of our study lies in its large sample size. In addition, because the National Health Insurance Program has 99% coverage in Taiwan, our study had minimal risk of selection bias.

In conclusion, this is the first study to investigate the risk of initial ischemic stroke in type 2 DM patients after HHS. It revealed that type 2 DM patients with HHS had an increased risk for developing ischemic stroke. It was not surprising that cardiovascular comorbidities, such as hypertension, coronary artery disease, atrial fibrillation, and chronic renal failure, were found to be important predictors for developing future ischemic stroke after HHS treatment. Therefore, interventions aimed at stroke prevention are extremely important in patients recovering from HHS who have such comorbidities.

Acknowledgments

This study is based partly on data from the National Health Insurance Research Database provided by the Bureau of National Health Insurance, Department of Health and managed by the National Health Research Institutes. The interpretation and conclusions contained herein do not represent those of aforementioned institutions.

Statement of responsibility: All authors had full access to the data, take responsibility for its integrity, and have read and agree to the manuscript as written.

Author Contributions

Conceived and designed the experiments: JYW CYW YSH PFC KYH PC WCL CCL. Analyzed the data: PC WCL CCL. Wrote the paper: JYW CYW.

References

1. Resnick HE, Shorr RI, Kuller L, Franse L, Harris TB (2001) Prevalence and clinical implications of American Diabetes Association-defined diabetes and other categories of glucose dysregulation in older adults: the health, aging and body composition study. J Clin Epidemiol 54: 869–876.
2. Beckman JA, Creager MA, Libby P (2002) Diabetes and atherosclerosis: epidemiology, pathophysiology, and management. JAMA 287: 2570–2581.
3. de Courten-Myers G, Myers RE, Schoolfield L (1988) Hyperglycemia enlarges infarct size in cerebrovascular occlusion in cats. Stroke 19: 623–630.
4. Nedergaard M (1987) Transient focal ischemia in hyperglycemic rats is associated with increased cerebral infarction. Brain Res 408: 79–85.
5. Bruno A, Biller J, Adams HP Jr., Clarke WR, Woolson RF, et al. (1999) Acute blood glucose level and outcome from ischemic stroke. Trial of ORG 10172 in Acute Stroke Treatment (TOAST) Investigators. Neurology 52: 280–284.
6. Moulin T, Tatu L, Crepin Leblond T, Chavot D, Berges S, et al. (1997) The Besancon Stroke Registry: an acute stroke registry of 2,500 consecutive patients. Eur Neurol 38: 10–20.
7. Fadini GP, de Kreutzenberg SV, Rigato M, Brocco S, Marchesan M, et al. (2011) Characteristics and outcomes of the hyperglycemic hyperosmolar non-ketotic syndrome in a cohort of 51 consecutive cases at a single center. Diabetes Res Clin Pract 94: 172–179.
8. Kitabchi AE, Nyenwe EA (2006) Hyperglycemic crises in diabetes mellitus: diabetic ketoacidosis and hyperglycemic hyperosmolar state. Endocrinol Metab Clin North Am 35: 725–751, viii.
9. Foster DW, McGarry JD (1983) The metabolic derangements and treatment of diabetic ketoacidosis. N Engl J Med 309: 159–169.
10. Lorber D (1995) Nonketotic hypertonicity in diabetes mellitus. Med Clin North Am 79: 39–52.
11. Capes SE, Hunt D, Malmberg K, Pathak P, Gerstein HC (2001) Stress hyperglycemia and prognosis of stroke in nondiabetic and diabetic patients: a systematic overview. Stroke 32: 2426–2432.
12. Cheng CL, Kao YH, Lin SJ, Lee CH, Lai ML (2011) Validation of the National Health Insurance Research Database with ischemic stroke cases in Taiwan. Pharmacoepidemiol Drug Saf 20: 236–242.
13. Lin HC, Lin YJ, Liu TC, Chen CS, Chiu WT (2007) Urbanization and stroke prevalence in Taiwan: analysis of a nationwide survey. J Urban Health 84: 604–614.
14. Engstrom G, Jerntorp I, Pessah-Rasmussen H, Hedblad B, Berglund G, et al. (2001) Geographic distribution of stroke incidence within an urban population: relations to socioeconomic circumstances and prevalence of cardiovascular risk factors. Stroke 32: 1098–1103.
15. McFadden E, Luben R, Wareham N, Bingham S, Khaw KT (2009) Social class, risk factors, and stroke incidence in men and women: a prospective study in the European prospective investigation into cancer in Norfolk cohort. Stroke 40: 1070–1077.
16. Chen CY, Liu CY, Su WC, Huang SL, Lin KM (2007) Factors associated with the diagnosis of neurodevelopmental disorders: a population-based longitudinal study. Pediatrics 119: e435–443.
17. Liu CY HY, Chung YL, Chen YJ, Weng WS, Liu JS, et al. (2006) Incorporating development stratification of Taiwan townships into sampling design of large scale health interview survey (in Chinese). J Health Manage: 1–22.
18. Stamler J, Vaccaro O, Neaton JD, Wentworth D (1993) Diabetes, other risk factors, and 12-yr cardiovascular mortality for men screened in the Multiple Risk Factor Intervention Trial. Diabetes Care 16: 434–444.
19. Chu CH, Lee JK, Lam HC, Lu CC (2001) Prognostic factors of hyperglycemic hyperosmolar nonketotic state. Chang Gung Med J 24: 345–351.
20. Ceriello A, Esposito K, Piconi L, Ihnat MA, Thorpe JE, et al. (2008) Oscillating glucose is more deleterious to endothelial function and oxidative stress than mean glucose in normal and type 2 diabetic patients. Diabetes 57: 1349–1354.
21. Jones SC, Saunders HJ, Qi W, Pollock CA (1999) Intermittent high glucose enhances cell growth and collagen synthesis in cultured human tubulointerstitial cells. Diabetologia 42: 1113–1119.
22. Quagliaro L, Piconi L, Assaloni R, Martinelli L, Motz E, et al. (2003) Intermittent high glucose enhances apoptosis related to oxidative stress in human umbilical vein endothelial cells: the role of protein kinase C and NAD(P)H-oxidase activation. Diabetes 52: 2795–2804.
23. Chiasson JL, Aris-Jilwan N, Belanger R, Bertrand S, Beauregard H, et al. (2003) Diagnosis and treatment of diabetic ketoacidosis and the hyperglycemic hyperosmolar state. CMAJ 168: 859–866.
24. Smeeth L, Thomas SL, Hall AJ, Hubbard R, Farrington P, et al. (2004) Risk of myocardial infarction and stroke after acute infection or vaccination. N Engl J Med 351: 2611–2618.
25. Pasticci MB, Paciaroni M, Floridi P, Malincarne L, Scavizzi M, et al. (2013) Stroke in patients with tuberculous meningitis in a low TB endemic country: an increasing medical emergency? New Microbiol 36: 193–198.
26. Kang JH, Ho JD, Chen YH, Lin HC (2009) Increased risk of stroke after a herpes zoster attack: a population-based follow-up study. Stroke 40: 3443–3448.
27. Majka J, Rog T, Konturek PC, Konturek SJ, Bielanski W, et al. (2002) Influence of chronic Helicobacter pylori infection on ischemic cerebral stroke risk factors. Med Sci Monit 8: CR675–684.
28. Liao CC, Su TC, Sung FC, Chou WH, Chen TL (2012) Does hepatitis C virus infection increase risk for stroke? A population-based cohort study. PLoS One 7: e31527.
29. Tseng CH (2004) Mortality and causes of death in a national sample of diabetic patients in Taiwan. Diabetes Care 27: 1605–1609.

13

Use of Antithrombotics after Hemorrhagic Transformation in Acute Ischemic Stroke

Joon-Tae Kim[1,2]*, Suk-Hee Heo[3], Man-Seok Park[1]*, Jane Chang[1], Kang-Ho Choi[1], Ki-Hyun Cho[1]

1 Department of Neurology, Cerebrovascular Center, Chonnam National University Hospital, Gwangju, Korea, **2** Biomedical Research Institute, Chonnam National University Hospital, Gwangju, Korea, **3** Department of Radiology, Chonnam National University Hwasun Hospital, Hwasun, Jeonnam, Korea

Abstract

Backgrounds: There have been neither appropriate guidelines nor clinical studies about the use of antithrombotics after hemorrhagic transformation (HT). We sought to find whether the use of antithrombotics after hemorrhagic infarction might be associated with aggravation of HT and neurological deterioration.

Methods: This retrospective study included prospectively registered consecutive patients with acute ischemic stroke and HT in our tertiary stroke center. We focused on the hemorrhagic infarction. Aggravation of HT was defined as either enlargement of the original HT or newly developed HT within the infarcted area by visual analysis. We analyzed relationships between antithrombotics and HT, and neurological deterioration after HT in patients with hemorrhagic infarction. In addition, we assessed composite outcomes including neurological deterioration, vascular events, and death at 1month after HT. We analyzed relationships between antithrombotics after discharge and composite outcomes within 1month after HT.

Results: 222 patients were finally analyzed. Of the 150 patients with hemorrhagic infarction, 75 (50.0%) were type 1. The use of warfarin after detection of hemorrhagic infarction more frequently increased aggravation of HT than did the use of antiplatelets (4 of 24 vs 3 of 69; $p = 0.094$), but neither warfarin nor antiplatelets caused more HT than no medication. In addition, the use of antithrombotics after hemorrhagic infarction was not significantly associated with neurological deterioration after HT. The frequency of composite events at 1months was significantly lower in patients treated with antithrombotics than those treated without ($p = 0.041$).

Conclusion: In conclusion, the results of this study suggest that antithrombotics can safely be used after hemorrhagic infarction and may not be associated with neurological deterioration and aggravation of HT. Further studies are needed to confirm our results.

Editor: Thiruma V. Arumugam, National University of Singapore, Singapore

Funding: This study was supported by a grant (CRI 12008-1) from Chonnam National University Hospital Research Institute of Clinical Medicine and a grant of the Korea Healthcare Technology R&D Project, Ministry of Health and Welfare, Republic of Korea (HI10C2020). The funders had no role in study design, data collection and analysis, decision to publish, or preparation of the manuscript.

Competing Interests: The authors have declared that no competing interests exist.

* E-mail: alldelight2@hanmail.net (JTK); mspark@jnu.ac.kr (MSP)

Introduction

Hemorrhagic transformation (HT) is an important complication of ischemic stroke. In particular, HT might be one of the most problematic complications after thrombolysis. However, the clinical implications of HT are still unclear, and recent studies have shown that asymptomatic HT could be associated with poor outcomes [1,2].

There have been neither appropriate guidelines nor clinical studies about the use of antithrombotics after HT. The American Heart Association/American Stroke Association's most recent guidelines suggest that HT within an ischemic stroke can be thought to have a different course and natural history from intracerebral hemorrhage (ICH) [3]. Therefore, the guidelines recommended that patients with cardioembolic stroke and hemorrhagic infarction continue anticoagulation treatment (Class IIb; Level of evidence C) [3]. However, many clinicians may still be reluctant to continue anticoagulation after HT.

There have been few studies on whether the use of antithrombotics after HT might enlarge hemorrhage in terms of size and extent, or aggravate clinical symptoms. A case series has shown that anticoagulation treatment after hemorrhagic infarction might be compatible with a stable clinical state and resolution of blood on follow-up imaging [4]. However, this should be cautiously interpreted due to the lack of large case series.

Therefore, we sought to investigate whether the use of antithrombotics after hemorrhagic infarction might be associated with aggravation of HT and neurological deterioration in acute ischemic stroke.

Materials and Methods

Subjects

This retrospective study included prospectively registered patients with acute ischemic stroke and HT in our tertiary stroke center who were admitted between August 2010 and March 2012. The patients complied from our stroke imaging protocol had ischemic lesions on diffusion-weighted imaging (DWI) and HT on brain images taken during admission. We excluded patients with (1) early loss of follow-up, including early death; (2) malignant infarction involving over two third of MCA territories; (3) bleeding complications such as hematuria; (4) history of recent bleeding or hemorrhagic disorders; and (4) brain surgery, such as decompression craniectomy.

Ethics Statement

This study was approved by the Institutional Review Board (IRB) of Chonnam National University Hospital. Written informed consent was not obtained from participants because of the retrospective design of this study; therefore, the IRB of the hospital waived the need for written informed consent from participants.

Demographic factors

Demographic and clinical data were collected from the prospective stroke registry. The following stroke risk factors were identified: age, sex, current cigarette smoking (cigarette smoking within the last 5 years), hypertension, diabetes mellitus, dyslipidemia, atrial fibrillation, and previous histories of stroke or transient ischemic attack. Baseline data collected from all patients included the National Institutes of Health Stroke Scales (NIHSS) scores and onset-to-visit times.

Imaging protocol

According to our stroke imaging protocol, patients underwent emergency MRI immediately after admission. The MRI protocol consisted of DWI, fluid-attenuated inversion recovery (FLAIR), gradient echo (GRE) imaging, and time-of-flight MR angiography (MRA) in sequence. Routine follow-up imaging was performed twice at 3 (±12 hours) and 5 (±12 hours) days (computed tomography [CT] angiography and DWI/GRE, respectively) after initial MRI. In addition, DWI/GRE was also performed if neurologic deterioration occurred. Another imaging protocol for thrombolysis included the following procedures: emergency CT, brain MRI immediately after intra-venous thrombolysis, follow-up DWI/GRE at 24 hours after thrombolysis and then routine follow-up protocol. In patients with hemorrhage, follow-up imaging studies were performed to examine the changes (resolution or aggravation) of the hemorrhage 3–5 days after HT detection.

Image analysis

HT cases were categorized as hemorrhagic infarcts (type 1 or 2) or parenchymal hematomas (type 1 or 2) according to the modified definitions established by a previous study [5]. We used GRE imaging for categorization of HT (Figure S1). A hemorrhagic infarct was defined as a petechial hemorrhage within the infarction area but with no space-occupying effect, while a parenchymal hemorrhage was defined as blood clots with the space-occupying effect. Aggravation of HT was defined as either enlargement of the original HT or newly developed HT within the infarcted area by visual analysis.

Clinical analysis

We assessed neurological statuses at admission and on each hospital day by using NIHSS scores. Although this study was retrospective, neurological deterioration was carefully assessed by frequent neurological examinations. Neurological deterioration (ND) after HT was defined as any neurological deterioration considered to be caused by aggravation of HT during admission periods. In addition, we assessed composite outcomes including neurological deterioration, vascular events, and death at 1 month (±7 days) after HT. ND was differently defined from early neurological deterioration in this study (END, END was usually defined as an increase in NIHSS scores by 2 or more points or the development of new neurological symptoms within 5 days of admission).

The timing of the use of antithrombotics was identified to investigate whether antithrombotics might be associated with aggravation of HT. In cases treated with thrombolysis, antithrombotics should be started 24 hours after thrombolysis, based on follow-up imaging results. Aspirin was used for antiplatelets (100 to 300 mg at physicians' discretion) and only warfarin (initially with bridging medication of aspirin) for anticoagulation. We also investigated antithrombotics both at discharge and at a follow-up of 1 month. We analyzed relationships between antithrombotics during admission and aggravation of HT/ND after HT in patients with hemorrhagic infarction. In addition, we analyzed relationships between antithrombotics after discharge and composite outcomes within 1month after HT.

Statistical analysis

Data are presented as mean ± SD or the frequency of categorical variables. Categorical variables were analyzed using the $\chi 2$ test and Fisher's exact test when appropriate. Continuous variables were analyzed using the independent sample *t* test or the Mann–Whitney *U* test when appropriate. We compared the frequency of HT, ND after HT, and composite outcomes within 1 month after HT between users and non-users of antithrombotics after HT in patients with hemorrhagic infarction. In order to evaluate the use of antithrombotics as a predictor of various types of outcomes (aggravation of HT), the use of antithrombotics was adjusted by age, NIHSS scores, and thrombolysis, in 150 patients with hemorrhagic infarction (model 1 by age and initial NIHSS, and model 2 by age, initial NIHSS, and thrombolysis). Odds ratios (ORs) and 95% confidence intervals (CIs) were calculated. A *p* value of <0.05 was considered statistically significant. All statistical analyses were performed using SPSS for Windows version 17 (SPSS Inc, Chicago, IL, USA).

Results

General characteristics of subjects

A total of 311 patients with HT within the infarcted area were screened during the study period. Of these patients, 89 were excluded: 56 were excluded due to malignant infarction. 29 were excluded due to loss of follow-up imaging studies (by early death or early loss of follow-up), and 4 were excluded due to surgeries, such as decompression craniectomy and hematoma removal. Ultimately, 222 patients (143 men; mean age, 70.45±11.42 years) were analyzed. Thrombolysis was performed on 104 of the 222 patients. One-hundred and thirty-four patients had atrial fibrillation.

Twenty-four (10.8%) patients had HT within the infarct area on initial MRI. The mean time between HT onset and hospital visit time was more delayed in patients with HT on initial MRI than in those without (1024.70 min vs 391.79 min, $p<0.001$) (Table S1).

Of the patients with HT on the initial imaging, 6 patients showed aggravation of HT, but none showed ND after HT.

Overall, patients with parenchymal hemorrhage (n = 72) had higher NIHSS scores than those with hemorrhagic infarction (n = 150) (11.0 vs 13.0, $p = 0.002$). Thrombolysis and END were more frequent in patients with parenchymal hemorrhage than in those with hemorrhagic infarction (Table 1).

Use of anti-thrombotics in patients with hemorrhagic infarction

Of the 150 patients with hemorrhagic infarction, 75 (50.0%) were of type 1. The characteristics of these 150 patients are shown in Table 1. Aggravation of HT (n = 15) was more frequently observed in type 2 than in type 1 (11 vs 5, $p = 0.185$), but the frequency of ND after HT was not significantly different between types 1 and 2 (4 vs 2, $p = 0.681$). Furthermore, ND after HT was not related to aggravation of HT (2 of 6). In the use of antithrombotics, the number of patients treated with 'no antithrombotics' were more frequent in type 2 than in type 1 and the number of patients treated with 'warfarin' were less frequent in type 2 than in type 1 (p for trends = 0.001). Changes in the use of antithrombotics after HT are shown in Figure S2 and S3. The use of warfarin after hemorrhagic infarction was more reduced in type 2 than in type 1. The use of antiplatelets was also more reduced after detection of type 2 (Figure S3) than in type 1 of hemorrhagic infarction. In addition, of the 93 patients with cardioembolism and hemorrhagic infarction, only 28 (30.1%) continued to use warfarin after hemorrhagic infarction. The use of antiplatelets was also reduced from 86.0% to 73.7% in patients with non-cardioembolism. At discharge, the use of antithrombotics was as follows: no antithrombotics in 27 patients (18.0%), antiplatelets in 89 patients (59.3%), and warfarin in 34 patients (22.7%) (Figure S2). The use of antithrombotics at discharge was maintained over the first month of follow-up.

Aggravation of HT/ND after HT/composite outcomes at 1month and the use of antithrombotics in hemorrhagic infarction

The use of warfarin after detection of hemorrhagic infarction more frequently increased aggravation of HT than did the use of antiplatelets (4 of 24 vs 3 of 69; $p = 0.094$), but neither warfarin nor antiplatelets caused more HT than no medication (Figure 1-A). In addition, the use of antithrombotics after hemorrhagic infarction was not significantly associated with ND after HT (Figure 1-B). Aggravation of HT was related to ND after HT in only 2 of the 16 patients ($p = 0.124$) and was not related to transition to parenchymal

Table 1. General characteristics of subjects with hemorrhagic transformation at initial MRI and all imaging.

	Patients with Hemorrhagic infarction			All patients with HT		
	HI-1 (N=75)	**HI-2 (N=75)**	**P**	**HI (N=150)**	**PH (N=72)**	**p**
Age (mean±SD)	71.17±10.89	71.13±12.40	0.276	71.15±11.63	69.01±10.90	0.192
Male (n, %)	50 (66.7)	49 (65.3)	>0.999	99(66.0)	44(61.1)	0.549
Risk factors (n, %)						
HTN	47 (62.7)	53 (70.7)	0.387	100 (66.7)	52 (72.2)	0.443
DM	28 (37.3)	17 (22.7)	0.074	45 (30.0)	19 (26.4)	0.637
Smoking	24 (32.0)	17 (22.7)	0.272	41(27.3)	20 (27.8)	>0.999
Dyslipidemia	20 (26.7)	19 (25.3)	>0.999	39 (26.0)	11 (15.3)	0.087
Previous stroke	10 (13.3)	11 (14.7)	>0.999	21(14.0)	9 (12.5)	0.836
Atrial fibrillation	46 (61.3)	47 (62.7)	>0.999	93(62.0)	41 (56.9)	0.558
Visit time after onset, min (mean±SD),	560.68±792.6	425.00±727.24	0.983	492.84±761.12	392.25±913.00	0.389
Baseline NIHSS (med, IQR)	9.0 (11.0)	11.0 (9.0)	0.089	11.0 (9.0)	13.0 (6.75)	0.002
Thrombolysis (n, %)			0.827			0.006
IV only	17 (22.7)	21 (28.0)		38 (25.3)	28 (38.9)	
IA or IV+IA	12 (16.0)	11 (14.7)		23 (15.3)	17 (23.6)	
First anti-thrombotics (before HT) (n, %)	N=68	N=65	0.167			<0.001
None	8 (11.8)	17 (26.2)		65 (43.3)	61 (84.7)	
Anti-platelet	241 (60.3)	31 (47.7)		52 (34.7)	9 (14.8)	
Anti-coagulation	119 (227.9)	17 (26.2)		33 (22.0)	2 (2.8)	
Anti-thrombotics after HT (n, %)			0.001			<0.001
None	15 (20.0)	35 (46.7)		50 (32.3)	68 (94.4)	
Anti-platelet	41 (54.7)	31 (41.2)		72 (48.0)	4 (5.6)	
Anti-coagulation	19 (25.3)	9 (12.0)		28 (18.7)	0	
Neurological deterioration after HT (n, %)	2 (2.7)	4 (5.3)	0.681	6 (4.0)	10 (13.9)	0.012
Aggravation of HT at FU imaging (n, %)	5 (6.7)	11 (14.7)	0.185	16 (10.7)	14 (19.4)	0.093
Composite events within 1month (n, %)	1 (1.3)	4 (5.3)	0.367	5 (3.3)	7 (10.8)*	0..047

HTN, hypertension; DM, diabetes mellitus; NIHSS, National Institutes of Health Stroke Scale; IV, intravenous; IA, intra-arterial; HT, hemorrhagic transformation; END, early neurological deterioration; FU, follow-up.
*N=65 (due to loss of follow-up).

hemorrhage from hemorrhagic infarction. Multivariate logistic regression analysis revealed that the use of antiplatelets after hemorrhagic infarction was negatively associated with aggravation of HT (Model 2: OR 0.153; 95% CI 0.036–0.657, $p = 0.012$), whereas the use of warfarin was not (Table 2). Furthermore, the use of antithrombotics (warfarin and antiplatelets) after hemorrhagic infarction was not associated with ND after HT (Table 3).

The frequency of composite events at 1months was significantly lower in patients treated with antithrombotics than those treated without (1.6% vs 11.1%, $p = 0.041$). In addition, by multivariate logistic regression, composite events at 1 month after HT were significantly associated with the use of antithrombotics after discharge (Model 1: OR 0.132; 95% CI 0.020–0.893; $p = 0.038$) (Table 4).

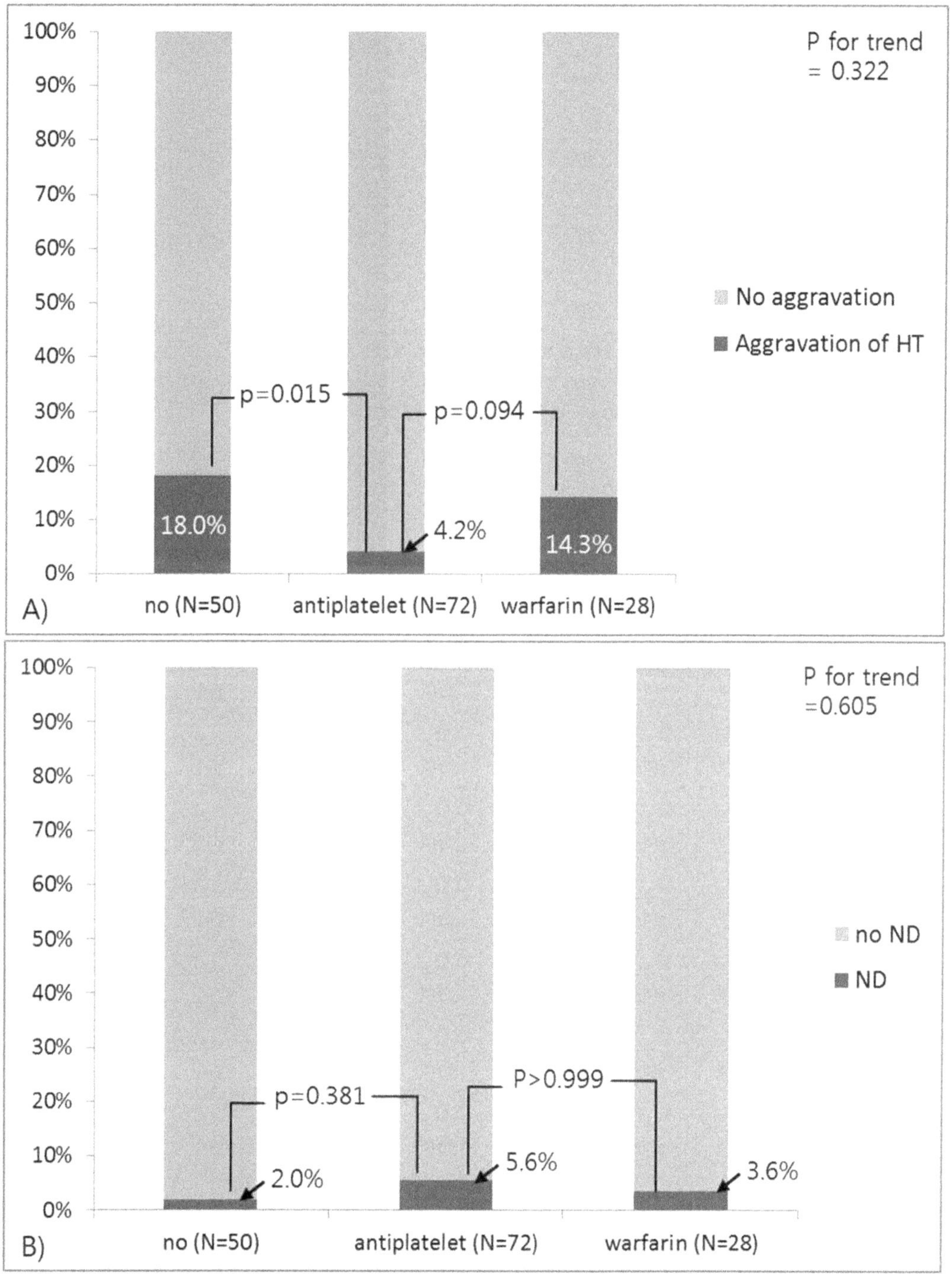

Figure 1. In hemorrhagic infarction (N = 150), a comparison of the development of HT aggravation (A) and neurological deterioration after HT (B) associated with the use of anti-thrombotic medication after HT. Abbreviations: HI, hemorrhagic infarction; HT, hemorrhagic transformation; ND, neurological deterioration after HT; END, early neurological deterioration.

Table 2. The associations between use of antithrombotics with aggravation of hemorrhagic transformation by multivariate logistic regression analysis in patients with hemorrhagic infarction (N = 150).

	Model 1	p	Model 2	p
Anti-thrombotics before HT		0.467		0.475
No med	Ref		Ref	
Antiplatelet	0.489 (0.117–2.049)	0.328	0.508 (0.120–2.147)	0.357
Warfarin	0.965 (0.199–4.679)	0.965	1.021 (0.206–5.053)	0.980
Anti-thrombotics after HT		0.038		0.041
No med	Ref		Ref	
Antiplatelet	0.150 (0.035–0.642)	0.011	0.153 (0.036–0.657)	0.012
Warfarin	0.517 (0.124–2.152)	0.365	1.186 (0.375–3.755)	0.771

Aggravation of HT; Model 1: Adjusted by age and initial NIHSS. Model 2: Adjusted by age, initial NIHSS, and thrombolysis.
END; adjusted by age, initial NIHSS and thrombolysis.

Aggravation of HT and the use of antithrombotics based on clinical situation in patients with hemorrhagic infarction

In patients treated with thrombolysis (n = 106), HT was mostly observed on 24-h GRE images obtained after thrombolysis (n = 96, 90.6%). Of the 106 thrombolysed patients, 61 developed hemorrhagic infarction. Of these 61 patients, 3 (9.4%) with type 2 hemorrhagic infarction developed ND after HT. There were no significant differences in aggravation of HT between types 1 and 2 (n = 3, 10.3% vs n = 4, 12.5%). After thrombolysis, 19 patients (31.1%) used no antithrombotics, 32 patients (52.5%) used antiplatelets, and 10 patients (16.4%) used warfarin, while after detection of hemorrhagic infarction, 1 user of warfarin and 6 users of antiplatelets stopped the use of antithrombotics. Aggravation of HT after the first use of antithrombotics was detected in 4 antiplatelet users, 2 warfarin users, and 1 patient who was not treated with antithrombotics (12.5% vs 20.0% vs 5.3%), without statistical significance. Therefore, the frequencies of aggravation HT after hemorrhagic infarction were 15.4% (4/26), 11.5% (3/26), and 0% (0/9) in non-users of antithrombotic, antiplatelet, or warfarin after HT, respectively (p for trends = 0.246), with no statistical significance (Table 5).

Eighty-nine of the 116 patients who did not undergo thrombolysis showed hemorrhagic infarction; only 33 patients (39.3%) showed hemorrhagic infarction on follow-up imaging within 2 days of initial MRI and the rest on follow-up imaging 3 days after initial MRI. Aggravation of HT was observed in 2 (4.3%) of the 46 patients with type 1 hemorrhagic infarction and 7 (16.3%) of the 43 patients with type 2 hemorrhagic infarction (p = 0.083). ND after HT was observed in 3 patients (2 patients in types 1 and 1 patient in type 2) (Table 5). Four (13.8%) of the 29 patients who used warfarin before HT showed aggravation of HT, all of whom continued to use warfarin after HT. However, ND after HT did not correlate with aggravation of HT (p = 0.277).

Discussion

Our study showed that although physicians may be reluctant to use antithrombotics after HT, even after hemorrhagic infarction, the use of antithrombotics after hemorrhagic infarction was not associated with ND after HT or aggravation of HT. In addition, although aggravation of HT was more frequently observed in patients with type 2 of hemorrhagic infarction than in those with type 1, the use of antithrombotics after hemorrhagic infarction was not associated with ND after HT or significant deleterious changes in the hemorrhagic infarction. Therefore, our study suggested that the use of antithrombotics after hemorrhagic infarction might be reasonable for prevention of subsequent ischemic stroke. However, because this was a retrospective study, further studies with a prospective design are needed to confirm our results.

In our study, about 66% of all patients used antithrombotics after hemorrhagic infarction, but only 30% of patients who required warfarin used warfarin after hemorrhagic infarction. The use of antiplatelets was reduced to about 73% in patients who had hemorrhagic infarction and non-cardioembolic stroke. Physicians were also reluctant to use antiplatelets after hemorrhagic infarction. Recent guidelines from the American Heart Association/American Stroke Association recommended that patients who need warfarin should continue to receive warfarin treatment regardless of hemorrhagic infarction (Class IIb; Level of evidence C) [3]. However, there is still a lack of evidence for this because only small case series have been conducted so far [4]. Our study, albeit a single-center retrospective study, demonstrates important factors physicians should consider when they detect HT in patients with acute ischemic stroke and the value of weighing the harms over the benefits of antithrombotics after HT.

Although the use of antiplatelets after HT has not been recommended in any trials, antiplatelet therapy should ideally be initiated within 24 to 48 hours of stroke onset [6]. Because patients with acute ischemic stroke do not generally receive follow-up imaging, asymptomatic HT may not easily be detected in actual practice. However, we were readily able to find asymptomatic HT

Table 3. The associations between use of antithrombotics with ND after HT by multivariate logistic regression analysis in patients with hemorrhagic infarction (N = 150).

	Model 1	p	Model 2	p
Use of antithrombotics after HT	2.332 (0.246–22.150)	0.461	2.503 (0.264–23.759)	0. 424
Initial NIHSS scores	0.964 (0.827–1.124)	0.639	0.938 (0.787–1.117)	0.470
Age	1.062 (0.963–1.171)	0.230	1.065 (0.965–1.175)	0.214
Thrombolysis	NA		2.228 (0.353–14.056)	0.394

Model 1: Adjusted by age and initial NIHSS. Model 2: Adjusted by age, initial NIHSS, and thrombolysis.

Table 4. The associations between use of antithrombotics with composite outcomes at 1 month by multivariate logistic regression analysis in patients with hemorrhagic infarction (N = 150).

	Model 1	p	Model 2	p
Use of antithrombotics after DC	0.132 (0.020–0.893)	0.038	0.128 (0.018–0.908)	0.040
Initial NIHSS scores	0.986 (0.835–1.165)	0.889	0.999 (0.847–1.177)	0.989
Age	1.019 (0.927–1.120)	0.700	1.016 (0.925–1.116)	0.743
Thrombolysis	NA		0.316 (0.033–3.061)	0.320

Model 1: Adjusted by age and initial NIHSS. Model 2: Adjusted by age, initial NIHSS, and thrombolysis.
DC; discharge.

by routine repetitive follow-up imaging studies in acute clinical setting. Our study showed that the acute use of antiplatelets after hemorrhagic infarction may be relatively safe. ND after HT was uncommon in the use of antithrombotics after hemorrhagic infarction. These results suggest that there may be no firm basis for physicians to reject to use antithrombotics after hemorrhagic infarction.

Asymptomatic HT is mainly considered to be an epiphenomenon of reperfusion into ischemic tissue without any clinical impact [7,8]. Only parenchymal hemorrhage (type 2) significantly increased the risk of early clinical deterioration and worse outcomes. Other types of HT, such as types 1 and 2 of hemorrhagic infarction, were not associated with deterioration after HT [9,10]. However, early anticoagulation after ischemic stroke could increase the risk of HT and is not recommended in the very early stage after ischemic stroke for patients with moderate to severe strokes [6]. Therefore, our results suggest that the cautious use of antithrombotics (continuation or temporarily discontinuation of the antithrombotics), was not related to the aggravation of HT and ND after HT even when hemorrhagic infarction is present on follow-up imaging. Discontinuing or continuing antithrombotics for a few days followed by repeat imaging to evaluate the stability of hemorrhagic infarction may then allow for the safe continuation of treatment. In our study, only 30% of patients with hemorrhagic infarction continue to use warfarin in acute ischemic stroke. The use of antithrombotics after hemorrhagic infarction can be supported by previous studies and ours.

We assessed the influence of the use of antithrombotics on composite events over early periods of follow-up. Even without aggravation of HT on follow-up imaging, 18% of patients did not use antithrombotics at the time of discharge. This may be due to higher risk of events in patients treated with no antithrombotics than in those treated with antithrombotics in the early periods. Although the use of antithrombotics after HT may raise concern about aggravation of HT, the risk of events may increase in patients treated without antithrombotics after HT. Therefore, the results of our study suggest that meticulous care may be needed over early periods after HT.

The results of this study are subject to some limitations. First, being a single-center, retrospective study that evaluated consecutive patients with HT according to our stroke protocol, further studies with a prospective design are needed to confirm our results. In particular, we could not confirm the efficacy of antithrombotics in patients with hemorrhagic infarction because they were neither randomly selected nor blinded to antithrombotics. However, in order to minimize a selection bias, we only analyzed patients with hemorrhagic infarction. In addition, since the number of warfarin

Table 5. Types of hemorrhagic infarction based on thrombolysis and clinical and imaging changes associated with use of antithrombotics.

	Before hemorrhagic infarction			After hemorrhagic infarction		
Thrombolysis (N = 61)	No med	Antiplatelet	Warfarin	No med	Antiplatelet	Warfarin
A) Hemorrhagic infarction type 1 (N = 29)	n = 7	n = 18	n = 4	n = 8	n = 15	n = 6
HT aggravation	1 (14.3)	2 (11.1)	0	2 (25.0)	1 (6.7)	0
ND after HT	0	0	0	0	0	0
B) Hemorrhagic infarction type 2 (N = 32)	n = 12	n = 14	n = 6	n = 18	n = 11	n = 3
HT aggravation	0	2 (14.3)	2 (33.3)	2 (11.1)	2 (18.2)	0
ND after HT	0	2 (14.3)	1 (16.7)	1 (5.6)	2 (18.2)	0
Non-thrombolysis (N = 89)						
A) Hemorrhagic infarction type 1 (N = 46)	n = 2	n = 26	n = 18	n = 7	n = 26	n = 13
HT aggravation	0	0	2 (11.1)	0	0	2 (15.4)
ND after HT	0	1 (3.8)	1 (5.6)	0	1 (3.8)	1 (7.7)
B) Hemorrhagic infarction type-2 (N = 43)	n = 10	n = 22	n = 11	n = 17	n = 20	n = 6
HT aggravation	3 (30.0)	2 (9.1)	2 (18.2)	5 (29.4)	0	2 (33.3)
ND after HT	0	1 (4.5)	0	0	1 (5.0)	0

HT, hemorrhagic transformation; ND, neurological deterioration.

users after hemorrhagic infarction was small, relationships between the use of warfarin after hemorrhagic infarction and aggravation of HT/ND after HT need to be further investigated through prospective studies. Furthermore, the effects of anti-thrombotic agents, either antiplatelet or anticoagulant, need at least 3 to 5 days to reach the optimal level, if not given loading dose initially. In our study, MR images were followed at 3–5 days after HT detection which may not be adequate time window to evaluate the drug effect on hematoma aggravation or other possible complications. We evaluated composite events at 1month after HT in order to overcome this limitation. Factors related to HT have been shown to be various clinical conditions, such as chronic kidney disease, high blood pressure, and infarct size. However, because we included only patients with HT in acute ischemic stroke in this study, these factors were excluded from the study. Finally, we excluded patients with malignant infarction over two-thirds of hemisphere. The risk of HT might be high in these patients. However, we considered that malignant infarction per se affect the safety and ND and thus should be excluded in this study.

In conclusion, the results of this study suggest that antithrombotics can safely be used after hemorrhagic infarction and may not be associated with ND after HT and aggravation of HT. However, many physicians are still reluctant to use antithrombotics when HT is detected by imaging, even in hemorrhagic infarction. Further studies are needed to confirm our results.

Supporting Information

Table S1 Characteristics of subjects with hemorrhagic transformation on initial imaging.

Figure S1 Types of hemorrhagic transformation according to the gradient echo imaging, modified by ECASS definition. A) Hemorrhagic infarction type 1. There are small petechiae along the margin of the infarct. B) Hemorrhagic infarction type 2. There are confluent petechiae within the infarcted area, but without space-occupying effect. C) Parenchymal hemorrhage type 1. There is a hematoma in 30% or less of infarcted area with some slight space-occupying effect. D) Parenchymal hematoma type 2. There is a dense hematoma over 30% of infarcted area with substantial space occupying effect, or as any hemorrhagic lesion outside infarcted area.

Figure S2 Changes in the use of anti-thrombotics before and after hemorrhagic infarction and at a follow-up of 1 month in patients with hemorrhagic infarction.

Figure S3 Changes in the use of anti-thrombotics before and after hemorrhagic infarction. Even after hemorrhagic infarction, use of anti-thrombotics decreased.

Author Contributions

Conceived and designed the experiments: JTK MSP SHH. Performed the experiments: JTK MSP. Analyzed the data: JTK MSP JC SHH. Contributed reagents/materials/analysis tools: JTK MSP JC SHH. Wrote the paper: JTK MSP JC. Critically revised the manuscript for important intellectual content: JTK MSP K.H. Choi K.H. Cho JC SHH. Provided statistical analysis: JTK MSP K.H. Choi K.H. Cho. Provided administrative, technical, or material support: K.H. Cho MSP.

References

1. Park JH, Ko Y, Kim WJ, Jang MS, Yang MH, et al. (2012) Is asymptomatic hemorrhagic transformation really innocuous? Neurology 78: 421–426.
2. Kent DM, Hinchey J, Price LL, Levine SR, Selker HP (2004) In acute ischemic stroke, are asymptomatic intracranial hemorrhages clinically innocuous? Stroke 35: 1141–1146.
3. Furie KL, Kasner SE, Adams RJ, Albers GW, Bush RL, et al. (2011) Guidelines for the prevention of stroke in patients with stroke or transient ischemic attack: a guideline for healthcare professionals from the american heart association/american stroke association. Stroke 42: 227–276.
4. Pessin MS, Estol CJ, Lafranchise F, Caplan LR (1993) Safety of anticoagulation after hemorrhagic infarction. Neurology 43: 1298–1303.
5. Hacke W, Kaste M, Fieschi C, von Kummer R, Davalos A, et al. (1998) Randomised double-blind placebo-controlled trial of thrombolytic therapy with intravenous alteplase in acute ischaemic stroke (ECASS II). Second European-Australasian Acute Stroke Study Investigators. Lancet 352: 1245–1251.
6. Adams HP Jr, del Zoppo G, Alberts MJ, Bhatt DL, Brass L, et al. (2007) Guidelines for the early management of adults with ischemic stroke: a guideline from the American Heart Association/American Stroke Association Stroke Council, Clinical Cardiology Council, Cardiovascular Radiology and Intervention Council, and the Atherosclerotic Peripheral Vascular Disease and Quality of Care Outcomes in Research Interdisciplinary Working Groups: the American Academy of Neurology affirms the value of this guideline as an educational tool for neurologists. Stroke 38: 1655–1711.
7. Fiehler J, Remmele C, Kucinski T, Rosenkranz M, Thomalla G, et al. (2005) Reperfusion after severe local perfusion deficit precedes hemorrhagic transformation: an MRI study in acute stroke patients. Cerebrovasc Dis 19: 117–124.
8. Molina CA, Alvarez-Sabin J, Montaner J, Abilleira S, Arenillas JF, et al. (2002) Thrombolysis-related hemorrhagic infarction: a marker of early reperfusion, reduced infarct size, and improved outcome in patients with proximal middle cerebral artery occlusion. Stroke 33: 1551–1556.
9. Berger C, Fiorelli M, Steiner T, Schabitz WR, Bozzao L, et al. (2001) Hemorrhagic transformation of ischemic brain tissue: asymptomatic or symptomatic? Stroke 32: 1330–1335.
10. Kablau M, Kreisel SH, Sauer T, Binder J, Szabo K, et al. (2011) Predictors and early outcome of hemorrhagic transformation after acute ischemic stroke. Cerebrovasc Dis 32: 334–341.

14

Neuroproteome Changes after Ischemia/Reperfusion Injury and Tissue Plasminogen Activator Administration in Rats: A Quantitative iTRAQ Proteomics Study

Zamir Merali[2], Meah MingYang Gao[1], Tim Bowes[1], Jian Chen[3], Kenneth Evans[3], Andrea Kassner[1,2]*

1 Department of Medical Imaging, University Of Toronto, Toronto, Ontario, Canada, **2** Physiology and Experimental Medicine, The Hospital For Sick Children, Toronto, Ontario, Canada, **3** Ontario Cancer Biomarker Network, Toronto, Ontario Canada

Abstract

The thrombolytic, recombinant tissue plasminogen activator (rt-PA) is the only approved therapy for acute ischemic stroke (AIS). When administered after AIS, rt-PA has many adverse pleiotropic actions, which are currently poorly understood. The identification of proteins showing differential expression after rt-PA administration may provide insight into these pleiotropic actions. In this study we used a 2D-LC MS/MS iTRAQ proteomic analysis, western blotting, and pathway analysis to analyze changes in protein expression 24-hours after rt-PA administration in the cortical brain tissue of 36 rats that underwent a sham or transient middle cerebral artery occlusion surgery. After rt-PA administration we reported alterations in the expressions of 18 proteins, many of which were involved in excitatory neurotransmitter function or cytoskeletal structure. The expression changes of GAD2 and EAAT1 were validated with western blot. The interactions between the identified proteins were analyzed with the IPA pathway analysis tool and three proteins: DPYSL2, RTN4, and the NF-kB complex, were found to have characteristics of being key proteins in the network. The differential protein expressions we observed may reflect pleiotropic actions of rt-PA after experimental stroke, and shine light on the mechanisms of rt-PA's adverse effects. This may have important implications in clinical settings where thrombolytic therapy is used to treat AIS.

Editor: Xiaoying Wang, Massachusetts General Hospital, United States of America

Funding: This work was supported by the Canada Research Chair Program (http://www.chairs-chaires.gc.ca/home-accueil-eng.aspx) and the Canadian Institutes of Health Research (94383, 111113) (http://www.cihr-irsc.gc.ca/e/193.html). The funders had no role in study design, data collection and analysis, decision to publish, or preparation of the manuscript.

Competing Interests: The authors have declared that no competing interests exist.

* E-mail: Andrea.kassner@utoronto.ca

Introduction

A thrombolytic agent, rt-PA (recombinant tissue plasminogen activator) is the only therapeutic used in the treatment of acute ischemic stroke (AIS) [1]. Numerous exclusion criteria, such as a narrow therapeutic window of 4.5 hrs, limit the number of patients receiving rt-PA. Even amongst eligible patients, rt-PA is substantially underused, with only 3% to 8.5% of potentially eligible patients receiving the drug [2]. The association of rt-PA with severe adverse effects has contributed to reluctance amongst emergency physicians to utilize the drug [3].

rt-PA is capable of both beneficial reperfusion due to its interaction with plasminogen, and neurotoxicity due to its pleiotropic effects on other brain tissue substrates [4]. While many of the pleiotropic effects are poorly characterized, the interaction between the N-methyl-D-aspartate (NMDA) receptor and rt-PA has received substantial experimental attention. In the presence of rt-PA, NMDA receptor signaling is potentiated, and the ensuing dysregulation of intracellular calcium levels contributes to neuron and glia death after stroke [5]. NMDA receptor antagonists were seen as promising neuroprotective agents for their ability to disrupt this process and perhaps mediate the harmful effects of rt-PA in an animal model [6]. The ultimate failure, however, of the NMDA receptor antagonists in clinical trials was demonstrative of the simplification of the NMDA receptor's role in the complex pathophysiology of stroke [7]. More broadly, it demonstrated the tendency to overemphasize the role of a single pathway in mediating a complex disease state. To achieve an understanding of how rt-PA contributes to the pathophysiology of AIS, it may not be sufficient to utilize a traditional biochemical approach, in which pathways are investigated in isolation [8–10].

With recent advances in proteomics technology, the overall protein expression of various samples can be compared within a single experiment. Analysis of these results with bioinformatics tools can generate a more comprehensive understanding of the involved pathways [11]. Neuroproteomic studies of AIS have varied in their methods, with many published before 2010 making use of the 2D-gel-based approach (2D-GE MS/MS) [12–15]. A small number of more recent studies have made use of LC MS/MS-based multi dimensional protein identification [9,10]. When combined with the multiplex isobaric tag for relative and absolute quantification (iTRAQ) method, the LC MS/MS approach can simultaneously quantify proteins in 4 or 8 samples [16]. A number of studies have successfully utilized neuroproteomic methods to analyze differentially expressed proteins after ischemic stroke, and these results have deepened our understanding of stroke pathophysiology. However, although rt-PA administration alters the pathophysiology of stroke in a clinically significant way, no study

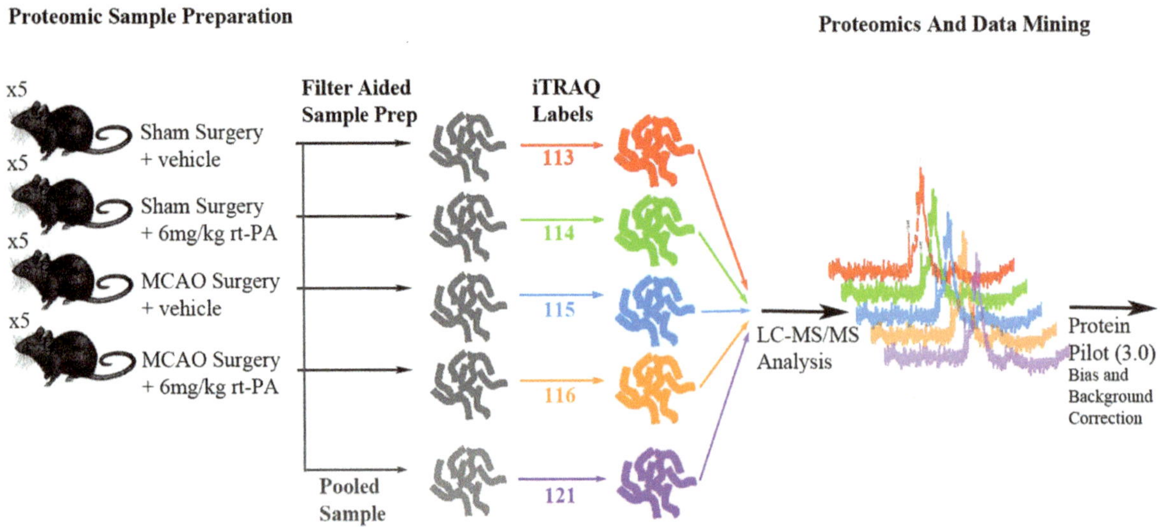

Figure 1. Schematic of 2D LC-MS/MS experimental design. Five iTRAQ labels were used: 113 for the Sham+distilled water injection. 114 for the Sham+rt-PA infusion. 115 for tMCAo+distilled water injection. 116 for tMCAo+rt-PA infusion. 121 for a pooled sample containing equal amounts from each group. Treated rats were given 6 mg/kg rt-PA 4 hrs after occlusion. All samples were pooled after iTRAQ labeling and subjected to mass spectrometric analysis.

that we are aware of has attempted to measure the proteome changes associated with rt-PA administration after AIS.

Since many of rt-PA's pleiotropic interactions are uncharacterized, the identification of proteins showing differential expression

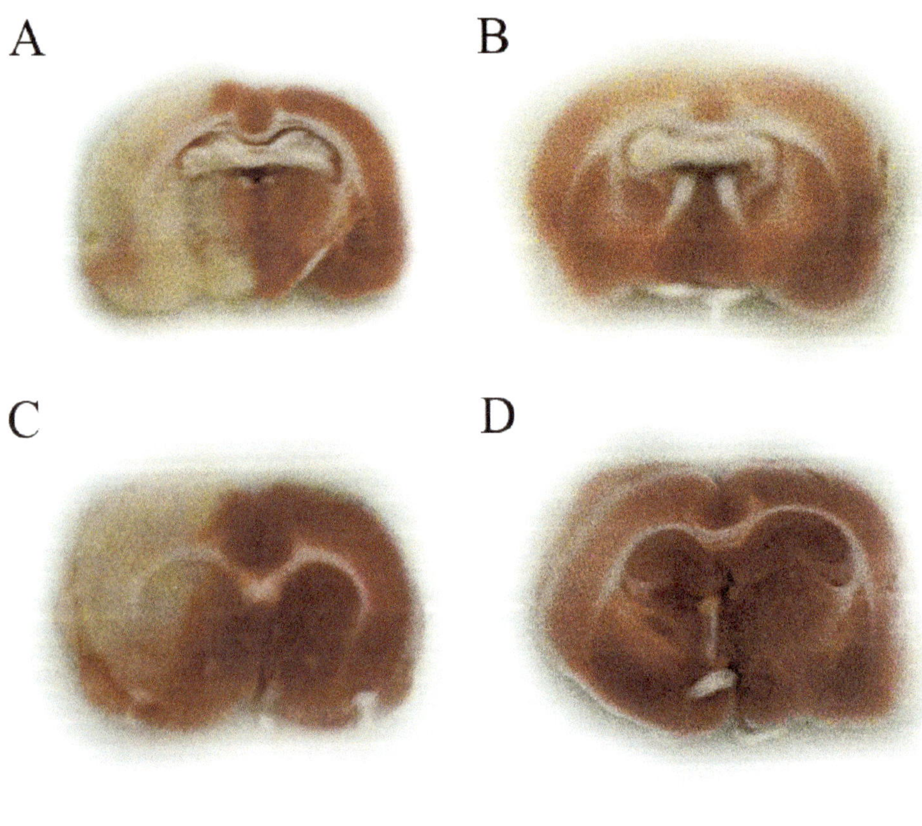

Figure 2. Representative tetrazolium chloride (TTC) stained sections of (A) transient middle cerebral artery occlusion (tMCAo)+rt-PA rats (B) sham+rt-PA rats (C) tMCAo+vehicle rats and (D) sham+vehicle rats. Dark areas reflect living viable tissue while white reflects infarcted tissue or areas of white matter. Infarcted areas occupy at least 50% of the right hemisphere in all tMCAo rats.

after rt-PA administration may shed light on the molecular mechanisms underlying rt-PA's adverse effects. We sought to apply 2D-LC MS/MS and iTRAQ proteomics directly to cortical brain tissue to analyze how rt-PA administration altered the proteome in a transient rodent stroke model. A further aim of this study was to probe the source of this protein regulation with a pathway analysis tool.

Materials and Methods

Reagents

All agents were purchased from Sigma-Aldrich (Oakville, Ontario) unless otherwise indicated.

Ethics Statement

The Hospital For Sick Children Animal Research Committee approved all procedures and protocols in accordance with the protocols of the Canadian Council of Animal Care. At the experimental endpoint all rats were humanely sacrificed with an intra-peritoneal euthanyl injection in accordance with the Canadian Council of Animal Care guidelines.

Proteomics Experimental Design

Sprague dawley rats (300–350 g males, Charles-River Laboratories, Sherbrooke, Canada), in pathogen free housing, were made use of. The experimental design for the iTRAQ proteomics analysis is as shown in Figure 1. Rats were randomized into one of four groups with a computerized random number generator (five per group). These groups were: a Sham group - rats receiving a sham surgery followed by IV sterile water infusion 4 hours after occlusion; Sham+rt-PA Group - rats receiving a sham surgery followed by a 10 minute intravenous infusion of 6 mg/kg rt-PA 4 hours after occlusion; tMCAo Group - rats receiving a 1 hr tMCAo followed by an IV sterile water infusion 4 hours after occlusion; and tMCAo+rt-PA Group, rats receiving a 1 hr tMCAo followed by a 10 minute intravenous infusion of 6 mg/kg rt-PA 4 hours after occlusion. An endpoint of 24-hours was chosen because in the tMCAo rodent model the risks of hemorrhage and neuronal death reach a peak at this time-point. In addition, this choice of end-point allowed for maximum comparability with previous results, as previous neuroproteomic studies have predominantly chosen an end-point of 24-hours. All rats were euthanized with an IP euthanyl injection. For the 2D LC-MS/MS iTRAQ analysis 5 biologic replicates for each experimental group and 1 injection was performed.

Transient Ischemia Model

A transient focal ischemia was induced in rats under isoflurane anesthesia with the transient middle cerebral artery occlusion (tMCAo) procedure as previously described [17]. A 0.39 mm diameter filament tip was used and the occlusion was maintained for 1 hr. For sham operations the carotid bifurcation was exposed, the external carotid was ligated, and the filament was inserted the correct distance before being immediately withdrawn. Core body

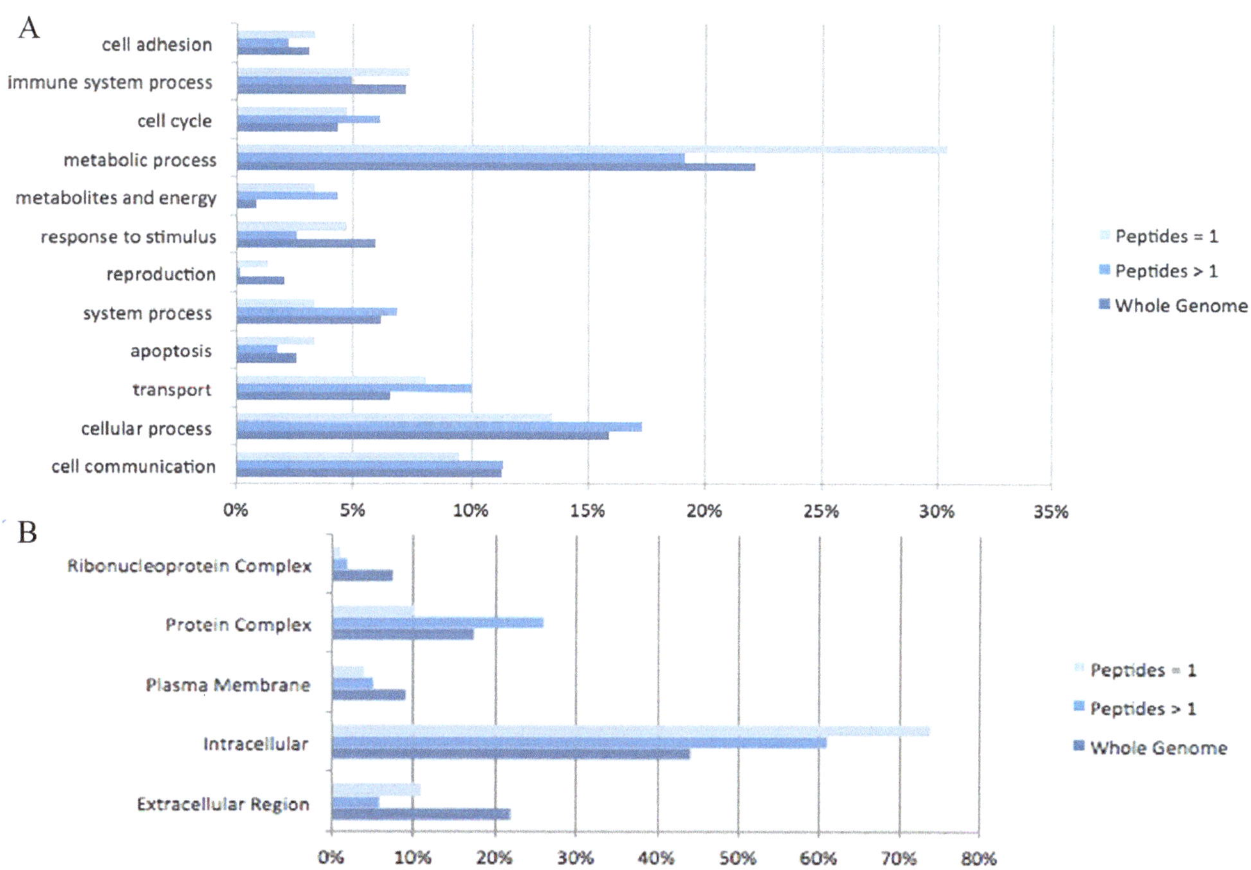

Figure 3. Functional distribution (A) and Sub-cellular distribution (B) of proteins identified with 1 peptide and 2 or more peptides compared to the entire Rattus norvegicus genome. Functional and spacial categories are those defined in the PANTHER database.

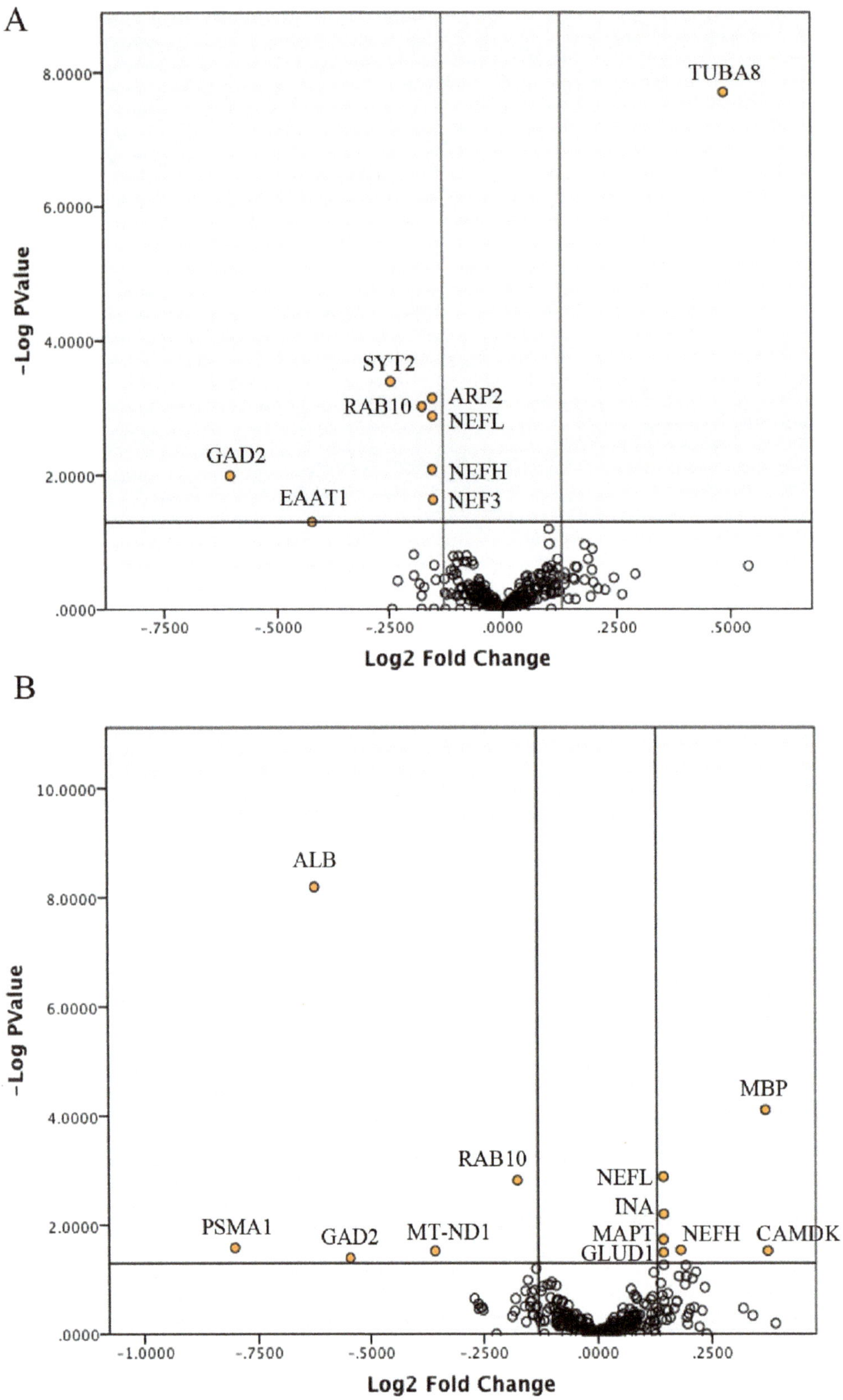

Figure 4. Volcano plots showing the distribution of significance and fold change of identified proteins in the (A) sham+rt-PA/sham comparison and (B) tMCAo+rt-PA/tMCAo comparison. All proteins with 2 or more peptides were plotted with fold change on the x-axis and p-value on the y-axis. Vertical lines mark a fold change of +/−10% and the horizontal line marks p =0.05. The 18 proteins marked in orange with text labels meet the criteria for having differential expression (>10% in either direction) and are significant (<p=0.05).

Table 1. Between group comparisons of protein expression fold changes after tMCAo and rt-PA administration meeting the criteria outlined in 'Statistical Analysis'.

Name	Uniprot ID	Peptides (95%)	control+rt-PA/ control	tMCAO/ control	tMCAO+rt-PA/tMCAO
			Fold Change	Fold Change	Fold Change
Actin-related protein-2	Q5M7U6	4	**−1.11**	−1.04	−1.09
Alpha-internexin	P23565	26	−1.03	1.09	**1.11**
Calcium/calmodulin-dependent protein kinase type II subunit delta	P15791	12	−1.09	**−1.48**	**1.29**
Excitatory amino acid transporter 1	P24942	4	**−1.34**	**−1.27**	1.07
Glutamate decarboxylase 2	Q05683	6	**−1.52**	**1.15**	**−1.46**
Glutamate dehydrogenase 1, mitochondrial	P10860	14	−1.03	−1.07	**1.10**
Microtubule-associated protein tau	P19332	5	−1.04	−1.08	**1.13**
Myelin basic protein S	P02688	20	1.03	**−1.22**	**1.29**
NADH dehydrogenase [ubiquinone] flavoprotein 2, mitochondrial	P19234	2	1.01	1.00	**−1.28**
Neurofilament heavy polypeptide	P16884	15	**−1.11**	**−1.20**	**1.19**
Neurofilament light polypeptide	P19527	32	**−1.11**	−1.09	**1.10**
Neurofilament medium polypeptide	P12839	27	**−1.11**	−1.07	−1.01
Proteasome subunit alpha type-2	P17220	2	−1.01	**1.16**	**−1.74**
Ras-related protein Rab-10	P35281	4	**−1.14**	**1.10**	**−1.16**
Serum Albumin	P02770	28	1.03	**1.89**	**−1.54**
Synapsin-2	Q63537	17	1.07	**1.14**	−1.09
Synaptotagmin-2	P29101	2	**−1.19**	**−1.25**	1.05
Tubulin alpha-8 chain	Q6AY56	55	**1.40**	1.00	−1.02

Fold changes in **bold** were significantly altered.

temperature was monitored continuously and kept constant at 37°C. Rats were given 0.03 mg/kg buprenorphine for post-surgical pain relief. At 5-hours after occlusion rats were given 2 mL of subcutaneous fluids. During the surgery heart rate, and breathing rate were monitored periodically.

Tissue Extraction

At 24-hours after euthanasia brains were quickly removed and sectioned into 2 mm slices over ice. The right hemisphere from a slice 0.3 mm anterior of bregma was carefully dissected under magnification over ice to isolate the cortical tissue. The cortical tissue was flash frozen in liquid nitrogen and stored at −80°C until proteomic analysis. The slices anterior and posterior to this slice were stained with Tetrazolium Chloride (TTC). Images of TTC stained sections were imported into the Image J software (NIH). The infarcted areas were manually traced, as were the total hemispheric areas. Rats with infarct sizes less than 40% cross-sectional area of the sampled right hemisphere sections were excluded from the proteomic analysis.

Proteomics Sample Preparation

The protocol used was the Filter Aided Sample Preparation (FASP) method originally developed by Matthial Mann [18]. FASP is able to reduce SDS and contaminant levels, and increase the yield of membrane bound and nuclear proteins. Cortical tissue was weighed and dissolved into 800 uL of lysis buffer (3% SDS, 5 mM TCEP, 0.1 M Tris-HCl at pH 7.6). After sonication the samples were heated at 95 C for 5 min. The samples were then centrifuged at 14000 g in a microcentrifuge for 10 minutes. The supernatants were isolated and protein content was measured using the Bio-Rad DC assay, having diluted 10 µL of sample into 1 mL of assay reagent buffer to reduce TCEP concentration to below acceptable assay thresholds. Once the concentrations of each sample were determined, 60 µg from each animal in the same treatment were pooled to a total of 300 µg. Following this, Nanosep 10 kDa filters (Pall Life Sciences, Ann Arbor, MI, USA) were rinsed with 100 µL deionized, distilled water, and spun through the filter. Then, the filters were rinsed with 100 µL of fresh urea buffer (8 M urea in 0.1 M Tris-HCl, pH 8.5), which was also spun through and discarded. 200 µg of sample was loaded onto each filter and spun through for 15 min at 14000 g. Following this, 100 µL of 50 mM iodoacetamide in urea buffer was applied to the filters and mixed for 1 min at 600 rpm. The filters were incubated at room temperature for 20 min and the buffer was removed by centrifugation at 14000 g for 15 min. The filters were then rinsed with 100 µL of urea buffer and then rinsed with 100 µL of 0.5 M TEAB removing buffer by centrifugation after each rinse. 40 uL of 1 µg Trypsin in 0.5 M TEAB was added and the filters were incubated at 37 C for 18 h. The digested samples were isolated by centrifugation, spinning through another 40 µL of 0.5 M TEAB to improve tryptic peptide yield. Peptide concentration was determined using a Nanospec (Nanolytik, Germany).

iTRAQ Labeling and 2D LC-MS/MS Analysis

The iTRAQ proteomics method provides extensive quantification coverage of around 88% with one technical replicate [19]. iTRAQ proteomics was performed using an 8-plex procedure

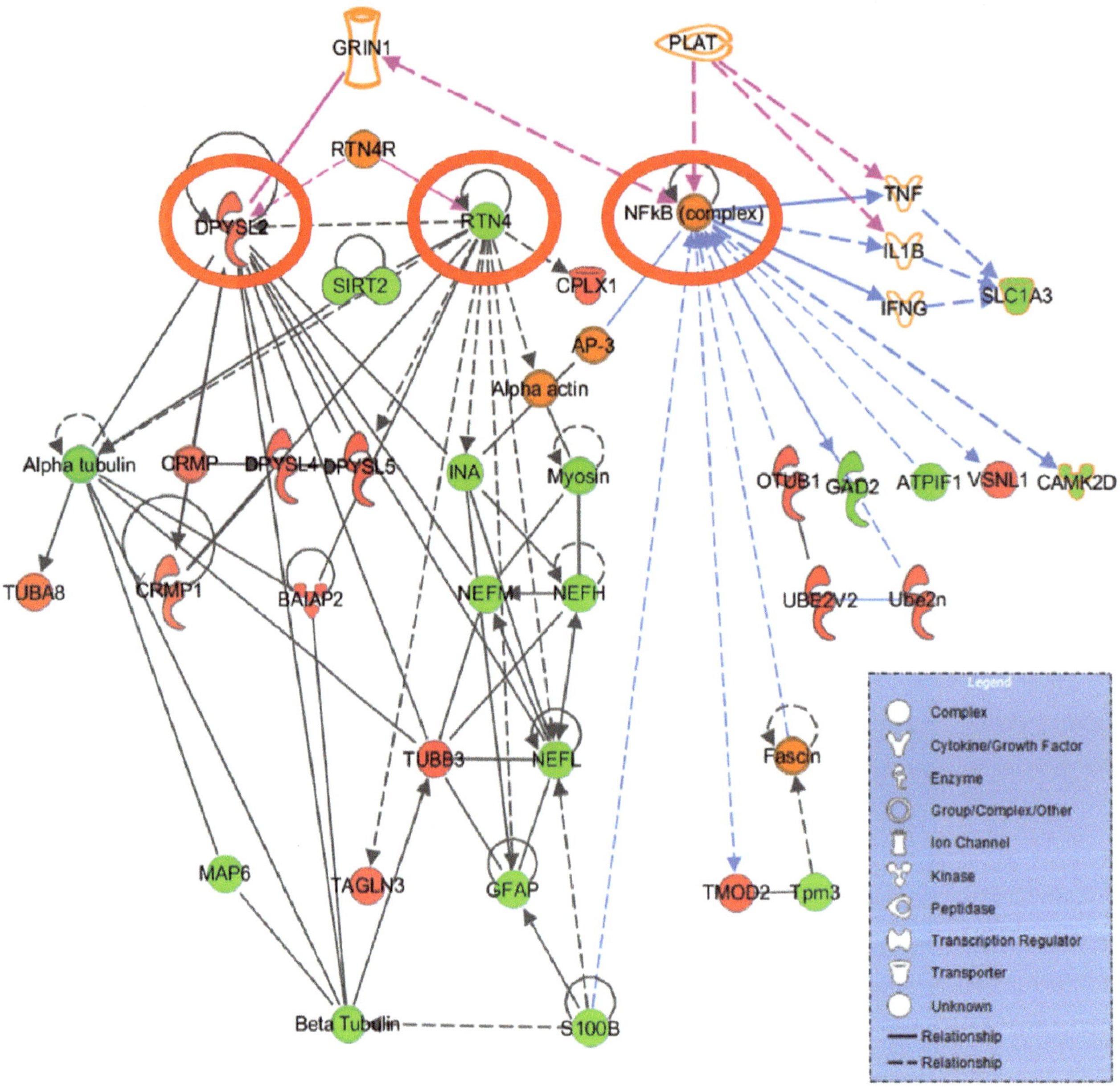

Figure 5. Results of an IPA pathway analysis of the tMCAo comparison. Encircled proteins are DPYSL2, RTN4, and NF-kB, which show a high centrality measure. Green nodes are up-regulated proteins, red nodes are down-regulated. A line between two nodes represents a direct or indirect interaction noted in the literature.

(only 5 samples were analyzed) so that all experimental samples were processed simultaneously. The iTRAQ labels for each group were as follows: 113 - sham surgery and vehicle, 114 – sham surgery and rt-PA, 115 – tMCAo surgery and vehicle, 116 – tMCAo surgery and rt-PA. Thirty µg of protein was used for iTRAQ labeling following the manufacturer's instructions with no modifications. Trypsin-digested and iTRAQ labeled samples were then pooled and subjected to strong cation exchange (SCX) fractionation on a Biobasic SCX column (4.6 mm I.D×15 cm L., Thermo, USA). Fifteen fractions were collected and injected into a nanoflow high-performance liquid chromatographer (HPLC) (Proxeon, Denmark), equipped with a 360 um filter and packed with Zorbax SB18-300 reversed phase (Agilent, USA). This HPLC set-up was coupled with a hybrid quadrupole/Time of flight MS (QStar Elite, AB Sciex, USA) and data was collected using Analyst QS 2.0 controlling software (AB Sciex, USA) through a nanospray ion source. ProteinPilot version 3.0 (AB Sciex, USA) was used for processing the raw acquired iTRAQ data files. The protein identification was performed by searching raw MS data against the Swissprot-Uniprot protein database (January, 2010), with species restriction to Rattus norvegicus. Default search parameters were predominantly used.

PANTHER Gene Ontology

The PANTHER classification system v8.1 (California) was used according to a published protocol [20]. The Uniprot IDs of the 209 proteins identified by 2 or more peptides and 113 proteins identified by 1 peptide were uploaded separately to the

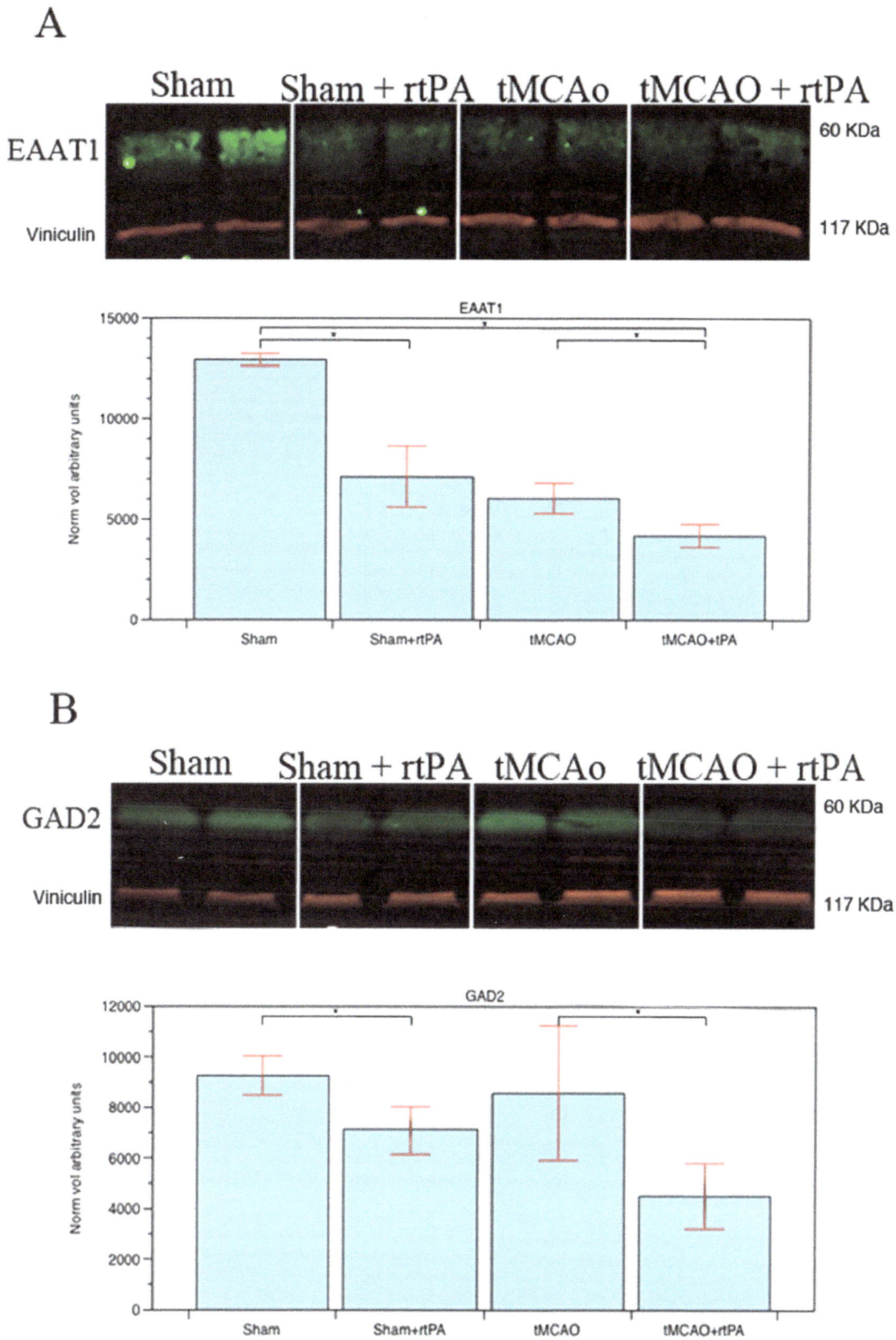

Figure 6. Quantification of protein expression by western blot. (A) Excitatory amino acid transporter 1 (EAAT1) and (B) Glutamate decarboxylase 2 (GAD2) expressions analyzed by western blot. Bands were quantified using scanned densitometry and normalized to viniculin expression. Vertical axis shows an arbitrary density unit. Asterisks mark significant changes ($p<0.05$, $n=4$).

PANTHER online tool. The Rattus norvegicus genome was chosen as the reference database. From the output report aggregate functional and sub-cellular location information was extracted. This was compared with the aggregate data from the entire Rattus norvegicus genome of 20966 proteins.

Pathway and Centrality Analysis

The Uniprot ID of the 403 proteins identified by 2D LC-MS/MS iTRAQ with an FDR<0.01 were uploaded to the Ingenuity Pathway Analysis (IPA) version 7.5 (Redwood City, CA) software. IPA allows for the identification of protein-protein interactions and network interactions based on a database of manually curated published protein interactions. We utilized a p-value cut-off at 0.05 and no fold change cut-off. Each Uniprot ID meeting this cut-off was mapped to the corresponding gene object in the Ingenuity pathway knowledge base. These genes are referred to as focus genes, and were overlaid onto the curated global molecular networks contained within the Ingenuity knowledge base. Next, networks of the focus genes were generated based on protein-protein interactions and each network was scored based on a Fisher test. The network score represented the relevance of the network to the input Uniprot IDs. The highest scoring network was chosen and was represented as a graph that indicated the interactions (direct or indirect) between proteins. The relative expression data from the tMCAo+rt-PA comparison was overlaid onto this network. Each node indicated a single protein, and the green or red color indicated up- or down- regulation as seen in the 2D LC-MS/MS iTRAQ analysis.

Lastly, the degree centrality for each protein in the network was calculated as previously described using the IPA software [11]. Briefly, the degree centrality is the simplest measure of centrality and represents the number of connections (direct or indirect) made by each protein in the network regardless of the direction of the connection. To determine the proteins that had the highest levels of centrality we used the standard cut-off of 5% [21]. Thus, the proteins with degree centrality measures in the top 5% of the distribution were identified as having high degree centrality.

Confirmation of Differentially Expressed Proteins by Western Blot

Separate animals were used for the western blot analysis (4 per group). At 24-hours after occlusion rats were euthanized with an IP euthanyl injection and the cortical tissue was extracted following the same procedure as for iTRAQ sample preparation. Whole-cell protein extracts were prepared from the cortical tissue. Primary antibodies used were: GAD2 (5834P, Cell Signalling), EAAT1 (5684P, Cell Signalling), and Vinculin (4650P, Cell Signalling). Infrared conjugated secondary antibodies (LI-COR) were used and luminescence was quantified using an Odyssey infrared imaging system.

Statistical Analysis

For data processing the ProteinPilot software v.3.0 (AB SCIEX, Framingham, USA) was used. The false discovery rate (FDR) for each protein was estimated using a concatenated target-decoy database as described by Elias and Gygi. [22] This generated a probability measure for each protein. To determine iTRAQ protein quantification the Pro Group algorithm within ProteinPilot was used to calculate a p-value of each relative expression change. Quantitation data for each protein was based on the underlying peptides that were determined to be unique by Pro Group. Within Pro Group, the null-hypothesis was taken as a lognormal distribution of unique peptide quantities and the p-value of the expression change was calculated from the standard deviation in logspace.

We imposed a strict set of criteria to reduce false positive expression changes. For a protein to be accepted as having a differential expression between treatment groups we used the following criteria: The protein must have been identified in all 5 iTRAQ preparations. Only proteins that were identified with at least 2 peptides with greater than 95% confidence were considered. Proteins with 10% increase or decrease in expression (iTRAQ ratios 114:113, 116:115, or 113:115 greater than 1.1 or less than −1.1) and a significant p-value ($p<0.05$), were considered to be differentially expressed.

The densitometry results of the western blot experiments were analyzed in the Excel program (Microsoft, 2013) with a two-tailed student's T-test and $p<0.05$ was taken as being significant.

Degree centrality data from the IPA analysis was also analyzed with the Excel program. Degree centrality data was taken to have a normal distribution and proteins with high levels of degree centrality were identified by calculating the standard deviation within the distribution.

Results

In total 44 rats underwent tMCAo or sham surgery and tissue extraction. Six rats died before the experimental end-point and were excluded from further analysis. Two rats had an insufficient stroke size (<40% hemispheric area) upon TTC staining and were also excluded from further analysis. This left 36 rats to undergo tissue analysis. Twenty of these rats underwent 2D LC-MS/MS iTRAQ analysis with 5 rats per experimental group. The remaining sixteen rats underwent western blotting experiments with 4 rats per experimental group.

Physiologic parameters and core body temperature did not differ between groups (data not shown). All rats that underwent further analysis had large strokes through the basal ganglia and cortical regions (Figure 2) occupying at least 40% of the hemispheric cross-sectional area.

Protein Identification and Relative Expression

Overall our analysis identified 1143 distinct proteins, of which 403 had an estimated global False Discovery Rate (FDR)<0.01 (Table S1). As an assessment of quality we compared the distributions of biologic functions of these 403 proteins (209 identified with 2 or more peptides and 113 identified by 1 peptide) with the entire Rattus norvegicus genome of 20966 proteins (Figure 3A). 12 functional categories were defined utilizing the PANTHER gene ontology database. Proteins identified with 2 or more peptides are comparable in distribution to the overall genome. Proteins identified with 1 peptide are over-represented in the metabolic process category.

We next compared the distribution based on sub-cellular location (Figure 3B). We have identified higher percentages of proteins from the cytoplasm, and lower percentages of proteins from the plasma membrane, extra cellular region, and nucleus. We chose to consider only proteins identified by 2 or more peptides in our comparative analysis, as there is higher reliability amongst these identifications [20]. The 115 and 113 labels in our 2D LC-MS/MS iTRAQ analysis are similar to a previous neuroproteomic study by Datta et al., which compared protein expression in rat brain 24-hours after tMCAo surgery with a sham group. Comparison of the 115 and 113 labelled proteins from our analysis, with the Datta et al study, revealed a 74% overlap between the two lists of identified proteins [10].

(Table 1) summarizes the expressions changes (fold changes) of protein pairs identified in the experimental groups. (Figure 4) illustrates the distribution of fold changes amongst the identified proteins. The main expression changes were seen in the tMCAo+ rt-PA comparison (Figure 4B), where 13 proteins were significantly up- or down-regulated. The same number of significant expression changes were seen in the tMCAo/sham comparison. Four proteins which were over-expressed after tMCAo were significantly down-regulated with tMCAo+rt-PA. These were glutamate decarboxylase 2 (GAD2), proteasome subunit alpha (PSMA2), Ras-related protein Rab-10 (RAB10), and Synapsin-2 (SYN2). Both the Myelin basic protein (MBP) and the Neurofilament heavy polypeptide (NEFH) were significantly down-regulated after tMCAo and significantly up-regulated after rt-PA administration following tMCAo.

Six proteins that were unaffected after tMCAo alone had their expressions significantly altered when rt-PA was administered after the tMCAO. These included 3 cytoskeletal proteins: (INA, MAPT, NEFL), a nucleotide phosphodiesterase (CNP1), and two dehydrogenases (GLDH1, NDUFV2).

Surprisingly there were four proteins affected by rt-PA administration in the sham group, which were unaffected by tMCAo, and rt-PA administration after tMCAo. These were the cytoskeletal proteins (ARP2, NEF3, TUBA8) and the phosphatase subunit PPP1CB. Only 2 proteins (GAD2 and RAB10) had their expressions significantly affected in the same direction when rt-PA was administered to the sham group as when rt-PA was administered to the tMCAo group. There were two cytoskeletal proteins (NEFH and NEFL) that showed opposite expression changes when rt-PA was given to the sham group compared to when it was given to the tMCAo group.

Pathway Analysis

(Figure 5) represents the output of the IPA analysis with relative expression information overlaid. In this network Dihydropyrimidinase-related protein 2 (DPYSL2), reticulon 4 (RTN4), and the nuclear factor-kappa B (NF-kB) complex had degree centralities in the upper 5% of the distribution. Both DPYSL2 and RTN4 connected to 11 identified proteins, the majority of which were related to cytoskeleton structure/maintenance. The NF-kB interacted with 10 identified proteins, many of which were related to excitatory neurotransmitter function.

Western Blot Validation

In order to confirm the results from the 2D LC-MS/MS experiment western blots were used to quantify the expression of GAD2 and EAAT1 (Figure 6). GAD2 and EAAT1 were chosen, as these are proteins that have previously been implicated in exacerbating cell death after AIS and may represent adverse pleiotropic actions of rt-PA. The western blot analysis of GAD2 and EAAT1 confirmed the iTRAQ data.

Discussion

Recombinant tissue plasminogen activator is the only medical agent used in the acute treatment of AIS, but because of its pleiotropic actions it is associated with severe adverse effects [23,24]. Since the extent of rt-PA's pleiotropic interactions are unknown, the identification of proteins that show differential expression after rt-PA administration may shed light on the molecular mechanisms underlying rt-PA's adverse effects. In this study we used a 2D LC-MS/MS iTRAQ proteomics approach to characterize the brain protein changes that result 24 hrs after rt-PA administration. We have identified 18 proteins showing differential expression after rt-PA administration to either sham rats or rats that underwent tMCAo. Many of these proteins were associated with either excitatory neurotransmitter function or cytoskeletal structure. By applying a pathway analysis tool to the results of the 2D LC-MS/MS iTRAQ analysis we identified 3 proteins: DPYSL2, RTN4, and the NF-kB complex as having characteristics of being key proteins in the interaction network. These results may provide insight into the potential mechanisms underlying the adverse effects of rt-PA use after AIS.

In this study, the rat tMCAo model and the iTRAQ MS analysis are potential sources of variation [15]. We utilized sample pooling, replicates, internal controls, and bioinformatic analyses to address these concerns, and assess their influence on the data, as these strategies have been validated [13,25,26]. The group of 209 proteins identified with 2 or more peptides showed similar functional and sub-cellular distributions to the entire Rattus norvegicus genome. The under-representation of nuclear and membrane bound proteins is an expected artifact, and our yield from these two compartments is comparable to another study utilizing the FASP protocol and exceeds that of studies which did not utilize FASP [27]. The comparable spacial and functional distributions yielded, as well as a high overlap between our results and the study by Datta et al. lend support to the reliability of our sample collection and analysis.

Excitatory neurotransmitter function is thought to become deregulated after stroke, leading to excitotoxic cell death through excessive activation of NMDA and AMPA type receptors [5,28]. Previous work has shown that after stroke, rt-PA potentiates glutamate activity at NMDA receptors by proteolytically cleaving the NR-2 subunit [29]. In addition, excitatory amino acid transporters can reverse transport direction under ischemic conditions, leading to a further increase in synaptic glutamate levels. [30] Our results indicated that after sham and tMCAo surgery, rt-PA had caused down-regulation of the EAAT1 and GAD2 proteins, both of which are responsible for reducing the levels of synaptic glutamate and other excitatory neurotransmitters. GAD2 is an enzyme that converts synaptic glutamate into the inhibitory GABA [31]. In an animal model, GAD2 was neuroprotective against excitotoxic damage by reducing levels of available glutamate in pre-synaptic neurons [32]. EAAT1 is the predominant transporter responsible for removing glutamate and aspartate from the synapse [33]. Like GAD2, EAAT1 activity is neuroprotective by reducing synaptic glutamate levels [34–36]. In addition, our results showed alterations in the expressions of synaptic vesicle proteins RAB10, SYN2, and SYT2. RAB10 is a key regulator of intra-cellular membrane trafficking, and may be responsible for recycling AMPA receptors from intracellular compartments to the synapse [37]. SYN2 and SYT2 are both involved in facilitating neurotransmitter release into the synapse. Previous studies have indicated that dysfunctions in the expression levels of the SYN and SYT families can markedly affect the extent of ischemic brain injury [38,39]. Our results also indicated that rt-PA had caused a change in the expression of the CaMK2δ, a protein responsible for sensing the rise in intracellular calcium levels due to excitatory neurotransmitter stimulation at the NMDA receptors [40]. Our results demonstrated that a number of proteins involved in excitatory neurotransmitter function were differentially expressed after rt-PA administration to sham and tMCAo rats. Many of these proteins have been previously implicated in neuronal damage after ischemic injury, and the observed differential expressions may reflect adverse pleiotropic effects of rt-PA administration.

Cytoskeletal structure is necessary for neurovascular integrity [41,42]. Alterations of cytoskeletal function and composition occur after ischemic stroke [43]. Our results indicated differential expression of cytoskeletal and cytoskeleton regulatory proteins after rt-PA administration to both sham and tMCAo rats. The family of neurofilament proteins is a major element of the neuronal cytoskeleton, regulating axonal structure and diameter. The increase in neurofilament proteins we observed with rt-PA administration in tMCAo rats may indicate increased axonal growth [44]. In addition, our observations indicated that the expression of cytoskeletal proteins such as ARP2, INA, MAPT, and TUBA8 may be highly sensitive to rt-PA administration after tMCAo, leading to alterations in cytoskeletal structure and function.

Pathway analysis has become a standard method to gain insight into the underlying biology of differentially expressed proteins identified by proteomic analyses [45]. We generated an interaction network from the results of our 2D LC-MS/MS iTRAQ experiment and used the IPA software to perform a centrality analysis on this network. In a previous study, proteins with high centrality were 3 times more likely to be biologically essential [46]. It therefore appears that DPYSL2, RTN4, and NF-kB complex, which all showed high centrality in our protein-protein interaction network, may serve important functions in this network. DPYSL2 is involved in neuronal regeneration and multiple studies have identified changes in DPYSL2 expression and function shortly after ischemic brain injury [47]. RTN4 is also involved in neuronal regeneration, and has been proposed as a potential therapeutic target because of its role in exacerbating damage after experimental stroke [48]. The NF-kB complex regulates the expression of many proteins and its activation is known to exacerbate ischemic brain injury while inhibition of the NF-kB complex is neuroprotective [49]. The NF-kB complex can be activated by rt-PA through a pathway involving annexin A2/CD11b and integrin-linked kinase [50]. In our model the activated NF-kB may go on to cause a subset of the protein expression changes noticed in the 2D LC-MS/MS iTRAQ analysis. It is important to note that our pathway analysis is limited to simply suggesting that DPYSL2, RTN4, or the NF-kB complex may be relevant to rt-PA's pleiotropic actions. Pathway analyses are limited in part by low-resolution knowledge databases, missing condition-specific interactions, and incomplete annotations. Despite this, however, these results may prompt further research into rt-PA's pleiotropic effects on the cortex. For example, we are currently examining the effect of rt-PA on various proteins under the control of the NF-kB complex after experimental stroke.

In conclusion, a 2D LC-MS/MS iTRAQ analysis identified 18 proteins with differential expression 24-hours after rt-PA administration to rats that underwent sham or tMCAo surgery. Many of the identified proteins have been previously implicated in ischemic brain injury. The differential protein expressions we observed may reflect pleiotropic actions of rt-PA on the cortex of rats. Although further focused work is required to investigate these protein regulations in isolation, the general overview of protein regulation presented in our study provides insight into the potential mechanisms of rt-PA's adverse pleiotropic actions. This work may guide future work and may have implications in clinical settings where rt-PA is used to treat AIS.

Supporting Information

Table S1 Output of false discovery rate (FDR) characteristics for identified peptides and proteins.

Table S2 Output of relative protein expression changes between iTRAQ labels 113/114 and 115/116.

Author Contributions

Conceived and designed the experiments: ZM MG TB AK JC KE. Performed the experiments: ZM MG TB. Analyzed the data: ZM MG TB AK JC KE. Contributed reagents/materials/analysis tools: ZM MG TB AK JC KE. Wrote the paper: ZM MG TB AK JC KE.

References

1. Jauch EC, Saver JL, Adams HP Jr, Bruno A, Connors JJ, et al. (2013) Guidelines for the early management of patients with acute ischemic stroke: A guideline for healthcare professionals from the american heart association/american stroke association. Stroke 44: 870–947.
2. Bambauer KZ, Johnston S, Bambauer DE, Zivin JA (2006) REasons why few patients with acute stroke receive tissue plasminogen activator. Archives of Neurology 63: 661–664.
3. Brown DL, Barsan WG, Lisabeth LD, Gallery ME, Morgenstern LB (2005) Survey of emergency physicians about recombinant tissue plasminogen activator for acute ischemic stroke. Ann Emerg Med 46: 56–60.
4. Yepes M, Roussel BD, Ali C, Vivien D (2009) Tissue-type plasminogen activator in the ischemic brain: More than a thrombolytic. Trends Neurosci 32: 48–55.
5. Kristián T, Siesjö BK (1998) Calcium in ischemic cell death. Stroke 29: 705–718.
6. Jeyaseelan K, Lim KY, Armugam A (2008) Neuroprotectants in stroke therapy. Expert Opin Pharmacother 9: 887–900.
7. Ikonomidou C, Turski L (2002) Why did NMDA receptor antagonists fail clinical trials for stroke and traumatic brain injury? Lancet Neurology 1: 383–386.
8. Amaral eSM, Vandresen-Filho S, Tavares C, Menegatti AO, Terenzi H, et al. (2013) Proteomic analysis of the mice hippocampus after preconditioning induced by N-methyl-d-aspartate (NMDA). Journal of Molecular Neuroscience 50: 154–164.
9. Datta A, Park JE, Li X, Zhang H, Ho ZS, et al. (2010) Phenotyping of an in vitro model of ischemic penumbra by iTRAQ-based shotgun quantitative proteomics. J Proteome Res 9: 472–484.
10. Datta A, Jingru Q, Khor TH, Teo MT, Heese K, et al. (2011) Quantitative neuroproteomics of an in vivo rodent model of focal cerebral ischemia/reperfusion injury reveals a temporal regulation of novel pathophysiological molecular markers. J Proteome Res 10: 5199–5213.
11. Kiran M, Nagarajaram HA (2013) Global versus local hubs in human Proteinâ€"Protein interaction network. J Proteome Res 12: 5436–5446.
12. Zhou Y, Bhatia I, Cai Z, He QY, Cheung PT, et al. (2008) Proteomic analysis of neonatal mouse brain: Evidence for hypoxia- and ischemia-induced dephosphorylation of collapsin response mediator proteins. J Proteome Res 7: 2507–2515.
13. White CN, Chan DW, Zhang Z (2004) Bioinformatics strategies for proteomic profiling. Clin Biochem 37: 636–641.
14. Sung JH, Cho EH, Kim MO, Koh PO (2009) Identification of proteins differentially expressed by melatonin treatment in cerebral ischemic injury–a proteomics approach. J Pineal Res 46: 300–306.
15. Focking M, Besselmann M, Trapp T (2006) Proteomics of experimental stroke in mice. Acta Neurobiol Exp (Wars) 66: 273–278.
16. Liu T, Hu J, Li H (2009) iTRAQ-based shotgun neuroproteomics. Methods Mol Biol 566: 201–216.
17. Uluç K, Miranpuri A, Kujoth GC, Aktüre E, Başkaya MK (2011) Focal cerebral ischemia model by endovascular suture occlusion of the middle cerebral artery in the rat.: e1978.
18. Winiewski JR, Zougman A, Nagaraj N, Mann M (2009) Filter-aided sample preparation (FASP) for MS-based proteomic analysis. Nature Methods 6.
19. Gan CS, Chong PK, Pham TK, Wright PC (2007) Technical, experimental, and biological variations in isobaric tags for relative and absolute quantitation (iTRAQ). J Proteome Res 6: 821–827.
20. Mi H, Muruganujan A, Thomas PD (2013) PANTHER in 2013: Modeling the evolution of gene function, and other gene attributes, in the context of phylogenetic trees. Nucleic Acids Research 41: D377–D386.
21. Han JJ, Bertin N, Hao T, Goldberg DS, Berriz GF, et al. (2004) Evidence for dynamically organized modularity in the yeast protein-protein interaction network. Nature 430: 88–93.
22. Elias JE, Gygi SP (2007) Target-decoy search strategy for increased confidence in large-scale protein identifications by mass spectrometry. Nat Methods 4: 207–214.
23. Anonymous (2003) TEnsions remain over tpa for stroke. JAMA 289: 1363–1364.
24. Donnan GA, Fisher M, Macleod M, Davis SM (2008) Stroke. Lancet 371: 1612–1623.

25. Diz AP, Truebano M, Skibinski DO (2009) The consequences of sample pooling in proteomics: An empirical study. Electrophoresis 30: 2967–2975.
26. Karp NA, Lilley KS (2009) Investigating sample pooling strategies for DIGE experiments to address biological variability. Proteomics 9: 388–397.
27. McDowell GS, Gaun A, Steen H (2013) iFASP: Combining isobaric mass tagging with filter-aided sample preparation. J Proteome Res 12: 3809–3812.
28. Hazell AS (2007) Excitotoxic mechanisms in stroke: An update of concepts and treatment strategies. Neurochem Int 50: 941–953.
29. Olivier N, Docagne F, Ali C, Margaill I, Carmeliet P, et al. (2001) The proteolytic activity of tissue-plasminogen activator enhances NMDA receptor-mediated signaling. Nat Med 7: 59–64.
30. Phillis JW, Ren J, O'Regan MH (2000) Transporter reversal as a mechanism of glutamate release from the ischemic rat cerebral cortex: Studies with dl-threo-Î^{2}-benzyloxyaspartate. Brain Res 868: 105–112.
31. Davalos A, Castillo J, Serena J, Noya M (1997) Duration of glutamate release after acute ischemic stroke. Stroke 28: 708–710.
32. Matthews CC, Zielke HR, Fishman PS, Remington MP, Bowen TG (2007) Glutamate decarboxylase protects neurons against excitotoxic injury. J Neurosci Res 85: 855–859.
33. Seal RP, Amara SG (1999) Excitatory Amino Acid Transporters: A family in flux. Annu Rev Pharmacol Toxicol 39: 431–456.
34. Douen AG, Akiyama K, Hogan MJ, Wang F, Dong L, et al. (2000) Preconditioning with cortical spreading depression decreases intraischemic cerebral glutamate levels and down-regulates excitatory amino acid transporters EAAT1 and EAAT2 from rat cerebal cortex plasma membranes. J Neurochem 75: 812–818.
35. Beschorner R, Simon P, Schauer N, Mittelbronn M, Schluesener HJ, et al. (2007) Reactive astrocytes and activated microglial cells express EAAT1, but not EAAT2, reflecting a neuroprotective potential following ischaemia. Histopathology 50: 897–910.
36. Beart PM, O'Shea RD (2007) Transporters for L-glutamate: An update on their molecular pharmacology and pathological involvement. Br J Pharmacol 150: 5–17.
37. Glodowski DR, Chen CC, Schaefer H, Grant BD, Rongo C (2007) RAB-10 regulates glutamate receptor recycling in a cholesterol-dependent endocytosis pathway. Mol Biol Cell 18: 4387–4396.
38. Bolay H, Gursoy-Ozdemir Y, Sara Y, Onur R, Can A, et al. (2002) Persistent defect in transmitter release and synapsin phosphorylation in cerebral cortex after transient moderate ischemic injury. Stroke 33: 1369–1375.
39. Iwakuma M, Anzai T, Kobayashi S, Ogata M, Kaneda Y, et al. (2003) Antisense in vivo knockdown of synaptotagmin I and synapsin I by HVJ-liposome mediated gene transfer modulates ischemic injury of hippocampus in opposing ways. Neurosci Res 45: 285–296.
40. Inagaki N, Nishizawa M, Arimura N, Yamamoto H, Takeuchi Y, et al. (2000) Activation of Ca2+/calmodulin-dependent protein kinase II within post-synaptic dendritic spines of cultured hippocampal neurons. J Biol Chem 275: 27165–27171.
41. Lee TY, Gotlieb AI (2003) Microfilaments and microtubules maintain endothelial integrity. Microsc Res Tech 60: 115–127.
42. Nag S (1995) Role of the endothelial cytoskeleton in blood-brain-barrier permeability to protein. Acta Neuropathol 90: 454–460.
43. Jia Z, Chen Q, Qin H (2012) Ischemia-induced apoptosis of intestinal epithelial cells correlates with altered integrin distribution and disassembly of F-actin triggered by calcium overload. J Biomed Biotechnol 2012: 617539.
44. Ueno Y, Chopp M, Zhang L, Buller B, Liu Z, et al. (2012) Axonal outgrowth and dendritic plasticity in the cortical peri-infarct area after experimental stroke. Stroke 43: 2221–2228.
45. Eisenberg D, Marcotte EM, Xenarios I, Yeates TO (2000) Protein function in the post-genomic era. Nature 405: 823–826.
46. Jeong H, Mason SP, Barabasi A, Oltvai ZN (2001) Lethality and centrality in protein networks. Nature 411: 41–42.
47. Indraswari F, Wong PT, Yap E, Ng YK, Dheen ST (2009) Upregulation of Dpysl2 and Spna2 gene expression in the rat brain after ischemic stroke. Neurochem Int 55: 235–242.
48. Kern F, Stanika RI, Sarg B, Offterdinger M, Hess D, et al. (2013) Nogo-A couples with apg-1 through interaction and co-ordinate expression under hypoxic and oxidative stress. Biochem J 455: 217–227.
49. Carroll JE, Hess DC, Howard EF, Hill WD (2000) Is nuclear factor-kappaB a good treatment target in brain ischemia/reperfusion injury? Neuroreport 11: R1–4.
50. Lin L, Wu C, Hu K (2012) Tissue plasminogen activator activates NF-kappaB through a pathway involving annexin A2/CD11b and integrin-linked kinase. J Am Soc Nephrol 23: 1329–1338.

15

Sequential Cohort Design Applying Propensity Score Matching to Analyze the Comparative Effectiveness of Atorvastatin and Simvastatin in Preventing Cardiovascular Events

Arja Helin-Salmivaara[1,2]*, Piia Lavikainen[1], Emma Aarnio[3,4], Risto Huupponen[1,3], Maarit Jaana Korhonen[1,5]

1 Department of Pharmacology, Drug Development and Therapeutics, University of Turku, Turku, Finland, **2** Unit of Primary Health Care, Hospital District of Helsinki and Uusimaa, Helsinki, Finland, **3** Department of Clinical Pharmacology, Tykslab, Turku University Hospital, Turku, Finland, **4** School of Pharmacy, University of Eastern Finland, Kuopio, Finland, **5** Department of Public Health, University of Turku, Turku, Finland

Abstract

Background: Sequential cohort design (SCD) applying matching for propensity scores (PS) in accrual periods has been proposed to mitigate bias caused by channeling when calendar time is a proxy for strong confounders. We studied the channeling of patients according to atorvastatin and simvastatin initiation in Finland, starting from the market introduction of atorvastatin in 1998, and explored the SCD PS approach to analyzing the comparative effectiveness of atorvastatin versus simvastatin in the prevention of cardiovascular events (CVE).

Methods: Initiators of atorvastatin or simvastatin use in the 45–75-year age range in 1998–2006 were characterized by their propensity of receiving atorvastatin over simvastatin, as estimated for 17 six-month periods. Atorvastatin (10 mg) and simvastatin (20 mg) initiators were matched 1:1 on the PS, as estimated for the whole cohort and within each period. Cox regression models were fitted conventionally, and also for the PS matched cohort and the periodically PS matched cohort, to estimate the hazard ratios (HR) for CVEs.

Findings: Atorvastatin (10 mg) was associated with a 11%–12% lower incidence of CVE in comparison with simvastatin (20 mg). The HR estimates were the same for a conventional Cox model (0.88, 95% confidence interval 0.85–0.91), for the analysis in which the PS was used to match across all periods and the Cox model was adjusted for strong confounders (0.89, 0.85–0.92), and for the analysis in which PS matching was applied within sequential periods (0.88, 0.84–0.92). The HR from a traditional PS matched analysis was 0.80 (0.77–0.83).

Conclusions: The SCD PS approach produced effect estimates similar to those obtained in matching for PS within the whole cohort and adjusting the outcome model for strong confounders, but at the cost of efficiency. A traditional PS matched analysis without further adjustment in the outcome model produced estimates further away from unity.

Editor: John Calvert, Emory University, United States of America

Funding: This study was funded by the Academy of Finland (www.aka.fi, decision number 138255). The Academy of Finland had no role in the design, analyses, interpretation of data, writing the report, or in the decision to submit the manuscript.

Competing Interests: The authors have read the journal's policy and have the following conflicts: AHS, MK and RH have been funded by the grants from the Social Insurance Institution and the Academy of Finland. EA was supported by state funding for university-level health research (Grant L 3820). She has received consultancy fees from ESiOR Ltd, which provides health economic and outcomes research services for pharmaceutical companies and hospitals. RH is a member of the Advisory Board for Social and Medical Affairs of the SII. He has conducted consultancy for Orion Corporation as an Independent External Member of a Data Monitoring and Safety Committee in a clinical trial, and assisted Santen Pharmaceutical Co in pharmacokinetic calculations. The authors declare no other financial or non-financial (professional or personal) conflict of interests.

* E-mail: arja.helin-salmivaara@utu.fi

Introduction

Comparative effectiveness analyses of pharmaceuticals in observational settings are prone to bias due to confounding and channeling. Channeling, the preferential prescribing of one drug over another for various reasons, may lead to confounding when selective prescribing is based on patient characteristics associated with the outcome of interest. When changes in channeling occur over time, calendar time itself is a potential confounder or is a proxy for other confounders [1,2]. Therefore, calendar time is a key component when the effects of a newly launched drug are compared with those of a pre-existing one. Sequential cohort design (SCD) applying propensity score (PS) matching has been proposed as a means of mitigating bias caused by channeling when calendar time is a proxy for strong confounders [1–3]. In this approach, PSs for receiving one treatment over another are first constructed for cohorts within a selected number of sequential periods. For each PS model, the effects of covariates on treatment selection may vary, and even different sets of covariates can be used according to the time and the availability of the covariates [1,2]. The persons in the comparison cohorts are then matched on PS. Matching according to PSs within study-specific periods increases the covariate balance [4] and hence enhances the comparability of the cohorts. Thereafter, analyses on exposure-outcome associations are conducted using period as a stratum.

Seeger at al. explored a similar design in comparing the incidence of myocardial infarction between initiators of statin therapy and non-initiators in a US health plan in the 1990's [2]. More recently, the design has been applied in comparative effectiveness studies on cancer chemotherapy [3] and second-generation antipsychotics [4], as well as in simulation studies on drug safety monitoring of drug therapies [5,6]. Applications of the design in settings outside US are scarce however.

In a previous study [7], we demonstrated that, during the first 4 years after its introduction into the Finnish market in 1998, atorvastatin was channeled to younger and healthier sectors of the population than simvastatin (introduced in the early 1990's) was. By 2004, however, the differences between atorvastatin and simvastatin initiators in the distributions of age and the number of cardiovascular drugs in use had disappeared [7]. In our present study, we have described the channeling of atorvastatin over simvastatin overall in 1998–2006 in Finland. We explored application of the SCD approach to analyzing the comparative effectiveness of atorvastatin versus simvastatin in the prevention of cardiovascular events (CVE) among new statin users. We assumed that, when used in equipotent doses, atorvastatin and simvastatin would be equally effective in preventing CVEs (i.e., the effect estimate would approach unity). Furthermore, by iterating the survival analysis stratified by the cohort accrual periods, we simulated accumulating data by time. The data were captured from nationwide health care registers.

Methods

Sources of Data

We used data from administrative health databases generated in Finland through the universal health care and drug reimbursement systems covering the 5.3 million residents. We identified prescription records since 1994 in the Prescription Register, which is managed by the Social Insurance Institution of Finland (SII) [8]. This register contains records of all reimbursed prescription drug purchases made by residents in non-institutional settings. For each purchase, the dispensing date, the Anatomical Therapeutic Chemical classification code of the WHO [9], the tablet strength, and the quantity dispensed are listed. Patients staying in a public nursing home or hospital without interruption for over 90 days are not eligible for drug reimbursement, and their purchases are not registered. We identified these patients from a separate SII register. For identifying patients entitled to higher rates of reimbursement because of certain severe, chronic conditions, we used the SII Special Reimbursement Register introduced in 1964. To be eligible for special reimbursement, a patient's condition must meet explicit predefined criteria, and a written certificate by a specialist physician is required.

We identified hospitalizations from the Finnish Care Register, managed by the National Institute for Health and Welfare. The register, covering all Finnish hospitals, includes individual-level administrative data on main and additional discharge diagnoses, as well as the admission and discharge dates. The 10th revision of the International Classification of Diseases (ICD-10) has been in use since 1 January 1996. The data from the databases were linked anonymously using encrypted personal identifiers.

Analyses

Synopsis. All initiators of atorvastatin or simvastatin use in 1998–2006 were characterized by the distributions of the covariates measured at baseline and the PSs for receiving atorvastatin over simvastatin estimated for each of 17 six-month periods. After restricting the cohort to those initiating atorvastatin (10 mg) or simvastatin (20 mg) use and with follow-up of at least 270 days since the initiation, we estimated the PSs for the entire period (1998–2006) and also for the 17 six-month periods. The atorvastatin and simvastatin initiators were matched 1:1 on the PS. Cox regression models were fitted both conventionally and for the PS matched cohorts to estimate the hazard ratios for CVEs occurring during the follow-up until 31 December 2008. Finally, hazard ratios were estimated cumulatively (simulating accruing data in real life) with a sequentially PS matched analysis and with conventional (unmatched) multivariable analyses. In these analyses, the follow-up was restricted to 730 days.

Cohorts. The initiators of statin therapy with simvastatin or atorvastatin between January 1998 and June 2006 and in the age range of 45–75 years were drawn from the SII Prescription Register. The initiation was defined as not having purchased any statin between 1 January 1994 and the date of the first simvastatin or atorvastatin purchase, which was set as the index date. Starting from the first half of 1998, the initiators were categorized into 17 cohorts according to the 6-month period of their index date. We estimated separate PSs for each period with a logistic regression by modeling the predicted probability of receiving atorvastatin as a function of covariates. The following covariates were used: demographic characteristics, number of hospital days in the preceding 365 days, prior cardiovascular disease in the preceding 7 years, comorbidities and medication used in the preceding 365 days, and the number of distinct drugs purchased during the 4 months prior to the initiation. A detailed list of the covariates, other than place of residence (categorized into 21 catchment areas of the secondary/tertiary care hospitals), is presented in Table 1. The covariates included in each PS model varied and reflected the time and changes in the availability of the covariates. The PS distributions of atorvastatin and simvastatin were compared within each period.

For the effectiveness analyses, the study population was restricted to the initiators with atorvastatin (10 mg) or simvastatin (20 mg). Atorvastatin in 10 mg doses has been reported to equal the potency of simvastatin in 20 mg doses [10] and simvastatin in 40 mg doses [11] in lowering the levels of low-density lipoprotein. We further restricted the population to those with a follow-up starting on the 270th day to avoid potential protopathic bias [12].

PS matching. After the restrictions were made, we estimated the PSs for the whole period (1998–2006) and for the 17 six-month periods by using the covariates. Within each period, an initiator with atorvastatin was matched to an initiator with simvastatin within a 0.01 caliper of propensity score, and the initiators without counterparts were excluded [13]. The balance of the key covariates was tested by calculating standardized mean differences [14]. The covariate distributions were displayed for the pooled cohorts.

Comparative effectiveness analyses. A survival analysis of time from the 270th day since the initiation or matching to CVE was estimated using Cox proportional hazard regression applying the intent-to-treat approach. The follow-up ended in death,

Table 1. Characteristics of the initiators of simvastatin and atorvastatin therapy between January 1998 and June 2006 in Finland.

	Initiators without matching			**Sequentially PS matched**		
	Simvastatin 20 mg	**Atorvastatin 10 mg**		**Simvastatin 20 mg**	**Atorvastatin 10 mg**	
	(*n* = 73 868)	(*n* = 96 995)		(*n* = 54 220)	(*n* = 54 220)	
	n (%)	*n* %	*P* value	*n* (%)	*n* %	*P* value
Female	36 612 (49.6)	50 107 (51.7)	<0.001	27 453 (50.6)	27 449 (50.6)	*
Age, mean (SD)	60.9 (8.0)	60.4 (8.0)	<0.001	60.7 (8.0)	60.7 (8.0)	*
Age category			<0.001			*
45–55 years	21 200 (28.7)	30 431 (31.4)		15 992 (29.5)	15 868 (29.3)	
56–65 years	29 252 (39.6)	37 674 (38.8)		21 400 (39.5)	21 338 (39.4)	
66–75 years	23 416 (31.7)	28 890 (29.8)		16 828 (31.0)	17 014 (31.4)	
Number of hospital days during 365 days prior to the initiation			<0.001			*
0	51 583 (69.8)	73 396 (75.7)		39 233 (72.4)	39 265 (72.4)	
1–7	14 202 (19.2)	15 908 (16.4)		9837 (18.1)	9835 (18.1)	
8–30	6790 (9.2)	6281 (6.5)		4262 (7.9)	4204 (7.8)	
31–365	1293 (1.8)	1410 (1.5)		888 (1.6)	916 (1.7)	
Comorbidities						
CVD, PTCA or CAPG in relation to the initiation			<0.001			*
None in preceding 7 years	63 469 (85.9)	82 625 (91.4)		48 130 (88.8)	48 166 (88.8)	
Only earlier than 30 days	3700 (5.0)	4791 (4.9)		2846 (5.3)	2833 (5.2)	
Only during the preceding 30 days	5743 (7.8)	2916 (3.0)		2705 (5.0)	2680 (4.9)	
Both prior to and during 30 days	956 (1.3)	663 (0.7)		539 (1.0)	541 (1.0)	
Hospitalized during 7 years prior to the initiation						
Diabetes	3589 (4.9)	4144 (4.3)	<0.001	2471 (4.6)	2493 (4.6)	*
Hypertension	5269 (7.1)	5933 (6.1)	<0.001	3593 (6.6)	3620 (6.7)	*
Stroke	3692 (5.0)	5755 (5.9)	<0.001	2972 (5.5)	2838 (5.2)	0.071
Cardiac insufficiency	990 (1.3)	814 (0.8)	<0.001	594 (1.1)	567 (1.1)	*
Atherosclerotic CVD	988 (1.3)	1195 (1.2)	0.054	710 (1.3)	711 (1.3)	*
Atherosclerosis in lower legs	416 (0.6)	507 (0.5)	0.258	295 (0.5)	288 (0.5)	*
	(*n* = 73 868)	(*n* = 96 995)		(*n* = 54 220)	(*n* = 54 220)	
	n (%)	*n* %	*P* value	*n* (%)	*n* %	*P* value
Hospitalized during 365 days prior to the initiation						
Atrial fibrillation	957 (1.3)	986 (1.0)	<0.001	655 (1.2)	614 (1.1)	*
Any cancer diagnosis	461 (0.6)	578 (0.6)	0.458	316 (0.6)	315 (0.6)	*
COPD/asthma	324 (0.4)	291 (0.3)	<0.001	207 (0.4)	207 (0.4)	*
Renal insufficiency	22 (0.0)	50 (0.1)	0.030	12 (0.0)	21 (0.0)	*
Dementia	36 (0.1)	35 (0.0)	0.204	19 (0.0)	21 (0.0)	*
Psychotic disease	180 (0.2)	206 (0.2)	0.177	127 (0.2)	123 (0.2)	*
Depression	189 (0.3)	202 (0.2)	0.041	124 (0.2)	126 (0.2)	*
Organ transplantation	8 (0.0)	13 (0.0)	0.634	3 (0.0)	4 (0.0)	*
Comorbidities based on the Special Reimbursement Register[#]						
Diabetes	8161 (11.1)	10 043 (10.4)	<0.001	5703 (10.5)	5760 (10.6)	*
Hypothyroidism	2494 (3.4)	3295 (3.4)	0.814	1866 (3.4)	1857 (3.4)	*
Psychotic disorders	2015 (2.7)	2319 (2.4)	<0.001	1345 (2.5)	1350 (2.5)	*
Severe psychotic disease	147 (0.2)	137 (0.1)	<0.001	96 (0.2)	97 (0.2)	*
Breast cancer	361 (1.0)	427 (0.9)	0.150	256 (1.0)	257 (1.0)	*
Prostate cancer	364 (0.9)	387 (0.9)	<0.001	243 (0.9)	242 (0.9)	*
Leukemia	227 (0.3)	229 (0.2)	0.005	145 (0.3)	140 (0.3)	*
Gynecologic cancers	42 (0.1)	68 (0.1)	0.285	34 (0.1)	27 (0.1)	*
Other cancers	85 (0.1)	89 (0.1)	0.135	45 (0.1)	48 (0.1)	*
Prior organ transplantation	69 (0.1)	139 (0.1)	0.003	56 (0.1)	52 (0.1)	*
Uremia with dialysis	40 (0.1)	104 (0.1)	<0.001	28 (0.0)	33 (0.1)	*

Table 1. Cont.

	Initiators without matching			Sequentially PS matched		
	Simvastatin 20 mg	Atorvastatin 10 mg		Simvastatin 20 mg	Atorvastatin 10 mg	
Use of interferon alpha	13 (0.0)	19 (0.0)	0.766	8 (0.0)	9 (0.0)	*
Cardiac insufficiency	2001 (2.7)	2181 (2.3)	<0.001	1341 (2.5)	1350 (2.5)	*
Rheumatic disease	2117 (2.9)	2559 (2.6)	<0.001	1492 (2.8)	1480 (2.7)	*
Asthma	5194 (7.0)	5867 (6.1)	<0.001	3576 (6.6)	3592 (6.6)	*
Chronic hypertension	22 723 (30.8)	30 214 (31.1)	0.085	16 776 (30.9)	16 819 (31.0)	*
	(*n* = 73 868)	(*n* = 96 995)		(*n* = 54 220)	(*n* = 54 220)	
	n (%)	*n* %	*P* value	*n* (%)	*n* %	*P* value
CAD	10 917 (14.9)	10 434 (10.8)	<0.001	7049 (13.0)	7034 (13.0)	*
Dysrhythmia	1707 (2.3)	2037 (2.1)	<0.001	1231 (2.3)	1223 (2.3)	*
Familial dyslipidemia	40 (0.1)	36 (0.0)	0.098	26 (0.1)	25 (0.1)	*
Dyslipidemia with CAD	3692 (5.0)	2927 (3.0)	<0.001	2256 (4.2)	2256 (4.2)	*
Clopidogrel use with CAD	74 (0.1)	43 (0.0)	<0.001	36 (0.1)	36 (0.1)	*
Clopidogrel use with other indications	235 (0.3)	220 (0.2)	<0.001	146 (0.3)	149 (0.3)	*
Use of anti-dementia drugs[§]	128 (0.2)	206 (0.2)	0.070	96 (0.2)	91 (0.2)	*
Parkinsonism	241 (0.3)	274 (0.3)	0.102	163 (0.3)	145 (0.3)	*
Epilepsy	847 (1.2)	1165 (1.2)	0.301	621 (1.2)	614 (1.1)	*
Medication						
Number of different preparations purchased during 4 months prior to the initiation			<0.001			
1–5	9571 (13.0)	7626 (7.9)		5675 (10.5)	5749 (10.6)	*
6–10	20 434 (27.7)	21 861 (22.5)		14 015 (25.9)	14 034 (25.9)	
11–15	17 596 (23.8)	22 806 (23.5)		13 108 (24.2)	13 087 (24.1)	
16–20	11 339 (15.4)	17 041 (17.6)		8828 (16.3)	8884 (16.4)	
>20	14 928 (20.2)	27 661 (28.5)		12 594 (23.2)	12 466 (23.0)	
At least one purchase during 365 days prior to the initiation						
Diabetes drugs	11 500 (15.6)	14 284 (14.7)	<0.001	8026 (14.8)	8027 (14.8)	*
Antithrombotic agents	8608 (11.7)	9850 (10.2)	<0.001	5887 (10.9)	5814 (10.7)	*
Organic nitrates and cardiac glycosides	15 772 (21.4)	15 877 (16.4)	<0.001	10 385 (19.2)	10 309 (19.0)	*
Centrally acting hypertension drugs	644 (0.9)	746 (0.8)	0.019	437 (0.8)	441 (0.8)	*
Diuretics	11 203 (15.2)	14 231 (14.7)	<0.001	8066 (14.9)	8050 (14.9)	*
Peripheral vasodilators	64 (0.1)	124 (0.1)	0.011	49 (0.1)	52 (0.1)	*
Beta-blocking agents	31 409 (42.5)	36 108 (37.2)	<0.001	21 906 (40.4)	21 915 (40.4)	*
Selective calcium channels blockers	12 678 (17.2)	16 133 (16.6)	<0.001	9203 (17.0)	9270 (17.1)	*
ACEI or ARB	26 292 (36.0)	30 162 (31.1)	<0.001	18 166 (33.5)	18 176 (33.5)	*
	(*n* = 73 868)	(*n* = 96 995)		(*n* = 54 220)	(*n* = 54 220)	
	n (%)	*n* %	*P* value	*n* (%)	*n* %	*P* value
Non-statin lipid-lowering drug	544 (0.7)	1573 (1.6)	<0.001	439 (0.8)	472 (0.9)	*
Drugs for obstructive airway diseases	7680 (10.4)	9293 (9.6)	<0.001	5361 (9.9)	5387 (9.9)	*
Anti-dementia drugs	79 (0.1)	111 (0.1)	0.645	59 (0.1)	54 (0.1)	*
Antidepressants	7086 (9.6)	9424 (9.7)	0.393	5232 (9.7)	5172 (9.5)	*
Antipsychotics	2088 (2.8)	2555 (2.6)	0.015	1430 (2.6)	1437 (2.7)	*
Antineoplastic agents	342 (0.5)	521 (0.6)	0.032	265 (0.5)	256 (0.5)	*

The study population restricted by the strength of the initiating drug and by the start of the follow-up at 270 days since the initiation is presented without and with the sequential matching by propensity score.

CVD, cardiovascular disease; PTCA, percutaneous transluminal coronary angioplasty; CAPG, coronary artery bypass craft surgery; COPD, chronic obstructive pulmonary disease; CAD, coronary artery disease; ACEI, angiotensin-converting-enzyme inhibitor; ABR, angiotensin receptor blocker.

[#]Eligibility to special reimbursement any time prior to the initiation.

[§]Use of donepezil, galantamine, memantine, or rivastigmine.

P values are based on Chi^2 test for categorical variables and Student's *t* test for continuous variables.

* >0.1.

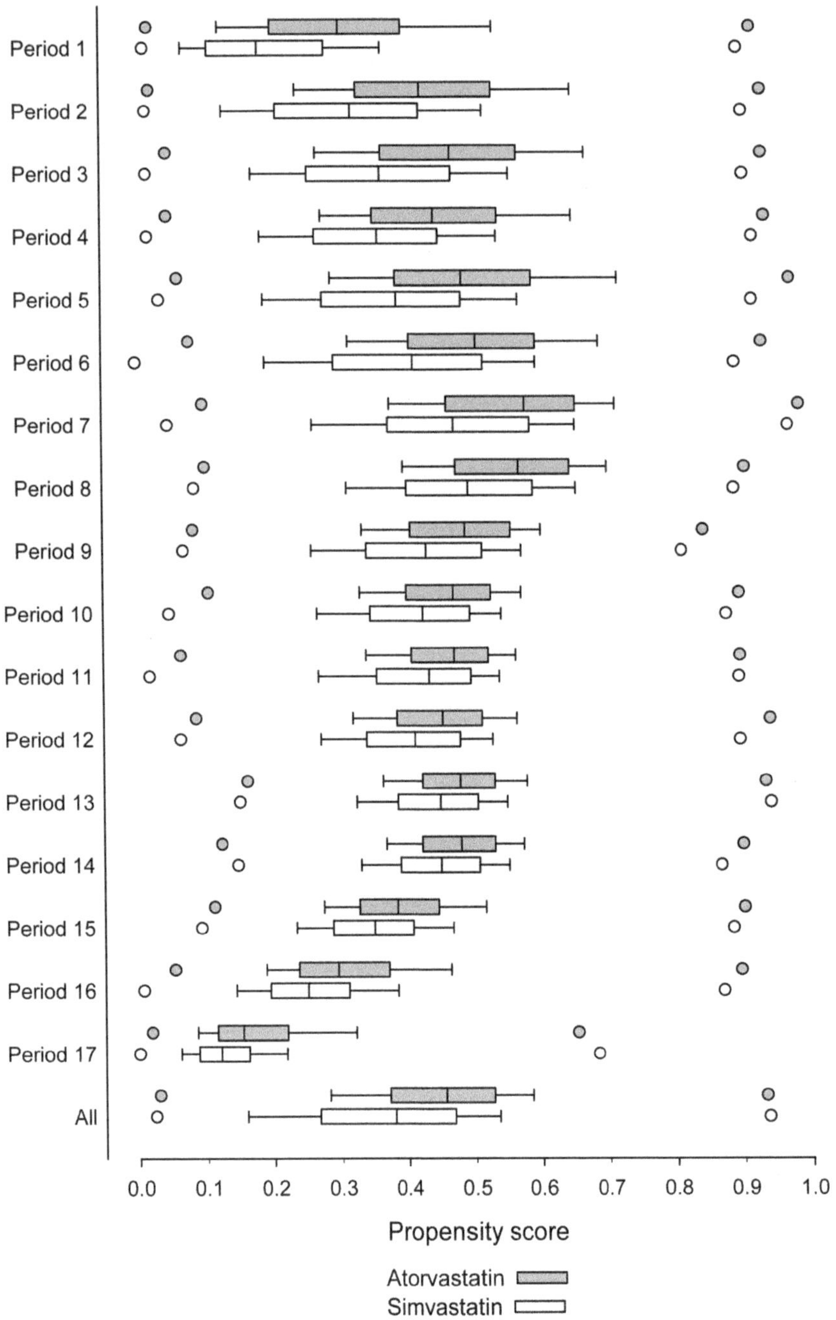

Figure 1. Distribution of propensity scores estimating the effect of initiating statin therapy with simvastatin versus atorvastatin in 1998–2006 in 6-month periods (1st = from 1 January 1998 to 30 June 1998; 17th = from 1 January 2006 to 30 June 2006). The boundary of the box closest to zero indicates the 25th percentile, a line within the box marks the median, and the boundary of the box farthest from zero indicates the 75th percentile. Whiskers (error bars) above and below the box indicate the 90th and 10th percentiles. In addition, the lowest and the highest values are presented by points.

institutionalization, 31 December 2008, or the outcome of interest, whichever came first. The primary outcome was a hospitalized CVE, a composite of acute myocardial infarction, ischemic cardiac disease (ICD codes I20.0, I20.1, I20.8, I20.9, I21.0–I21.9, I22.0, I22.1, I22.8, I22.9, I23.0–I23.5, I23.8, I24.0, I24.1, I24.8, I24.9), percutaneous coronary intervention or coronary artery bypass surgery, and ischemic stroke (I63, I64). Both the main and additional diagnoses were selected. The validity of the measures in the Care Register has been reported to be fairly good in that, when myocardial infarction and unstable angina pectoris diagnoses combined were compared with the population-based FINAMI register, the positive predictive value was 76% for males and 69% for females in 1998–2002 [15]. The positive predictive value of the first stroke diagnosis in the Care Register compared with the population-based FINSTROKE register was 85% for 1996–2002 [16].

Hazard ratios were estimated with Cox models using the following three different PS approaches: 1) a PS estimated across all periods combined (period included in the logistic regression model for PS) and used for matching, 2) a PS estimated across all periods combined and used for matching as above and the outcome model adjusted for variables strongly predicting the outcome ($p<0.001$), and 3) a PS estimated and used for matching within the cohort accrual periods. Furthermore, conventional outcome models using the same covariates as in the logistic model for the PS were fitted.

Cumulative Analyses. To simulate real life, we added the subsequent matched cohort to the previous ones and iterated the survival analysis stratified by the cohort accrual periods 16 times. For the unmatched accrual cohorts, Cox proportional regression models were adjusted for the same covariates as included in the PSs. In these analyses, the follow-up was restricted to between the 270th and 730th days since the initiation.

We used SAS software (version 9.2, SAS Institute, Inc., Cary, NC, USA) for the statistical analyses.

Ethics Statement. Data were obtained from the databases hosted by the SII and the National Institute for Health and Welfare, Helsinki, Finland that are not public repositories. The SII, the National Institute for Health and Welfare, and the national data protection agency (Office of the Data Protection Ombudsman) approved the study protocol.

There was no legal requirement for an ethics committee approval because researchers used only de-identified register data and the persons in the registers were not contacted (the Finnish legislation at: http://www.finlex.fi/fi/laki/ajantasa/1999/19990488 - not available in English). No written consent from patients was required either. Data were de-identified by the SII after the record linkage. De-identified data can be shared by permission only.

Results

All Initiators

Between January 1998 and June 2006 in Finland, 118 623 persons initiated atorvastatin use and 180 238 began simvastatin therapy. The mean age of the atorvastatin initiators was 60.3 (SD 8.0) years and that of simvastatin initiators was 61.4 (SD 8.0) years (Table S1). The initiators of atorvastatin tended to have slightly fewer comorbid conditions than their comparison group when the persons in all of the periods were pooled (Table S1). Over the periods, however, the prevalence of prior CVD identified in the discharge register changed remarkably. In the first half of 1998, 80.8% of the initiators with atorvastatin and 67.7% with simvastatin did not have prior CVD. In the first half of 2006, the respective proportions were 83.3% and 90.97%. As shown in Figure 1, the medians of the PSs for the atorvastatin and simvastatin initiators were the closest in period 11 (the first half of 2003) (i.e., 0.47 and 0.44, respectively). The overlap of the distributions started increasing in the first half of 2001.

Restrictions and Matching

After restrictions according to the strength of the initiating statin and the start of the follow-up, the atorvastatin cohort included 96 995 persons, and the simvastatin cohort had 73 868 persons. The mean age of the atorvastatin initiators was 60.4 (SD 8.0) years, and that of the simvastatin initiators was 60.9 (SD 8.0) (Table 1). As in the cohort containing all of the initiators, the persons with atorvastatin tended to have slightly fewer comorbid conditions. After the PS matching across all of the cohorts combined, 128 540 persons from both groups retained; 66.2% of the restricted atorvastatin cohort and 87% of the respective simvastatin cohort. After sequential PS matching, 54 220 persons were retained in each group (55.9% of the restricted atorvastatin cohort and 73.4% of the respective simvastatin cohort, the proportions varying across the periods) (Table S2). The covariate balance increased after the restrictions and PS matching (Table 1, Table S3).

Comparative Effectiveness Analyses

During the 256 060 person-years of the atorvastatin (10 mg) initiators followed-up since the 270th day after the initiation until censoring or experiencing an event, 3795 CVEs were observed, yielding a crude incidence of 15/1000 person-years. For the simvastatin (20 mg) initiators, 4261 CVEs in 253 278 person-years yielded an incidence of 17/1000 person-years. The larger person-time of the atorvastatin initiators was mainly due to the larger number of deaths among simvastatin initiators (4.01% versus 4.26%).

Atorvastatin (10 mg) was associated with an 11%–12% lower incidence of CVE in comparison with simvastatin (20 mg). The hazard ratio (HR) estimated with a conventionally adjusted Cox model was the same as the one obtained in the analysis in which the PS was used for matching across all periods and the Cox model was adjusted for strong predictors of the outcome, as well as the one from the analysis in which the PS matching was applied within sequential periods: 0.88, 0.89, and 0.88 with nearly identical confidence intervals (CI) (95% CI 0.85–0.91, 0.85–0.92, and 0.84–0.92, respectively) (Table 2). However, the HR from the analysis in which PS matching was used across all of the periods without further adjustment of the outcome model for confounders produced an HR of 0.80 (95% CI 0.77–0.83).

Cumulative Analyses

For each period, the HRs estimated with conventional models tended to be slightly closer to one than the HRs from the models applying PS matching, with the exception of the first two periods (Table 3).

Discussion

The difference in the characteristics of the atorvastatin and simvastatin initiators overall was shown by the distribution of the PSs, a sum function of the covariates measured at treatment initiation. According to the PSs, the covariates were extremely well balanced after sequential matching in the cohorts restricted by the strength of the initiating statin and by the start of the follow-up. Our comparative effectiveness analysis indicated that atorvastatin (10 mg) was more effective than simvastatin (20 mg) for the prevention of CVEs. The HRs estimated with the Cox proportional hazard models were the same whether derived from the sequential cohort approach or the conventional model. No substantial difference in the effect estimates was found between the sequential cohort and conventional approaches when the accumulation of data was extrapolated to real life and the follow-up was restricted to 2 years.

Channeling

As PS is a relative sum function, the interpretation of our findings is challenging. Since the first half of 2001 (period 7), the interquartile range of the PS distributions increasingly overlapped, although a common trend for the PSs can be found. The distribution of the PSs was visually classified into the following three phases; the phase of increasing scores from 1998 to 2001, a stable phase between 2002 and 2004, and a phase of decreasing scores since 2005 (Figure 1). The start of the plateau phase coincides with the withdrawal of cerivastatin from the market [17].

Table 2. Comparative effectiveness of atorvastatin (10 mg) versus simvastatin (20 mg).

Models	HR (95% CI)
Conventional outcome models	
Unadjusted (*n* = 170 763)	0.70 (0.68–0.73)
Adjusted (*n* = 170 763)[2]	0.88 (0.85–0.91)
PS models	
Matched by PS, unadjusted (*n* = 128 540)[3]	0.80 (0.77–0.83)
Matched by PS, adjusted (*n* = 128 540)[4]	0.89 (0.85–0.92)
Sequentially matched by PS (*n* = 108 440)[5]	0.88 (0.84–0.92)

The analyses included initiators between January 1998 and June 2006 in Finland. Hazard ratios for a composite of cardiovascular events[1] were estimated with different Cox proportional hazard regression models.
HR = hazard ratio; CI = confidence interval; PS = propensity score.
[1]Cardiovascular events; hospitalized acute myocardial infarction ischemic cardiac disease (ICD-10 codes I20–I24), percutaneous coronary intervention or coronary artery bypass surgery, and stroke (I63, I64).
[2]Adjusted for all covariates included in the propensity scores, including the period.
[3]Period included in the propensity score. Matching within the whole cohort within a 0.01 caliber.
[4]Adjusted for the covariates strongly associated with the outcome.
[5]Matching conducted within each of the 17 six-month periods since January 1998.

The withdrawal hardly directly affects the preferential prescribing of either statin or, consequently, the PSs. The absolute number of initiators of both statins, however, decreased during the period following the withdrawal (period 8 in Table S2). This decrease possibly reflects mistrust towards the safety of statin drugs. The end of the plateau phase coincided with a substantial decrease in the prices of the generic simvastatin products [18]. Generic substitution was launched in Finland in April 2003. We assume that the price gradient between the branded atorvastatin and generic simvastatin (and other generic statins) was great enough to affect prescribing practices as late as 2005. During the last three periods (Table S2), initiations clearly shifted toward simvastatin products. A policy change restricting reimbursement for atorvastatin was implemented in October 2006; however, the fact that this change was forthcoming was not made known until the preceding June.

Comparative Effectiveness

The effect estimate did not reach unity in any of our comparative effectiveness analyses. The strengths of atorvastatin (10 mg) and simvastatin (20 mg) may not compare equally. For feasible analyses we had, however, too few of those initiating simvastatin (40 mg) use in the first years of the study. In a systematic review [11], the percentage of reduction in serum low-density lipoprotein by simvastatin (20 mg) was 32% and that for atorvastatin (10 mg) was 37%, yielding a potency ratio of 0.86, near the HRs in our exploratory comparative effectiveness analyses.

We compared, however, the effectiveness of atorvastatin (10 mg) versus simvastatin (40 mg) in the whole cohort of initiators; that is, we estimated a PS across all periods combined and used the PS for matching within the whole cohort. In this analysis, HRs approached the unity (HR 0.94; 95% CI 0.84–1.06) (Table S4).

As the analyses were all intention-to-treat, neither switching between statins, changes in the doses, nor discontinuation of, or

Table 3. Comparative effectiveness of atorvastatin (10 mg) versus simvastatin (20 mg) estimated cumulatively.

	Sequentially matched by PS[2]	Conventional[3]
Period	**HR (95% CI)**	**HR (95% CI)**
1	0.88 (0.54–1.43)	0.85 (0.56–1.30)
2	1.02 (0.75–1.40)	1.11 (0.85–1.44)
3	0.89 (0.70–1.12)	0.89 (0.73–1.09)
4	0.85 (0.70–1.03)	0.88 (0.75–1.04)
5	0.83 (0.71–0.98)	0.83 (0.72–0.96)
6	0.76 (0.66–0.88)	0.77 (0.68–0.88)
7	0.77 (0.68–0.88)	0.78 (0.70–0.88)
8	0.78 (0.69–0.88)	0.80 (0.72–0.89)
9	0.78 (0.70–0.87)	0.80 (0.72–0.88)
10	0.80 (0.72–0.89)	0.82 (0.75–0.90)
11	0.80 (0.72–0.88)	0.81 (0.75–0.89)
12	0.81 (0.73–0.89)	0.82 (0.75–0.89)
13	0.83 (0.75–0.90)	0.83 (0.77–0.90)
14	0.83 (0.76–0.91)	0.84 (0.78–0.90)
15	0.86 (0.79–0.93)	0.86 (0.80–0.92)
16	0.87 (0.80–0.94)	0.87 (0.81–0.93)
17	0.86 (0.80–0.93)	0.87 (0.81–0.93)

The analyses included the initiators between January 1998 and June 2006 in Finland; hazard ratios of a composite of cardiovascular events[1] estimated cumulatively in the sequentially matched cohorts and in conventional Cox proportional hazard regression models. The follow-up was restricted to between 270 and 730 days since initiation.
HR = hazard ratio; CI = confidence interval; PS = propensity score.
[1]Cardiovascular events: hospitalized acute myocardial infarction (ICD-10 codes I20–I24), percutaneous coronary intervention or coronary artery bypass surgery, and stroke (I63, I64).
[2]Matching conducted within each of the 17 six-month periods since January 1998.
[3]Adjusted for all of the covariates included in the propensity scores, including the period.

adherence to statin therapy was accounted for. Therefore, a misclassification of person-time was possible.

Head-to-head comparisons of the effects of atorvastatin versus simvastatin on cardiovascular outcomes are scarce. In the only large enough comparative randomized trial, 75% of the participants had pre-randomization statin therapy, which diluted the possible difference [19]. In several observational studies conducted among privately insured or employer insured populations in the US at the beginning of the 2000's, the initiators of atorvastatin (10/20 mg) use tended to have a lower risk of cardiovascular outcomes than those initiating simvastatin (20/40 mg] use during a few years of follow-up [20–23]. In the conventionally adjusted predictive models, the HRs ranged from 0.87 [21] to 0.98 [22]. In a study in which PS matching was applied to the whole cohort, the relative risk was 0.91 ($p = 0.02$) [23].

Analyses of Comparative Effectiveness

For valid effect estimates, correct specification of the PS model is essential. If the associations between the covariates and the exposure substantially differ across subgroups, applying cohort-wide PS in subgroup analyses may lead to biased estimates. In our exploration, the effect estimates from the cohort-wide PS analysis improved (i.e., approached unity) when we added strong predictors of the outcome (i.e., age, sex, prior CVD, drugs used for the modification of CVD risks, number of hospital days, and number of different drugs redeemed) to the outcome model (Table 2). Actually, the estimate became identical to the one from the sequential cohort model. Correct matching for PS, on the other hand, can be estimated by covariate balance. In our study, the balance of the key patient characteristics predicting CVEs, calculated as the standardized mean difference, improved after cohort-wide PS matching when compared with that of the unmatched study population. The balance was, however, further improved after matching within periods (Table S3). It must be noted that, due to the limitations of the register data, we did not have access to information on many important risk factors for CVEs. We did not have data on lipid profiles, family history of CVD, lifestyle-related risk factors nor on the use of acetylsalicylic acid of the study population.

We reached the same results with the conventional regression model applying standard adjustments as we did with the period-stratified (sequential cohort) model and the cohort-wide PS matched model adjusted for strong predictors of the outcome. Our period-stratified model could probably not discriminate between the characteristics of the atorvastatin and simvastatin initiators and other factors associated with calendar time. Although period was a weak confounder, we did, however, find prescribing dynamics over time as the odds ratios of some of the covariates (number of hospital days, prior CVD, diabetes) varied across the PS models. Furthermore, omitting period from the conventional Cox model did not affect the HR of the outcome. However, a traditional PS matched analysis produced an effect estimate that was the furthest from unity.

In a recent analysis of the effect estimates of cancer chemotherapies that applied a calendar time-specific PS approach [3], a clear confounding effect of the calendar time was found. The definition of the periods was based on drug policy events. Policy events may substantially affect the cost of relatively expensive cancer drugs and thus modify the selection of a therapy. In our study, the length of the accrual periods was based on calendar time, and only one substantial policy change took place during the study period. Although we could identify channeling of the atorvastatin and simvastatin after the policy event, calendar time did not act as a strong confounder in our comparative effectiveness analyses.

This study expands upon the previous work of Rassen et al. [24], who compared the effect estimates for subgroups from the outcome models by applying a PS estimated for a full cohort and also within the subgroups. They observed practically the same effect estimates for the subgroups in the subgroup-specific PS models as in the full cohort PS models. The model for the full cohort PS included interaction terms between the subgroups and strong confounders. When the subgroups were large enough, the validity of the full cohort PS approach was not threatened, and it was more efficient than the stratified analyses. The calendar-time-specific PS matched approach in an analysis of the effectiveness of second-generation antipsychotics on cardiovascular outcomes yielded the same effect estimates as the conventional PS matched approach [4]. Furthermore, preliminary results on the effectiveness of inhaled, long-acting beta-agonists on asthma exacerbations [25] showed that the effect estimates were the same whether or not they were derived from the model using a PS estimated for the entire study period or a PS estimated for specific years and used for matching in the models.

Conclusions

Clinically, atorvastatin (10 mg) was more effective than simvastatin (20 mg) in preventing CVEs. From the analytical point of view, when accrued data are analyzed, the sequential cohort approach applying PS matching may produce a similar, and as valid, effect estimates as matching for PS within a whole cohort and adjusting the outcome model for strong confounders, at the cost of efficiency. However, without further adjustment, the traditional matching for the cohort-wide PS may lead to less valid estimates. The feasibility of the approach is worth testing in other settings.

Supporting Information

Table S1 Characteristics of the initiators of simvastatin and atorvastatin therapy between January 1998 and June 2006 in Finland.

Table S2 Number of all initiators of simvastatin and atorvastatin therapy between January 1998 and June 2006 in Finland by 6-month periods, number of those restricted by the first tablet strength (simvastatin, 20 mg, and atorvastatin, 10 mg) and by the start of the follow-up at 270 days since initiation, and those matched by propensity score in each period.

Table S3 Covariate balance within selected periods and across all periods, presented as the standardized difference.

Table S4 Comparative effectiveness among initiators of atorvastatin (10 mg) versus simvastatin (40 mg) between January 1998 and June 2006 in Finland; hazard ratios for a composite of cardiovascular events[1] estimated with different Cox proportional hazard regression models.

Author Contributions

Conceived and designed the experiments: AHS PL EA MK RH. Analyzed the data: AHS MK. Wrote the paper: AHS PL EA MK RH.

References

1. Schneeweiss S, Gagne JJ, Glynn RJ, Ruhl M, Rassen JA (2011) Assessing the comparative effectiveness of newly marketed medications: methodological challenges and implications for drug development. Clin Pharmacol Ther 90: 777–790.
2. Seeger JD, Williams PL, Walker AM (2005) An application of propensity score matching using claims data. Pharmacoepidemiol Drug Saf 14: 465–476.
3. Mack CD, Glynn RJ, Brookhart MA, Carpenter WR, Meyer AM, et al. (2013) Calendar time-specific propensity scores and comparative effectiveness research for stage III colon cancer chemotherapy. Pharmacoepidemiol Drug Saf 22: 810–818. DOI: 10.1002/pds.3386.
4. Dusetzina SB, Mack CD, Stürmer T (2013) Propensity score estimation to address calendar time-specific channeling in comparative effectiveness research of second generation antipsychotics. PLoS One 8: e63973. DOI: 10.1371/journal.pone.0063973.
5. Wahl PM, Gagne JJ, Wasser TE, Eisenberg DF, Rodgers JK, et al. (2012) Early steps in the development of a claims-based targeted healthcare safety monitoring system and application to three empirical examples. Drug Saf 2012 35: 407–416.
6. Gagne JJ, Rassen JA, Walker AM, Glynn RJ, Schneeweiss S (2012) Active safety monitoring of new medical products using electronic healthcare data: selecting alerting rules. Epidemiology 23: 238–246. DOI: 10.1097/EDE.0b013e3182459d7d.

7. Halava H, Helin-Salmivaara A, Junnila J, Huupponen R (2009) Selective prescribing of simvastatin and atorvastatin by patient characteristics at treatment initiation over a 7-year period in Finland. Eur J Clin Pharmacol 65: 927–933.
8. Furu K, Wettermark B, Andersen M, Martikainen JE, Almarsdottir AB, et al. (2009) The Nordic countries as a cohort for pharmacoepidemiological research. Basic Clin Pharmacol Toxicol 106: 86–94. DOI: 10.1111/j.1742-7843.2009.00494.x.
9. WHO. About the ATC/DDD system. Available http://www.whocc.no/atcddd/. Accessed 15 Aug 2013.
10. Weng TC, Yang YH, Lin SJ, Tai SH (2010) A systematic review and meta-analysis on the therapeutic equivalence of statins. J Clin Pharmacol Ther 35: 139–151. DOI: 10.1111/j.1365-2710.2009.01085.x.
11. Law MR, Wald NJ, Rudnicka AR (2003) Quantifying effect of statins on low density lipoprotein cholesterol, ischaemic heart disease, and stroke: systematic review and meta-analysis. BMJ 326: 1423–1430.
12. Korhonen MJ, Huupponen R, Ruokoniemi P, Helin-Salmivaara A (2009) Protopathic bias in observational studies on statin effectiveness. Eur J Clin Pharmacol 65: 1167–1168.
13. Parsons LS. Using SAS software to perform a case-control match on propensity score in an observational study. Paper 225-25. Available: http://www2.sas.com/proceedings/sugi25/25/po/25p225.pdf. Accessed 15 Aug 2013.
14. Austin P (2009) Balance diagnostics for comparing the distribution of baseline covariates between treatment groups in propensity-score matched samples. Statist Med 28: 3083–3107. DOI: 10.1002/sim.3697.
15. Pajunen P, Koukkunen H, Ketonen M, Jerkkola T, Immonen-Räihä P, et al. (2005) The validity of the Finnish Hospital Discharge Register and Causes of Death Register data on coronary heart disease. Eur J Cardiovasc Prev Rehabil 12: 132–137.
16. Tolonen H, Salomaa V, Torppa J, Sivenius J, Immonen-Räihä P, et al. (2007) FINSTROKE register. The validation of the Finnish Hospital Discharge Register and Causes of Death Register data on stroke diagnoses. Eur J Cardiovasc Prev Rehabil 14: 380–385.
17. European Medicines Agency. Cerivastatin. Available: http://www.ema.europa.eu/ema/index.jsp?curl=pages/medicines/human/referrals/Cerivastatin/human_referral_000108.jsp. Accessed 15 Aug 2013.
18. Martikainen JE, Saastamoinen LK, Korhonen MJ, Enlund H, Helin-Salminen A (2010) Impact of restricted reimbursement on the use of statins in Finland - a register-based study. Med Care 48: 761–766.
19. Pedersen TR, Faergeman O, Kastelein JJ, Olsson AG, Tikkanen MJ, et al. (2005) High-dose atorvastatin vs usual-dose simvastatin for secondary prevention after myocardial infarction: the IDEAL study: a randomized controlled trial. JAMA 294: 2437–2445.
20. Foody JM, Joyce AT, Rudolph AE, Liu LZ, Benner JS (2008) Cardiovascular outcomes among patients newly initiating atorvastatin or simvastatin therapy: a large database analysis of managed care plans in the United States. Clin Ther 30: 195–205.
21. Jacobson TA, Wertz DA, Hoy T, Kuznik A, Grochulski D, et al. (2008) Comparison of cardiovascular event rates in patients without cardiovascular disease in whom atorvastatin or simvastatin was newly initiated. Mayo Clin Proc 83: 1316–1325.
22. Wilke RA, Berg RL, Linneman JG, Zhao C, McCarty CA, et al. (2008) Characterization of low-density lipoprotein cholesterol-lowering efficacy for atorvastatin in a population-based DNA biorepository. Basic Clin Pharmacol Toxicol 103: 354–359.
23. Simpson RJ, Jr., Signorovitch J, Birnbaum H, Ivanova J, Connolly C, et al. (2009) Cardiovascular and economic outcomes after initiation of lipid-lowering therapy with atorvastatin vs simvastatin in an employed population. Mayo Clin Proc 84: 1065–1072.
24. Rassen JA, Glynn RJ, Rothman KJ, Setoguchi S, Schneeweiss S (2012) Applying propensity scores estimated in a full cohort to adjust for confounding in subgroup analyses. Pharmacoepidemiol Drug Saf 21: 697–709. DOI: 10.1002/pds.2256.
25. Dilokthornsakul P, Chaiyakunapruk N, Schumock GT, Lee TA (2012) Estimating time-specific propensity scores: a case study of the effectiveness of inhaled long-acting beta-agonists on asthma exacerbations. Poster number 146. 28th International Conference on Pharmacoepidemiology & Therapeutic Risk Management, August 23–26, 2012 CCIB Barcelona, Spain.

16

Increased Risk of Stroke after Septicaemia: A Population-Based Longitudinal Study in Taiwan

Jiunn-Tay Lee[1]*, Wen Ting Chung[2], Jin-Ding Lin[3], Giia-Sheun Peng[1], Chih-Hsin Muo[4,5], Che-Chen Lin[5], Chi-Pang Wen[6], I-Kuan Wang[7,8,9], Chun-Hung Tseng[8,10], Chia-Hung Kao[11,12], Chung Y. Hsu[7]

1 Department of Neurology, Tri-Service General Hospital, National Defense Medical Center, Taipei, Taiwan, Republic of China, **2** Graduate Institute of Clinical Medicine, Taipei Medical University, Taipei, Taiwan, Republic of China, **3** School of Public Health, National Defense Medical Center, Taipei, Taiwan, Republic of China, **4** Department of Public Health, China Medical University Hospital, Taichung, Taiwan, Republic of China, **5** Management Office for Health Data, China Medical University Hospital, Taichung, Taiwan, Republic of China, **6** Institute of Population Health Sciences, National Health Research Institutes, Zhunan, Taiwan, Republic of China, **7** Graduate Institute of Clinical Medical Science, China Medical University, Taichung, Taiwan, Republic of China, **8** Department of Internal Medicine, College of Medicine, China Medical University, Taichung, Taiwan, Republic of China, **9** Division of Kidney Disease, China Medical University Hospital, Taichung, Taiwan, Republic of China, **10** Department of Neurology, China Medical University Hospital, Taichung, Taiwan, Republic of China, **11** Graduate Institute of Clinical Medicine Science and School of Medicine, College of Medicine, China Medical University, Taichung, Taiwan, Republic of China, **12** Department of Nuclear Medicine and PET Center, China Medical University Hospital, Taichung, Taiwan, Republic of China

Abstract

Inflammation and infection have been noted to increase stroke risk. However, the association between septicaemia and increased risk of stroke remains unclear. This population-based cohort study, using a National Health Insurance database, aimed to investigate whether patients with septicaemia are predisposed to increased stroke risk. The study included all patients hospitalised for septicaemia for the first time between 2000 and 2003 without prior stroke. Patients were followed until the end of 2010 to evaluate incidence of stroke. An age-, gender- and co-morbidities-matched cohort without prior stroke served as the control. Cox's proportional hazards regressions were used to assess differences in stroke risk between groups. Based on hazard ratios (HRs), patients with septicaemia had greater stroke risk, especially in the younger age groups (age <45: HR = 4.16, 95% CI: 2.39–7.24, $p<0.001$; age 45–64: HR = 1.76, 95% CI: 1.41–2.19, $p<0.001$; age ≥ 65: HR = 1.05, 95% CI: 0.91–1.22, $p>0.05$). Haemorrhagic stroke was the dominant type (ischaemic stroke: HR = 1.20, 95% CI: 1.06–1.37, $p<0.01$; haemorrhagic stroke: HR = 1.82, 95% CI: 1.35–2.46, $p<0.001$) and patients without co-morbidities were at slightly higher risk (without co-morbidities: HR = 1.49, 95% CI: 1.02–2.17, $p<0.05$; with co-morbidities: HR = 1.24, 95% CI: 1.10–1.41, $p<0.001$). The impact of septicaemia on stroke risk was highest within 6 months of the event and gradually declined over time. Our results suggest that septicaemia is associated with an increase in stroke risk, which is greatest in haemorrhagic stroke. Closer attention to patients with history of septicaemia may be warranted for stroke preventive measures, especially for younger patients without co-morbidities.

Editor: David P. Burgner, Murdoch Childrens Research Institute, Australia

Funding: This study was supported in part by the Tri-Service General Hospital grants (TSGH-C98-11-S02; TSGH-C99-010-11-S02; TSGH-C100-006-010-11-S02), Ministry of Health and Welfare grant (DOH101-TD-B-111-004), Academia Sinica Taiwan Biobank - Stroke Biosignature Project (BM102021169), Tseng-Lien Lin Foundation, Taiwan Brain Disease Foundation and Katsuzo and Kiyo Aoshima Memorial Funds, Japan. The funders had no role in study design, data collection and analysis, decision to publish, or preparation of the manuscript.

Competing Interests: The authors have declared that no competing interests exist.

* E-mail: jiunntay@gmail.com

Introduction

Stroke is an important cause of death and disability worldwide. Improving stroke prevention is more cost-effective than developing effective stroke therapy. In Taiwan, stroke is the leading cause of adult disability, the third leading cause of death, and the second highest healthcare expenditure for adults aged 65 and older [1,2]. Analysis of the national stroke profile and data maintained by the Taiwan Stroke Registry [2] shows that the Get with the Guidelines (GWTG) Program of the American Heart Association and American Stroke Association [3,4] is applicable in Taiwan. In addition to setting performance standards, the GWTG Program aims to improve stroke prevention and reduce healthcare expenditures by promoting public and professional awareness of risk factors for stroke [3,4]. The major risk factors for stroke have been established, and identification of these can help in the development of preventive measures. However, up to 40% of stroke patients may have health conditions other than the established stroke risk factors, that predispose a selected population to stroke [5,6]. Exploration of selected health conditions to develop a more comprehensive list of stroke risk factors may improve stroke prevention.

Acute infection may have a short-term impact as a trigger of stroke [7–12]. However, the causal role of inflammation/infection in stroke pathogenesis has not been firmly established [13]. Although evidence points to acute and chronic infections acting in combination with conventional risk factors to increase risk of stroke, it has not yet been determined whether an acute infection such as septicaemia (acute and serious systemic infection) could independently increase risk of stroke in the absence of established stroke risk factors. In addition to classic risk factors for stroke, it is important to explore the impact of acute inflammation and infection, especially severe episodes such as septicaemia, on stroke risk, since there is currently no definitive association reported between acute infection and stroke except for a short-term increase in stroke risk [7,8].

The availability of a large database from the Taiwan National Health Insurance program which represents 98% of the population in Taiwan provided an opportunity for us to investigate the relationship between hospitalisation for septicaemia and subsequent stroke. The purpose of this study was to explore whether a history of septicaemia is accompanied by a subsequent increase in the risk for developing stroke.

Methods

Database

This study used the Longitudinal Health Insurance Database (LHID) released by the Taiwan National Health Research Institute in 2011. LHID contains data from original claims of one million beneficiaries, randomly sampled from the registry for the Beneficiaries of the National Health Insurance Research Database (NHIRD) where more than 23 million individuals are enrolled into the National Health Insurance (NHI) program, the universal payer for healthcare in Taiwan [14]. The LHID contains records on inpatient, outpatient and ambulatory care services, covering the period from 1996 to 2010. The disease diagnosis accepted by the NHI is the International Classification of Diseases, Ninth Revision, Clinical Modification (ICD-9-CM). NHI has a rigorous monitoring system to ensure that the claims for reimbursement for healthcare are based on valid diagnoses. NHI randomly audits the healthcare records to validate medical claims for diagnosis and treatment. Previous reports have shown the reliability of the diagnosis coding in the LHID [15,16]. This epidemiological research project was approved by China Medical University Institute Review Board (CMU-REC-101-012). Because data in the LHID is de-identified, the signed informed consent of participants was waived.

Study Samples

The study group and a control cohort were selected from the LHID. The diagnoses of septicaemia and stroke were the basis for claims for reimbursement for relevant services rendered by the hospitals and physicians. NHI maintains stringent regulations and periodically audits the claims field for reimbursement. The study group comprised all patients who had been hospitalised for septicaemia based on ICD-9-CM codes 003.1, 036.2 and 038 for the first time from 2000 to 2003 (N = 7,611). Patients admitted for treatment of septicaemia before 2000 were excluded to increase the likelihood of identifying new cases. We also excluded patients with diagnosis of stroke (ICD-9-CM codes 430 to 438) before the diagnosis of septicaemia (N = 1,288). Patients who were hospitalised with septicaemia and who died during hospitalisation or within 7 days after discharge (N = 1,695) were also excluded. We excluded patients who died within 7 days of discharge, since based on Taiwanese customs, a large percentage of Taiwanese patients prefer to die at home, rather than in a hospital. We therefore presumed that patients who died within 7 days of discharge were in the same category as patients who died during hospitalisation. The final study group contained 4,628 cases. The first hospitalisation from the beginning of 2000 to the end of 2003 during which a patient was diagnosed with septicaemia, was set as the index date. We randomly selected 18,399 subjects (a sample size 4-fold that of the septicaemia group), frequency matched with the study cohort in terms of age, gender and co-morbidities including hypertension, diabetes, ischaemic heart diseases, atrial fibrillation and dyslipidaemia and index date. Each patient was then followed up from the index date until the occurrence of stroke. For those who did not have stroke, the last day of follow-up was defined as the date of insurance withdrawal or the last day of the study period (December 31, 2010).

Definitions of Stroke Subtypes by ICD Classification

Stroke subtypes were classified into haemorrhagic stroke (ICD-9-CM codes 430–432) and ischaemic stroke (ICD-9-CM codes 433–437). Computed tomography (CT) or magnetic resonance imaging (MRI) was used to further confirm the diagnosis of stroke and to confirm that the patient was a new stroke case rather than somebody with a history of stroke. If the patient only had ICD codes of stroke but no procedure coding of CT or MRI, the diagnosis of stroke was not made. Co-morbidities that are also stroke risk factors were established before the index date based on outpatient and inpatient data with the following ICD codes: hypertension (ICD-9-CM codes 401–405), diabetes (ICD-9-CM code 250), ischaemic heart diseases (ICD-9-CM codes 410–414), dyslipidaemia (ICD-9-CM code 272) and atrial fibrillation (ICD-9-CM code 427.3).

Statistical Analysis

Continuous variables were presented as mean ± SD and categorical variables as frequencies and percentages. Differences between study group and control cohort in the distribution of demographic characteristics (age and gender) and co-morbidities (hypertension, diabetes, ischaemic heart diseases, dyslipidaemia and atrial fibrillation) were examined by Pearson chi-square test. Cox's proportional hazard regression analysis was performed to calculate crude and adjusted hazard ratios (HR), with 95% confidence intervals (CI), for the impact of septicaemia on developing stroke. To investigate the interaction of covariates in relation to the association of septicaemia and stroke, we also calculated crude and adjusted HR stratified by age (<45, 45 to 64, ≥65 years), gender, co-morbidities, and follow-up time. We also tested the relationship between Schoenfeld residuals for septicaemia and follow-up time in the Cox's proportional hazard model for assessing the risk of stroke. All statistical analyses were performed with SAS software version 9.2 (SAS Institute Inc., Cary, NC). A two-tailed p value less than 0.05 was considered statistically significant.

Results

Baseline characteristics of the study group and the control cohort are shown in Table 1. There were no significant differences in distribution of age, gender, and co-morbidities between the two groups. There were no significant differences in baseline characteristics between the study group with septicaemia and the control cohort. Over the course of a 7–10 year follow-up period, there were 335 (incidence: 16.06/1,000 person-years) and 1,593 (incidence: 14.32/1,000 person-years) stroke events in the study group and the control cohort, respectively (Table 2). In the subgroup analysis, patients with septicaemia had a consistently higher cumulative incidence of stroke compared to those in the control cohort. The age-adjusted HR for developing stroke of any type among patients with septicaemia was 1.27 (95% CI: 1.13–1.43, p<0.001). The age-adjusted HRs were 1.20 (95% CI: 1.06–1.37, p<0.01) and 1.82 (95% CI: 1.35–2.46, p<0.001) for developing ischaemic and haemorrhagic stroke, respectively.

Table 1. Baseline characteristics of the septicaemia group and the control cohort.

	Patients with Septicaemia† (N = 4,628)		(N = 18,399)		Control Cohort
Variables	**n**	**%**	**n**	**%**	***p*-value**
Age, years					0.96
<45	1344	29	5362	29.1	
45–64	1215	26.3	4853	26.4	
≥65	2069	44.7	8184	44.5	
Mean ± SD	55.4	−25.2	55.1	−24.9	0.54
Gender					0.93
Male	2483	53.6	9885	53.7	
Female	2145	46.4	8514	46.3	
Co-morbidities					
Hypertension	2193	47.4	8718	47.4	>0.99
Diabetes	1472	31.8	5819	31.6	0.81
Ischaemic Heart Diseases	1343	29	5310	28.9	0.83
Atrial Fibrillation	215	4.65	780	4.24	0.22

†ICD9 003.1, 036.2 & 038.
Chi-square test.

The age-adjusted HR for stroke of any type was higher in the septicaemia group with co-morbidities as compared to the control cohort with co-morbidities (HR = 1.24, 95% CI: 1.10–1.41, $p <$ 0.001), and patients in the co-morbidities group with ischaemic stroke had an HR of 1.19 (95% CI: 1.05–1.37, $p<0.01$) compared to patients with haemorrhagic stroke (HR = 1.71, 95% CI: 1.22–2.40, $p<0.01$) (Table 2). The age-adjusted HR for stroke of any type was also higher in the septicaemia group without co-morbidities as compared to the control cohort without co-morbidities (HR = 1.49, 95% CI: 1.02–2.17, $p<0.05$), and patients without co-morbidities who had ischaemic stroke had an HR of 1.20 (95% CI: 0.75–1.91, $p>0.05$) compared to patients with haemorrhagic stroke (HR = 2.32, 95% CI: 1.21–4.43, $p<0.05$) (Table 2). The impact reflected by HRs appears slightly greater among those without co-morbidities. However, because of smaller case numbers, the confidence intervals were wider in the groups without co-morbidities (Table 2).

Table 3 presents results of further analysis of patient data stratified by age (<45 years; 45–64 years; ≥65 years) and gender. The risk for developing stroke was inversely associated with age (interaction $p<0.05$). The HR for developing stroke of any type was significantly higher in the septicaemia group than in the control cohort in the <45 years age group (HR = 4.16, 95% CI: 2.39–7.24, $p<0.001$). Patients in this group with ischaemic stroke had a significantly lower HR (2.08, 95% CI: 1.02–4.25, $p<0.05$), compared to those with haemorrhagic stroke (HR = 28.6, 95% CI: 6.46–127, $p<0.001$). The impact of septicaemia on stroke risk declined in the 45–64 years age group (stroke of any type, HR = 1.76, 95% CI: 1.41–2.19, $p<0.001$; ischaemic stroke, HR = 1.77, 95% CI: 1.39–2.25, $p<0.001$; haemorrhagic stroke, HR = 1.68, 95% CI: 0.98–2.90, $p>0.05$), and shows no significant difference between the septicaemia group and the control cohort with age ≥65 years (stroke of any type, HR = 1.05, 95% CI: 0.91–1.22, $p>0.05$; ischaemic stroke, HR = 1.03, 95% CI: 0.88–1.20, $p>0.05$; haemorrhagic stroke, HR = 1.34, 95% CI: 0.88–2.04, $p>$ 0.05). The interaction p value between age and septicaemia was < 0.05 for all types of stroke, ischaemic and haemorrhagic stroke. The interaction p value between gender and septicaemia was 0.042 for haemorrhagic stroke, but >0.05 for all types of stroke and ischaemic stroke. In addition, the adjusted HR for developing haemorrhagic stroke in patients with septicaemia compared with controls was 1.10 (95% CI: 0.65–1.87) among females ($p>0.05$) and 2.08 among males (95% CI: 1.45–3.00, $p<0.001$).

Figure 1 shows the impact of time on the risk of developing stroke. A time-dependent decline was noted. The stroke risk was highest within the first 6 months of the septicaemia episode (stroke of any type, HR = 1.97, 95% CI: 1.46–2.68, $p<0.001$; ischaemic stroke, HR = 1.75, 95% CI: 1.24–2.46, $p = 0.001$; haemorrhagic stroke, HR = 3.27, 95% CI: 1.68–6.40, $p<0.001$). Beyond 6 months, there was a significant increase in stroke risk for haemorrhagic stroke within 2 years of the septicaemia episode (HR = 2.04, 95% CI: 1.13–3.70, $p<0.05$). Beyond 2 years (up to 10 years), there was no significant difference in overall stroke risk between the septicaemia group and the control cohort. The decline in stroke risk over time was significant ($p<0.05$) based on the relationship between Schoenfeld residuals for septicaemia and follow-up time in the Cox's proportional hazard model.

Discussion

This population-based longitudinal study was performed to assess whether septicaemia, an acute systemic infection, was associated with an increased risk for developing stroke. We showed that patients with septicaemia had a higher risk for developing ischaemic or haemorrhagic stroke. Comparison of the effect estimates (HRs) of stroke between the septicaemia and control groups showed significantly higher HRs in patients without co-morbidities compared with those with co-morbidities (established stroke risk factors including hypertension, diabetes, ischaemic heart diseases, atrial fibrillation and dyslipidaemia). It is worth noting that the risk for developing haemorrhagic stroke was higher than that for ischaemic stroke.

Septicaemia is a serious systemic infection characterized by intense inflammation intertwined with profound alteration of vascular function, often followed by a state of relative immune paralysis [17]. Although case-control studies suggested that recent

Table 2. Hazard ratios for development of stroke associated with septicaemia.

	Patients with Septicaemia				Control Cohort
Variable	No. of events	Incidence, per 1,000 person-years	No. of events	Incidence, per 1,000 person-years	Age-adjusted HR (95% CI)
Overall					
All Strokes	335	16.06	1593	14.32	1.27 (1.13–1.43)***
Ischaemic Stroke	278	13.53	1425	12.81	1.20 (1.06–1.37)**
Haemorrhagic Stroke	57	2.77	184	1.65	1.82 (1.35–2.46)***
With co-morbidities					
All Strokes	296	27.51	1452	23.12	1.24 (1.10–1.41)***
Ischaemic Stroke	257	23.89	1314	20.92	1.19 (1.05–1.37)**
Haemorrhagic Stroke	44	4.09	152	2.42	1.71 (1.22–2.40)**
Without co-morbidities					
All Strokes	34	3.47	141	2.91	1.49 (1.02–2.17)*
Ischaemic Stroke	21	2.14	111	2.29	1.20 (0.75–1.91)
Haemorrhagic Stroke	13	1.33	32	0.66	2.32 (1.21–4.43)*

HR: hazard ratio, CI: confidence interval.
*$p<0.05$; **$p<0.01$; ***$p<0.001$.

Table 3. Hazard ratios for the development of stroke associated with septicaemia by age and gender.

	Patients with Septicaemia				Control Cohort
Variable	No. of events	Incidence, per 1,000 person-years	No. of events	Incidence, per 1,000 person-years	HR (95% CI)
Age, years					
<45					
All Strokes	24	2.87	26	0.69	4.16 (2.39–7.24)***
Ischaemic Stroke	11	1.32	24	0.63	2.08 (1.02–4.25)*
Haemorrhagic Stroke	13	1.56	2	0.05	28.6 (6.46–127)***
45–64					
All Strokes	105	18.45	330	10.54	1.76 (1.41–2.19)***
Ischaemic Stroke	89	15.64	279	8.91	1.77 (1.39–2.25)***
Haemorrhagic Stroke	17	2.99	55	1.76	1.68 (0.98–2.90)
≥65					
All Strokes	201	30.92	1237	29.43	1.05 (0.91–1.22)
Ischaemic Stroke	178	27.39	1122	26.69	1.03 (0.88–1.20)
Haemorrhagic Stroke	27	4.15	127	3.02	1.34 (0.88–2.04)
Gender					
Male					
All Strokes	171	15.89	841	13.99	1.13 (0.95–1.33)
Ischaemic Stroke	744	12.38	134	12.45	1.00 (0.83–1.20)
Haemorrhagic Stroke	40	3.72	105	1.75	2.08 (1.45–3.00)***
Female					
All Strokes	159	16.24	752	14.71	1.10 (0.95–1.30)
Ischaemic Stroke	144	14.71	744	12.38	1.10 (0.92–1.31)
Haemorrhagic Stroke	17	1.74	79	1.55	1.10 (0.65–1.87)

HR: hazard ratio, CI: confidence interval; *$p<0.05$; **$p<0.01$; ***$p<0.001$.
The interaction p between age and septicaemia was <0.05 for all strokes, ischaemic and haemorrhagic stroke.
The interaction p between gender and septicaemia was 0.042 for haemorrhagic stroke but interaction p for all strokes and ischaemic stroke was >0.05.

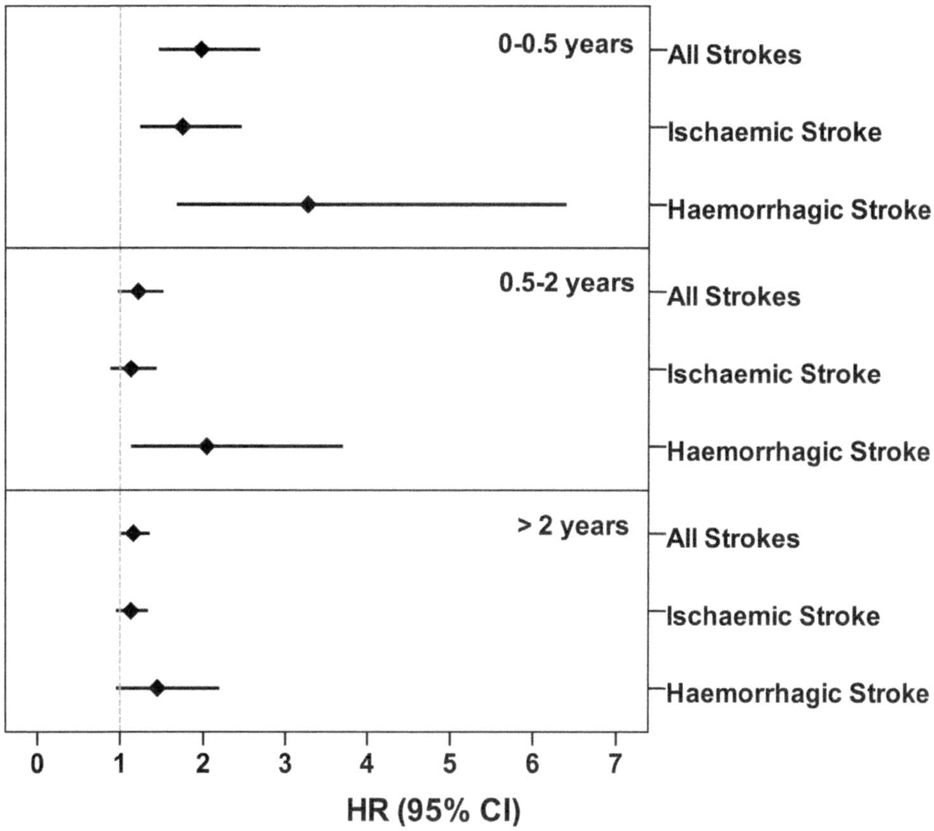

Figure 1. Age-, gender- and co-morbidities-adjusted hazard ratios for development of stroke following septicaemia at various time intervals.

infection (within 1 week) may be a trigger of stroke [9–12], results from the present study showed that septicaemia may have a sustained impact in increasing stroke risk especially in the first 6 months after septicaemia.

We showed that the young age group (<45 years) was more vulnerable to developing stroke compared to the middle aged group (45–64 years) which in turn was more vulnerable than the elderly (≥65 years) group. This was especially true for the haemorrhagic type that patients with septicaemia in the young age group had 28.6 times of risk for developing stroke compared to the control cohort, which was extremely higher to that of other types. Because of smaller case numbers in the young age group and in the group without co-morbidities, wider confidence intervals were noted. Male patients with septicaemia showed an increased risk of haemorrhagic stroke, around 2.1 times compared to the control cohort. The impact of septicaemia on stroke risk was greatest within 6 months of the septicaemia episode, and then declined gradually over time. These findings suggested that septicaemia increased the risk of developing stroke, especially the haemorrhagic type. We showed that the impact of septicaemia on stroke risk was more prominent in the younger population. This was consistent with studies showing that age is the most important risk factor for stroke [18–21]. Our data suggested that the greater effect size seen with septicaemia in younger patients could be due to the lower prevalence of established stroke risk factors in this group.

Inflammation and infection are gaining awareness and interest as potential conditions that increase stroke risk [22]. Systemic infections with resultant immune/inflammatory processes are related to stroke aetiology and pathology [23].

Chronic inflammation may influence the formation of atherosclerotic plaque [13,24] and lipid metabolism, which are known to play a role in atherothrombotic diseases including stroke [25–27], and chronic inflammation has been added to the list of established risk factors for stroke [13].

Prior acute infections with *Mycoplasma pneumoniae, Helicobacter pylori, Chlamydia pneumoniae,* herpes virus, and cytomegalovirus are thought to contribute to the pathogenesis of ischaemic stroke, possibly resulting from the infectious burden, aberrant activation of the coagulation process, and endothelial dysfunction [28–32]. Systemic respiratory tract infections were shown to significantly increase the risk of stroke and myocardial infarction, especially during the first three days, supporting the notion that acute infections result in a transient increase in risk of vascular events [7]. These results were consistent with another study showing that individuals hospitalised for infections had an increased risk for stroke, with a higher risk within a short interval after infection [8]. Acute infections have been reported to increase plasma fibrinogen and CRP levels, which may affect the risk of stroke [33]. Acute respiratory tract and urinary tract infections have also been reported to independently increase the risk for ischaemic stroke [28]. The neuropathology of septic shock in a report on 23 patients who had died of this condition included cerebral haemorrhage, hypercoagulability syndrome, micro-abscesses, multifocal necrotising leukoencephalopathy, and ischaemia [34]. These studies suggest that identification of treatable infectious diseases associated with stroke risk may lead to more effective stroke prevention [28].

Based on these studies and our present results, we hypothesise that septicaemia may initiate an intense systemic inflammatory reaction and disordered coagulation process, resulting in structural changes in the cerebral vasculature, thereby increasing the risk for developing stroke. Septicaemia-induced structural changes in cerebral blood vessels may accelerate the pathogenic processes that culminate in earlier onset of stroke. The observation that septicaemia is associated with a higher risk for developing haemorrhagic stroke is also consistent with the contention that structural vascular changes associated with septicaemia could be the culprit. It will be interesting to further explore the pathogenic mechanisms underlying septicaemia-associated increase in stroke risk especially the haemorrhagic type.

An important strength of this study was the use of a population-based data set that allowed for inclusion of a large number of septicaemia patients, a sizeable number of whom eventually developed stroke during the follow-up period. We were able to obtain a well-matched control group without septicaemia from the same population for a long follow-up period of 7–10 years. The large sample sizes allowed subgroup analysis, which showed 1) a greater risk for developing haemorrhagic than ischaemic stroke following septicaemia, 2) a trend for the younger age group to be more vulnerable than the older group and 3) a significant decline in stroke risk over time.

Limitations

This study has several limitations. First, data used in the present study did not include medications or lifestyle factors such as smoking, alcohol consumption, exercise habits and diet that may influence the risk of stroke. Second, data from a large dataset of this type may also include unidentified recurrent patients who may have had septicaemia and stroke before 1996 when NIH was started. Future prospective studies of patients with septicaemia will be necessary to expand and confirm our present results. The caveat associated with smaller case numbers in selected groups (young age groups, the groups without co-morbidities) should also be recognised. Finally, results presented in this study show only an association without establishing causality.

Conclusion

In conclusion, to our knowledge, this is the first report to explore a possible association between septicaemia and stroke in a large nationwide population-based study. Septicaemia was associated with an increased risk of developing stroke, especially haemorrhagic stroke, particularly within the first 6 months of the septicaemia episode, with declining impact over time. Young patients (age <45 years) with septicaemia were more vulnerable to developing stroke, especially the haemorrhagic type, than the older group. Patients with septicaemia, who did not have the conventional stroke risk factors (co-morbidities) had a slightly higher risk for developing stroke, in particular the haemorrhagic type, than the control cohort. These findings suggest that stroke preventive measures could be improved by paying closer attention to subgroups of patients, particularly patients <45 years old who have no co-morbidities, within 6 months of a septicaemia episode.

Author Contributions

Conceived and designed the experiments: JTL. Performed the experiments: JTL WTC. Analyzed the data: JDL JTL WTC CHM CYH CCL. Contributed reagents/materials/analysis tools: CYH JTL GSP CPW IKW CHT CHK. Wrote the paper: JTL.

References

1. Jeng JS, Su TC (2007) Epidemiological studies of cerebrovascular diseases and carotid atherosclerosis in Taiwan. Acta Neurol Taiwan 16: 190–202.
2. Hsieh FI, Lien LM, Chen ST, Bai CH, Sun MC, et al. (2010) Get With the Guidelines-Stroke performance indicators: surveillance of stroke care in the Taiwan Stroke Registry: Get With the Guidelines-Stroke in Taiwan. Circulation 122: 1116–1123.
3. Fonarow GC, Reeves MJ, Zhao X, Olson DM, Smith EE, et al. (2010) Age-related differences in characteristics, performance measures, treatment trends, and outcomes in patients with ischemic stroke. Circulation 121: 879–891.
4. Silva GS, Schwamm LH (2013) Review of stroke center effectiveness and other get with the guidelines data. Curr Atheroscler Rep 15: 350.
5. Whisnant JP (1997) Modeling of risk factors for ischemic stroke. The Willis Lecture. Stroke 28: 1840–1844.
6. Donnan GA, Fisher M, Macleod M, Davis SM (2008) Stroke. Lancet 371: 1612–1623.
7. Smeeth L, Thomas SL, Hall AJ, Hubbard R, Farrington P, et al. (2004) Risk of myocardial infarction and stroke after acute infection or vaccination. N Engl J Med 351: 2611–2618.
8. Elkind MS, Carty CL, O'Meara ES, Lumley T, Lefkowitz D, et al. (2011) Hospitalization for infection and risk of acute ischemic stroke: the Cardiovascular Health Study. Stroke 42: 1851–1856.
9. Bova IY, Bornstein NM, Korczyn AD (1996) Acute infection as a risk factor for ischemic stroke. Stroke 27: 2204–2206.
10. Syrjanen J, Valtonen VV, Iivanainen M, Kaste M, Huttunen JK (1988) Preceding infection as an important risk factor for ischaemic brain infarction in young and middle aged patients. Br Med J (Clin Res Ed) 296: 1156–1160.
11. Grau AJ, Buggle F, Heindl S, Steichen-Wiehn C, Banerjee T, et al. (1995) Recent infection as a risk factor for cerebrovascular ischemia. Stroke 26: 373–379.
12. Grau AJ, Buggle F, Becher H, Zimmermann E, Spiel M, et al. (1998) Recent bacterial and viral infection is a risk factor for cerebrovascular ischemia: clinical and biochemical studies. Neurology 50: 196–203.
13. Lindsberg PJ, Grau AJ (2003) Inflammation and infections as risk factors for ischemic stroke. Stroke 34: 2518–2532.
14. Database NHIR (2012).
15. Cheng CL, Kao YH, Lin SJ, Lee CH, Lai ML (2011) Validation of the National Health Insurance Research Database with ischemic stroke cases in Taiwan. Pharmacoepidemiol Drug Saf 20: 236–242.
16. Kang JH, Chen YH, Lin HC (2010) Comorbidity profiles among patients with ankylosing spondylitis: a nationwide population-based study. Ann Rheum Dis 69: 1165–1168.
17. Bernard AM, Bernard GR (2012) The immune response: targets for the treatment of severe sepsis. Int J Inflam 2012: 697592.
18. Olesen JB, Lip GY, Hansen ML, Hansen PR, Tolstrup JS, et al. (2011) Validation of risk stratification schemes for predicting stroke and thromboembolism in patients with atrial fibrillation: nationwide cohort study. BMJ 342: d124.
19. Marinigh R, Lip GY, Fiotti N, Giansante C, Lane DA (2010) Age as a risk factor for stroke in atrial fibrillation patients: implications for thromboprophylaxis. J Am Coll Cardiol 56: 827–837.
20. Brown RD, Whisnant JP, Sicks JD, O'Fallon WM, Wiebers DO (1996) Stroke incidence, prevalence, and survival: secular trends in Rochester, Minnesota, through 1989. Stroke 27: 373–380.
21. Wolf PA, D'Agostino RB, O'Neal MA, Sytkowski P, Kase CS, et al. (1992) Secular trends in stroke incidence and mortality. The Framingham Study. Stroke 23: 1551–1555.
22. Goldstein LB (2000) Novel risk factors for stroke: homocysteine, inflammation, and infection. Curr Atheroscler Rep 2: 110–114.
23. McColl BW, Allan SM, Rothwell NJ (2009) Systemic infection, inflammation and acute ischemic stroke. Neuroscience 158: 1049–1061.
24. Maekawa T, Takahashi N, Tabeta K, Aoki Y, Miyashita H, et al. (2011) Chronic oral infection with Porphyromonas gingivalis accelerates atheroma formation by shifting the lipid profile. PLoS One 6: e20240.
25. Ross R (1999) Atherosclerosis–an inflammatory disease. N Engl J Med 340: 115–126.
26. Pearson TA, Mensah GA, Alexander RW, Anderson JL, Cannon RO 3rd, et al. (2003) Markers of inflammation and cardiovascular disease: application to clinical and public health practice: A statement for healthcare professionals from the Centers for Disease Control and Prevention and the American Heart Association. Circulation 107: 499–511.
27. O'Keefe JH, Carter MD, Lavie CJ (2009) Primary and secondary prevention of cardiovascular diseases: a practical evidence-based approach. Mayo Clin Proc 84: 741–757.
28. Palm F, Urbanek C, Grau A (2009) Infection, its treatment and the risk for stroke. Curr Vasc Pharmacol 7: 146–152.

29. Kang JH, Ho JD, Chen YH, Lin HC (2009) Increased risk of stroke after a herpes zoster attack: a population-based follow-up study. Stroke 40: 3443–3448.
30. Mattila KJ, Valtonen VV, Nieminen MS, Asikainen S (1998) Role of infection as a risk factor for atherosclerosis, myocardial infarction, and stroke. Clin Infect Dis 26: 719–734.
31. Grau AJ (1997) Infection, inflammation, and cerebrovascular ischemia. Neurology 49: S47–51.
32. Elkind MS, Ramakrishnan P, Moon YP, Boden-Albala B, Liu KM, et al. (2010) Infectious burden and risk of stroke: the northern Manhattan study. Arch Neurol 67: 33–38.
33. Emsley HC, Hopkins SJ (2008) Acute ischaemic stroke and infection: recent and emerging concepts. Lancet Neurol 7: 341–353.
34. Sharshar T, Annane D, de la Grandmaison GL, Brouland JP, Hopkinson NS, et al. (2004) The neuropathology of septic shock. Brain Pathol 14: 21–33.

17

Impact of Coexisting Coronary Artery Disease on the Occurrence of Cerebral Ischemic Lesions after Carotid Stenting

Kuo-Lun Huang[1,2], Yeu-Jhy Chang[1,2], Chien-Hung Chang[1,2,3], Ting-Yu Chang[1,2], Chi-Hung Liu[1,2], I-Chang Hsieh[2,4], Ho-Fai Wong[2,5], Yau-Yau Wai[2,5], Yu-Wei Chen[6,7,8], Bak-Sau Yip[9], Tsong-Hai Lee[1,2]*

1 Stroke Center and Department of Neurology, Linkou Chang Gung Memorial Hospital, Taoyuan, Taiwan, **2** College of Medicine, Chang Gung University, Taoyuan, Taiwan, **3** Department of Electrical Engineering, Chang Gung University, Taoyuan, Taiwan, **4** Department of Internal Medicine, Section of Cardiology, Linkou Chang Gung Memorial Hospital, Taoyuan, Taiwan, **5** Department of Medical Imaging and Intervention, Linkou Chang Gung Memorial Hospital, Taoyuan, Taiwan, **6** Department of Neurology, Landseed Hospital, Taoyuan, Taiwan, **7** Department of Neurology, National Taiwan University Hospital, Taipei City, Taiwan, **8** Department of Computer Science and Information Engineering, National Central University, Zhongli City, Taiwan, **9** Department of Neurology, National Taiwan University Hospital Hsinchu Branch, Hsinchu, Taiwan

Abstract

Background: Coronary artery disease (CAD) may coexist with extracranial carotid artery stenosis (ECAS), but the influence of CAD on procedure-related complications after carotid artery stenting (CAS) has not been well investigated. The study aimed to determine the impact of CAD on the occurrence of peri-CAS cerebral ischemic lesions on diffusion-weighted imaging (DWI) scanning.

Methods: Coronary angiography was performed within six months before CAS. DWI scanning was repetitively done within 1 week before and after CAS. Clinical outcome measures were stroke, angina, myocardial infarction and death within 30 days.

Results: Among 126 patients (69.5±9.0 years) recruited for unilateral protected CAS, 33 (26%) patients had peri-CAS DWI-positive lesions. CAD was noted in 79% (26 in 33) and 48% (45 in 93) of patients with and without peri-CAS DWI-positive lesions (OR, 4.0; 95% CI, 1.6–10.0; $P = .0018$), and the number of concomitant CAD on coronary angiography was positively correlated with the risk for peri-CAS DWI-positive lesions ($P = .0032$). In patients with no CAD (n = 55), asymptomatic CAD (n = 41) and symptomatic CAD (n = 30), the occurrence rates of peri-CAS DWI-positive lesions were 13%, 41% and 30% ($P = .0048$), and the peri-CAS stroke rates were 2%, 7% and 0% ($P = .2120$).

Conclusions: The severity of morphological CAD and the presence of either symptomatic or asymptomatic CAD are associated with the occurrence of peri-CAS cerebral ischemic lesions.

Editor: Carmine Pizzi, University of Bologna, Italy

Funding: This study was carried out with financial support from the National Science Council, Taiwan (grant number 102-2314-B-182A-114-) and Chang Gung Memorial Hospital, Taiwan (grant CMRPG350733, CMRPG390821, CMRPG3B0612, CMRPG3A0352, and CMRPG3B0111). The funders had no role in study design, data collection and analysis, decision to publish, or preparation of the manuscript.

Competing Interests: The authors have declared that no competing interests exist.

* E-mail: thlee@adm.cgmh.org.tw

Introduction

Extracranial carotid artery stenosis (ECAS) is a risk factor for cerebral ischemic stroke by causing cerebral embolism and cerebral hypoperfusion as well [1]. Carotid endarterectomy (CEA) is the current standard treatment for significant ECAS, and carotid artery stenting (CAS) is an alternative for high-risk patients, such as those with coronary artery disease (CAD), history of neck radiotherapy, and bilateral carotid artery stenosis [2]. Even though the long-term treatment outcome is similar between the two treatment choices [3], a recent randomized study has shown that there are more procedure-related cerebral ischemic lesions on diffusion-weighted imaging (DWI) scanning in patients receiving CAS than CEA [4].

Atherosclerosis is a chronic and multi-territory disease. In patients with ECAS, CAD is the most common concomitant vascular disease with the concurrence rate as high as 57% to 77% [5,6,7]. Although the presence of concomitant CAD has been shown to be associated with the long-term major cardiac events after CAS [8], there are limited studies investigating the impact of CAD on the occurrence of peri-CAS cerebral ischemic lesions. In a recent study by Chung *et al*, the presence of CAD was associated with increased amount of emboli production captured by embolic protection devices (EPDs) during CAS [9]. However, whether these emboli would lead to the occurrence of cerebral ischemic lesions or even stroke remains unanswered [10,11]. Furthermore, only 39% to 59% of patients with concomitant ECAS and CAD had overt manifestations of myocardial ischemia [6,7]. Therefore, patients with asymptomatic CAD may be unrecognized during the pre-CAS evaluation of stroke risk.

Considering the high prevalence rate of CAD in patients with ECAS, the present study aimed to determine whether the presence of morphological CAD on coronary angiography is a risk for peri-CAS cerebral ischemic lesions on DWI scanning, and also would like to investigate the influence of both asymptomatic and symptomatic CAD on the risk for peri-CAS cerebral DWI-positive lesions.

Methods

Subjects

From December 2005 to December 2012, we included patients with 1) age ≥50 years, 2) significant ECAS ≥50% by NASCET criteria on cerebral angiography [12], and 3) receiving CAS with EPDs. The exclusion criteria were 1) lack of serial MRI scanning within 1 week before and within 1 week after CAS, 2) lack of coronary angiography study before CAS, or 3) receiving bilateral CAS. A total of 126 patients fulfilled the selection criteria (Figure 1), and there was no significant difference in demographic factors or ECAS severity between patients included and excluded. The patient data and procedure results were prospectively collected and retrospectively analyzed from our stroke registry databank [13]. All patients or next of kin gave written informed consent to angiography and MRI examinations and CAS treatment. To obtain clinical information from the stroke registry databank for analysis, patient records were anonymized and de-identified prior to data retrieval and analysis. The Institute Ethics Committee of Chang Gung Memorial Hospital approved the study protocol and data retrieval process.

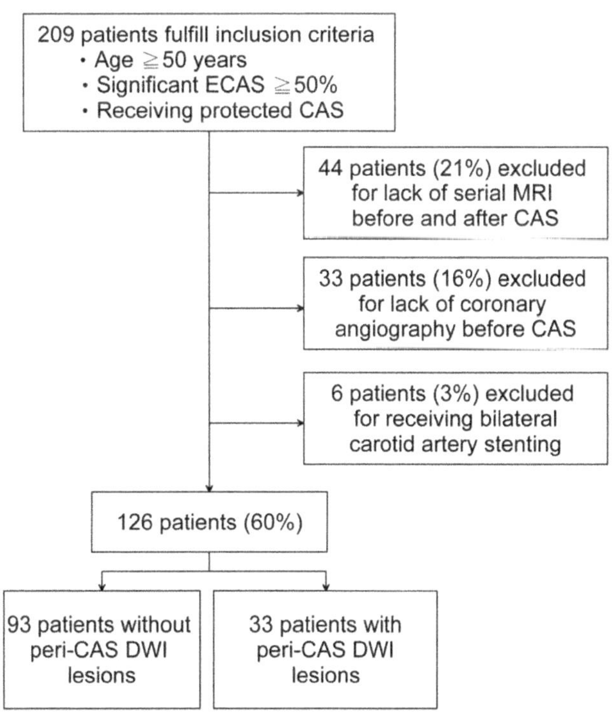

Figure 1. Flow chart for patient collection. The number of patients receiving unilateral protected CAS with coronary angiography and serial MRI evaluation (ECAS, extracranial carotid artery stenosis; CAS, carotid artery stenting; DWI, diffusion-weighted imaging; MRI, magnetic resonance imaging).

Evaluation of coronary artery disease and concomitant stenosis in other arteries

Coronary angiography and aortogram were reviewed for the study if they were performed within six months before or simultaneously with cerebral angiography prior to CAS [8]. Coronary artery disease and stenosis of extracranial vertebral artery, subclavian artery and iliac artery were defined as having artery diameter narrowing ≥50% in the projection showing the greatest severity [5]. Patients having evidence of CAD on coronary angiography were further divided into asymptomatic and symptomatic CAD by history of angina, myocardial infarction, or coronary revascularization in medical records [14].

Carotid artery stenting procedure

Carotid artery stenting was performed with WALLSTENT (Boston Scientific Corp, Natick, MA) or Zilver stent (Cook Medical, Bloomington, IN). EPI FilterWire (Boston Scientific Corp, Natick, MA), post-stenting angioplasty with balloon dilation and intra-procedural heparinization were applied in all patients. A combination of aspirin (100 mg/day) and clopidogrel (75 mg/day) was routinely administered 72 hours before CAS, and clopidogrel was prescribed for 3 months and aspirin was maintained indefinitely after CAS. Patients were evaluated 1 day before and 1 day and 30 days after CAS by independent neurologists [15].

MRI studies

Brain MRI was repeatedly performed within 1 week before and after CAS. MRI was obtained at a 1.5 Tesla scanner (Symphony, Siemens) with 5-mm slice thickness and 0.5-mm interslice gap for all sequences, including axial T1-weighted (T1W) sequence (spin-echo; repetition time [TR]/echo time [TE] = 449/12 ms; matrix 256×256), axial T2-weighted (T2W) sequence (fast spin-echo; TR/TE = 4000/90), fluid-attenuated inversion recovery sequence (TR/TE/TI = 9416/90/2200), and DWI sequence (single-shot spin-echo echo-planar technique; TR/TE = 2812/60; b values of 0, 500, and 1000 s/mm^2). Peri-CAS acute ischemic events were defined as the occurrence of hyperintensity lesions on the post-CAS DWI scanning which were not observed in the pre-CAS MRI studies [15].

Statistical analysis

All variables were summated using mean ± standard deviation for continuous variables and frequency distribution for categorical variables. Comparisons between groups were conducted with the Student's t test or analysis of variance (ANOVA) with Bonferroni adjustment where appropriate for continuous variables, and the chi-square test or Fisher's exact test for categorical variables. Logistic regression method with cumulative logit modeling for ordinal response variables was applied to obtain odds ratio (OR) and 95% confidence interval (CI) when response variables had more than 2 categories, and it was also applied to adjust for confounding factors [15]. SAS version 9.0 or higher was used for analyses, and $p<0.05$ was considered significant.

Results

Patient and procedural data

The study recruited 126 patients receiving unilateral protected CAS. The mean age of patients was 69.5±9.0 years, and 112 of them (89%) were men. The stenosis severity values of the treated and non-treated carotid arteries were 76.1±11.2% and 35.1±32%, respectively, and 47 of the 126 patients (37%) had symptomatic carotid stenosis. Of the 126 carotid artery stents, 122 were WALLSTENT and the rest were Zilver stent. EPI FilterWire was attempted in all patients except one treated carotid artery due to difficulty in anatomical approach. Within 30 days after CAS, 4 patients had minor ischemic stroke with the increase of NIH stroke scale <4, and no peri-procedural myocardial infarction or mortality was observed.

Thirty three of the 126 patients (26%) had new cerebral DWI-positive lesions on DWI scanning after CAS. Comparing to patients without peri-CAS DWI-positive lesions, patients with DWI-positive lesions had a higher frequency of concomitant CAD on coronary angiography (OR, 4.0; 95% CI, 1.6–10.0; $P = .0018$), but there was no difference in conventional vascular risk factors or ECAS severity between the two groups ($P > .05$, Table 1). The frequencies of concomitant arterial stenosis in vertebral artery, iliac artery and subclavian artery were 44%, 22% and 13%, and their presence was not related to the occurrence of peri-CAS DWI-positive lesions.

Relationship between morphological CAD and peri-CAS ischemic lesions

In the 55 patients without CAD, there were 7 having peri-CAS DWI lesions and 1 having peri-CAS stroke, and in the 71 patients with CAD, there were 26 having peri-CAS DWI lesions (OR, 4.0; 95% CI, 1.6–10.0; $P = .0018$) and 3 having peri-CAS stroke (OR, 2.4; 95% CI, 0.2–23.6; $P = .6313$). In patients with 0-vessel, 1-vessel, 2-vessel and 3-vessel CAD, the frequencies of peri-CAS DWI-positive lesions were 13%, 23%, 52% and 33% ($P = .0032$; 1-vessel versus 0-vessel OR, 2.1 with 95% CI, 0.7–6.7; 2-vessel versus 0-vessel OR, 7.3 with 95% CI, 2.5–21.6; 3-vessel versus 0-vessel OR, 3.4 with 95% CI, 0.8–11.4), and the frequencies of peri-CAS manifesting stroke were 2%, 3%, 7% and 0% ($P = .6470$; OR is not provided because the maximum likelihood estimate may not exist), respectively.

Relationship between symptomatology of CAD and peri-CAS ischemic lesions

Seventy one patients (56%) had concomitant CAD on coronary angiography, and 41 of them (58%) were asymptomatic CAD. Considering the composite findings on coronary angiography and the relevant cardiac symptoms and signs, there were 55 patients without CAD (Group I), 41 patients with asymptomatic CAD (Group II), and 30 patients with symptomatic CAD (Group III) (Table 2). In Group III, there were 27 patients with angina, 9 with myocardial infarction, 17 with prior coronary revascularization, 9 with ischemic changes on echocardiography, 10 with ischemic changes on treadmill or thallium stress tests, and 4 with congestive heart failure of New York Function Class III or IV. In Group I, there were 8 patients with previous neck radiation therapy, 10 with contralateral carotid artery stenosis >70%, and 5 with age >80 years. The rest patients of Group I preferred CAS to CEA even after well explanation of the benefits and risks between the two interventional choices.

Peri-CAS DWI-positive lesions were found in 13%, 41%, and 30% of patients ($P = .0048$; Group II versus Group I OR, 4.9 with 95% CI, 1.8–13.3; Group III versus Group I OR, 2.9 with 95% CI, 1.0–8.9), and peri-CAS manifesting stroke was found in 2%, 7%, and 0% of patients from Groups I to III, respectively ($P = .212$; OR is not provided because the maximum likelihood

Table 1. Baseline characteristics of patients according to the occurrence of peri-CAS DWI-positive lesions.

	Without DWI-positive lesions	With DWI-positive lesions	*P*
N	93	33	
Continuous factors, mean (SD)*			
Age, years	69.3 (9.5)	69.8 (7.5)	0.7915
Stenosis severity of treated carotid arteries, %	75.7 (11.7)	77.1 (10.0)	0.5401
Stenosis severity of non-treated carotid arteries, %	35.4 (32.0)	34.3 (32.6)	0.8665
Left ventricular ejection fraction, %	64.3 (11.3)	65.7 (12.3)	0.5610
Serum creatinine, mg/dL	1.01 (0.28)	1.07 (0.34)	0.3740
Categorical factors, N (%)†			
Gender, male	82 (88)	30 (91)	1.0000
Symptomatic carotid artery stenosis	35 (38)	12 (36)	0.8967
Diabetes mellitus	32 (34)	14 (42)	0.4142
Hypertension	75 (81)	28 (85)	0.5854
Dyslipidemia	67 (72)	22 (67)	0.5632
Findings on coronary angiography or aortogram			
Concomitant CAD	45 (48)	26 (79)	0.0018‡
Concomitant vertebral artery stenosis	41 (44)	15 (45)	0.8919
Concomitant iliac artery stenosis	19 (20)	9 (27)	0.4237
Concomitant subclavian artery stenosis	12 (13)	4 (12)	1.0000
Peri-CAS manifesting stroke	0 (0)	4 (12)	0.0041
History of anti-platelet medication over 90 days before CAS	56 (60)	22 (67)	0.5095

*Comparison with two-group t test.
†Comparison with chi-square test or Fisher's exact test.
‡p<0.01 after adjustment for age, gender, LVEF, creatinine level, symptomatic carotid stenosis and anti-platelet medication history.
CAS, carotid artery stenting; DWI, diffusion-weighted imaging; CAD, coronary artery disease.

Table 2. Clinical and imaging characteristics of patients with no CAD, asymptomatic CAD and symptomatic CAD.

	No CAD, Group I	Asymptomatic CAD, Group II	Symptomatic CAD, Group III	*P*
N	55	41	30	
Continuous factors, mean (SD)*				
Age, years	67.5 (9.4)	70.4 (8.9)	71.9 (7.8)	0.0722
Stenosis severity of treated carotid arteries, %	75.7 (12.0)	76.8 (10.5)	75.6 (11.2)	0.8812
Stenosis severity of non-treated carotid arteries, %	33.3 (32.8)	32.6 (28.7)	42.0 (34.7)	0.4093
Left ventricular ejection fraction, %	67.0 (8.8)	65.3 (12.6)	59.4 (13.0)‡	0.0127
Serum creatinine, mg/dL	0.95 (0.25)	1.08 (0.34)	1.09 (0.29)	0.0294
Categorical factors, N (%)†				
Gender, male	48 (87)	37 (90)	27 (90)	0.9360
Symptomatic carotid artery stenosis	24 (44)	17 (41)	6 (20)	0.0658
Diabetes mellitus	16 (29)	15 (37)	15 (50)	0.1638
Hypertension	40 (73)	36 (88)	27 (90)	0.0675
Dyslipidemia	38 (69)	24 (59)	27 (90)	0.0091
Atrial fibrillation	3 (5)	2 (5)	4 (13)	0.3738
Number of CAD on coronary angiography				<0.0001§
No CAD	–	–	–	
1-vessel CAD	–	26 (64)	4 (13)	
2-vessel CAD	–	12 (29)	17 (57)	
3-vessel CAD	–	3 (7)	9 (30)	
Peri-CAS cerebral DWI-positive lesions	7 (13)	17 (41)	9 (30)	0.0048‖
Peri-CAS manifesting stroke	1 (2)	3 (7)	0 (0)	0.2120
History of anti-platelet medication over 90 days before CAS	25 (45)	23 (56)	30 (100)	<0.0001

*Comparison with ANOVA test.
†Comparison with chi-square test or Fisher's exact test.
‡p<0.05 versus patients with no CAD by Bonferroni post hoc analysis.
§Comparison between patients with asymptomatic and symptomatic CAD.
‖p<0.01 after adjustment for age, gender, LVEF, creatinine level, symptomatic carotid stenosis, hypertension, dyslipidemia and anti-platelet medication history.
CAS, carotid artery stenting; DWI, diffusion-weighted imaging; CAD, coronary artery disease.

estimate may not exist). Patients with symptomatic CAD (Group III) had tendency toward older age (*P* = .0722), worse left ventricular ejection fraction (LVEF) (*P* = .0127) and creatinine (*P* = .0294), a lower percentage of symptomatic ECAS (*P* = .0658; Group II versus Group I OR, 0.92 with 95% CI, 0.40–2.07; Group III versus Group I OR, 0.32 with 95% CI, 0.11–0.92), and higher percentages of hypertension (*P* = .0675; Group II versus Group I OR, 2.70 with 95% CI, 0.89–8.17; Group III versus Group I OR, 3.38 with 95% CI, 0.89–12.79), dyslipidemia (*P* = .0091; Group II versus Group I OR, 0.63 with 95% CI, 0.27–1.47; Group III versus Group I OR, 4.03 with 95% CI, 1.07–15.12) and anti-platelet medication over 90 days before CAS (*P*<.0001; OR is not provided because the maximum likelihood estimate may not exist) than the other two groups, and they also had greater number of diseased coronary artery than patients with asymptomatic CAD (*P* = <.0001). After adjusting for age, gender, LVEF, creatinine level, symptomatic carotid stenosis, hypertension, dyslipidemia and anti-platelet medication history, patients with either asymptomatic (OR, 4.9; 95% CI, 1.7–14.0; *P* = .0031) or symptomatic CAD (OR, 3.5; 95% CI, 0.9–12.9; *P* = .0639) had a moderate to significant risk for the occurrence of peri-CAS DWI-positive lesions comparing to patients with no CAD. Among patients with CAD (Groups II & III), the history of taking anti-platelet medication over 90 days was associated with the presence of symptomatic ECAS (OR, 0.26; 95% CI, 0.08–0.80; *P* = .0175).

Discussion

Coronary artery disease is the most common concomitant vascular disease in patients with ECAS, and their coexistence has been shown to be associated with carotid plaque composition and characteristics of peri-CAS emboli captured on EPDs [9]. Our previous report has noticed that the presence of CAD might influence the occurrence of peri-CAS silent cerebral ischemic lesions on DWI scanning [15]. However, most of the studies diagnosed CAD by clinical history and did not examine the coronary angiographic findings [9,16,17]. Furthermore, it is not studied if symptomatic and asymptomatic CAD would carry a similar risk for peri-CAS DWI-positive lesions, as asymptomatic CAD comprises a substantial proportion of patients with ECAS [7,18]. In the present series, the diagnosis of CAD, either symptomatic or asymptomatic, was documented on coronary angiography before undertaking protected CAS. Our study demonstrated that the risk for peri-CAS cerebral DWI-positive lesions was higher in patients with CAD, especially those with asymptomatic CAD.

CAS is preferred to CEA in patients with significant ECAS when there is concomitant CAD. On the other hand, the presence of CAD is also regarded as a major risk factor for peri-operative stroke, but only limited studies focused on the influence of CAD on the peri-CAS cardiac and neurological risks [8,19]. Although the presence of CAD on angiography is reported to be associated with long-term cardiac and all-cause mortality [8], our study showed the 30-day risk for myocardial infarction or angina after CAS was relatively low, which is concordant with the recent report [19]. In our study, the frequencies of concomitant stenosis in coronary artery, vertebral artery, iliac artery and subclavian artery were 56%, 44%, 22% and 13% respectively, and the frequency order was compatible with Wu *et al*'s report [7]. On the other hand, the non-treated carotid artery stenosis severity and the frequencies of concomitant stenosis in other arteries were similar between patients with and without CAD (Table S1). As to the relationship between peri-CAS cerebral emboli and CAD, Chung *et al* reported that patients with prior myocardial infarction had a greater number of peri-CAS embolic particles with smaller minimum size (109±71 μm in diameter) than patients without prior myocardial infarction (212±200 μm in diameter) [9], and debris particles smaller than the filter pores of the EPDs may have the chance to pass through embolic protection devices [20]. However, the association between the coexisting CAD and the occurrence of peri-CAS cerebral ischemic lesions was not investigated. In our study, only the concomitant CAD imposed adverse effects on the occurrence of peri-CAS ischemic lesions (Table 1). Such findings may suggest that the higher risk for peri-CAS DWI-positive lesions in CAD patients can possibly be related to the fact that CAD is a marker of more diffuse atherosclerosis.

Both CAD and ECAS are the consequence of systematic atherosclerosis. Systematic inflammation may destabilize carotid plaques in patients with unstable angina [21], and administration of low-dose aspirin over 3 months may be capable of stabilizing carotid plaques through its anti-inflammatory and anti-atherogenic effects [22]. In our study, patients with symptomatic CAD had a higher percentage of taking anti-platelet medication than asymptomatic CAD, and the history of taking anti-platelet medication over 90 days was associated with the presence of symptomatic ECAS ($P = .0175$) in patients with CAD. It is speculated that carotid plaques could be more labile in patients without anti-platelet medication, and that may in part explain why asymptomatic CAD had a higher risk for peri-CAS cerebral vascular events in our study.

Although the presence of CAD is one of the indications in choosing CAS for carotid revascularization [23], we found that it should be more precautious when performing CAS in patients with coexisting CAD since they may also have a higher risk for peri-CAS cerebral ischemic lesions comparing to those without coexisting CAD. However, the optimal pre-operation survey for CAD remains a debate in patients with ECAS. Although both our and the previous studies showed that simultaneous diagnostic coronary angiography with CAS carried little additional risk for procedure-related complications [6], the invasive characteristics of coronary angiography limit its widespread application for the CAD survey in routine clinical practice. Several non-invasive imaging modalities, including multi-detector computed tomography (MDCT) angiography and contrast-enhanced cardiac MRI, have been proposed to evaluate the presence of CAD in patients with ECAS [18,24]. In a recent study comparing the diagnostic performance for detecting CAD between the coronary MDCT and MR angiography based on the findings of the coronary conventional angiography, Liu *et al* found coronary MR angiography has favorable ability in detecting significant stenosis than MDCT angiography, with the sensitivity and specificity of 75~83% and 71~81% respectively [25]. Such finding suggests that the non-invasive imaging survey for the presence of CAD is feasible and may be helpful for stratifying the risk of peri-CAS cerebral ischemic lesions.

The application of EPDs in patients receiving CAS has been reported to reduce the occurrence of procedure-related stroke [26], but there are still a certain proportion of patients, from 17% to 73%, having silent cerebral DWI-positive lesions after protected CAS [4,11]. In our study, only one type of protection device (FilterWire) was used in all patients, which can avoid the variation in protection effect of different filter types. The occurrence rate of cerebral DWI-positive lesions after protected CAS was 26% (33 in 126 patients), and it was similar to previous reports. Although most peri-CAS DWI-positive lesions are clinically silent [27], they may impose adverse effects on the cognitive function after carotid revascularization [15,28]. Therefore, patients having peri-CAS DWI-positive lesions may need long-term follow-up for cognitive function evaluation.

There were several limitations in our study. First, not every CAS patient routinely received both cerebral MRI and coronary angiography. Even though there was no difference in the demographic data between patients with and without both imaging studies, a selection bias may still be present. Moreover, the study was administered in a single medical institute with limited case numbers, and further recruitment of patients will strengthen the statistical power. Second, the presence of concurrent CAD is the major risk factor for the occurrence of peri-CAS cerebral ischemic lesions in our study, but its underlying mechanism was not well evaluated. Since carotid atherosclerosis has been demonstrated to be associated with the severity of CAD [29], to adopt carotid MRI or ultrasound would be helpful in analyzing the correlation between carotid plaque composition features and risks for peri-CAS cerebral ischemic lesions among patients with varying severity of CAD. Third, the study was conducted in Chinese population with male predominance, and the carotid plaque characteristics would vary among ethnic [30] and gender [31], and the current study results should be verified before further application. Finally, the study mainly focused on the peri-operative neurological complications, and the effect of CAD on the long-term post-CAS neurological manifestations should be monitored in further studies.

Conclusions

Both symptomatic and asymptomatic CAD can be commonly found in patients with ECAS, and patients with CAD may carry a higher risk for the occurrence of peri-CAS cerebral DWI-positive lesions than patients without CAD. Our study suggests the importance to identify patients with concomitant CAD before undertaking CAS, especially the asymptomatic CAD, and the benefit of CAS should be balanced with the increased risk for peri-operative cerebral ischemic injuries in patients with concomitant CAD.

Supporting Information

Table S1 Comparing the clinical data between patients with and without CAD. The demographic and imaging characteristics of patients with and without CAD.

Acknowledgments

We would like to thank Shu-Yu Chou for her technical assistance.

Author Contributions

Conceived and designed the experiments: KLH YJC CHC TYC CHL ICH YWC BSY THL. Performed the experiments: KLH YJC CHC TYC CHL ICH HFW THL. Analyzed the data: KLH YJC CHC TYC CHL ICH HFW THL. Contributed reagents/materials/analysis tools: KLH CHC TYC CHL ICH HFW YYW YWC BSY THL. Wrote the paper: KLH YJC TYC ICH THL.

References

1. Sztriha LK, Nemeth D, Sefcsik T, Vecsei L (2009) Carotid stenosis and the cognitive function. J Neurol Sci 283: 36–40.
2. Yadav JS, Wholey MH, Kuntz RE, Fayad P, Katzen BT, et al. (2004) Protected carotid-artery stenting versus endarterectomy in high-risk patients. N Engl J Med 351: 1493–1501.
3. Brott TG, Hobson RW, Howard G, Roubin GS, Clark WM, et al. (2010) Stenting versus endarterectomy for treatment of carotid artery stenosis. N Engl J Med 363: 11–23.
4. Bonati LH, Jongen LM, Haller S, Flach HZ, Dobson J, et al. (2010) New ischaemic brain lesions on MRI after stenting or endarterectomy for symptomatic carotid stenosis: a substudy of the International Carotid Stenting Study (ICSS). Lancet Neurol 9: 353–362.
5. Hsieh MJ, Chen CC, Lee TH, Lee CH, Wen MS, et al. (2009) Metabolic syndrome and homocysteine level as predictors of the severity of coronary artery disease in patients with carotid stenosis. Am J Med Sci 338: 447–452.
6. Hofmann R, Kypta A, Steinwender C, Kerschner K, Grund M, et al. (2005) Coronary angiography in patients undergoing carotid artery stenting shows a high incidence of significant coronary artery disease. Heart 91: 1438–1441.
7. Wu YW, Lin MS, Lin YH, Chao CL, Kao HL (2007) Prevalence of concomitant atherosclerotic arterial diseases in patients with significant cervical carotid artery stenosis in Taiwan. Int J Cardiovasc Imaging 23: 433–439.
8. Hofmann R, Kypta A, Steinwender C, Kammler J, Kerschner K, et al. (2006) Mid-term outcome after carotid artery stenting depends on presence of coronary artery disease. Ann Med 38: 137–143.
9. Chung C, Shah TR, Shin H, Han D, Marin ML, et al. (2010) Determinants of embolic risk during angioplasty and stenting: neurologic symptoms and coronary artery disease increase embolic risk. Ann Surg 252: 618–624.
10. Maleux G, Demaerel P, Verbeken E, Daenens K, Heye S, et al. (2006) Cerebral ischemia after filter-protected carotid artery stenting is common and cannot be predicted by the presence of substantial amount of debris captured by the filter device. Am J Neuroradiol 27: 1830–1833.
11. Pinero P, Gonzalez A, Mayol A, Martinez E, Gonzalez-Marcos JR, et al. (2006) Silent ischemia after neuroprotected percutaneous carotid stenting: a diffusion-weighted MRI study. Am J Neuroradiol 27: 1338–1345.
12. North American Symptomatic Carotid Endarterectomy Trial Collaborators (1991) Beneficial effect of carotid endarterectomy in symptomatic patients with high-grade carotid stenosis. N Engl J Med 325: 445–453.
13. Lee TH, Chang CH, Chang YJ, Chang KC, Chung J (2011) Establishment of electronic chart-based stroke registry system in a medical system in Taiwan. J Formos Med Assoc 110: 543–547.
14. Kastrup A, Nagele T, Groschel K, Schmidt F, Vogler E, et al. (2006) Incidence of new brain lesions after carotid stenting with and without cerebral protection. Stroke 37: 2312–2316.
15. Huang KL, Ho MY, Chang CH, Ryu SJ, Wong HF, et al. (2011) The impact of silent ischemic lesions on cognition following carotid artery stenting. Eur Neurol 66: 351–358.
16. Jeng JS, Chung MY, Yip PK, Hwang BS, Chang YC (1994) Extracranial carotid atherosclerosis and vascular risk factors in different types of ischemic stroke in Taiwan. Stroke 25: 1989–1993.
17. Kastrup A, Groschel K, Schnaudigel S, Nagele T, Schmidt F, et al. (2008) Target lesion ulceration and arch calcification are associated with increased incidence of carotid stenting-associated ischemic lesions in octogenarians. J Vasc Surg 47: 88–95.
18. Bruder O, Goricke S, Hunold P, Lowitsch M, Barkhausen J, et al. (2009) Myocardial scars are an underestimated cardiovascular burden in patients with internal carotid artery stenosis. Cerebrovasc Dis 28: 80–87.
19. Abbott AL, Adelman MA, Alexandrov AV, Barber PA, Barnett HJM, et al. (2013) Why calls for more routine carotid stenting are currently inappropriate: an international, multispecialty, expert review and position statement. Stroke 44: 1186–1190.
20. Muller-Hulsbeck S, Jahnke T, Liess C, Glass C, Paulsen F, et al. (2002) In vitro comparison of four cerebral protection filters for preventing human plaque embolization during carotid interventions. J Endovasc Ther 9: 793–802.
21. Lombardo A, Biasucci LM, Lanza GA, Coli S, Silvestri P, et al. (2004) Inflammation as a possible link between coronary and carotid plaque instability. Circulation 109: 3158–3163.
22. Wehinger A, Tancevski I, Seiler R, Frotschnig SM, Frantz S, et al. (2009) Influence of aspirin on SR-BI expression in human carotid plaques. Atherosclerosis 206: 234–238.
23. Xavier AR, Chaturvedi S (2008) Carotid stenting for patients with coexisting carotid and coronary disease. Arch Neurol 65: 1670–1672.
24. Zelinger A, Wayhs R, Graboys TB, Tavel ME (2002) Asymptomatic coronary artery disease. Chest 121: 1684–1687.
25. Liu X, Zhao X, Huang J, Francois CJ, Tuite D, et al. (2007) Comparison of 3D free-breathing coronary MR angiography and 64-MDCT angiography for detection of coronary stenosis in patients with high calcium scores. Am J Roentgenol 189: 1326–1332.
26. Kastrup A, Groschel K, Krapf H, Brehm BR, Dichgans J, et al. (2003) Early outcome of carotid angioplasty and stenting with and without cerebral protection devices: a systematic review of the literature. Stroke 34: 813–819.
27. Hammer FD, Lacroix V, Duprez T, Grandin C, Verhelst R, et al. (2005) Cerebral microembolization after protected carotid artery stenting in surgical high-risk patients: results of a 2-year prospective study. J Vasc Surg 42: 847–853.
28. Capoccia L, Speziale F, Gazzetti M, Mariani P, Rizzo A, et al. (2010) Comparative study on carotid revascularization (endarterectomy vs stenting) using markers of cellular brain injury, neuropsychometric tests, and diffusion-weighted magnetic resonance imaging. J Vasc Surg 51: 584–591.
29. Zhao X, Zhao Q, Chu B, Yang Y, Li F, et al. (2010) Prevalence of compositional features in subclinical carotid atherosclerosis determined by high-resolution magnetic resonance imaging in Chinese patients with coronary artery disease. Stroke 41: 1157–1162.
30. Saam T, Cai JM, Cai YQ, An NY, Kampschulte A, et al. (2005) Carotid plaque composition differs between ethno-racial groups: An MRI pilot study comparing Mainland Chinese and American Caucasian patients. Arterioscler Thromb Vasc Biol 25: 611–616.
31. Underhill H, Yuan C, Terry J, Chen H, Espeland M, et al. (2008) Differences in carotid arterial morphology and composition between individuals with and without obstructive coronary artery disease: A cardiovascular magnetic resonance study. J Cardiovasc Magn Reson 10: 31.

18

The SNP rs1883832 in CD40 Gene and Risk of Atherosclerosis in Chinese Population

Yan Yun, Chi Ma, XiaoChun Ma*

School of Medicine, Shandong University, Ji'nan, Shandong, People's Republic of China

Abstract

Background: The complications of atherosclerosis such as coronary and cerebrovascular disease, are the most prevalent causes of mortality and morbidity worldwide. A single nucleotide polymorphism (SNP) rs1883832 (-1C/T) in CD40 gene has been recently suggested to contribute to the susceptibility to atherosclerosis in Chinese population; however, previous genetic association studies yielded inconsistent results.

Methods: A meta-analysis of eligible studies reporting the association between rs1883832 and atherosclerosis in Chinese population was carried out.

Results: Pooling 7 eligible case-control studies involving 2129 patients and 1895 controls demonstrated a significant association between rs1883832 and atherosclerosis under dominant model [odds ratio (OR) = 1.631, 95% confidence interval [CI] [1.176, 2.260] in Chinese population with evident heterogeneity. Meta-regression analysis indicated that the heterogeneity could be completely explained by disease category. In subgroup analysis, rs1883832 conferred ORs of 2.866 (C/C versus T/T, 95%CI [2.203, 3.729]) and 1.680 (C/T versus T/T, 95%CI [1.352, 2.086]) for coronary artery disease (CAD) under co-dominant model without heterogeneity. Similar results were obtained for acute coronary syndrome (ACS) (C/C versus T/T, 3.674, 95%CI [2.638, 5.116]; C/T versus T/T, 1.981, 95%CI [1.483, 2.646]). The other genetic models including dominant, recessive and additive models, yielded consistent results without heterogeneity for CAD and ACS, respectively. However, a protective role was found for C allele in ischemic stroke (IS) under recessive model (0.582, 95%CI [0.393, 0.864]) and additive model (0.785, 95%CI [0.679, 0.909]) with reduced heterogeneity.

Conclusions: This meta-analysis provided evidence of association of rs1883832 C allele with an overall increased risk of atherosclerosis but distinct effect of C allele on CAD (including ACS) and IS in Chinese population, respectively.

Editor: Waldo Belloso, Hospital Italiano de Buenos Aires, Argentina

Funding: The authors have no support or funding to report.

Competing Interests: The authors have declared that no competing interests exist.

* E-mail: mxcmxc2008@163.com

Introduction

Atherosclerosis, with clinical consequences including coronary artery disease (CAD) and ischemic stroke (IS), is one of the leading causes of death worldwide [1]. Accumulating evidence has suggested a pivotal role of CD40-CD40L interaction in the pathogenesis of atherosclerosis [2,3]. CD40, a 50-kDa cell surface transmembrane glycoprotein receptor of the tumor necrosis factor receptor (TNFR) superfamily, which is expressed on the surface of immune cells as well as non-immune cells, determines T cell responses to antigen presentation and B cells immunoglobulin isotype switching [4]. A C/T single nucleotide polymorphism (SNP) (rs1883832) in the 5′ untranslated region of CD40 gene located at the -1 position within the Kozak sequence has been recently associated with CD40 protein expression and susceptibility to atherosclerotic diseases in Chinese population [5–7]. However, consistent results were not obtained from previous genetic association studies.

We undertook the present meta-analysis of relevant literature to evaluate the association of rs1883832 (-1C/T) in CD40 gene with atherosclerosis (overall, CAD, acute coronary syndrome [ACS] and IS) in Chinese population, with the following objectives: A) to estimate C allele frequencies in controls; B) to assess if the effect of rs1883832 on atherosclerosis (overall, CAD, ACS and IS, respectively) is statistically significant in Chinese population; if so, C) to estimate the magnitude of effect of C allele and determine the most appropriate genetic model (s) for atherosclerosis (overall, CAD, ACS and IS, respectively) in Chinese population.

Materials and Methods

Eligibility Criteria

We sought eligible studies which met the following criteria: (1) published studies based on case-control design assessing the association between rs1883832 (CD40 gene -1C/T) and atherosclerosis; (2) involving subjects restricted to Chinese ethnicity; (3) providing sufficient data for calculating genotypic odds ratio (OR) with corresponding 95% confidence interval (95% CI). Non-English language studies were excluded, as were review articles, case reports, editorial comments and animal studies. It inevitably introduces a source of bias when a meta-analysis incorporates the genetic association studies from the same or different research group(s) utilizing duplicate samples. Thereby, it is obligatory to exclude in advance those repetitive publications to avoid the duplicate-study effects on our meta-analysis. The recruiting periods and hospitals were checked thoroughly for all the included studies. Additionally, the corresponding authors were contacted directly via email to confirm whether or not there were duplicate results to be eliminated.

Search Strategy

MEDLINE and EMBASE were independently searched by two reviewers (Xiaochun Ma and Chi Ma) for potentially eligible studies from the earliest available date to August 2013. The search terms used either alone or in combination included "rs1883832-1C/T, CD40, TNFRSF5, atherosclerosis, coronary artery disease, acute coronary syndrome, ischemic stroke and cerebral infarction". Reference lists from retrieved articles were also manually searched for articles meeting our criteria. Abstracts identified using our search strategies were reviewed separately by two reviewers (Xiaochun Ma and Yan Yun). The full-text articles that potentially met criteria were then reviewed in duplicate to determine the inclusion in the analysis. Then all the authors further critically reviewed the studies upon which the 2 reviewers disagreed. Either the inclusion or exclusion of a certain study was agreed upon by all the authors finally.

Data Extraction

Data extraction was performed independently by two reviewers (Xiaochun Ma and Chi Ma). In the process of data abstraction, the two authors were blinded to the information of each research group conducting the study. Extracted data included: (1) author's name, year of publication and journal; and (2) study design, sample size, characteristics of cases and controls (geographic

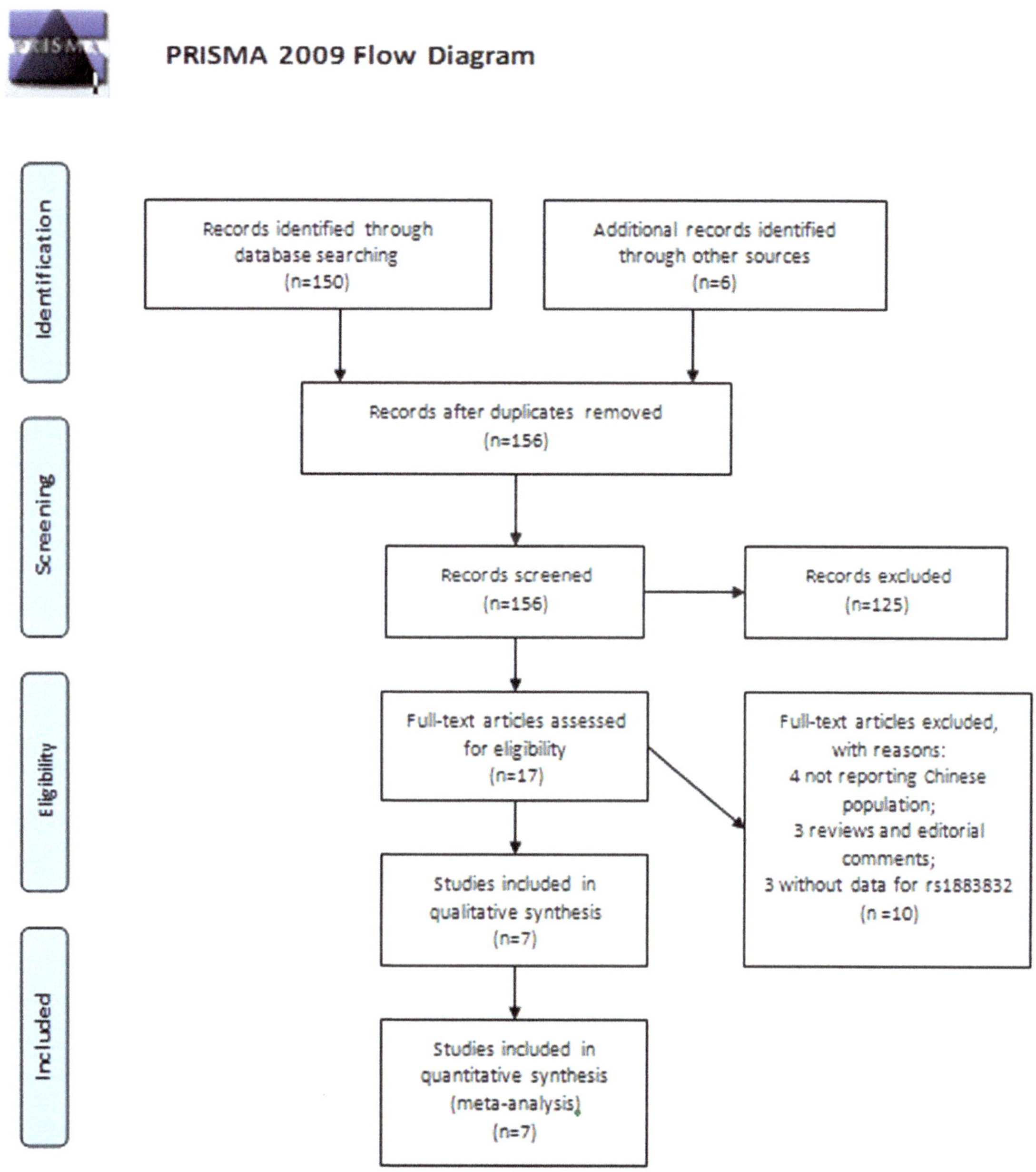

Figure 1. The PRISMA recommended flow-diagram depicting the methodology of article selection for this meta-analysis.

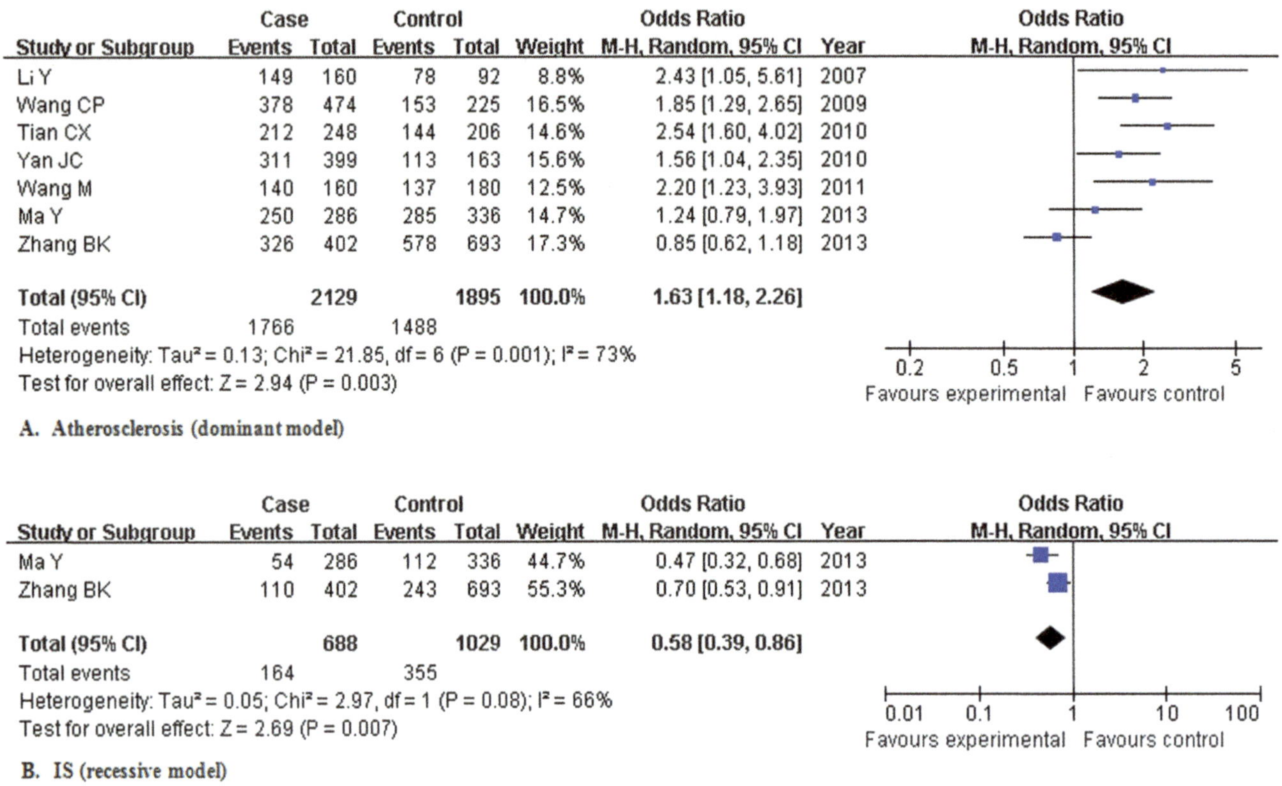

Figure 2. Meta-analysis for the association of rs1883832 with atherosclerosis and ischemic stroke in Chinese population. Abbreviation: IS, ischemic stroke; M-H, Mantel-Haenszel method.

location or ethnicity of study population, control source, male/female rate and mean age), genotyping method, distribution of genotypes and alleles in cases and controls. The quality of studies was assessed with the Newcastle-Ottawa scale (NOS) for observational studies [8]. Eight items, in each of which a series of response options is provided, are categorized into three perspectives in NOS: four for the Selection of the study group (S), one for the Comparability (C) of the groups and three for Exposure of interest (E). A 'star system' is utilized for the assessment of study quality, such that a study can be awarded a maximum of one star for each numbered item within the Selection and Exposure categories while a maximum of two stars can be assigned for Comparability. The NOS scores from zero to nine stars [9].

Statistical Analysis

Hardy-Weinberg equilibrium was assessed again for each study by goodness-of-fit x^2 test (P>0.05) only in control groups. Pooled frequency of the A allele was estimated using the inverse variance method previously described by Thakkinstian et al. [10] in which random-effects or fixed-effects model was applied, depending on whether or not there is evident heterogeneity for allele frequencies across studies. Random-effects model introduces a 'weight term' that accounts for between-study variation and weight adjustment. Three crude ORs with corresponding 95% CIs, i.e. crude OR1 (C/C versus T/T), crude OR2 (C/T versus T/T) and crude OR3 (C/C versus C/T) were calculated for rs1883832. Cochran's Q statistic and the I^2 metric for heterogeneity were also estimated separately for crude OR1, OR2 and OR3. Three modified ORs and various genetic models would be measured afterwards only if there was no evident heterogeneity. For the Q statistic, a p value of less than 0.1 was considered statistically significant. For the I^2 metric, $I^2>50\%$ indicates significant heterogeneity [11]. If heterogeneity was evident for at least one of the 3 crude ORs, a meta-regression model was employed to explore possible sources of heterogeneity across studies. Subgroup analysis was then conducted on the basis of the results of meta-regression analysis. If there was no heterogeneity, logistic regression analysis was performed for determining the gene effect, which protected against inflated type I error in the context of multiple tests. The overall gene effect was evaluated using likelihood ratio (LR) test. If the main effect of the genotype was statistically significant, three modified ORs, i.e. OR1 (C/C versus T/T), OR2 (C/T versus T/T), and OR3 (C/C versus C/T) were further calculated using logistic regression model. Three pairs of crude and modified ORs were then utilized to suggest the most appropriate or ideal genetic model previously described by Thakkinstian et al. [10,12] as follows:

If $OR1 = OR3 \neq 1$ and $OR2 = 1$, then a recessive model is suggested.

If $OR1 = OR2 \neq 1$ and $OR3 = 1$, then a dominant model is suggested.

If $OR1>OR2>1$ and $OR1>OR3>1$ (or $OR1<OR2<1$ and $OR1<OR3<1$), then a co-dominant model is suggested.

Besides the finest genetic model, several other possible genetic models were also assessed: co-dominant model (modified OR1 and OR2), (C/C versus T/T) and (C/T versus T/T); dominant model (OR4), (C/C and C/T) versus T/T; recessive model, C/C versus (C/T and T/T) (OR5); additive model (OR6) (table S1). For additive model, scores of 0, 1, and 2 were assigned to genotype CC, CT, and TT respectively and per-allele ORs were calculated by logistic regression model. Sensitivity analysis was performed to assess the effects of each study (especially the studies which do not

Study or Subgroup	Case Events	Case Total	Control Events	Control Total	Weight	Odds Ratio M-H, Random, 95% CI	Year
Li Y	45	56	12	26	6.9%	4.77 [1.73, 13.16]	2007
Wang CP	121	217	35	107	30.3%	2.59 [1.60, 4.21]	2009
Yan JC	95	183	26	76	23.1%	2.08 [1.19, 3.62]	2010
Tian CX	96	132	42	104	23.7%	3.94 [2.28, 6.81]	2010
Wang M	53	73	41	84	15.9%	2.78 [1.42, 5.43]	2011
Total (95% CI)		**661**		**397**	**100.0%**	**2.87 [2.20, 3.75]**	
Total events	410		156				

Heterogeneity: Tau² = 0.00; Chi² = 3.73, df = 4 (P = 0.44); I² = 0%
Test for overall effect: Z = 7.74 (P < 0.00001)

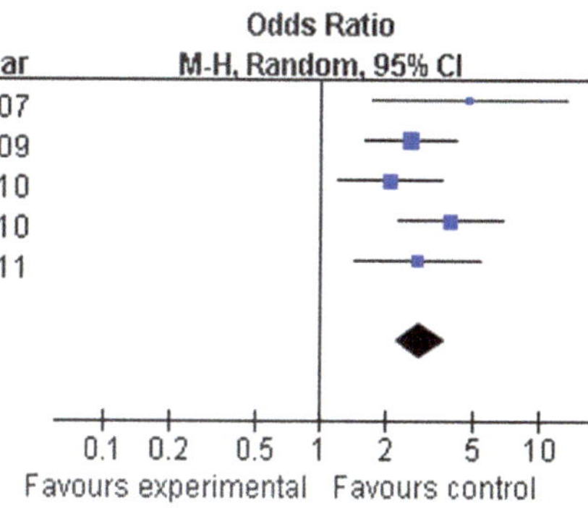

A. CAD (co-dominant model OR1)

Study or Subgroup	Case Events	Case Total	Control Events	Control Total	Weight	Odds Ratio M-H, Random, 95% CI	Year
Li Y	104	115	66	80	6.7%	2.01 [0.86, 4.68]	2007
Wang CP	257	353	118	190	34.0%	1.63 [1.12, 2.38]	2009
Tian CX	116	152	102	164	20.0%	1.96 [1.20, 3.19]	2010
Yan JC	216	304	87	137	26.2%	1.41 [0.92, 2.16]	2010
Wang M	87	107	96	139	13.1%	1.95 [1.06, 3.57]	2011
Total (95% CI)		**1031**		**710**	**100.0%**	**1.69 [1.36, 2.10]**	
Total events	780		469				

Heterogeneity: Tau² = 0.00; Chi² = 1.44, df = 4 (P = 0.84); I² = 0%
Test for overall effect: Z = 4.70 (P < 0.00001)

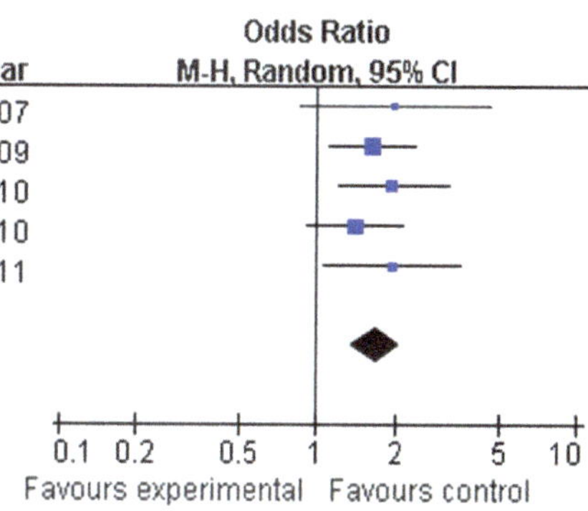

B. CAD (co-dominant model OR2)

Figure 3. Meta-analysis for the association of rs1883832 with coronary artery disease in Chinese population. Abbreviation: CAD, coronary artery disease; OR, odds ratio; M-H, Mantel-Haenszel method.

Study or Subgroup	Case Events	Case Total	Control Events	Control Total	Weight	Odds Ratio M-H, Random, 95% CI	Year
Li Y	45	56	12	26	10.8%	4.77 [1.73, 13.16]	2007
Tian CX	96	132	42	104	37.0%	3.94 [2.28, 6.81]	2010
Yan JC	65	97	26	76	27.5%	3.91 [2.07, 7.37]	2010
Wang M	53	73	41	84	24.8%	2.78 [1.42, 5.43]	2011
Total (95% CI)		**358**		**290**	**100.0%**	**3.68 [2.64, 5.13]**	
Total events	259		121				

Heterogeneity: Tau² = 0.00; Chi² = 1.02, df = 3 (P = 0.80); I² = 0%
Test for overall effect: Z = 7.67 (P < 0.00001)

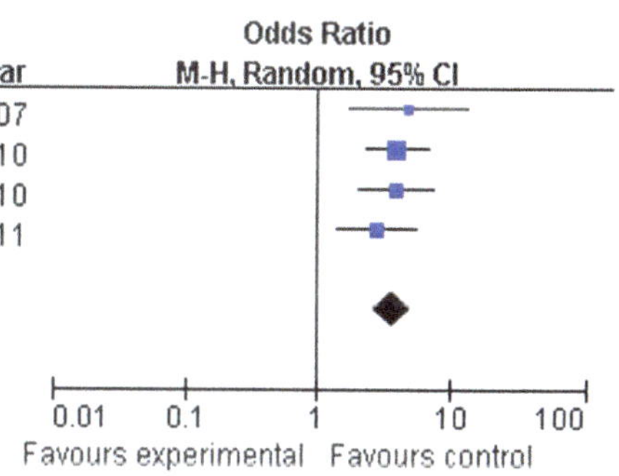

A. ACS (co-dominant model OR1)

Study or Subgroup	Case Events	Case Total	Control Events	Control Total	Weight	Odds Ratio M-H, Random, 95% CI	Year
Li Y	104	115	66	80	11.7%	2.01 [0.86, 4.68]	2007
Yan JC	113	145	87	137	30.5%	2.03 [1.20, 3.43]	2010
Tian CX	116	152	102	164	35.0%	1.96 [1.20, 3.19]	2010
Wang M	87	107	96	139	22.9%	1.95 [1.06, 3.57]	2011
Total (95% CI)		**519**		**520**	**100.0%**	**1.98 [1.48, 2.65]**	
Total events	420		351				

Heterogeneity: Tau² = 0.00; Chi² = 0.01, df = 3 (P = 1.00); I² = 0%
Test for overall effect: Z = 4.64 (P < 0.00001)

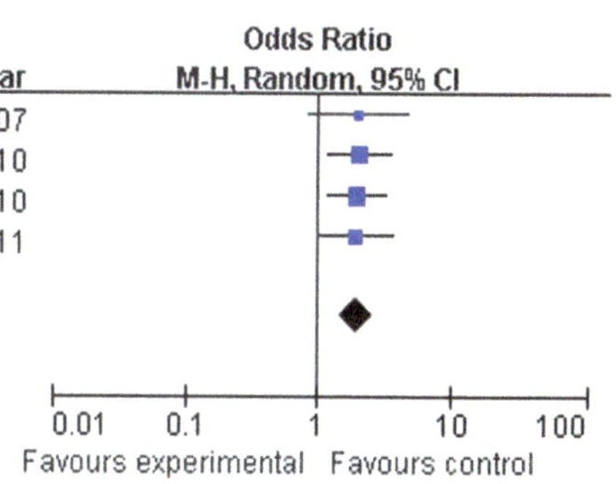

B. ACS (co-dominant model OR2)

Figure 4. Meta-analysis for the association of rs1883832 with acute coronary syndrome in Chinese population. Abbreviation: ACS, acute coronary syndrome; OR, odds ratio; M-H, Mantel-Haenszel method.

observe HWE), on the pooled results. Publication bias was assessed using the Funnel plot method with Egger's test. Random-effects models were chosen for pooling data and a p value of less than 0.05 was considered statistically significant for all estimates except for Q tests of heterogeneity. Agreement assessment between reviewers was evaluated using the Cohen k statistic. Stata 12.0 and Reviewer Manager 5.1 were utilized for performing the meta-analysis.

Results

Eligible Studies

A total of 156 potential eligible citations were identified with the literature search, among which there were no articles written and published in languages other than English and Chinese. The titles of these citations were reviewed and 125 were rejected leaving 31 potentially eligible studies. After review of abstracts, an additional 14 were rejected. Seventeen studies were then retrieved in full-text to determine the inclusion. Assessment agreement of study selection between the two reviewers led to a k score of 0.84 (95% CI [0.79, 0.89]). Then a further discussion was conducted among all the authors with regard to the studies upon which the 2 reviewers disagreed. Finally, corporate critical review of full-text excluded 4 studies for not reporting Chinese population, 3 studies for being reviews and editorial comments, 3 studies for without data for rs1883832 (figure 1). All the included studies in this meta-analysis were written and published in English. Furthermore, there is currently no genetic association study concerning rs1883832 in atherosclerosis in other ethnicities, based on our search result.

Study Characteristics

Ultimately, 7 studies (5 on coronary artery disease [CAD] and 2 on ischemic stroke [IS]) involving a total of 4024 subjects (2129 patients and 1895 controls) met our criteria and were included in this meta-analytical study [6,7,13–17]. The corresponding authors of our included studies were contacted and they confirmed that there were no duplicate results utilized in multiple studies to be deleted. Characteristics of the included studies are detailed in table 1. The distributions of genotypes and alleles in the individual studies for rs1883832 were shown in table 2. Within 7 included studies, one study was inconsistent with HWE [14]. All the studies we included gained a score of S3C1E3 based on the Newcastle-Ottawa scale.

Pooled Frequency of C allele in Control Groups

The pooled frequency of the C allele in Chinese controls was 46.8% (95% CI [41.1%–52.5%]) under random-effects model. Heterogeneity was statistically significant (p heterogeneity<0.001, $I^2 = 91.5\%$) (table 3). When pooled separately, the frequency of the C allele in the studies on CAD was 45.1% (95% CI 42.7%–47.4%) under fixed-effects model without evident heterogeneity (p heterogeneity = 0.156, $I^2 = 39.7\%$) (table 4) while the frequency in the studies on IS was 49.9% (95% CI 31.9%–67.8%) under random-effects model with extreme heterogeneity (p heterogeneity<0.001, $I^2 = 98.4\%$) (table 5).

Meta-analysis of Association between rs1883832 and Atherosclerosis

For atherosclerosis, the 7 studies (n = 4024, 2129 patients and 1895 controls) were pooled for three crude ORs and Cochran's Q statistic and the I^2 metric indicated heterogeneity for OR1 and OR3 but not for OR2. To explore potential sources of between-study heterogeneity, a meta-regression model was employed using the data for crude OR1. After initially running an empty regression [18] (in which no variable was introduced) to evaluate the baseline value for tau^2 ($tau^2 = 0.5276$), a univariate model was then performed by adding disease category (CAD and IS), which reduced the tau^2 value to 0 (adjusted R^2 value 100%, p = 0.001). It indicated that the heterogeneity could be totally explained by category of atherosclerotic diseases. Pooling all the 7 studies yielded crude OR1 of 1.926 (1.044, 3.555), OR2 of 1.502 (1.212, 1.862) and OR3 of 1.214 (0.758, 1.942). Logistic regression showed that the overall gene effect was statistically significant, with the modified OR1, OR2, and OR3 being 1.896 (1.183, 3.041), 1.474 (1.239, 1.753), and 1.255 (0.841, 1.873), respectively. Those results suggested a dominant model of gene effect on atherosclerosis (OR4 1.631, 95% CI [1.176, 2.260]) (figure 2A). Several other possible genetic models were also estimated: co-dominant model, OR1 and OR2 being 1.896 (1.183, 3.041) and 1.474 (1.239, 1.753); recessive model, OR5 being 1.370 (0.821, 2.287); additive model, OR6 being 1.361 (0.981, 1.889). All the potential genetic models showed evidence of significant heterogeneity (table 3). Subgroup analysis by disease category was thus further performed for CAD, IS and ACS, respectively.

For CAD, in subgroup analysis, pooling the 5 studies (n = 2307, 1441 patients and 866 controls) yielded crude OR1 of 2.869 (2.197, 3.746), OR2 of 1.691 (1.359, 2.105) and OR3 of 1.688 (1.352, 2.109) without heterogeneity. Logistic regression showed that the overall gene effect was statistically significant, with the

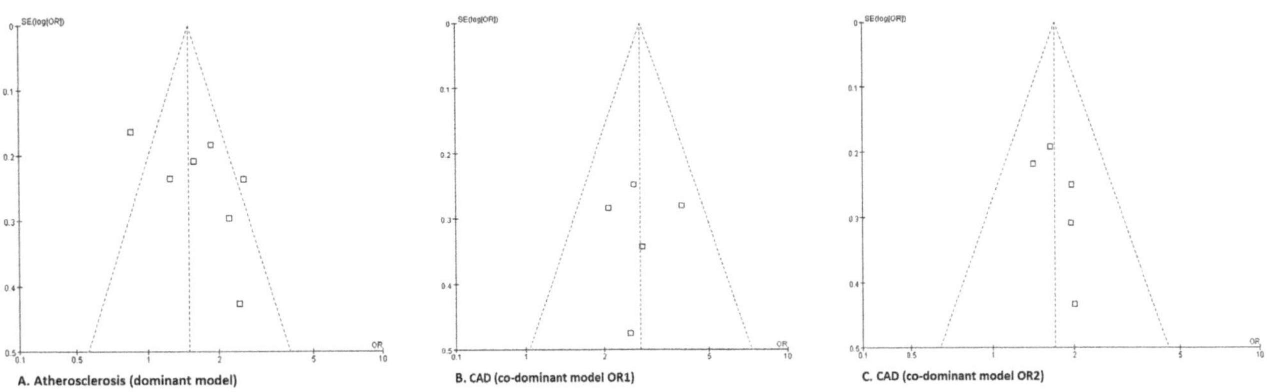

Figure 5. Funnel plots for the publication bias of atherosclerosis (A, dominant model) and coronary artery disease (B and C, co-dominant model). Abbreviation: CAD, coronary artery disease; OR, odds ratio.

Table 1. The characteristics of the studies included in the meta-analysis for the association of rs1883832 with atherosclerosis.

First author, Published year	Ethnicity	Control source	Study type	Genotyping method	Disease category	Case/ Control	Male/female ratio		Mean age	
							Case	Control	Case	Control
Li Y, 2007*	Chinese	Population based	Replication	PCR-RFLP	ACS	160/92	3.57	3.60	64.0	59.0
Wang CP, 2009*	Chinese	Patients angiographically normal	Replication	PCR-RFLP	CAD	474/225	2.04	2.08	63.5	62.4
Tian CX, 2010*	Chinese	Population based	Replication	PCR-RFLP	ACS	248/206	1.76	1.94	63.8	59.8
Yan JC, 2010*	Chinese	Population based	Replication	PCR-RFLP	ACS, SA	399/163	3.53	3.41	63.8	62.8
Wang M,2011*	Chinese	Population based	Replication	PCR-RFLP	ACS	160/180	3.57	3.62	64.4	60.7
Ma Y, 2013#	Chinese Han	Population based	Replication	PCR-RFLP	IS	286/336	1.55	1.20	66.1	67.5
Zhang BK,2013#	Chinese Han	Population based	Replication	PCR-RFLP	CI	402/693	2.14	1.14	63.2	50.5

Abbreviation: PCR-RFLP, polymerase chain reaction-restriction fragment length polymorphism; ACS, acute coronary syndrome; CAD coronary artery disease; SA, stable angina; IS, ischemic stroke; CI, cerebral infarction.
Symbols: '*' indicates the study on coronary artery disease; '#' indicates the study on ischemic disease.

modified OR1, OR2, and OR3 being 2.866 (2.203, 3.729), 1.680 (1.352, 2.086), and 1.707 (1.366, 2.132), respectively. Those results suggested a co-dominant model of gene effect on CAD (figure 3A and 3B). Several other possible genetic models were also estimated for references: dominant model, OR4 being 1.965 (1.594, 2.423); recessive model, OR5 being 1.971 (1.594, 2.438); additive model, OR6 being 1.689 (1.480, 1.927). No genetic model presented significant heterogeneity (table 4).

For IS, in subgroup analysis, pooling the 2 studies (n = 1717, 688 patients and 1029 controls) demonstrated crude OR1 of 0.684 (0.506, 0.926), OR2 of 1.216 (0.749, 1.974) and OR3 of 0.556 (0.341, 0.907) with marginal heterogeneity for OR2, evident heterogeneity for OR3 and no heterogeneity for OR1. Logistic regression showed that the overall gene effect was statistically significant, with the modified OR1, OR2, and OR3 being 0.666 (0.477, 0.930), 1.190 (0.866, 1.635), and 0.562 (0.402, 0.787), respectively. Those results suggested a recessive protective model of gene effect on IS (OR5 0.582 95% CI [0.393, 0.864]) (figure 2B). Several other possible genetic models were also estimated: co-dominant model, OR1 and OR2 being 0.666 (0.477, 0.930) and 1.190 (0.866, 1.635); dominant model, OR4 being 0.992 (0.691, 1.423); additive model, OR6 being 0.785 (0.679, 0.909). Recessive and co-dominant models showed significant heterogeneity (table 5).

For ACS, 4 studies (n = 1967, 1281 patients and 686 controls) were pooled to yield crude OR1 of 3.679 (2.637, 5.133), OR2 of 1.983 (1.485, 2.649) and OR3 of 1.852 (1.423, 2.409) without heterogeneity. Logistic regression showed that the overall gene effect was statistically significant, with the modified OR1, OR2, and OR3 being 3.674 (2.638, 5.116), 1.981 (1.483, 2.646), and 1.854 (1.428, 2.408), respectively. Those results suggested a co-dominant model of gene effect on ACS (figure 4A and 4B). Results under several other possible genetic models were also estimated: dominant model, OR4 being 2.421 (1.835, 3.193); recessive model, OR5 being 2.211 (1.719, 2.844); additive model, OR6 being 1.909 (1.619, 2.251). No genetic models showed evidence of significant heterogeneity (table 6).

Sensitivity Study

Sensitivity study was conducted to assess the effects of each study on the pooled results of dominant model for atherosclerosis, co dominant model for CAD and recessive model for IS, respectively. As showed in table 7, no single study, especially the one which does not observe HWE, significantly altered the pooled ORs with corresponding 95%CI, indicating the robustness of the current results. As well, the effects of each study on the pooled results of additive model for CAD and IS were evaluated, respectively. Results were similar before and after removal of each study (table 7).

Publication Bias

The funnel plots and the Egger's tests demonstrated that there was no publication bias in the dominant model for atherosclerosis (p for Egger's test: p dominant model = 0.151; p additive model = 0.108) and co-dominant model and additive model for CAD (p for Egger's test: p dominant model [OR1] = 0.397; p dominant model [OR2] = 0.253; p additive model = 0.379) (figure 5). Attempt has been made at identifying studies not in the published literature. However, we did not obtain any unpublished results.

Discussion

In the current meta-analysis, pooling the data from 7 published case-control studies indicated a significant association between a

Table 2. Distribution of genotypes and alleles in the individual study.

First author, published year	Genotype							Gene allele				Allele frequency		HWE for controls	
	Case			Control				Case		Control		Case	Control		
	CC	CT	TT	CC	CT	TT	Total	C	T	C	T	C	C	x2	P
Li Y, 2007	45	104	11	12	66	14	252	194	126	90	94	0.61	0.49	17.45	2.956E-05
Wang CP, 2009	121	257	96	35	118	72	699	499	449	188	262	0.53	0.42	1.37	0.242
Tian CX, 2010	96	116	36	42	102	62	454	308	188	186	226	0.62	0.45	1.6788E-05	0.997
Yan JC, 2010	95	216	88	26	87	50	562	406	392	139	187	0.51	0.43	1.35	0.245
Wang M,2011	53	87	20	41	96	43	340	193	127	178	182	0.60	0.49	0.80	0.370
Ma Y, 2013	54	196	36	112	173	51	622	304	268	397	275	0.53	0.59	1.41	0.234
Zhang BK,2013	110	216	76	243	335	115	1095	436	368	821	565	0.54	0.59	6.38E-04	0.980

Abbreviation: HWE, Hardy-Weinberg equilibrium.

Table 3. Meta-analysis for the association of rs1883832 with atherosclerosis.

Genetic model	OR 95% CI	P	P heterogeneity	I^2
C/C versus T/T	Crude OR1: 1.926 (1.044, 3.555)	0.036	<0.001	88.5%
	Modified OR1: 1.896 (1.183, 3.041)	0.008	–	–
C/T versus T/T	Crude OR2: 1.502 (1.212, 1.862)	<0.001	0.183	32.1%
	Modified OR2: 1.474 (1.239, 1.753)	<0.001	–	–
C/C versus C/T	Crude OR3: 1.214 (0.758, 1.942)	0.42	<0.001	87.7%
	Modified OR3: 1.255 (0.841, 1.873)	0.265	–	–
Dominant model (C/C and C/T) versus T/T	OR4: 1.631 (1.176, 2.260)	0.003	0.001	72.5%
Recessive model C/C versus (C/T and T/T)	OR5: 1.370 (0.821, 2.287)	0.228	<0.001	90.5%
Additive model	OR6: 1.361 (0.981, 1.889)	0.065	<0.001	90.4%

Included publications: CAD: Li Y, 2007; Wang CP, 2009; Tian CX, 2010; Yan JC, 2010; Wang M, 2011; IS or CI: Ma Y, 2013; Zhang BK, 2013.
Likelihood ratio test: LR = 23.82, P<0.001.
Pooled C allele frequency: 46.8% (41.1%–52.5%), P heterogeneity<0.001, I^2 = 91.5%.
Abbreviation: ACS, acute coronary syndrome; CAD coronary artery disease; IS, ischemic stroke; CI, cerebral infarction; OR, odds ratio; 95% CI, 95% confidence interval.

single nucleotide polymorphism (SNP) rs1883832 in CD40 gene and atherosclerosis under dominant model in Chinese population. Subgroup analysis presented that C allele of rs1883832 conferred a higher risk for CAD or ACS under all genetic models, with co-dominant model potentially being the most appropriate model. However, a protective role of gene effect was noted for C allele in ischemic stroke (IS) under recessive and additive models. Our results demonstrated that rs1883832 contributed to an overall increased risk of atherosclerosis and provided clear evidence of distinct effect of rs1883832 on CAD (ACS) and IS in Chinese population, respectively. To our knowledge, this study was the first performed to pool published case-control studies to obtain estimates for association of rs1883832 with atherosclerosis in populations of Chinese ethnicity.

Genetic association studies with case-control design usually have a lack of power to replicate the associations from genome-wide association studies (GWAS). The difficulty of replication occurs partially due to the modest effect of those SNPs in complex

Table 4. Meta-analysis for the association of rs1883832 with coronary artery disease.

Genetic model	OR 95%CI	P	P heterogeneity	I^2
C/C versus T/T	Crude OR1: 2.869 (2.197, 3.746)	<0.001	0.444	0%
	Modified OR1: 2.866 (2.203, 3.729)	<0.001	–	–
C/T versus T/T	Crude OR2: 1.691 (1.359, 2.105)	<0.001	0.838	0%
	Modified OR2: 1.680 (1.352, 2.086)	<0.001	–	–
C/C versus C/T	Crude OR3: 1.688 (1.352, 2.109)	<0.001	0.684	0%
	Modified OR3: 1.707 (1.366, 2.132)	<0.001	–	–
Dominant model (C/C and C/T) versus T/T	OR4: 1.965 (1.594, 2.423)	<0.001	0.58	0%
Recessive model C/C versus (C/T and T/T)	OR5: 1.971 (1.594, 2.438)	<0.001	0.603	0%
Additive model	OR6: 1.689 (1.480, 1.927)	<0.001	0.403	0.6%

Included publications: Li Y, 2007; Wang CP, 2009; Tian CX, 2010; Yan JC, 2010; Wang M, 2011.
Likelihood ratio test: LR = 63.73, P<0.001.
Pooled C allele frequency: 45.1% (42.7%–47.4%), P heterogeneity = 0.156, I^2 = 39.7%.
Abbreviation: ACS, acute coronary syndrome; CAD coronary artery disease; IS, ischemic stroke; CI, cerebral infarction; OR, odds ratio; 95% CI, 95% confidence interval.

Table 5. Meta-analysis for the association of rs1883832 with ischemic stroke.

Genetic model	OR 95%CI	P	P heterogeneity	I^2
C/C versus T/T	Crude OR1: 0.684 (0.506, 0.926)	0.014	0.933	0%
	Modified OR1: 0.666 (0.477, 0.930)	0.017	–	–
C/T versus T/T	Crude OR2: 1.216 (0.749, 1.974)	0.429	0.093	64.6%
	Modified OR2: 1.190 (0.866, 1.635)	0.283	–	–
C/C versus C/T	Crude OR3: 0.556 (0.341, 0.907)	0.019	0.04	76.4%
	Modified OR3: 0.562 (0.402, 0.787)	0.001	–	–
Dominant model (C/C and C/T) versus T/T	OR4: 0.992 (0.691, 1.423)	0.965	0.188	42.3%
Recessive model C/C versus (C/T and T/T)	OR5: 0.582 (0.393, 0.864)	0.007	0.085	66.3%
Additive model	OR6: 0.785 (0.679, 0.909)	0.001	0.550	0%

Included publications: Ma Y, 2013; Zhang BK,2013.
Likelihood ratio test: LR = 22.04, P<0.001.
Pooled C allele frequency: 49.9% (31.9%–67.8%), P heterogeneity<0.001, I^2 = 98.4%.
Abbreviation: IS, ischemic stroke; OR, odds ratio; 95%CI, 95% confidence interval.

diseases. Additionally, the overestimation of genetic effect may render replication studies underpowered and possibly fail because the necessary sample size is underestimated based on the original data from GWAS, a phenomenon known as the "winner's curse" [19]. Our pooled results demonstrated a relatively high frequency of C allele in controls and large magnitudes of effect of C allele on atherosclerosis in Chinese. And our studies had an adequate sample size and 100% study power to evaluate the precise effect of rs1883832 on atherosclerosis in Chinese population. On the basis of the methods proposed by Thakkinstian et al. [10,12], dominant model was probably the ideal mode of inheritance for atherosclerosis and suggested a positive association between C allele and an excess risk for atherosclerosis. Though between-study heterogeneity was obvious for dominant model, the following meta-regression analysis attributed the heterogeneity totally to disease category. Subsequent subgroup analysis for CAD and ACS suggested a potential co-dominant model as the finest mode. The dominant model showed an approximate 2-fold and 2.5-fold higher risk for CAD and ACS in individuals carrying at least one C allele than in ones with TT genotype, respectively. Furthermore, each additional C allele led to an average of nearly 1.7-fold and 1.9-fold increase in risk for CAD and ACS under additive model, respectively. Heterogeneity was completely removed for all estimates for CAD and ACS. However, subgroup analysis for IS presented an inverse outcome that C allele was associated with a reduction of nearly 40% risk for IS in 2 C allele carriers than in ones with CT and TT genotypes under recessive model, and each additional C allele lowered a 20% risk for IS on average under additive model. Heterogeneity in the subgroup analysis for IS was removed for additive model and reduced for recessive model. In our study, LR test was applied to gauge that the overall gene effect was statistically significant given an inflated type I error in the context of multiple tests. Further modified ORs were produced using logistic regression analysis to better estimate effect sizes and we found only subtle quantitative changes in modified ORs compared to respective crude ORs calculated by the traditional method. Due to the heterogeneity for atherosclerosis (overall and IS) and the inclusion of one study that did not observe HWE, sensitivity analysis was carried out to assess the stability of the estimates for the most appropriate genetic models for atherosclerosis (overall, CAD and IS, respectively) and additive models for CAD and IS. No single study markedly altered the estimates of the effect sizes and statistical differences remained significant before and after removal of each study, suggesting high robustness of our estimates. As well, we observed no publication bias in our meta-analysis.

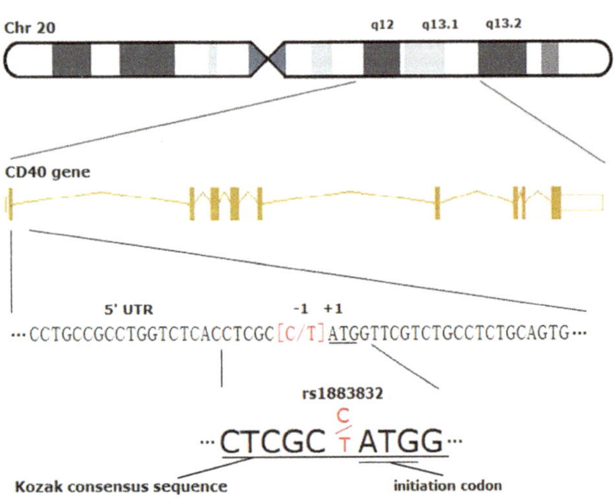

Figure 6. The specific position of rs1883832. Abbreviation: Chr, Chromosome; 5′ UTR, 5′ untranslated region.

CD40-CD40L interaction has recently been linked with the pathogenesis of atherosclerosis. Previous studies demonstrated the elevation of serum-soluble CD40L levels which may serve as one key indicator of an independent, increased risk of major adverse cardiovascular events in patients with unstable CAD. The expression of the CD40-CD40L system on platelets and B lymphocytes was as well found to be up-regulated in patients with ACS [15,20–22]. In addition, soluble CD40L is potentially applied as a biomarker for atherosclerotic plague activity [14,23]. The involvement of CD40-CD40L interaction in the inflammatory responses aggravates the development of atherosclerotic diseases and destabilization of plaques, which may ultimately renders vulnerable plagues susceptible to rupture and initiate lethal thrombosis and stenosis in ACS [24,25]. The SNP rs1883832 maps in the functional region of the CD40 gene, i.e. the kozak consensus sequence (figure 6) and has recently been associated with ACS risk independent of the traditional risk factors such as

Table 6. Meta-analysis for the association of rs1883832 with acute coronary syndrome.

Genetic model	OR 95%CI	P	P heterogeneity	I^2
C/C versus T/T	Crude OR1: 3.679 (2.637, 5.133)	<0.001	0.796	0%
	Modified OR1: 3.674 (2.638, 5.116)	<0.001	–	–
C/T versus T/T	Crude OR2: 1.983 (1.485, 2.649)	<0.001	1	0%
	Modified OR2: 1.981 (1.483, 2.646)	<0.001	–	–
C/C versus C/T	Crude OR3: 1.852 (1.423, 2.409)	<0.001	0.642	0%
	Modified OR3: 1.854 (1.428, 2.408)	<0.001		–
Dominant model (C/C and C/T) versus T/T	OR4: 2.421 (1.835, 3.193)	<0.001	0.985	0%
Recessive model C/C versus (C/T and T/T)	OR5: 2.211 (1.719, 2.844)	<0.001	0.615	0%
Additive model	OR6: 1.909 (1.619, 2.251)	<0.001	0.714	0%

Included publications: Li Y, 2007; Tian CX, 2010; Yan JC, 2010; Wang M, 2011.
Likelihood ratio test: LR = 62.64, P<0.001.
Abbreviation: ACS, acute coronary syndrome; OR, odds ratio; 95%CI, 95% confidence interval.

Table 7. Sensitivity analysis.

Atherosclerosis		
Study omitted	**Dominant model**	**Additive model**
	Crude OR4 95%CI	**Crude OR6 95%CI**
Li Y, 2007	1.570(1.111,2.218)	1.275(0.905,1.796)
Wang CP, 2009	1.602(1.086,2.360)	1.324(0.911,1.926)
Tian CX, 2010	1.503(1.079,2.093)	1.274(0.908,1.787)
Yan JC, 2010	1.657(1.118,2.456)	1.353(0.924,1.981)
Wang M,2011	1.565(1.096,2.235)	1.324(0.918,1.909)
Ma Y, 2013	1.719(1.175,2.513)	1.511(1.078,2.119)
Zhang BK,2013	1.825(1.475,2.259)	1.493(1.082,2.060)
Combined	1.631(1.176,2.260)	1.361(0.981,1.889)
IS		
Study omitted	**Recessive model**	**Additive model**
	Crude OR5 95%CI	**Crude OR6 95%CI**
Ma Y, 2013	0.698(0.533,0.913)	0.810(0.677,0.968)
Zhang BK,2013	0.466(0.320,0.676)	0.737(0.571,0.951)
Combined	0.582(0.393,0.864)	0.785(0.678,0.909)
CAD		
Study omitted	**Co-dominant model**	**Additive model**
	Crude OR1 95%CI Crude OR2 95%CI	**Crude OR6 95%CI**
Li Y, 2007	2.762(2.095,3.643) 1.670(1.332,2.095)	1.654(1.443,1.896)
Wang CP, 2009	3.013(2.124,4.274) 1.721(1.315,2.253)	1.730(1.443,2.074)
Tian CX, 2010	2.600(1.915,3.529) 1.630(1.276,2.082)	1.607(1.383,1.868)
Yan JC, 2010	3.161(2.332,4.286) 1.804(1.398,2.327)	1.773(1.525,2.060)
Wang M,2011	2.913(2.093,4.056) 1.655(1.309,2.093)	1.711(1.444,2.028)
Combined	2.869(2.197,3.746) 1.691(1.359,2.105)	1.689(1.480,1.927)

Abbreviation: OR, odds ratio; 95%CI, 95% confidence interval; IS, is chemic stroke; CAD, coronary artery disease.

hypertension and diabetes mellitus [7,13]. Alteration of Kozak sequence which comprises 6 to 8 nucleotides before and after the initiation codon, may have an impact on the initiation of transcriptional activity and final gene expression [26,27]. In Grave's disease, up-regulation of CD40 by rs1883832 places an individual at an increased disease risk [28]. Similarly, C allele appeared to contribute to the over-expression of CD40 on not only platelets which are central to the formation of thrombosis in ACS patients, but also B lymphocytes and monocytes [7,15,17]. C allele is also positively associated with an increased risk of rupture of complex coronary atherosclerotic plagues underlying ACS [17]. Of note, CD40-CD40L interaction and rs1883832 may not promote the disease progression of stable angina (SA). Yan et al. [7]. reported no significant difference in C allele frequency or genotype distribution between the SA group and controls. The same study team demonstrated similar CD40-CD40L system expression levels of SA group and controls. Moreover, C allele frequency and genotype distribution in the group with stable plagues underlying SA was comparable with those of controls [17]. Thus rs1883832 is hypothesized to impact primarily on plague vulnerability rather than the initiation and development of atherosclerosis. We noted in our study the larger magnitudes for ACS risk than those for CAD risk, which might be consistent with the above assumption. However, C allele was negatively associated with the susceptibility to IS in our study. It might be a dissimilar genetic or etiologic contribution of rs1883832 to IS. It was indicated that altered CD40-CD40L interaction affected thrombus composition and its pattern of lyses. Another possibility was that aberrant CD40 isoforms might result in the changes in CD40-CD40L binding dynamics and tighter platelet-leukocyte adhesion, which increased IS risk [29]. Zhang et al. presented that TT genotype carriers showed higher CD40 expression and serum-soluble CD40 concentration in male IS patients [16]. Moreover, geographic variation and genetic heterogeneity may explain partially the different allele frequencies between CAD (ACS) and IS patients, and the high heterogeneity of allele frequencies in controls between different studies observed in our study. For genetic association studies, the same or different research groups occasionally utilize repetitive samples (especially controls). When a meta-analysis is conducted incorporating duplicate publications, a seemingly significant result may be obtained whereas the association is not robustly reproduced with a truly lower sample size. Besides, it may lead to a deviated estimate of the gene effects. Thus the potential duplicate-study effects were carefully examined and finally excluded in our analysis.

Limitations

We wish to point out a few limitations of the present meta-analysis that readers should consider when interpreting the study results. First, inclusion of retrospective observational studies based on case-control design inevitably introduced a source of potential bias that inherently exists in non-randomized, unblinded design. Second, we failed to eliminate the heterogeneity in the subgroup analysis for IS. Third, atherosclerosis is a complex disorder triggered by multiple susceptibility genes and environmental factors. However, lacking of further evaluation of gene-gene and gene-environment interactions may have a diluting influence on the estimates for rs1883832. Fourth, other SNPs within or near CD40 gene, including rs1535045, rs3765459, rs4810485, rs3092952 and rs3092920, could be constructed statistically with rs1883832 to form multi-SNP haplotypes, which fine-map this region and are potentially more informative than individual SNP. Linkage disequilibrium (LD) pattern of this region should as well be determined using genotyping data of these SNPs [30–33]. It is likely that rs1883832 is a marker SNP in strong LD with the genuine causal loci. Thus the causal variants conferring an increased risk of atherosclerosis may remain unclearly determined. In addition, distinct LD patterns exist in different ethnicities whereas our meta-analysis did not analyze the association of rs1883832 with atherosclerosis in other populations. Although it might introduce less heterogeneity between the study populations, the restriction to Chinese ethnicity is a limitation in terms of the generalizability of our finding. Genetic association studies in other populations and multi-ethnic meta-analysis for this association are expected to be performed in near future. Fifth, only a portion of atherosclerotic diseases were investigated in our study. Thus risk of other diseases, such as peripheral or renal artery diseases and overall risk of atherosclerosis need to be further clarified.

Conclusions

Our meta-analysis suggests that C allele rs1883832 in CD40 gene is positively associated with susceptibility to atherosclerosis, CAD and ACS whereas C allele appears to contribute to a decreased risk of IS in Chinese population. In the future, large scale case-control studies with rigorous design are called for in different ethnicities to replicate the association between rs1883832 and atherosclerosis and various atherosclerotic diseases. Further efforts for fine-mapping of CD40 gene region and functional analysis are required to identify causal variants and elucidate detailed mechanisms of CD40 polymorphisms in atherosclerosis.

Supporting Information

Table S1 Genetic models tested in this meta-analysis. Abbreviation: OR, odds ratio.

Checklist S1 PRISMA checklist for this meta-analysis.

Author Contributions

Conceived and designed the experiments: YY CM XM. Performed the experiments: YY CM XM. Analyzed the data: YY CM XM. Contributed reagents/materials/analysis tools: YY CM XM. Wrote the paper: YY CM XM.

References

1. Weber C, Noels H (2011) Atherosclerosis: current pathogenesis and therapeutic options. Nat Med 17: 1410–1422.
2. Phipps RP (2000) Atherosclerosis: the emerging role of inflammation and the CD40-CD40 ligand system. Proc Natl Acad Sci U S A 97: 6930–6932.
3. Urbich C, Dimmeler S (2004) CD40 and vascular inflammation. Can J Cardiol 20: 681–683.
4. Chen K, Huang J, Gong W, Zhang L, Yu P, et al. (2006) CD40/CD40L dyad in the inflammatory and immune responses in the central nervous system. Cell Mol Immunol 3: 163–169.
5. Wu T, Guo R, Zhang B (2012) [Developments in the study of CD40/CD40L gene and its polymorphism in atherosclerosis]. Zhong Nan Da Xue Xue Bao Yi Xue Ban 37: 413–418.
6. Ma Y, Wang SX, Liu Y, Peng GG, Wang XM, et al. (2013) Single nucleotide polymorphism of CD40 in the 5′-untranslated region is associated with ischemic stroke. Gene 10.1016/j.gene.2013.07.086.
7. Yan J, Wang C, Du R, Liu P, Chen G (2010) Association analysis of CD40 gene polymorphism with acute coronary syndrome. Clinical and experimental medicine 10: 253–258.
8. http://www.ohri.ca/programs/clinical_epidemiology/oxford.asp.

9. Stang A (2010) Critical evaluation of the Newcastle-Ottawa scale for the assessment of the quality of nonrandomized studies in meta-analyses. European journal of epidemiology 25: 603–605.
10. Thakkinstian A, McEvoy M, Minelli C, Gibson P, Hancox B, et al. (2005) Systematic review and meta-analysis of the association between {beta}2-adrenoceptor polymorphisms and asthma: a HuGE review. American journal of epidemiology 162: 201–211.
11. Liu X, Zhu R, Li L, Deng S, Li Q, et al. (2013) Genetic polymorphism in PDE4D gene and risk of ischemic stroke in Chinese population: a meta-analysis. PloS one 8: e66374.
12. Thakkinstian A, McElduff P, D'Este C, Duffy D, Attia J (2005) A method for meta-analysis of molecular association studies. Statistics in medicine 24: 1291–1306.
13. Li Y, Tian CX, Wang M, Xia ZE (2007) [Correlation of CD40 gene polymorphisms with acute coronary syndrome, hypertension and diabetes]. Zhonghua Yi Xue Za Zhi 87: 690–694.
14. Wang C, Yan J, Yang P, Du R, Chen G (2010) The relationship between CD40 gene polymorphism and unstable coronary atherosclerotic plaques. Clin Cardiol 33: E55–60.
15. Tian C, Qin W, Li L, Zheng W, Qiu F (2010) A common polymorphism in CD40 Kozak sequence (-1C/T) is associated with acute coronary syndrome. Biomed Pharmacother 64: 191–194.
16. Zhang B, Wu T, Song C, Chen M, Li H, et al. (2013) Association of CD40-1C/T polymorphism with cerebral infarction susceptibility and its effect on sCD40L in Chinese population. Int Immunopharmacol 16: 461–465.
17. Wang M, Li Y, Li W, Xia ZE, Wu Q (2011) The CD40 gene polymorphism rs1883832 is associated with risk of acute coronary syndrome in a Chinese case-control study. DNA Cell Biol 30: 173–178.
18. Zheng X, Wang L, Zhu Y, Guan Q, Li H, et al. (2012) The SNP rs961253 in 20p12.3 is associated with colorectal cancer risk: a case-control study and a meta-analysis of the published literature. PloS one 7: e34625.
19. Zhong H, Prentice RL (2010) Correcting "winner's curse" in odds ratios from genomewide association findings for major complex human diseases. Genetic epidemiology 34: 78–91.
20. Yan JC, Wu ZG, Kong XT, Zong RQ, Zhan LZ (2004) Relation between upregulation of CD40 system and complex stenosis morphology in patients with acute coronary syndrome. Acta Pharmacol Sin 25: 251–256.
21. Yan JC, Zhu J, Gao L, Wu ZG, Kong XT, et al. (2004) The effect of elevated serum soluble CD40 ligand on the prognostic value in patients with acute coronary syndromes. Clin Chim Acta 343: 155–159.
22. Yan J, Wu Z, Huang Z, Li L, Zhong R, et al. (2002) Clinical implications of increased expression of CD40L in patients with acute coronary syndromes. Chin Med J (Engl) 115: 491–493.
23. Aukrust P, Muller F, Ueland T, Berget T, Aaser E, et al. (1999) Enhanced levels of soluble and membrane-bound CD40 ligand in patients with unstable angina. Possible reflection of T lymphocyte and platelet involvement in the pathogenesis of acute coronary syndromes. Circulation 100: 614–620.
24. Yan JC, Wu ZG, Kong XT, Zong RQ, Zhang LZ (2003) Effect of CD40-CD40 ligand interaction on diacylglycerol-protein kinase C signal transduction pathway and intracellular calcium in cultured human monocytes. Acta Pharmacol Sin 24: 687–691.
25. Yan JC, Wu ZG, Kong XT, Zong RQ, Zhan LZ (2003) Effect of CD40-CD40 ligand interaction on diacylglycerol-protein kinase C and inositol trisphosphate-Ca(2+) signal transduction pathway in human umbilical vein endothelial cells. Clin Chim Acta 337: 133–140.
26. Kozak M (1991) An analysis of vertebrate mRNA sequences: intimations of translational control. J Cell Biol 115: 887–903.
27. Kozak M (1991) Structural features in eukaryotic mRNAs that modulate the initiation of translation. J Biol Chem 266: 19867–19870.
28. Jacobson EM, Huber AK, Akeno N, Sivak M, Li CW, et al. (2007) A CD40 Kozak sequence polymorphism and susceptibility to antibody-mediated autoimmune conditions: the role of CD40 tissue-specific expression. Genes Immun 8: 205–214.
29. del Rio-Espinola A, Fernandez-Cadenas I, Rubiera M, Quintana M, Domingues-Montanari S, et al. (2010) CD40-1C>T polymorphism (rs1883832) is associated with brain vessel reocclusion after fibrinolysis in ischemic stroke. Pharmacogenomics 11: 763–772.
30. Burdon KP, Langefeld CD, Beck SR, Wagenknecht LE, Carr JJ, et al. (2006) Variants of the CD40 gene but not of the CD40L gene are associated with coronary artery calcification in the Diabetes Heart Study (DHS). American heart journal 151: 706–711.
31. Garcia-Bermudez M, Gonzalez-Juanatey C, Lopez-Mejias R, Teruel M, Corrales A, et al. (2012) Study of association of CD40-CD154 gene polymorphisms with disease susceptibility and cardiovascular risk in Spanish rheumatoid arthritis patients. PloS one 7: e49214.
32. Niu T, Qin ZS, Xu X, Liu JS (2002) Bayesian haplotype inference for multiple linked single-nucleotide polymorphisms. American journal of human genetics 70: 157–169.
33. Niu T (2004) Algorithms for inferring haplotypes. Genetic epidemiology 27: 334–347.

Efficacy and Safety of Vitamin K-Antagonists (VKA) for Atrial Fibrillation in Non-Dialysis Dependent Chronic Kidney Disease

Judith Kooiman[1]*, Nienke van Rein[1,2], Bas Spaans[1], Koen A. J. van Beers[1], Jonna R. Bank[1], Wilke R. van de Peppel[1], Antonio Iglesias del Sol[3], Suzanne C. Cannegieter[4], Ton J. Rabelink[5], Gregory Y. H. Lip[6], Frederikus A. Klok[1], Menno V. Huisman[1]

1 Department of Thrombosis and Hemostasis, Leiden University Medical Center, Leiden, The Netherlands, **2** Einthoven Laboratory of Experimental Vascular Medicine, Leiden University Medical Center, Leiden, The Netherlands, **3** Department of Internal Medicine, Rijnland Hospital, Leiderdorp, The Netherlands, **4** Department of Clinical Epidemiology, Leiden University Medical Center, Leiden, The Netherlands, **5** Department of Nephrology, Leiden University Medical Center, Leiden, The Netherlands, **6** Haemostasis, Thrombosis, and Vascular Biology Unit, University of Birmingham Centre for Cardiovascular Sciences, City Hospital, Birmingham, United Kingdom

Abstract

Background: Essential information regarding efficacy and safety of vitamin K-antagonists (VKA) treatment for atrial fibrillation (AF) in non-dialysis dependent chronic kidney disease (CKD) is still lacking in current literature. The aim of our study was to compare the risks of stroke or transient ischemic attack (TIA) and major bleeds between patients without CKD (eGFR >60 ml/min), and those with moderate (eGFR 30–60 ml/min), or severe non-dialysis dependent CKD (eGFR <30 ml/min).

Methods: We included 300 patients without CKD, 294 with moderate, and 130 with severe non-dialysis dependent CKD, who were matched for age and sex. Uni- and multivariate Cox regression analyses were performed reporting hazard ratios (HRs) for the endpoint of stroke or TIA and the endpoint of major bleeds as crude values and adjusted for comorbidity and platelet-inhibitor use.

Results: Overall, 6.2% (45/724, 1.7/100 patient years) of patients developed stroke or TIA and 15.6% (113/724, 4.8/100 patient years) a major bleeding event. Patients with severe CKD were at high risk of stroke or TIA and major bleeds during VKA treatment compared with those without renal impairment, HR 2.75 (95%CI 1.25–6.05) and 1.66 (95%CI 0.97–2.86), or with moderate CKD, HR 3.93(1.71–9.00) and 1.86 (95%CI 1.08–3.21), respectively. These risks were similar for patients without and with moderate CKD. Importantly, both less time spent within therapeutic range and high INR-variability were associated with increased risks of stroke or TIA and major bleeds in severe CKD patients.

Conclusions: VKA treatment for AF in patients with severe CKD has a poor safety and efficacy profile, likely related to suboptimal anticoagulation control. Our study findings stress the need for better tailored individualised anticoagulant treatment approaches for patients with AF and severe CKD.

Editor: Kathrin Eller, Medical University of Graz, Austria

Funding: The authors have no support or funding to report.

Competing Interests: The authors have declared that no competing interests exist.

* E-mail: j.kooiman@lumc.nl

Introduction

About one-third of atrial fibrillation (AF) patients suffer from chronic kidney disease (CKD) [1–3], a condition that by itself increases the risk of stroke, even in the absence of AF. Inversely, AF in CKD patients is associated with progression of CKD, cardiovascular morbidity and mortality [4–6].

Antithrombotic treatment is very effective in preventing stroke or a transient ischemic attack (TIA) in patients with AF, both in patients with normal renal function and in those with CKD in terms of a relative risk reduction [7–9]. However, CKD increases a patient's risk of major bleeding complications during antithrombotic treatment [8,10]. The extent to which non-dialysis dependent CKD increases the risk of stroke and major bleeds in AF patients during VKA treatment is understudied, as the main focus in research in this area has been on patients with end-stage-renal disease requiring dialysis. However, these patients comprise less than 1% of the AF population [8,11]. The few studies that have focussed on risks of stroke and/or major bleeding in AF patients with non-dialysis dependent CKD were limited by their small sample size [10,12,13], the absence of information on eGFR levels [8], exclusion of patients with severe CKD [7], or a divergent patient cohort with various indications for VKA treatment [14]. Knowledge about these risks would most certainly provide relevant insights into treatment outcomes in a patient group that frequently attends both cardiology and internal medicine practices. Moreover, with the emergence of novel oral anticoagulants, understanding the risks of stroke and major bleeding events in AF patients with various stages of CKD is essential when evaluating whether these new agents would provide a more favourable risk-benefit ratio than the traditional vitamin K-antagonists (VKA) for this specific patient population [11].

Therefore, the aim of our study was to compare risks of stroke or TIA and major bleeds in patients with moderate or severe CKD and AF treated with VKAs with patients without renal impairment. Second, we assessed the influence of quality of anticoagulation control on the risks of stroke or TIA and major bleeds.

Methods

Patients diagnosed with new onset valvular or non-valvular AF starting VKA treatment between 1997 and 2005 at the Leiden anticoagulation clinic were included in a previously described study cohort [3]. This anticoagulation clinic serves one academic (Leiden University Medical Center, Leiden) and two non-academic teaching hospitals (Diaconessenhuis, Leiden, and Rijnland Hospital, Leiderdorp). Within this cohort of 5039 AF patients, 3316 had no CKD (eGFR >60 ml/min), 1557 (eGFR 30–60 ml/min) had moderate CKD, and 166 patients severe CKD (eGFR <30 ml/min), as measured at start of VKA therapy. For the current analysis, we excluded fourteen patients from the severe CKD group who had acute kidney injury at time of VKA therapy initiation, after which renal function recovered to a less critical CKD stage, thus leaving 152 patients with severe CKD. Since reviewing medical records of all 1557 moderate and 3316 non-CKD patients would be an effort not offsetting the statistical gain, we sampled 300 patients without CKD and 294 patients with moderate CKD for inclusion, matched for age and gender to those with severe CKD. Patients treated with VKA via the Leiden anticoagulation clinic for <7 days were excluded from the study cohort and replaced by others of the same age, gender, and level of renal impairment. Patients on dialysis at start of VKA therapy were also excluded, but were not replaced. Patients were treated with either phenprocoumon (Marcoumar) or acenocoumarol. The study was approved by the ethics committee of the three participating hospitals (ethics committee Leiden University Medical Center, Leiden, the Netherlands) that waived the need for informed consent.

Chart review

Medical records from two sources (i.e. the participating hospitals and the Leiden anticoagulation clinic) were searched for information on patient characteristics at baseline, comorbidity, use of platelet-inhibitors, International Normalized Ratios (INRs) and study outcomes. Renal function was assessed using the abbreviated modification of diet in renal disease (MDRD) formula, as it accurately estimates renal function in elderly patients and the mean age of our study population was high [15,16].

Study outcomes and definitions

Primary outcomes of this study were the combined endpoint of stroke or TIA and the occurrence of major bleeding events. Major bleeding was defined by the International Society of Thrombosis and Hemostasis criteria (i.e. fatal bleeding, any bleeding causing a drop in hemoglobin level ≥1.24 mmol/L and/or requiring transfusion of ≥2 units of whole blood or red cells and/or a symptomatic bleeding in a critical area/organ (intracranial, intraspinal, intraocular, pericardial, or intramuscular with compartment syndrome)) [17]. Secondary endpoints were major adverse cardiovascular events (MACE), fatal MACE and fatal bleeding. MACE was defined as stroke or TIA, myocardial infarction, intermittent claudication, unstable angina, carotid endarterectomy, coronary artery bypass graft, peripheral arterial bypass or angioplasty [18]. Other variables of interest were time within therapeutic range (TTR) and INR-variability; both established risk factors for MACE and major bleeding complications during VKA treatment [19–23]. INR-values were measured using HepatoQuick (Roche Diagnostics, Mannheim, Germany) and serum creatinine values by using Roche Diagnostics Analyzers (Mannheim, Germany).

Follow- up

Duration of follow-up was defined as time elapsed between the day of initiation and permanent discontinuation of VKA treatment, occurrence of the endpoint of interest, or death, or December 31, 2010. Only the first stroke or TIA, MACE or major bleeding event that occurred was recorded in the database, although some patients had more than one episode of the endpoints. For non-acute MACE such as intermittent claudication, carotid endarterectomy, coronary artery bypass graft, peripheral arterial bypass or angioplasty, the day of diagnosis or intervention was recorded as the date of MACE occurrence.

Statistical analysis

Incidence rates (i.e. events/100 patient years (py)) of primary outcomes were reported with corresponding 95% confidence intervals (CI). As patients with moderate or without CKD were matched for age and gender to those with severe CKD, incidence rates of our study endpoints in the first two patient groups reflect the incidences of these endpoints for the population with this age and sex distribution, rather than that of the overall AF population. Nonetheless, this design allowed us to study relative risks of stroke or TIA and major bleeds between patients with severe or moderate CKD and those without renal impairment, which was our main research question. This analysis was performed using uni- and multivariate Cox regression analyses reporting hazard ratios (HRs) as crude values and as values corrected for age, gender, concomitant use of platelet-inhibitors or non-steroidal anti-inflammatory drugs, hypertension, diabetes mellitus, and congestive heart failure. As for secondary analysis, TTR and INR-variability were calculated using the *Rosendaal* method and the formula by *Cannegieter*, respectively [23,24]. INR-variability and TTR were compared between patients with moderate or severe CKD and non-CKD patients, using first a Kruskal Wallis and second a Mann Whitney U-test, as these values had a non-parametric distribution among the population.

Mediation analysis

A mediation analysis was performed to assess whether the expected increased risks of stroke or TIA, major bleeds and MACE in patients with moderate and severe CKD compared with non-CKD patients were mediated via TTR or INR-variability. This analysis was performed for the three endpoints and the combined endpoint of MACE and major bleeds in a nested case-control study [24]. We chose this design as the duration of follow-up needed to be matched for cases and controls. Cases were patients developing the endpoint of interest. For each case, a maximum of four controls was selected from the total study population of 724 patients who were treated during the same period with VKA while not developing this specific endpoint at the time that the case did (incidence density sampling). A control could be selected for more than one case. INR-variability and TTR were calculated over the entire treatment period, for the last six and the last three months prior to the outcome of interest. For each time frame, only patients with sufficient follow-up were selected for that specific analysis [24]. Crude odds ratios (OR) were then computed for the risks of the four outcomes comparing severe and moderate CKD with non-CKD patients. Next, these ORs were first adjusted for comorbidity, and second for either INR-variability, TTR, or both for each individual time frame.

All statistical analyses were performed in SPSS 20.0 (IBM SPSS statistics, IBM Corp, Somers, NY).

Results

Serum creatinine values were available in 5039 out of 6933 patients with new onset AF at start of VKA therapy. Of those, 733 matched subjects were selected for inclusion for this present study, comprising all patients with non-dialysis depended severe CKD, and a sample of those with moderate or without CKD. Registered duration of VKA treatment in the Leiden anticoagulation clinic was less than seven days in 52 patients who were excluded and replaced by 43 patients of similar gender, age, and level of renal impairment. The remaining nine severe CKD patients could not be replaced (Figure 1). Thus, 724 patients were included in this study, 300 without CKD (eGFR >60 ml/min), 294 with moderate (eGFR 30–60 ml/min) and 130 with severe CKD (eGFR < 30 ml/min). Patient characteristics at baseline are reported in Table 1. Compared with patients without CKD, those with moderate or severe CKD were more likely to have congestive heart failure, hypertension, diabetes mellitus, or a previous episode of major bleeds before initiation of VKA therapy. Median follow-up time was 2.1 years (2.5–97.5percentile 0.0–10.0) for the endpoint of stroke or TIA and 2.3 years (2.5–97.5percentiles 0.0–10.0) for major bleeding events.

Stroke or TIA and MACE

During follow-up for the primary endpoint, 6.2% (45/724, 1.67/100 py) of patients developed a stroke (29 patients) or TIA (16 patients). The risk of stroke or TIA was increased in those with severe CKD compared with patients without renal dysfunction (HR 2.75, 95%CI 1.25–6.05) or those with moderate CKD (HR 3.93, 95%CI 1.71–9.00, Table 2). The risk of stroke or TIA was similar for patients with moderate and without CKD.

Overall, 14.8% (107/724) of patients developed MACE of whom 28 patients had a stroke, 15 a TIA, 28 a myocardial infarction, 17 an unstable angina pectoris, 11 patients underwent coronary artery bypass grafting, and 8 patients had developed peripheral artery disease (one patient developed a stroke and another patient a TIA after the occurrence of an earlier MACE). Patients with severe CKD were at increased risk of MACE compared with non-CKD patients (adjusted HR 3.57, 95%CI 2.10–6.06) and those with moderate CKD (adjusted HR 3.40, 95%CI 2.05–5.64). MACE risk was similar for those without and with moderate CKD. Twenty-three of 724 patients had a fatal MACE, of whom 14 (60.9%) developed a myocardial infarction and 9 (39.1%) a stroke. Although non-significant, moderate and severe CKD were associated with a 60–90% increased risk of fatal MACE compared with non-CKD patients, respectively.

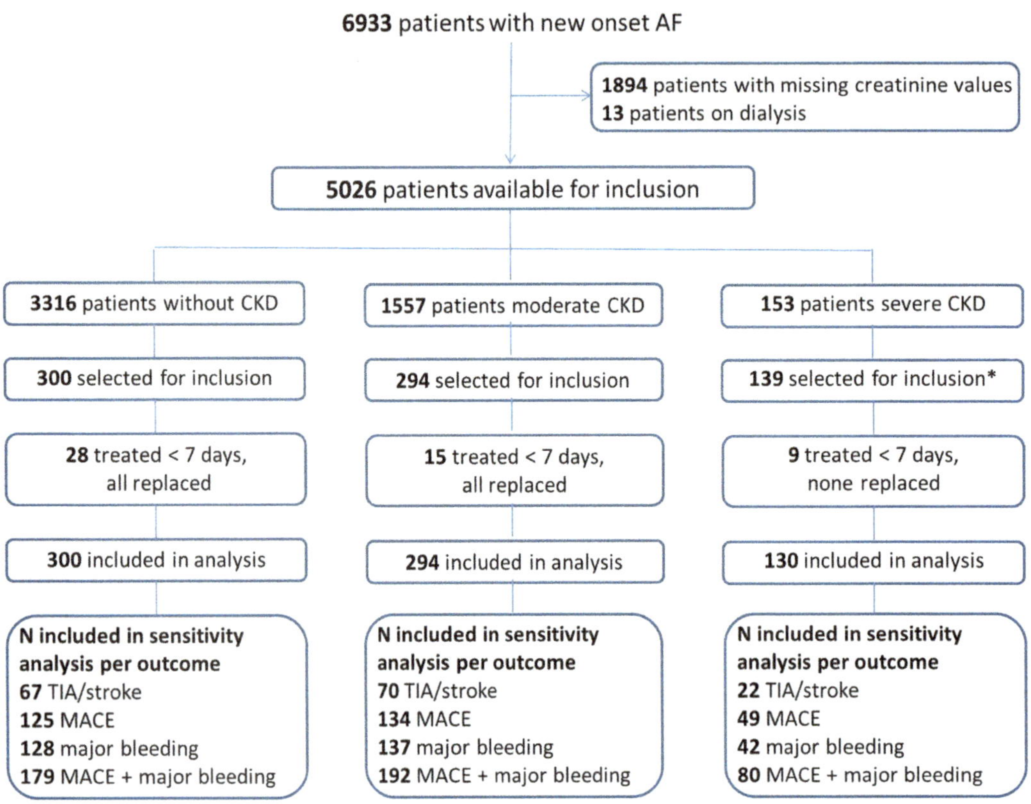

Figure 1. Flow chart. Abbreviations: CKD = Chronic kidney disease, TIA = transient ischemic attack, MACE = major adverse cardiovascular event. * Fourteen patients from the severe CKD group had acute kidney injury at time of VKA therapy initiation, after which renal function recovered to a less critical CKD stage.

Table 1. Patient characteristics at baseline of the total population.

	No CKD eGFR>60 ml/min	Moderate CKD eGFR 30–60 ml/min	Severe CKD eGFR<30 ml/min
N	**300**	**294**	**130**
Mean age (SD)	74(10)	75(10)	76(9)
Gender, m/f	171/129	165/129	73/57
Mean eGFR (SD)	92(37)	46(8)	21(7)
Diabetes Mellitus	35(11.7)	50(17.0)	38(29.2)
Hypertension	138(46.0)	181(61.6)	80(61.5)
Concomitant use of platelet inhibitors	26(8.7)	35(11.9)	7(5.4)
Previous stroke or TIA	47(15.7)	59(20.1)	21(16.2)
Previous major bleeding	14(4.7)	21(7.1)	10(7.7)
Congestive heart failure	50(17.0)	105(35.7)	54(41.5)
INR target range*			
2.0–3.0	1(0.3)	0(0.0)	1(0.8)
2.5–3.5	287(98.6)	280(97.9)	116(97.5)
3.0–4.0	3(1.0)	6(2.1)	2(1.7)
Acenocoumarol**	13(4.3)	15(5.1)	9(7.0)
Phenprocoumon	287(95.7)	278(94.6)	120(93.0)

Data is presented as n, % unless stated otherwise.
CKD = chronic kidney disease, eGFR = estimated glomerular filtration rate, SD = standard deviation, TIA = transient ischemic attack.
* Lacking in 30 patients, ** lacking in one patient.

Major bleeding complications

Major bleeding complications occurred in 15.6% of patients (113/724, 4.8/100 py). Although non-significant, severe CKD was associated with an increased risk of major bleeds compared with patients without renal impairment (adjusted HR 1.66, 95%CI0.97–2.86), and those with moderate CKD (HR 1.86, 95%CI1.08–3.21). Major bleeding risks were similar for those without and with moderate CKD. The most frequent locations of major bleeding were gastrointestinal (34.5%) and intracranial (27.4%) in the total population. Patients with severe CKD were more likely to develop gastrointestinal bleeding (63.6%), yet less frequently developed intracranial haemorrhages (13.6%).

Fatal bleeding occurred in 2.9% of patients (21/724). Severe CKD might be associated with an increased risk of fatal bleeding events compared with non-CKD patients (HR 1.52, 95%CI0.46–5.02, Table 2), and those with moderate CKD (HR 1.90, 95%CI0.57–6.41).

TTR and INR variability

Compared with patients without CKD, TTR was higher in those with moderate CKD (75.1%, $p<0.01$) whereas TTR was similar in patients with severe CKD (70.3%, $p = 0.41$, Table 3). The proportion of time spent above target range was higher for all CKD stages compared with patients without renal impairment, and higher for those with severe compared with moderate CKD. Median INR-variability during the entire treatment period significantly increased with each stage of CKD, with median values of 0.5 in patients without CKD, 0.7 ($p = 0.03$) in those with moderate, and 0.9 ($p<0.001$) in those with severe CKD. For all three groups, the degree of INR variability can be regarded as below average or unstable anticoagulant control according to previous research [25].

Mediation analysis

Mediation analyses were performed on the influence of TTR and INR-variability on the increased risks of stroke or TIA, MACE and major bleeding complications in severe CKD compared with non-CKD patients. TTR and INR-variability were analysed as continuous and categorical variables (based on 33rd and 66th percentiles) in separate models demonstrating similar results. For all four outcomes, the results demonstrated a decrease in the odds ratio towards unity in severe CKD compared with non-CKD patients, when corrected for either INR-variability or TTR (Table 4 and 5). However, the effect of INR-variability and TTR in the three months prior to combined endpoint of stroke or TIA and to the endpoint of MACE was less pronounced. This might be the result of the low number of INR measurements during this short timeframe (median 5.0, 2.5–97.5 percentile 2.0–10.5), which might not be sufficient for adequate assessment of TTR and INR-variability. Simultaneous correction for both INR-variability and TTR did not result in a further decrease towards unity for any of the endpoints comparing severe and moderate CKD to non-CKD patients, indicating no additive effect of TTR over INR-variability, and vice versa. This indicates that the increased risks in patients with severe CKD for stroke or TIA, major bleeds and MACE were mediated via suboptimal anticoagulation control.

Discussion

Our study has three important findings. First, risks of stroke or TIA, MACE and major bleeding complications during VKA therapy were high in AF patients with severe non-dialysis dependent CKD, when compared to those without renal impairment, or with moderate CKD. Second, stroke or TIA, MACE and major bleeding risks were similar for patients with moderate CKD and those with normal renal function. Third, patients with CKD spent more time above INR target range and

Table 2. Risk of stroke, TIA, MACE and major bleeding events during vitamin K-antagonist treatment stratified by renal function within the entire population.

Endpoint	No. of events	N/100 py‡ (95% CI)	Crude HR (95% CI)	Adjusted HR (95% CI)
Stroke or TIA				
No CKD	19	1.62(1.03–2.54)	ref	ref
Moderate CKD	15	1.20(0.71–1.99)	0.72(0.36–1.41)	0.70(0.35–1.41)
Severe CKD	11	4.24(2.30–7.53)	2.40(1.13–5.07)	2.75(1.25–6.05)
Overall MACE*				
No CKD	36	3.48(2.51–4.80)	ref	ref
Moderate CKD	41	3.79(2.80–5.12)	1.06(0.68–1.67)	1.05(0.66–1.67)
Severe CKD	30	15.4(10.95–21.16)	3.78(2.31–6.19)	3.57(2.10–6.06)
Fatal MACE†				
No CKD	7	0.64(0.28–1.35)	ref	ref
Moderate CKD	12	1.05(0.58–1.85)	1.68(0.66–4.27)	1.64(0.64–4.17)
Severe CKD	4	1.67(0.50–4.38)	2.09(0.60–7.23)	1.92(0.55–6.67)
Overall major bleeding*				
No CKD	46	4.45(3.34–5.89)	ref	ref
Moderate CKD	45	4.11(3.07–5.46)	0.91(0.60–1.37)	0.90(0.59–1.37)
Severe CKD	22	8.84(5.85–13.07)	1.88(1.13–3.14)	1.66(0.97–2.86)
Fatal bleeding†				
No CKD	9	0.83(0.41–1.59)	ref	ref
Moderate CKD	8	0.70(0.33–1.40)	0.85(0.33–2.21)	0.82(0.32–2.13)
Severe CKD	4	1.67(0.50–4.38)	1.62(0.49–5.33)	1.52(0.46–5.02)

Definitions: no-CKD = estimated glomerular filtration rate (eGFR) >60 ml/min, moderate CKD = eGFR 30–60 ml/min, severe CKD = eGFR <30 ml/min.
Abbreviations: CKD = chronic kidney disease, PY = patient years, CI = confidence interval, HR = hazard ratio, MACE = major adverse cardiovascular event, TIA = transient ischemic attack.
‡Reported incidences for patients with an eGFR 30–60 or eGFR >60 ml/min are influenced by sampling of patients matched for age and gender to those with an eGFR <30 ml/min.
* HR adjusted for age, gender, hypertension, the use of platelet-inhibitors, diabetes mellitus and congestive heart failure.
†HR adjusted for age and gender. Further correcting resulted in non-converging coefficients.

had a higher INR-variability. Consequently, in a nested case-control study we have shown additionally that poor anticoagulation control was associated with increased risks of stroke or TIA, MACE and major bleeds in severe CKD patients. Our study therefore provides important insights into the efficacy and safety of VKA treatment in patients with CKD and AF.

CKD is a common comorbid condition in AF patients and increases a patient's risk for both stroke and major bleeds. Suggested mechanisms for this higher stroke and bleeding risk are endothelial dysfunction, hypercoagulability, and chronic inflammation [8,11,12]. We demonstrated in a nested case-control study that impaired anticoagulation control might be an important additional determinant. Interestingly, within the total study population of 724 patients, CKD patients were spending more time above INR target range and had a higher INR variability compared with non-CKD patients, despite frequent INR monitoring. We hypothesize several explanations for this observation. CKD by itself may affect the quality of anticoagulant treatment. First, renal impairment might influence hepatic VKA metabolism, as has been shown in animal models for hepatic cytochrome P-450 metabolism [26,27]. Second, CKD influences the pharmacokinetic characteristics of VKA, as warfarin half-life was reported to be shorter in CKD compared with non-CKD patients with a greater unbound warfarin fraction [28,29]. Third, we cannot exclude that anticoagulant control is impaired in patients with CKD by poor patient compliance. Regardless of the mechanism by which CKD influences the quality of VKA therapy, our nested case-control study indicates that the increased risks of stroke or TIA, MACE and major bleeding complications in severe CKD patients are mediated through suboptimal anticoagulation control. This suggests that although warfarin has been shown to be effective in preventing stroke in CKD patients with AF in two observational and one randomized study [7,8,12], there is a great need for better tailored anticoagulant treatment approaches for this specific population, involving either better INR control, or the use of anticoagulants other than VKAs.

The use of computer-assisted dosage programs surveying both INR-variability and TTR during VKA treatment may help to identify patients with poor anticoagulant control in order to prevent them from developing stroke, TIA or major bleeding events [30]. Further, patient education and self-monitoring of INRs might improve patient compliance [31].

The novel oral anticoagulants have demonstrated less inter- and intra-individual variability in their pharmacokinetic properties compared with VKA. Within the Phase-3 trials, subgroup analyses have been performed for the efficacy and safety of these new agents compared with standard warfarin or aspirin treatment in AF patients with moderate CKD (i.e. eGFR >25 or >30 ml/min) [32]. These analyses demonstrated either a reduced risk of stroke and systemic thromboembolism compared with warfarin (Dabigatran 150 mg twice daily) or aspirin (Apixaban 5 mg twice daily), or a similar efficacy compared with warfarin treatment for AF

Table 3. Time within therapeutic range and INR variability within the entire population of 724 patients with atrial fibrillation.

	No CKD	Moderate CKD	P-value comparison	Severe CKD	P-value comparison	P-value comparison with
	eGFR>60 ml/min	eGFR 30-60 ml/min	with no CKD patients	eGFR<30 ml/min	with no CKD patients	moderate CKD patients
Time spend within therapeutic range, %						
First six weeks of VKA therapy	39.4(13.2–73.5)	49.7(24.1–81.3)	0.01	44.1(26.4–77.9)	0.10	0.60
First eighteen weeks of VKA therapy	57.9(29.8–79.3)	65.5(42.1–83.9)	0.01	60.7(39.4–80.6)	0.37	0.19
First twenty-six weeks of VKA therapy	61.5(38.7–79.8)	67.1(46.7–82.4)	0.02	64.7(41.5–75.6)	0.92	0.07
Entire treatment period	67.0(43.1–81.1)	75.1(57.8–82.9)	<0.01	70.3(49.2–81.1)	0.41	0.10
Time under target range (entire treatment), %	8.7(2.6–35.5)	6.2(2.1–13.0)	<0.001	5.5(2.3–12.9)	0.001	0.77
Time above target range (entire treatment), %	11.7(3.9–21.2)	15.2(9.8–24.0)	<0.001	20.8(11.7–32.7)	<0.001	<0.01
INR variability (2.5-97.5 percentiles)						
First six weeks of VKA therapy	0.5(0.1–1.6)	0.6(0.2–1.6)	0.10	0.7(0.4–2.3)	0.001	0.03
First eighteen weeks of VKA therapy	0.4(0.2–1.3)	0.6(0.2–1.5)	0.08	0.8(0.4–1.8)	<0.001	0.01
First twenty-six weeks of VKA therapy	0.5(0.3–1.2)	0.7(0.4–1.2)	0.24	0.8(0.4–1.8)	<0.001	<0.01
Entire treatment period	0.5(0.3–1.2)	0.7 (0.4–1.2)	0.03	0.9(0.5–1.8)	<0.001	<0.01

Data are presented as median, (Interquartile range), P-values were computed using Mann-Whitney test, after proof of significant differences between groups using a Kruskal-Wallis test.
CKD = chronic kidney disease, VKA = vitamin K-antagonists, eGFR = estimated glomerular filtration rate, INR = international normalized ratio.

Table 4. Mediation analysis on effect of INR-variability on the increased risks of major adverse cardiovascular events and major bleeding complications in patients with chronic kidney disease in a nested case-control study.

Outcome	Crude OR (95% CI)	Adjusted OR 1 (95% CI)	Adjusted OR 2 (95% CI)	Adjusted OR 3 (95% CI)	Adjusted OR 4 (95% CI)
Stroke or TIA					
No CKD (N = 91, of whom 67 unique)	ref	ref	ref	ref	ref
Moderate CKD (N = 90, of whom 70 unique)	0.76(0.36–1.61)	0.76(0.35–1.67)	0.79(0.36–1.76)	1.06(0.41–2.75)	1.02(0.40–2.56)
Severe CKD (N = 25, of whom 22 unique)	2.98(1.17–7.60)	2.56(0.92–7.10)	2.23(0.73–6.84)	1.96(0.50–7.74)	2.50(0.69–9.07)
MACE					
No CKD (N = 210, of whom 125 unique)	ref	ref	ref	ref	ref
Moderate CKD (N = 205, of whom 134 unique)	1.21(0.74–1.98)	1.14(0.68–1.93)	1.15(0.66–1.99)	1.05(0.58–1.91)	1.10(0.62–1.96)
Severe CKD (N = 58, of whom 49 unique)	5.18(2.76–9.70)	5.07(2.57–10.02)	5.37(2.58–11.19)	3.58(1.59–8.03)	3.77(1.71–8.32)
Major bleeding					
No CKD (N = 211, of whom 128 unique)	ref	ref	ref	ref	ref
Moderate CKD (N = 245, of whom 137 unique)	0.81(0.51–1.28)	0.76(0.47–1.23)	0.74(0.45–1.22)	0.88(0.52–1.52)	0.83(0.49–1.40)
Severe CKD (N = 60, of whom 42 unique)	2.08(1.12–3.85)	1.77(0.91–3.43)	1.82(0.93–3.56)	1.55(0.70–3.44)	1.57(0.72–3.40)
Major bleeding or MACE					
No CKD (N = 361, of whom 179 unique)	ref	ref	ref	ref	ref
Moderate CKD (N = 419, of whom 192 unique)	0.87(0.62–1.25)	0.85(0.59–1.24)	0.87(0.59–1.27)	0.93(0.61–1.41)	0.88(0.59–1.34)
Severe CKD (N = 122, of whom 80 unique)	2.92(1.88–4.54)	2.61(1.64–4.16)	2.67(1.64–4.34)	2.49(1.40–4.41)	2.31(1.33–4.03)

Model 1 includes age, gender, hypertension, the use of platelet-inhibitors, diabetes mellitus and congestive heart failure.
Model 2 includes model 1 + INR VAR entire treatment period, Model 3 includes model 1 + INR variability over six months prior to event.
Model 4 includes model 1 + INR variability over three months prior to event.
Abbreviations: CKD = chronic kidney disease, MACE = major adverse cardiovascular event, OR = odds ratio, TIA = transient ischemic attack.

Table 5. Mediation analysis on effect of time within therapeutic range on the increased risks of major adverse cardiovascular events and major bleeding complications in patients with chronic kidney disease in a nested case-control study.

Outcome	Crude OR (95% CI)	Adjusted OR 1 (95% CI)	Adjusted OR 2 (95% CI)	Adjusted OR 3 (95% CI)	Adjusted OR 4 (95% CI)
Stroke or TIA					
No CKD (N = 91, of whom 67 unique)	ref	ref	ref	ref	ref
Moderate CKD (N = 90, of whom 70 unique)	0.76(0.36–1.61)	0.76(0.35–1.67)	0.94(0.41–2.13)	1.31(0.52–3.37)	1.01(0.40–2.56)
Severe CKD (N = 25, of whom 22 unique)	2.98(1.17–7.60)	2.56(0.92–7.10)	1.95(0.64–5.88)	2.49(0.65–9.55)	2.46(0.68–8.88)
MACE					
No CKD (N = 210, of whom 125 unique)	ref	ref	ref	ref	ref
Moderate CKD (N = 205, of whom 134 unique)	1.21(0.74–1.98)	1.14(0.68–1.93)	1.16(0.67–2.01)	1.06(0.58–1.93)	1.11(0.62–1.98)
Severe CKD (N = 58, of whom 49 unique)	5.18(2.76–9.70)	5.07(2.57–10.02)	4.98(2.42–10.23)	3.26(1.45–7.34)	3.42(1.55–7.55)
Major bleeding					
No CKD (N = 211, of whom 128 unique)	ref	ref	ref	ref	ref
Moderate CKD (N = 245, of whom 137 unique)	0.81(0.51–1.28)	0.76(0.47–1.23)	0.73(0.44–1.21)	0.87(0.51–1.50)	0.83(0.49–1.41)
Severe CKD (N = 60, of whom 42 unique)	2.08(1.12–3.85)	1.77(0.91–3.43)	1.55(0.79–3.07)	1.48(0.67–3.29)	1.50(0.68–3.28)
Major bleeding or MACE					
No CKD (N = 361, of whom 179 unique)	ref	ref	ref	ref	ref
Moderate CKD (N = 419, of whom 192 unique)	0.87(0.62–1.25)	0.85(0.59–1.24)	0.93(0.62–1.40)	0.96(0.63–1.46)	0.93(0.62–1.40)
Severe CKD (N = 122, of whom 80 unique)	2.92(1.88–4.54)	2.61(1.64–4.16)	2.22(1.27–3.88)	2.37(1.33–4.21)	2.22(1.27–3.88)

Model 1 includes age, gender, hypertension, the use of platelet-inhibitors, diabetes mellitus and congestive heart failure.
Model 2 includes model 1 + time within therapeutic range over entire treatment period, Model 3 includes model 1 + time within therapeutic range over six months prior to event, Model 4 includes model 1 + time within therapeutic range over three months prior to event.
Abbreviations: CKD = chronic kidney disease, MACE = major adverse cardiovascular event, OR = odds ratio, TIA = transient ischemic attack.

(rivaroxaban 20 mg per day, or apixaban 5 mg twice daily). In terms of safety, the Aristotle trial demonstrated a lower risk of major bleeds in the apixaban compared with the warfarin group, whereas for all other novel oral anticoagulants, bleeding risks were comparable with the risks on warfarin or aspirin treatment [32]. Though, it is unknown whether these new agents would provide a better tailored anticoagulant treatment strategy compared with warfarin in severe CKD patients as they have been excluded systematically from the Phase-3 trials [33–35]. In terms of renal clearance, apixaban (25%) and betrixaban (17%) might be most suitable for use in patients with CKD. Although betrixaban has not been studied yet in a Phase-3 trial for stroke prevention in AF, the results of the Phase-2 trial, in which only CKD patients on dialysis were excluded, were promising in terms of a lower risk of bleeding compared with standard warfarin treatment in the group receiving the lowest betrixaban dose (i.e. 40 mg daily) [36]. However, the use of novel oral anticoagulants may not be advisable when the insufficient anticoagulant control in the CKD population is caused by poor patient compliance, which might even more be difficult to manage when laboratory monitoring of anticoagulant therapy is no longer required.

Our study has limitations. First, we had no information on alterations in renal function during follow-up, which might have led to misclassification of patients and consequently a misestimation of the reported hazard ratios. Second, events were recorded from chart review given the design of the study and we cannot fully exclude that some events were missed. However, our endpoints of stroke or TIA, MACE and major bleeding were clearly defined and are both serious medical events, requiring evaluation in a hospital setting and are thus likely to be reported in medical charts. Third, our primary and secondary outcomes were not adjudicated by an independent committee. Fourth, our sample size was too small to make further subdivisions in the stages of CKD other than moderate and severe CKD, or to demonstrate statistical differences in fatal MACE and bleeding rates. Fifth, we did not investigate the influence of co-medication interacting with VKAs on study outcomes. However, the majority of medication used by severe CKD patients is not known for interactions with VKAs. Sixth, we missed serum creatinine values at time of VKA initiation in 1894 of 9633 patients (19.6%) but we selected all patients with severe CKD (for whom serum creatinine values are highly unlikely to be lacking) and sampled controls matched for age and gender with moderate or without CKD. As patients without serum creatinine values are unlikely to have severe CKD it is implausible that lacking creatinine values in 1894 patients influenced the reported HRs on study outcomes.

In conclusion, patients with severe non-dialysis dependent CKD (i.e. eGFR <30 ml/min) are at higher risk for stroke or TIA, MACE and major bleeding complications during VKA treatment for AF, compared with those with moderate CKD (i.e. eGFR 30–60), or without renal impairment. Our study suggests that suboptimal anticoagulation control is a determinant in their poor cardiovascular prognosis. These study findings stress the need for more advanced tailored anticoagulant treatment approaches for AF patients with severe CKD. Whether the use of computer-assisted VKA dosage programs monitoring both INR-variability and TTR, or the use of novel oral anticoagulants are the answer to this issue remains to be studied.

Acknowledgments

The authors thank Dr. T.J. Römer (Department of Cardiology, Diaconessenhuis, Leiden, the Netherlands) for his help with data collection.

Author Contributions

Conceived and designed the experiments: JK NVR SCC TJR GYHL MVH. Performed the experiments: JK BS KAJVB JRB WRVDP AIDS SCC. Analyzed the data: JK NVR BS KAJVB JRB WRVDP AIDS SCC TJR GYHL MVH. Contributed reagents/materials/analysis tools: JK BS KAJVB JRB WRVDP AIDS. Wrote the paper: JK NVR SCC TJR GYHL MVH FAK. Interpretation of study results: FAK.

References

1. Koren-Morag N, Goldbourt U, Tanne D (2006) Renal dysfunction and risk of ischemic stroke or TIA in patients with cardiovascular disease. Neurology 67: 224–228. 67/2/224 [pii];10.1212/01.wnl.0000229099.62706.a3 [doi].
2. Tsukamoto Y, Takahashi W, Takizawa S, Kawada S, Takagi S (2012) Chronic kidney disease in patients with ischemic stroke. J Stroke Cerebrovasc Dis 21: 547–550. S1052-3057(10)00277-6 [pii];10.1016/j.jstrokecerebrovasdis.2010.12.005 [doi].
3. Kooiman J, van de Peppel WR, van der Meer FJ, Huisman MV (2011) Incidence of chronic kidney disease in patients with atrial fibrillation and its relevance for prescribing new oral antithrombotic drugs. J Thromb Haemost 9: 1652–1653. 10.1111/j.1538-7836.2011.04347.x [doi].
4. McManus DD, Rienstra M, Benjamin EJ (2012) An update on the prognosis of patients with atrial fibrillation. Circulation 126: e143–e146. 126/10/e143 [pii];10.1161/CIRCULATIONAHA.112.129759 [doi].
5. Herzog CA, Asinger RW, Berger AK, Charytan DM, Diez J, et al. (2011) Cardiovascular disease in chronic kidney disease. A clinical update from Kidney Disease: Improving Global Outcomes (KDIGO). Kidney Int 80: 572–586. ki2011223 [pii];10.1038/ki.2011.223 [doi].
6. Winkelmayer WC (2013) More evidence on an abominable pairing: atrial fibrillation and kidney disease. Circulation 127: 560–562. 127/5/560 [pii];10.1161/CIRCULATIONAHA.112.000640 [doi].
7. Hart RG, Pearce LA, Asinger RW, Herzog CA (2011) Warfarin in atrial fibrillation patients with moderate chronic kidney disease. Clin J Am Soc Nephrol 6: 2599–2604. CJN.02400311 [pii];10.2215/CJN.02400311 [doi].
8. Olesen JB, Lip GY, Kamper AL, Hommel K, Kober L, et al. (2012) Stroke and bleeding in atrial fibrillation with chronic kidney disease. N Engl J Med 367: 625–635. 10.1056/NEJMoa1105594 [doi].
9. Camm AJ, Lip GY, De CR, Savelieva I, Atar D, et al. (2012) 2012 focused update of the ESC Guidelines for the management of atrial fibrillation: an update of the 2010 ESC Guidelines for the management of atrial fibrillation—developed with the special contribution of the European Heart Rhythm Association. Europace 14: 1385–1413. eus305 [pii];10.1093/europace/eus305 [doi].
10. Abdelhafiz AH, Myint MP, Tayek JA, Wheeldon NM (2009) Anemia, hypoalbuminemia, and renal impairment as predictors of bleeding complications in patients receiving anticoagulation therapy for nonvalvular atrial fibrillation: a secondary analysis. Clin Ther 31: 1534–1539. S0149-2918(09)00228-8 [pii];10.1016/j.clinthera.2009.07.015 [doi].
11. Ng KP, Edwards NC, Lip GY, Townend JN, Ferro CJ (2013) Atrial Fibrillation in CKD: Balancing the Risks and Benefits of Anticoagulation. Am J Kidney Dis. S0272-6386(13)00784-1 [pii];10.1053/j.ajkd.2013.02.381 [doi].
12. Lai HM, Aronow WS, Kalen P, Adapa S, Patel K, et al. (2009) Incidence of thromboembolic stroke and of major bleeding in patients with atrial fibrillation and chronic kidney disease treated with and without warfarin. Int J Nephrol Renovasc Dis 2: 33–37.
13. Roldan V, Marin F, Fernandez H, Manzano-Fernandez S, Gallego P, et al. (2013) Renal impairment in a "real-life" cohort of anticoagulated patients with atrial fibrillation (implications for thromboembolism and bleeding). Am J Cardiol 111: 1159–1164. S0002-9149(12)02648-3 [pii];10.1016/j.amjcard.2012.12.045 [doi].
14. Wieloch M, Jonsson KM, Sjalander A, Lip GY, Eriksson N, et al. (2013) Estimated glomerular filtration rate is associated with major bleeding complications but not thromboembolic events, in anticoagulated patients taking warfarin. Thromb Res 131: 481–486. S0049-3848(13)00008-X [pii];10.1016/j.thromres.2013.01.006 [doi].
15. Levey AS, Coresh J, Greene T, Stevens LA, Zhang YL, et al. (2006) Using standardized serum creatinine values in the modification of diet in renal disease study equation for estimating glomerular filtration rate. Ann Intern Med 145: 247–254. 145/4/247 [pii].
16. Pottelbergh van G, Van HL, Mathei C, Degryse J (2010) Methods to evaluate renal function in elderly patients: a systematic literature review. Age Ageing 39: 542–548. afq091 [pii];10.1093/ageing/afq091 [doi].
17. Schulman S, Kearon C (2005) Definition of major bleeding in clinical investigations of antihemostatic medicinal products in non-surgical patients. J Thromb Haemost 3: 692–694. JTH1204 [pii];10.1111/j.1538-7836.2005.01204.x [doi].

18. Klok FA, Zondag W, van Kralingen KW, van Dijk AP, Tamsma JT, et al. (2010) Patient outcomes after acute pulmonary embolism. A pooled survival analysis of different adverse events. Am J Respir Crit Care Med 181: 501–506. 200907-1141OC [pii];10.1164/rccm.200907-1141OC [doi].
19. Amouyel P, Mismetti P, Langkilde LK, Jasso-Mosqueda G, Nelander K, et al. (2009) INR variability in atrial fibrillation: a risk model for cerebrovascular events. Eur J Intern Med 20: 63–69. S0953-6205(08)00136-2 [pii];10.1016/j.ejim.2008.04.005 [doi].
20. Cannegieter SC, Rosendaal FR, Wintzen AR, van der Meer FJ, Vandenbroucke JP, et al. (1995) Optimal oral anticoagulant therapy in patients with mechanical heart valves. N Engl J Med 333: 11–17. 10.1056/NEJM199507063330103 [doi].
21. Hylek EM, Go AS, Chang Y, Jensvold NG, Henault LE, et al. (2003) Effect of intensity of oral anticoagulation on stroke severity and mortality in atrial fibrillation. N Engl J Med 349: 1019–1026. 10.1056/NEJMoa022913 [doi];349/11/1019 [pii].
22. Reynolds MW, Fahrbach K, Hauch O, Wygant G, Estok R, et al. (2004) Warfarin anticoagulation and outcomes in patients with atrial fibrillation: a systematic review and metaanalysis. Chest 126: 1938–1945. 126/6/1938 [pii];10.1378/chest.126.6.1938 [doi].
23. Rosendaal FR, Cannegieter SC, van der Meer FJ, Briet E (1993) A method to determine the optimal intensity of oral anticoagulant therapy. Thromb Haemost 69: 236–239.
24. Leeuwen van Y, Rosendaal FR, Cannegieter SC (2008) Prediction of hemorrhagic and thrombotic events in patients with mechanical heart valve prostheses treated with oral anticoagulants. J Thromb Haemost 6: 451–456. JTH2874 [pii];10.1111/j.1538-7836.2007.02874.x [doi].
25. Ibrahim S, Jespersen J, Poller L (2013) The clinical evaluation of International Normalized Ratio variability and control in conventional oral anticoagulant administration by use of the variance growth rate. J Thromb Haemost 11: 1540–1546. 10.1111/jth.12322 [doi].
26. Dreisbach AW, Lertora JJ (2003) The effect of chronic renal failure on hepatic drug metabolism and drug disposition. Semin Dial 16: 45–50. 3011 [pii].
27. Leblond F, Guevin C, Demers C, Pellerin I, Gascon-Barre M, et al. (2001) Downregulation of hepatic cytochrome P450 in chronic renal failure. J Am Soc Nephrol 12: 326–332.
28. Bachmann K, Shapiro R, Mackiewicz J (1976) Influence of renal dysfunction on warfarin plasma protein binding. J Clin Pharmacol 16: 468–472.
29. Bachmann K, Shapiro R, Mackiewicz J (1977) Warfarin elimination and responsiveness in patients with renal dysfunction. J Clin Pharmacol 17: 292–299.
30. Ibrahim S, Jespersen J, Poller L (2013) The clinical evaluation of International Normalized Ratio variability and control in conventional oral anticoagulant administration by use of the variance growth rate. J Thromb Haemost 11: 1540–1546. 10.1111/jth.12322 [doi].
31. Beyth RJ, Quinn L, Landefeld CS (2000) A multicomponent intervention to prevent major bleeding complications in older patients receiving warfarin. A randomized, controlled trial. Ann Intern Med 133: 687–695. 200011070-00010 [pii].
32. Hart RG, Eikelboom JW, Brimble KS, McMurtry MS, Ingram AJ (2013) Stroke prevention in atrial fibrillation patients with chronic kidney disease. Can J Cardiol 29: S71–S78. S0828-282X(13)00222-5 [pii];10.1016/j.cjca.2013.04.005 [doi].
33. Connolly SJ, Ezekowitz MD, Yusuf S, Eikelboom J, Oldgren J, et al. (2009) Dabigatran versus warfarin in patients with atrial fibrillation. N Engl J Med 361: 1139–1151. NEJMoa0905561 [pii];10.1056/NEJMoa0905561 [doi].
34. Patel MR, Mahaffey KW, Garg J, Pan G, Singer DE, et al. (2011) Rivaroxaban versus warfarin in nonvalvular atrial fibrillation. N Engl J Med 365: 883–891. 10.1056/NEJMoa1009638 [doi].
35. Granger CB, Alexander JH, McMurray JJ, Lopes RD, Hylek EM, et al. (2011) Apixaban versus warfarin in patients with atrial fibrillation. N Engl J Med 365: 981–992. 10.1056/NEJMoa1107039 [doi].
36. Connolly SJ, Eikelboom J, Dorian P, Hohnloser SH, Gretler DD, et al. (2013) Betrixaban compared with warfarin in patients with atrial fibrillation: results of a phase 2, randomized, dose-ranging study (Explore-Xa). Eur Heart J 34: 1498–1505. eht039 [pii];10.1093/eurheartj/eht039 [doi].

Effect of HDL-Raising Drugs on Cardiovascular Outcomes

Navjot Kaur[1¶], Avaneesh Pandey[1¶], Harish Negi[1¶], Nusrat Shafiq[1*], Srinivas Reddy[2], Harpreet Kaur[3], Neelima Chadha[4], Samir Malhotra[1]

1 Department of Pharmacology, Post Graduate Institute of Medical Education & Research, Chandigarh, India, **2** Department of Cardiology, Post Graduate Institute of Medical Education & Research, Chandigarh, India, **3** ICMR- Advanced centre for evidence based child health, Advance Paediatric Centre, Post Graduate Institute of Medical Education & Research, Chandigarh, India, **4** Dr. Tulsi Das Library, Post Graduate Institute of Medical Education & Research, Chandigarh, India

Abstract

Background: Substantial residual cardiovascular risk remains after optimal LDL lowering in patients of established coronary artery disease. A number of therapeutic agents that raise HDL-C have been tested in clinical trials to cover this risk. However, the results of clinical trials are conflicting.

Objectives: To determine whether raising HDL-C with pharmacologic therapies translates into beneficial cardiovascular outcomes and to find out if this change was proportional to the percentage change in HDL levels.

Methods: Electronic and printed sources were searched up to August, 2013 for randomised controlled trials (RCTs) using at least one of the HDL raising therapies for secondary prevention of adverse cardiovascular events over optimal LDL levels. Data from eligible studies were pooled for the following outcomes: all cause mortality, cardiovascular disease mortality, hospitalization for unstable angina, non-fatal myocardial infarction, coronary revascularization and ischemic stroke. Mantel Haensnzel fixed effect model was used preferentially. Meta-regression was done to see the correlation of change in HDL levels and cardiovascular outcomes. Pooled odds ratios with 95% confidence interval (CI) were calculated.

Results: A total of 12 RCTs including 26,858 patients with follow up period ranging from 1 year to 6.2 years were included in the analysis. Pooled analysis showed no significant difference in all-cause mortality between the treatment and control group (Pooled OR 1.07; 95% CI 0.98–1.16, $p = 0.15$). No significant difference was found between the groups for any of the secondary outcomes. Similarly no correlation was seen between percentage change in HDL and adverse cardiovascular outcomes on meta-regression analysis.

Conclusion: Increasing HDL levels via pharmacological manipulation beyond optimal lipid lowering therapy for secondary prevention is not beneficial.

Editor: Christina Bursill, Heart Research Institute, Australia

Funding: The authors have no support or funding to report.

Competing Interests: The authors have declared that no competing interests exist.

* E-mail: nusha.pgl2302@yahoo.com

¶ These authors contributed equally to this work.

Introduction

High level of low density lipoprotein cholesterol (LDL) is a well-established risk factor for increased cardiovascular morbidity and mortality. Lowering of LDL levels with pharmacotherapeutic agents leads to a significant reduction in cardiovascular events. However, even after lowering LDL levels to currently recommended targets; patients still remain at a substantial residual cardiovascular risk [1]. Further, low levels of high density lipoprotein (HDL) cholesterol (defined as <40 mg/dl in men and <50 mg/dl in women) have been identified as another critical risk factor for cardiovascular events independent of plasma LDL levels. As early as 1976, the Framingham heart study [2] showed an association between low HDL levels and increased cardiovascular mortality. This was supported by a large number of prospective epidemiological studies conducted thereafter. It has been shown that for every 1 mg/dl rise in HDL- cholesterol, the risk of developing cardiovascular diseases decreases by 2–3% [3–6].

Though regular exercise and moderate alcohol consumption which are reported to be atheroprotective, do increase HDL levels; this increase is modest [7,8]. Among drugs statins, fibrates and niacin raise HDL-C to the extent of about 5–10%, 10–20% and 30–40% respectively [9]. Statins are prescribed both for primary and secondary prevention of IHD, but the beneficial effects cannot be segregated to be accomplished by a decrease in LDL or an increase in HDL levels. Regular exercise is an integral component of lifestyle modification advised for primary and secondary prevention. Alcohol consumption on a chronic basis cannot be a part of the recommendations because of its ancillary effects. Therefore, intense research efforts have been devoted to develop therapeutic agents to primarily raise HDL-C with the therapeutic intent of covering the residual cardiovascular risk. Most important agents among these are the Cholesteryl ester transfer protein (CETP) Inhibitors (eg. anacetrapib, evacetrapib) which raise the plasma HDL levels to the extent of about 72–138% and some are currently in advanced stages of clinical development [10]. But the recent failure of AIM-HIGH trial, CETP inhibitors (torcetrapib, dalcetrapib) in large phase III clinical trials have put a question mark on the clinical utility of therapies aimed at raising HDL [12,13,21]. To find an answer to whether therapies raising HDL cholesterol (including niacin, fibrates and CETP inhibitors) confers cardiovascular benefit or not in patients with a history of cardiovascular disease, we conducted a systematic review and metanalysis. We performed a meta-analysis of all published RCTs which used HDL raising therapeutic agents (niacin, fibrates and CETP inhibitors) as monotherapy or co-administered with statins versus standard lipid lowering therapy in patients at high cardiovascular risk. Effects on mortality and other cardiovascular outcomes were evaluated. We also intended to further determine if this change was proportional to the percentage change in HDL levels for which we conducted a meta-regression analysis.

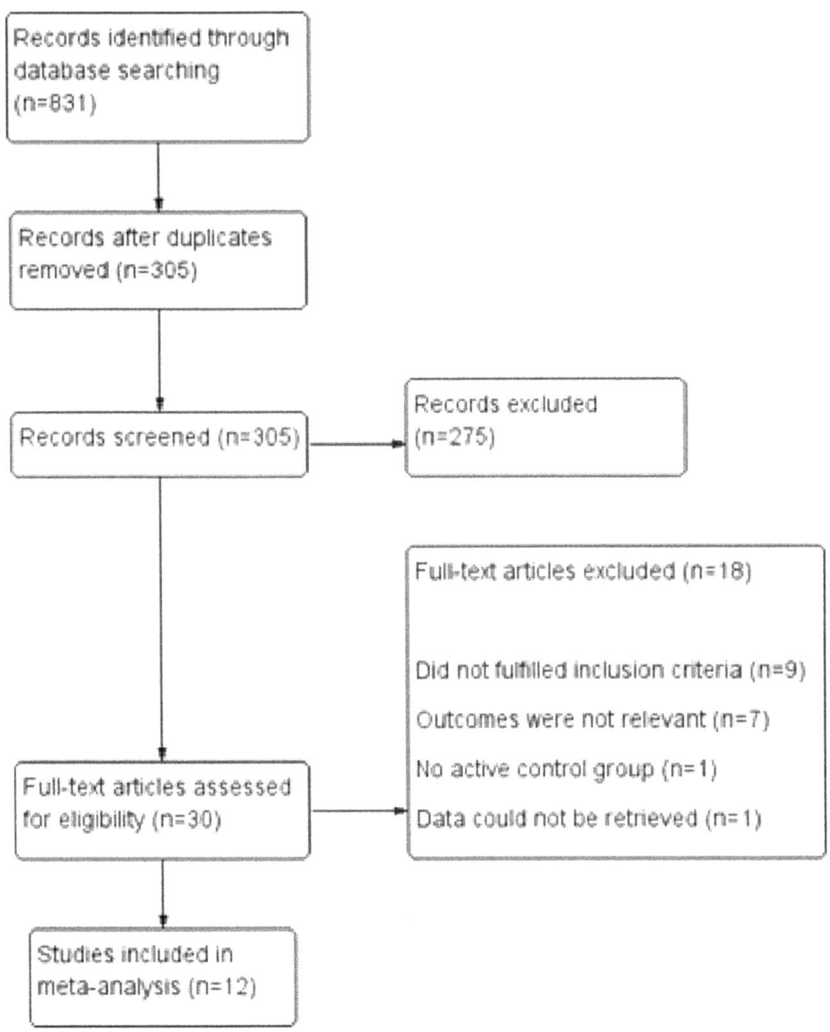

Figure 1. Study flow diagram.

Materials and Methods

Data sources, search strategy, and selection criteria

Randomized controlled trials using at least one of the HDL raising therapies for secondary prevention of adverse cardiovascular events over optimal LDL levels were eligible for inclusion in our meta-analysis. The search was limited to English-language literature only. Relevant trials were identified with the following procedure:

(1) **Electronic searches.** We searched the electronic databases Pubmed (File S1), EmBase, Ovid and the Cochrane Central Register of Controlled Trials for articles to a time limit of August 2013, using "niacin", "clofibrate", "fenofibrate", "gemfibrozil", "bezafibrate", "CETP inhibitors", "torcetrapib", "dalcetrapib", "evacetrapib", "anacetrapib", "cardiovascular disease" and "randomized controlled trial" as the search terms. All reference lists from reports on non-randomized controlled trials were searched manually for additional eligible studies.

(2) **Other sources.** In addition, we searched for ongoing randomized controlled trials, which had been registered as completed but not yet published, in the Meta Register of Controlled Trials. Medical subject headings and methods, patient population, and intervention were used to identify

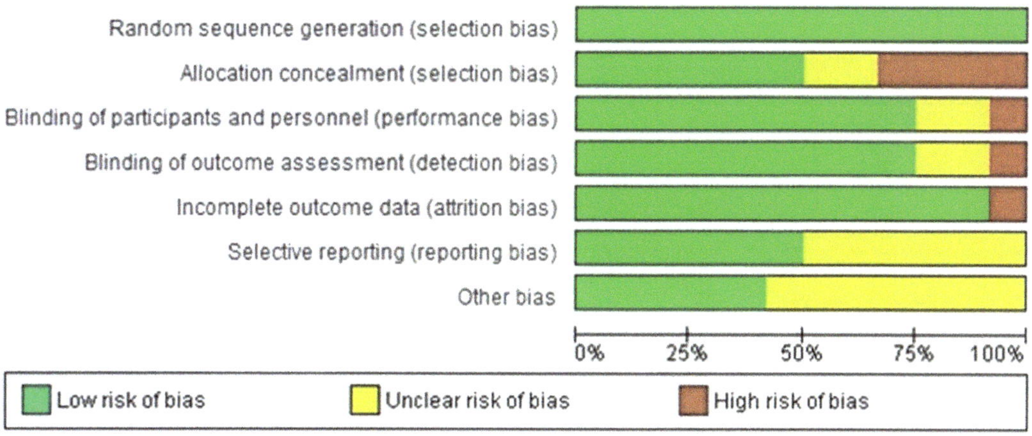

Figure 2. Risk of bias graph.

relevant trials. This review was conducted and reported according to the PRISMA (Preferred Reporting Items for Systematic Reviews and Meta-Analysis) Statement issued in 2009 [11].

The literature search was undertaken independently by two authors (H.K, N.C) with a standardized approach, and any disagreement between these 2 authors was settled by a third author (N.K) until a consensus was reached. Only those randomized clinical trials were included in the study in which patients with a history of cardiovascular disease received at least one of the HDL raising agents for prevention of cardiovascular events.

Inclusion/Exclusion criteria

Only those randomized clinical trials were included in the study in which patients with a history of cardiovascular disease received at least one of the HDL raising agents for prevention of cardiovascular events. The control arm should have had an intervention which would permit appropriate attribution of the results to HDL targeting drug. The included participants should have had LDL levels not warranting drug therapy or were lowered to the current optimum by use of statins.

Exclusion criteria were the following:

(i) Studies not reporting cardiovascular events as an outcome,
(ii) Primary prevention trials,
(iii) Studies where a combination of HDL raising drugs was used,
(iv) Studies where LDL levels were not considered/mentioned in the inclusion criteria.

Data extraction

Data extraction forms were used to obtain the following information: characteristics of study participants, number of participants, type of intervention (dose, duration), randomization, blinding, study outcomes and duration of follow-up. The data were extracted independently by two investigators and compiled by a third investigator. Differences in data extraction were resolved by consensus, referring back to the original article.

For trials in which data were not expressed in desired format for pooling, such information was extracted from data given in the published report. An attempt was made to obtain the data from authors if this could not be carried out.

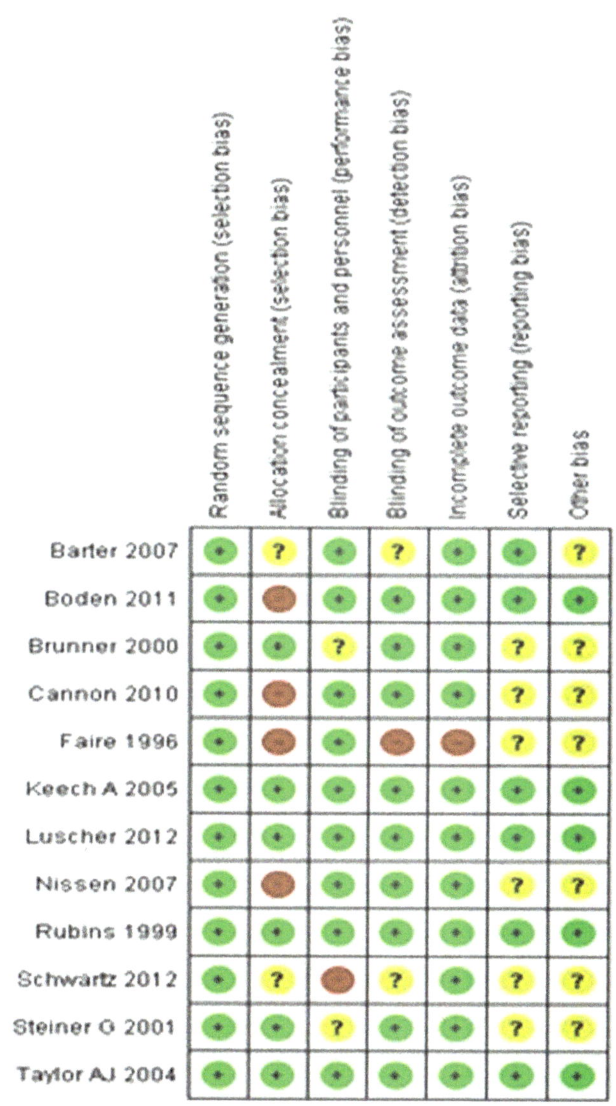

Figure 3. Risk of bias summary.

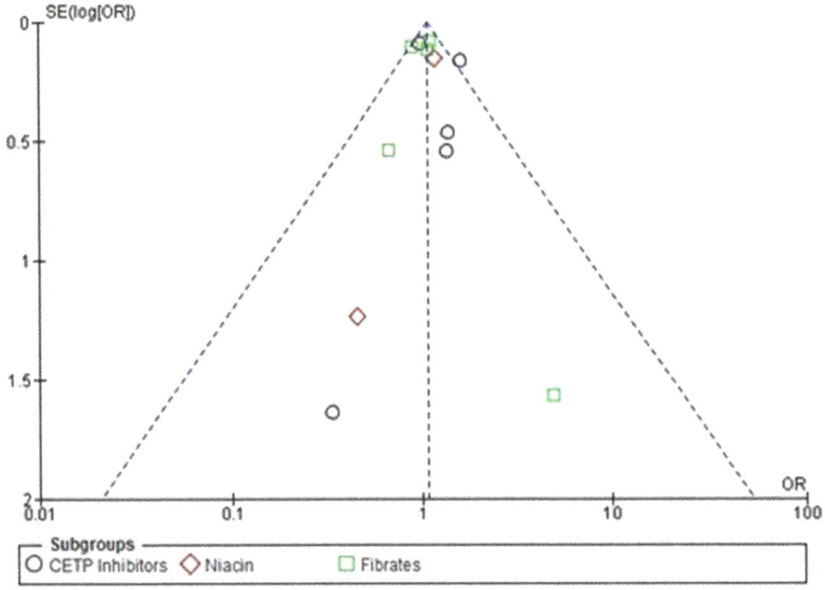

Figure 4. Funnel plot of primary endpoint (total mortality).

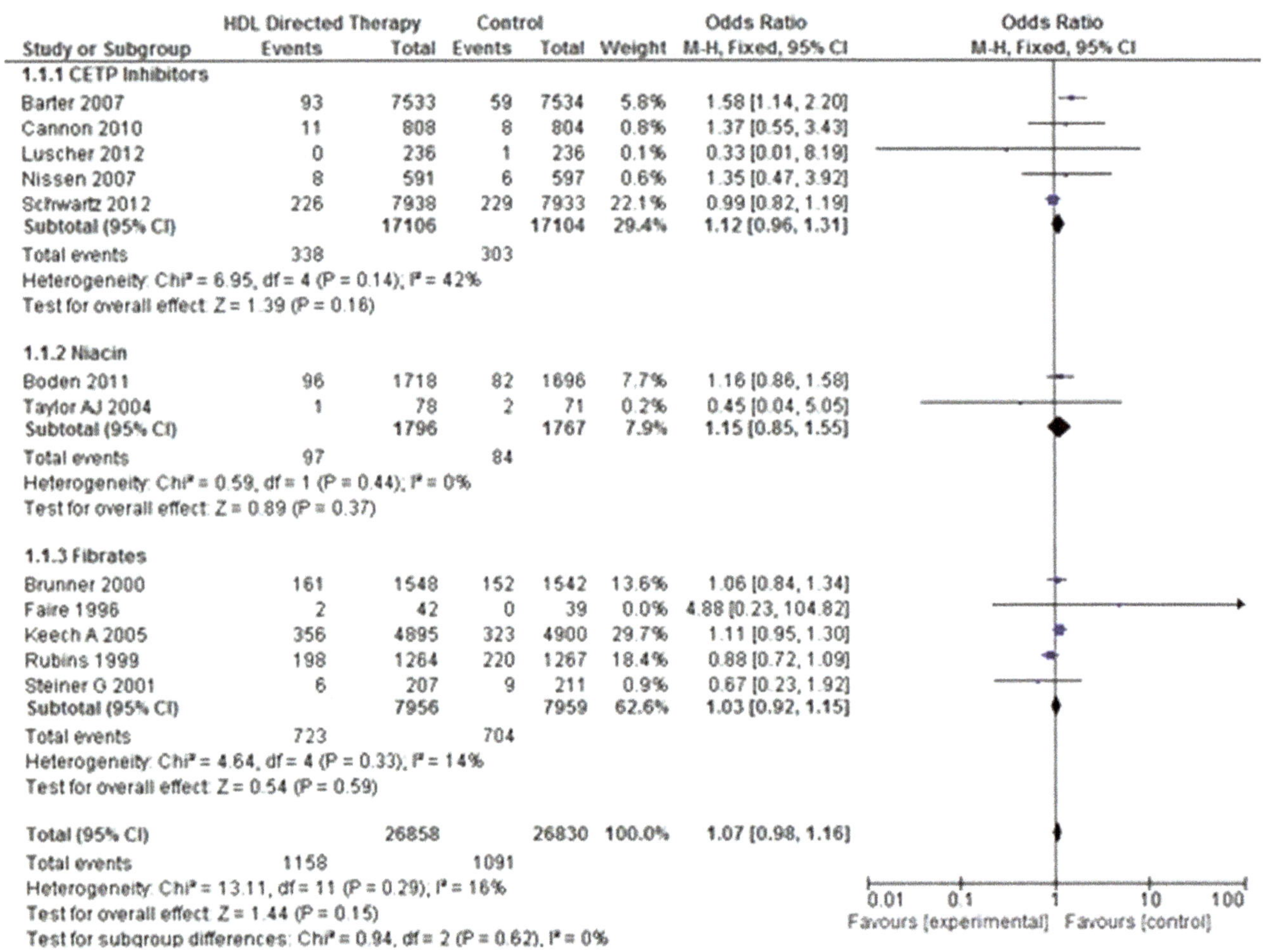

Figure 5. Total mortality in HDL targeted therapies versus control group using pooled odds ratio.

Study outcomes

The primary endpoint for our study was total mortality (death due to any cause). Secondary outcomes included cardiovascular mortality, non-fatal myocardial infarction, hospitalization for unstable angina, coronary revascularization and ischaemic stroke.

For all evaluated variables, subgroup analysis was undertaken as per the class of HDL raising agents. Meta-regression was done to see the effect of percentage change in HDL levels and its impact on hard cardiovascular end points.

Assessment of Study Quality

The quality of included RCTs was assessed based on Cochrane handbook of systematic reviews, by recording seven items of bias risk: random sequence generation, allocation concealment, blinding of participants and personnel, blinding of outcome assessment, incomplete outcome data addressed, free of selective reporting, and free of other bias. Each of the seven items is scored as "low risk," "unclear risk," or "high risk."

Data Analysis

Quantitative variables were expressed as mean ± S.D, while qualitative variables were expressed as n (%). Authors were contacted if some data was missing or not in the form to be pooled. The data from various studies were pooled and expressed as odds ratio (OR) with 95% confidence interval (CI). The separate forest plots were constructed for pooled study outcomes. Pooling of data was planned if two or more studies had used the same outcome and expressed the data in the format to enable pooling. To avoid potential clinical heterogeneity we formed homogeneous groups of studies according to class of HDL raising agents and used these as subcategories. Statistical heterogeneity was assessed with chi square test and the magnitude of heterogeneity was assessed with I^2 statistics. $I^2 \geq 50\%$ was considered to be representative of high heterogeneity. Sensitivity analysis was performed by excluding the high risk studies from analysis. The data were pooled by random effect model in case of significant heterogeneity otherwise fixed effect model was used. The meta-analysis was performed by Review Manager (REVMAN) software, version 5.2 (The Cochrane Collaboration, Denmark). Publication bias was assessed by visual inspection of the inverted funnel plot.

For meta-regression, percentage HDL change was calculated in both control and treatment group and expressed as odds ratio (OR) with 95% confidence limit. Separate meta-regression plots were generated to assess the impact of percentage change in HDL over cardiovascular outcomes. Random effect analysis was preferred to overcome any possibility of residual heterogeneity. Meta-regression was performed by MetaAnalyst 3.1 beta.

Study or Subgroup	HDL Directed Therapy Events	Total	Control Events	Total	Weight	Odds Ratio M-H, Fixed, 95% CI
1.2.1 CETP inhibitors						
Barter 2007	40	7533	33	7534	5.4%	1.21 [0.76, 1.93]
Cannon 2010	4	808	1	804	0.2%	4.00 [0.45, 35.82]
Luscher 2012	0	236	1	236	0.2%	0.33 [0.01, 8.19]
Nissen 2007	1	591	1	597	0.2%	1.01 [0.06, 16.19]
Schwartz 2012	118	7938	125	7933	20.2%	0.94 [0.73, 1.21]
Subtotal (95% CI)		**17106**		**17104**	**26.2%**	**1.01 [0.81, 1.26]**
Total events	163		161			
Heterogeneity: Chi² = 2.86, df = 4 (P = 0.58); I² = 0%						
Test for overall effect: Z = 0.11 (P = 0.91)						
1.2.2 Niacin						
Boden 2011	96	1718	82	1696	12.8%	1.16 [0.86, 1.58]
Taylor AJ 2004	1	78	2	71	0.3%	0.45 [0.04, 5.05]
Subtotal (95% CI)		**1796**		**1767**	**13.1%**	**1.15 [0.85, 1.55]**
Total events	97		84			
Heterogeneity: Chi² = 0.59, df = 1 (P = 0.44); I² = 0%						
Test for overall effect: Z = 0.89 (P = 0.37)						
1.2.3 Fibrates						
Brunner 2000	95	1548	88	1542	13.6%	1.08 [0.80, 1.46]
Faire 1996	1	42	0	39	0.1%	2.86 [0.11, 72.19]
Keech A 2005	140	4895	127	4900	20.3%	1.11 [0.87, 1.41]
Rubins 1999	146	1264	184	1267	26.7%	0.77 [0.61, 0.97]
Subtotal (95% CI)		**7749**		**7748**	**60.7%**	**0.95 [0.82, 1.10]**
Total events	382		399			
Heterogeneity: Chi² = 5.84, df = 3 (P = 0.12); I² = 49%						
Test for overall effect: Z = 0.63 (P = 0.53)						
Total (95% CI)		**26651**		**26619**	**100.0%**	**0.99 [0.89, 1.11]**
Total events	642		644			
Heterogeneity: Chi² = 10.49, df = 10 (P = 0.40); I² = 5%						
Test for overall effect: Z = 0.09 (P = 0.93)						
Test for subgroup differences: Chi² = 1.20, df = 2 (P = 0.55), I² = 0%						

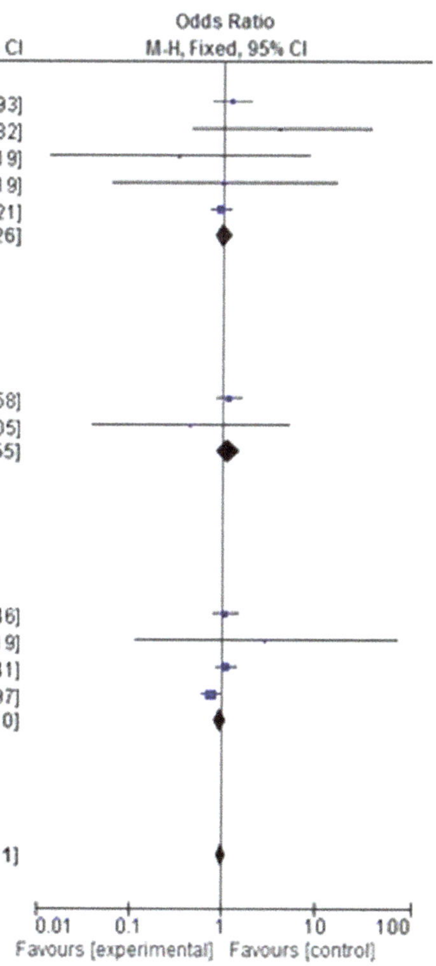

Figure 6. Cardiovascular disease mortality in HDL targeted therapies versus control group using pooled odds ratio.

Results

Description of included studies

831 hits were obtained after combining search of all selected databases. After excluding duplicate articles, thorough screening of titles & abstracts and searching of cross-references; 30 studies were found suitable for full text search. Out of these, 12 studies were considered for data extraction and quality assessment [12–23]. Other studies were excluded for following reasons: 9 studies did not fulfil the inclusion criteria, in 7 studies, outcomes were not relevant, one study did not have active control and from one study data could not be retrieved for analysis. (Figure 1) The included studies (n = 12) involved evaluation of 17,106 patients with CETP inhibitors, 1796 with niacin and 7956 with fibrates. The follow up period ranged from 1 year to 6.2 years. Characteristics of included studies are presented in (Table S1). The included studies involved 3 types of HDL raising agents (Niacin = 2, Fibrates = 5, CETP Inhibitor = 5). HDL raising agents were used as monotherapy in 6 studies, while in another 6 these were co-administered with statins.

Quality assessment results

According to quality assessment based on Cochrane handbook, we found that the studies largely had low or medium risk of bias except the study conducted by Faire et al, which had risk due to bias arising from allocation and blinding [16]. Irrespective of high risk study; sensitivity analysis revealed that this had no major influence on outcomes of analysis. The risk of bias graph and summary of included studies is given in Figure 2 and Figure 3. From the funnel plot, the presence of publication bias could not be ruled out. (Figure 4).

Primary Endpoint

1. *Total Mortality (Death due to any cause).* Twelve studies, including 53,721 participants were included in this analysis. No statistical heterogeneity was observed between studies. There was no significant difference in incidence of total mortality between treatment group and control group (Pooled OR 1.07; 95% CI 0.98–1.16, p = 0.15). In subgroup analysis no significant difference was observed with any class of drugs. (Figure 5).

Secondary Endpoints

1. *Cardiovascular Disease Mortality.* Eleven studies were included for this analysis. There was no significant difference in incidence of cardiovascular disease mortality between treatment group and control group (Pooled OR 0.99; 95% CI 0.89–1.11, p = 0.93). None of the subgroups indicated any significant difference in the outcome. (Figure 6).

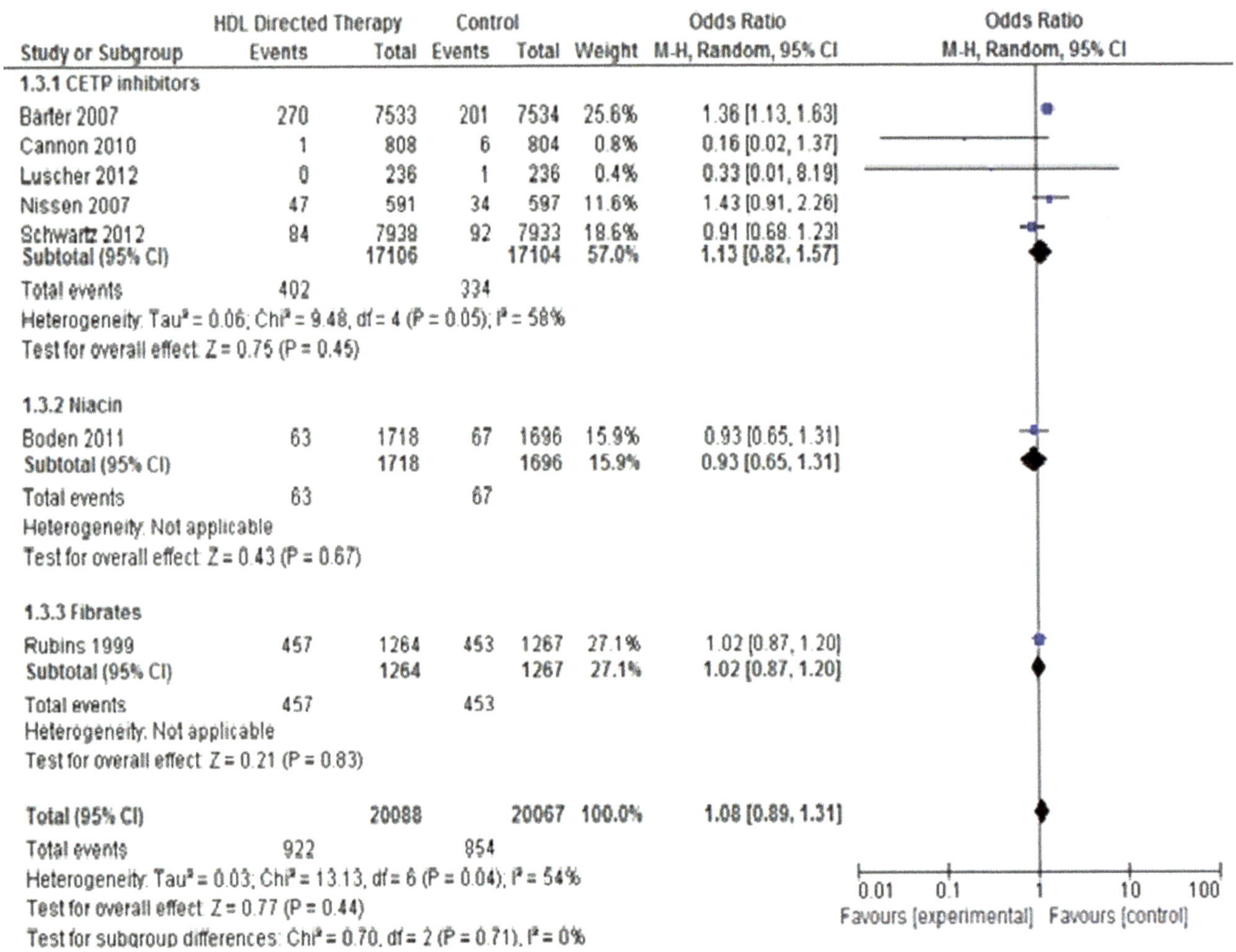

Figure 7. Hospitalizations for unstable angina in HDL targeted therapies versus control group using pooled odds ratio.

2. *Hospitalization for Unstable Angina.* Seven studies were included in this outcome. There was no significant difference between the treatment group and control group (Pooled OR 1.08; 95% CI 0.89–1.31, p = 0.44). No significant difference was found with any of the subgroups. (Figure 7).

3. *Nonfatal myocardial infarction.* Ten studies were included for this analysis. No significant difference was found in the incidence of non-fatal myocardial infarction between control and treatment group (Pooled OR 0.93; 95% CI 0.86–1.02, p = 0.11). Subgroup analysis, however, favoured fibrates for this outcome (Pooled OR 0.79; 95% CI 0.69–0.90, p = 0.0003). (Figure 8).

4. *Coronary revascularization.* Eight studies were included for this analysis. There was no significant difference in the incidence of total mortality between treatment group and control group (Pooled OR 0.93; 95% CI 0.77–1.12, p = 0.44). However, on subgroup analysis, significant difference was found favouring treatment group in Fibrate treated subjects (Pooled OR 0.85; 95% CI 0.72–1.00, p = 0.05). Two studies, Boden 2011 and Luscher 2012, showed no difference between the placebo group and the treatment group. In a study conducted by Boden 2011, 167 patients had coronary or cerebral revascularization in the treatment group as compared to 168 in the control group while in study by Luscher 2012, 9 had coronary and non-coronary revascularization in the treatment group and 7 in the control group. These studies were not pooled in the analysis because combined data were given for coronary revascularization with cerebral revascularizations and non-coronary revascularizations. (Figure 9).

5. *Ischemic stroke.* Six studies were included in this analysis. The pooled OR for ischemic stroke was (Pooled OR 1.00; 95% CI 0.78–1.30, p = 0.97) which shows no statistically significant difference between control and treatment group. In subgroup analysis, significant difference was found between two groups favouring treatment group in fibrate treated subjects (Pooled OR 0.79; 95% CI 0.69–0.92, p = 0.002). One study, Taylor 2004, could not be pooled because the author had not mentioned whether the stroke was ischemic or hemorrhagic. (Figure 10).

Sensitivity analysis

Sensitivity analysis of primary endpoint revealed no significant difference in incidence of total mortality between control and treatment group (Pooled OR 1.07; 95% CI 0.96–1.19, p = 0.21), therefore nullifying the impact of excluded study on primary analysis.

Correlation of percentage change in HDL with cardiovascular outcome

In the 13 trials included in the primary analysis, reporting outcome data for total mortality, only 6 were found suitable for random-effect meta-regression analysis as they provided a baseline

Study or Subgroup	HDL Directed Therapy Events	HDL Directed Therapy Total	Control Events	Control Total	Weight	Odds Ratio M-H, Fixed, 95% CI
1.4.1 CETP inhibitors						
Barter 2007	142	7533	118	7533	10.3%	1.21 [0.94, 1.54]
Cannon 2010	6	808	9	804	0.8%	0.66 [0.23, 1.87]
Luscher 2012	2	236	3	236	0.3%	0.66 [0.11, 4.01]
Nissen 2007	13	591	16	597	1.4%	0.82 [0.39, 1.71]
Schwartz 2012	414	7938	407	7933	34.2%	1.02 [0.88, 1.17]
Subtotal (95% CI)		**17106**		**17103**	**46.9%**	**1.05 [0.93, 1.18]**
Total events	577		553			
Heterogeneity: Chi² = 2.88, df = 4 (P = 0.58); I² = 0%						
Test for overall effect: Z = 0.72 (P = 0.47)						
1.4.2 Niacin						
Boden 2011	96	1718	82	1696	6.9%	1.16 [0.86, 1.58]
Subtotal (95% CI)		**1718**		**1696**	**6.9%**	**1.16 [0.86, 1.58]**
Total events	96		82			
Heterogeneity: Not applicable						
Test for overall effect: Z = 0.99 (P = 0.32)						
1.4.3 Fibrates						
Brunner 2000	150	1548	172	1542	13.8%	0.85 [0.68, 1.08]
Faire 1996	1	42	3	39	0.3%	0.29 [0.03, 2.94]
Keech A 2005	158	4895	207	4900	17.7%	0.76 [0.61, 0.93]
Rubins 1999	146	1264	184	1267	14.4%	0.77 [0.61, 0.97]
Subtotal (95% CI)		**7749**		**7748**	**46.2%**	**0.79 [0.69, 0.90]**
Total events	455		566			
Heterogeneity: Chi² = 1.37, df = 3 (P = 0.71); I² = 0%						
Test for overall effect: Z = 3.64 (P = 0.0003)						
Total (95% CI)		**26573**		**26547**	**100.0%**	**0.93 [0.86, 1.02]**
Total events	1128		1201			
Heterogeneity: Chi² = 16.42, df = 9 (P = 0.06); I² = 45%						
Test for overall effect: Z = 1.59 (P = 0.11)						
Test for subgroup differences: Chi² = 12.23, df = 2 (P = 0.002), I² = 83.7%						

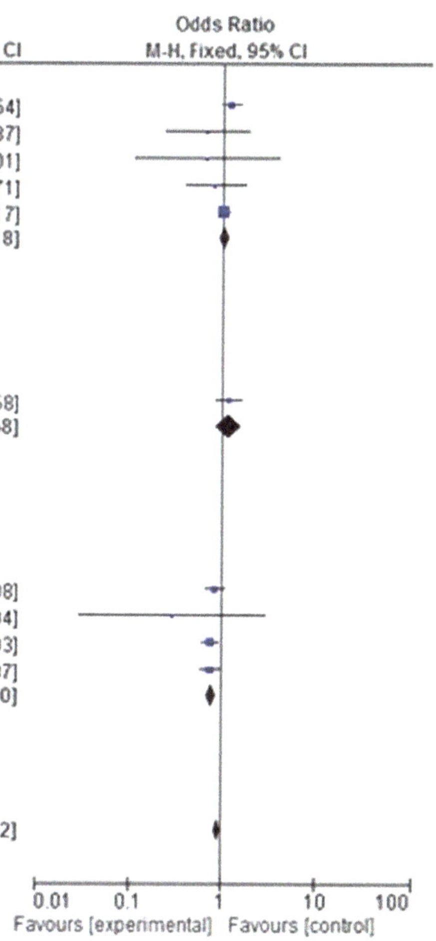

Figure 8. Non-fatal myocardial infarction in HDL targeted therapies versus control group using pooled odds ratio.

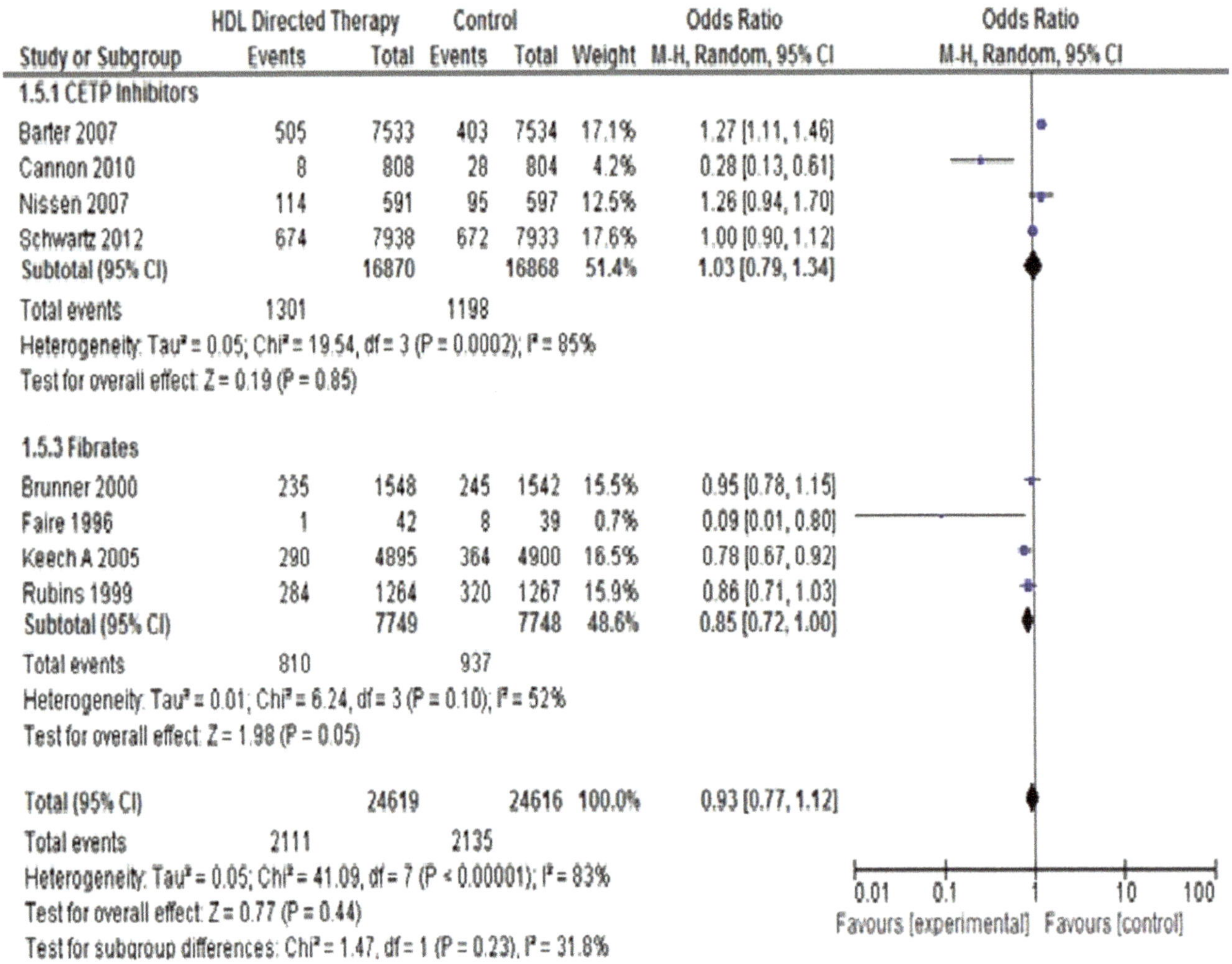

Figure 9. Coronary revascularisation in HDL targeted therapies versus control group using pooled odds ratio.

and post treatment measures of HDL [12,13,15,17,19,23]. No significant association was found between the percentage change in HDL and the odds ratio for total mortality (B = 0.004, p = 0.345). (Figure 11) 6 studies reported outcome data for cardiovascular mortality thus included for random-effect meta-regression analysis [12,13,15,17,19,21]. (Figure 12) For the above studies no significant correlation was found between the percentage change in HDL and cardiovascular mortality (B = 0.011, p = 0.43). The Meta - regression analysis included only 5 studies for non-fatal myocardial infarction [12,13,15,17,19]. (Figure 13) Similar absence of correlation was noted for this outcome as well (B = −0.002, p = 0.54).

Adverse Events

Adverse events could not be pooled for analysis as the included studies defined and reported these differently. Among the CETP inhibitors, however hypertension was the most important adverse event associated with torcetrapib use as compared to the control arm (18.7% vs 7.5%; p = 0.001) [12]. Such adverse events were not significantly associated with other CETP inhibitors i.e. dalcetrapib and anacetrapib [15,18]. Use of niacin led to significantly higher number of discontinuation of study drug and need of dose reductions as compared to the control arm due to higher incidences of skin flushing or itching (341 vs 436; p = 0.001) [12]. Among fibrates, use of fenofibrate was found to be associated with higher risk of pancreatitis (23 vs 40; p = 0.031), pulmonary embolism (32 vs 53; p = 0.022) and deep vein thrombosis (48 vs 67; p = 0.074), [16] while gemfibrozil led to significantly higher number of complaints of dyspepsia as compared to control arm (34% vs 40%; p = 0.002) [20].

Discussion

A number of epidemiological and experimental studies showed a consistent inverse relationship between the HDL and adverse cardiovascular outcomes [3–6]. Since then, a number of clinical trials have been conducted with HDL raising therapies to manage the residual cardiovascular risk that remains beyond the optimal statin therapy. However, the clinical trial results were conflicting to each other e.g. the Coronary Drug Project supported that niacin can reduce adverse cardiovascular events including mortality [25], whereas the AIM-HIGH trial was prematurely terminated on grounds of futility and concerns regarding increased risk of stroke with niacin [13]. Similar results were seen with a novel class of HDL raising therapies i.e. CETP inhibitors, two of which (Torcetrapib and Dalcetrapib), not only failed to reduce cardiovascular risk, but on the other hand, increased cardiovascular morbidity and mortality [12,21]. These contrary and conflicting

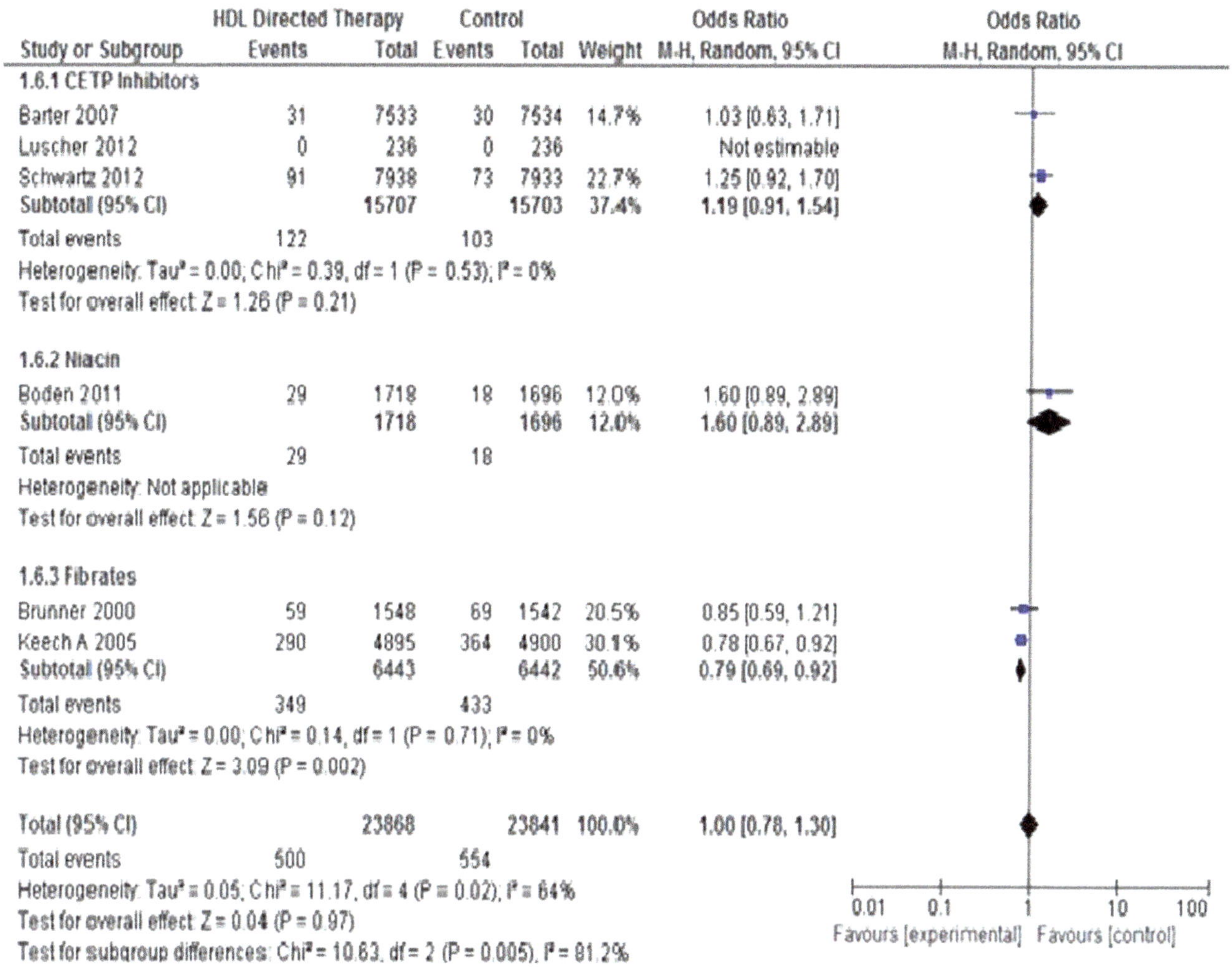

Figure 10. Ischaemic stroke in HDL targeted therapies versus control group using pooled odds ratio.

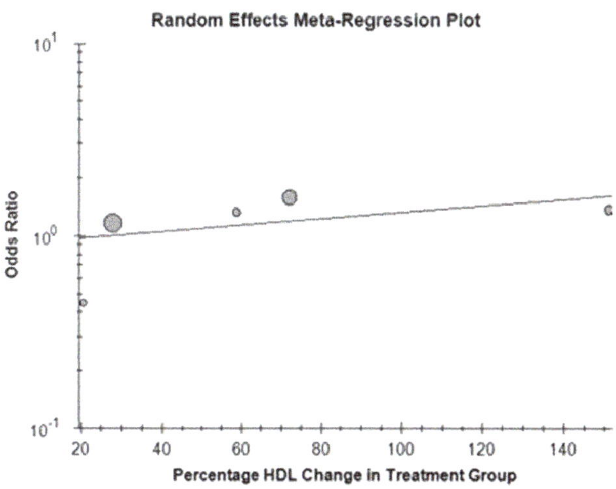

Figure 11. Total morality with percentage change in HDL.

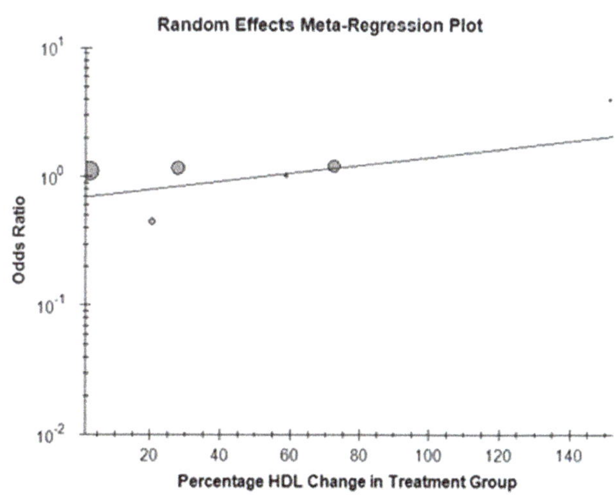

Figure 12. Cardiovascular mortality with percentage change in HDL.

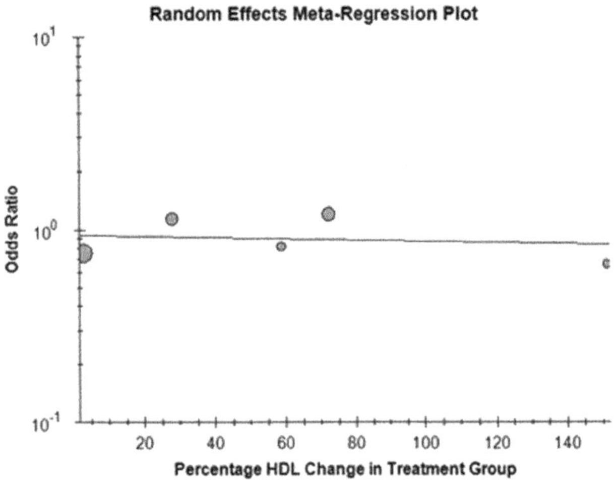

Figure 13. Non-fatal myocardial infarction with percentage change in HDL.

results from large clinical trials have raised a debate on how good is good cholesterol.

The present meta-analysis is important and relevant as it answers that whether increasing HDL levels (surrogate marker) through varied pharmacological interventions, actually translate into some clinically beneficial outcome for the patient or not (true endpoint) based on the currently available evidence. Previous reviews too addressed this question [24–26]. These were either only narrative reviews [24] or addressed different research questions like analysing the lipid modifying effects of different classes of HDL raising therapies separately [25,26] and also did not assess the effect of such change on hard cardiovascular endpoints which are more relevant for the clinician to make informed decisions for improving individual patient care [26].

In our study, we found no statistically significant difference on primary endpoint of all cause mortality in the control group versus the intervention group. Similar results were found in subgroup analysis for different classes of HDL raising agents versus the total mortality. For secondary outcomes, including cardiovascular mortality, hospitalization for unstable angina, non-fatal MI, coronary revascularisation and ischemic stroke; we found no significant differences between the two groups. However, subgroup analysis revealed that use of fibrates is associated with significantly lower incidence of non- fatal MI, coronary revascularisation and ischaemic stroke. The benefits of fibrates could be due to the additional benefit of fibrates in triglycerides. This could be a possibly because two of the included studies were exclusively in diabetic patients [17,22]. On the other hand, CETP inhibitors besides failing to demonstrate any benefit were associated with increased incidence of hospitalization due to unstable angina. The reasons for such an observation could be an increase in the incidence of hypertension and electrolyte imbalance that were reported in the torcetrapib group previously [12]. Similarly dalcetrapib was also reported to increase median C reactive protein levels to an extent of 18%, which might indicate a pro-inflammatory treatment effect in itself [21]. It has been suggested that inhibition of CETP might generate HDL particles that are either non-functional or proatherogenic. Another possibility is that HDL particles are protective in healthy individuals, but their composition is altered in individuals with cardiovascular disease in such a way that they remain no more productive at high levels or after therapeutic intervention [21].

There was possible heterogeneity in the combined estimate of cardiovascular outcomes due to some pre-specified subgroups of different classes of HDL raising agents. Although more appropriate information was obtained by the use of random effect model wherever statistical heterogeneity existed. Our sensitivity analysis, done by removing one study [16] demonstrated no difference on cardiovascular outcomes, hence making the findings of primary analysis more robust. Included studies in the present analysis were conducted between the time span of fifteen years from 1996 to 2012, and the importance of HDL cholesterol as a significant risk factor has been considered during this period. While the NCEP ATP II guidelines recommended HDL cholesterol level of <35 mg/dL as major and independent risk factor of coronary heart disease, ATP III recommends raising categorically low HDL cholesterol to <40 mg/dL.

Regarding adverse effect profile, CETP inhibitors were always a focus of concern due to possibility of their other off-target effects or per-se adverse effects of CETP inhibition. Torcetrapib was mainly associated with increased systolic blood pressure, but the differences were not statistically significant. Its specific molecular structure could be responsible for BP elevation along with CETP inhibition, as similar effects were not observed with other molecules of same class such as dalcetrapib and anacetrapib [27]. Study using niacin revealed higher number of discontinuation of study drug and need of dose reduction in treatment group. Amongst reason for discontinuation flushing, itching, increased glucose level and gastrointestinal symptoms were found significant. Although fenofibrate and gemfibrozil were generally well tolerated and appeared safe in included studies, it is important to monitor their long term safety profiles. Apart from pancreatitis, which is already reported with fenofibrate, small excess of venous thromboembolic events were observed in one of the included study [17].

In our exploratory meta-regression analysis, we found no significant association between the percentage rise in HDL levels and a reduction in adverse cardiovascular outcomes. Thus, we conclude that increasing HDL levels via pharmacological manipulation over and above optimal lipid therapy with statins is not beneficial in terms of reducing adverse cardiovascular outcomes. Large numbers of trials are recommended for meta-regression to be scientifically useful [28]. This may hence be considered as a limitation of our study. Results from ongoing large phase III trials of anacetrapib and evacetrapib are still awaited. How the results of these trials would alter the current evidence base needs to be seen in the future.

Though not evaluated in our study some explanations exist for the lack of association of increase in HDL and cardiovascular outcomes. It has been noted that functionality and change in HDL sub-fractions may be more important determinants of cardiovascular risk [29]. Analysis of the same was not the objective of our study. However, this may be undertaken as more evidence appears for the same.

Supporting Information

Table S1 Characteristics of included studies.

Checklist S1 PRISMA 2009 Checklist.

File S1 Search strategy.

Author Contributions

Conceived and designed the experiments: NS SM. Performed the experiments: NK NS AP HN HK NC SR SM. Analyzed the data: NK NS AP HN SR SM. Contributed reagents/materials/analysis tools: NK NS AP HN HK NC SR SM. Wrote the paper: NK AP HN NS SM.

References

1. Lim S, Park YM, Sakuma I, Koh KK (2013) How to control residual cardiovascular risk despite statin treatment: focusing on HDL-cholesterol. Int J Cardiol 166: 8–14.
2. Gordon T, Castelli WP, Hjortland MC, Kannel WB, Dawber TR (1977) High density lipoprotein as a protective factor against coronary heart disease. The Framingham Study. Am J Med 62: 707–714.
3. Gordon DJ, Probstfield JL, Garrison RJ, Neaton JD, Castelli WP, et al. (1989) High-density lipoprotein cholesterol and cardiovascular disease. Four prospective American studies. Circulation 79: 8–15.
4. Barter P, Gotto AM, LaRosa JC, Maroni J, Szarek M, et al. (2007) HDL cholesterol, very low levels of LDL cholesterol, and cardiovascular events. N Engl J Med 357: 1301–1310.
5. Assmann G, Schulte H (1988) The Prospective Cardiovascular Munster (PROCAM) study: prevalence of hyperlipidemia in persons with hypertension and/or diabetes mellitus and the relationship to coronary heart disease. Am Heart J 116: 1713–1724.
6. Toth PP (2005) Cardiology patient page. The "good cholesterol": high-density lipoprotein. Circulation 111: e89–91.
7. Blazek A, Rutsky J, Osei K, Maiseyeu A, Rajagopalan S (2013) Exercise-mediated changes in high-density lipoprotein: impact on form and function. Am Heart J 166: 392–400.
8. De Oliveira ESER, Foster D, McGee Harper M, Seidman CE, Smith JD, et al. (2000) Alcohol consumption raises HDL cholesterol levels by increasing the transport rate of apolipoproteins A-I and A-II. Circulation 102: 2347–2352.
9. Mahley RW, Bersot TP (2011) Drug therapy for hypercholesterolemia and dyslipidemia. In: Bruton L, Lazo JS, Parker KL, editors. Goodman and Gilman's The Pharmacological Basis of Therapeutics.Newyork: McGraw Hill Companies. p949.
10. Shinkai H (2012) Cholesteryl ester transfer-protein modulator and inhibitors and their potential for the treatment of cardiovascular diseases. Vasc Health Risk Manag 8: 323–331.
11. Moher D, Liberati A, Tetzlaff J, Altman DG (2009) Preferred reporting items for systematic reviews and meta-analyses: the PRISMA statement. PLoS Med 6: e1000097.
12. Barter PJ, Caulfield M, Eriksson M, Grundy SM, Kastelein JJ, et al. (2007) Effects of torcetrapib in patients at high risk for coronary events. N Engl J Med 357: 2109–2122.
13. Boden WE, Probstfield JL, Anderson T, Chaitman BR, Desvignes-Nickens P, et al. (2011) Niacin in patients with low HDL cholesterol levels receiving intensive statin therapy. N Engl J Med 365: 2255–2267.
14. Brunner D, Agmon J, Kaplinsky E (2000) Secondary prevention by raising HDL cholesterol and reducing triglycerides in patients with coronary artery disease. Circulation 102: 21–27.
15. Cannon CP, Shah S, Dansky HM, Davidson M, Brinton EA, et al. (2010) Safety of anacetrapib in patients with or at high risk for coronary heart disease. N Engl J Med 363: 2406–2415.
16. de Faire U, Ericsson CG, Grip L, Nilsson J, Svane B, et al. (1996) Secondary preventive potential of lipid-lowering drugs. The Bezafibrate Coronary Atherosclerosis Intervention Trial (BECAIT). Eur Heart J 17 Suppl F: 37–42.
17. Keech A, Simes RJ, Barter P, Best J, Scott R, et al. (2005) Effects of long-term fenofibrate therapy on cardiovascular events in 9795 people with type 2 diabetes mellitus (the FIELD study): randomised controlled trial. Lancet 366: 1849–1861.
18. Luscher TF, Taddei S, Kaski JC, Jukema JW, Kallend D, et al. (2012) Vascular effects and safety of dalcetrapib in patients with or at risk of coronary heart disease: the dal-VESSEL randomized clinical trial. Eur Heart J 33: 857–865.
19. Nissen SE, Tardif JC, Nicholls SJ, Revkin JH, Shear CL, et al. (2007) Effect of torcetrapib on the progression of coronary atherosclerosis. N Engl J Med 356: 1304–1316.
20. Rubins HB, Robins SJ, Collins D, Fye CL, Anderson JW, et al. (1999) Gemfibrozil for the secondary prevention of coronary heart disease in men with low levels of high-density lipoprotein cholesterol. Veterans Affairs High-Density Lipoprotein Cholesterol Intervention Trial Study Group. N Engl J Med 341: 410–418.
21. Schwartz GG, Olsson AG, Abt M, Ballantyne CM, Barter PJ, et al. (2012) Effects of dalcetrapib in patients with a recent acute coronary syndrome. N Engl J Med 367: 2089–2099.
22. Steiner G, Hamsten A, Hosking J, Stewart D, Mclaughlin P, et al. (2001) Effect of fenofibrate on progression of coronary-artery disease in type 2 diabetes: the Diabetes Atherosclerosis Intervention Study, a randomised study. Lancet 357: 905–910.
23. Taylor AJ, Sullenberger LE, Lee HJ, Lee JK, Grace KA (2004) Arterial Biology for the Investigation of the Treatment Effects of Reducing Cholesterol (ARBITER) 2: a double-blind, placebo-controlled study of extended-release niacin on atherosclerosis progression in secondary prevention patients treated with statins. Circulation 110: 3512–3517.
24. Wright RS (2013) Recent clinical trials evaluating benefit of drug therapy for modification of HDL cholesterol. Curr Opin Cardiol 28: 389–398.
25. Birjmohun RS, Hutten BA, Kastelein JJ, Stroes ES (2005) Efficacy and safety of high-density lipoprotein cholesterol-increasing compounds: a meta-analysis of randomized controlled trials. J Am Coll Cardiol 45: 185–197.
26. Li C, Zhang W, Zhou F, Chen C, Zhou L, et al. (2013) Cholesteryl ester transfer protein inhibitors in the treatment of dyslipidemia: a systematic review and meta-analysis. PLoS One 8: e77049.
27. Forrest MJ, Bloomfield D, Briscoe RJ, Brown PN, Cumiskey AM, et al. (2008) Torcetrapib-induced blood pressure elevation is independent of CETP inhibition and is accompanied by increased circulating levels of aldosterone. Br J Pharmacol 154: 1465–1473.
28. Thompson SG, Higgins JP (2002) How should meta-regression analyses be undertaken and interpreted? Stat Med 21: 1559–1573.
29. Pirillo A, Norata GD, Catapano AL (2013) High-density lipoprotein subfractions—what the clinicians need to know. Cardiology 124: 116–125.

Brain Remodelling following Endothelin-1 Induced Stroke in Conscious Rats

Hima C. S. Abeysinghe[2]*, Laita Bokhari[1,3], Gregory J. Dusting[4,5], Carli L. Roulston[1]

1 Neurotrauma Research team, Department of Medicine, St Vincent's Campus, University of Melbourne, Victoria, Australia, 2 Department of Surgery, St Vincent's Campus, University of Melbourne, Victoria, Australia, 3 Department of Biochemistry and Molecular Biology, Bio21 Molecular Science and Biotechnology Institute, University of Melbourne, Victoria, Australia, 4 Cytoprotection Pharmacology Program, Centre for Eye Research, The Royal Eye and Ear Hospital Melbourne, Victoria, Australia, 5 Department of Opthamology, Faculty of Medicine, University of Melbourne, Victoria, Australia

Abstract

The extent of stroke damage in patients affects the range of subsequent pathophysiological responses that influence recovery. Here we investigate the effect of lesion size on development of new blood vessels as well as inflammation and scar formation and cellular responses within the subventricular zone (SVZ) following transient focal ischemia in rats ($n = 34$). Endothelin-1-induced stroke resulted in neurological deficits detected between 1 and 7 days ($P<0.001$), but significant recovery was observed beyond this time. MCID image analysis revealed varying degrees of damage in the ipsilateral cortex and striatum with infarct volumes ranging from 0.76–77 mm^3 after 14 days, where larger infarct volumes correlated with greater functional deficits up to 7 days ($r = 0.53$, $P<0.05$). Point counting of blood vessels within consistent sample regions revealed that increased vessel numbers correlated significantly with larger infarct volumes 14 days post-stroke in the core cortical infarct ($r = 0.81$, $P<0.0001$), core striatal infarct ($r = 0.91$, $P<0.005$) and surrounding border zones ($r = 0.66$, $P<0.005$; and $r = 0.73$, $P<0.05$). Cell proliferation within the SVZ also increased with infarct size ($P<0.01$) with a greater number of Nestin/GFAP positive cells observed extending towards the border zone in rats with larger infarcts. Lesion size correlated with both increased microglia and astrocyte activation, with severely diffuse astrocyte transition, the formation of the glial scar being more pronounced in rats with larger infarcts. Thus stroke severity affects cell proliferation within the SVZ in response to injury, which may ultimately make a further contribution to glial scar formation, an important factor to consider when developing treatment strategies that promote neurogenesis.

Editor: Thiruma V. Arumugam, National University of Singapore, Singapore

Funding: This study was supported in part by grants from the National Heart Foundation Australia (NHF G07M3237, http://www.heartfoundation.org.au); The Bethlehem Griffiths Foundation (http://www.bethlehemgrf.com.au/); and the National Health and Medical Research Council Australia for project grant (NHMRC project grant 628767, http://www.nhmrc.gov.au/), and fellowship to Professor Dusting (No. 1003113). The funders had no role in study design, data collection and analysis, decision to publish, or preparation of the manuscript.

Competing Interests: The authors have declared that no competing interests exist.

* E-mail: himaa@student.unimelb.edu.au

Introduction

The degree of brain injury varies between each stroke victim and infarct volume has been shown to directly correlate with functional improvements 90 days post-stroke [1]. A number of events including excitotoxicity, oxidative stress, inflammation and apoptosis are initiated during and following stroke that contribute to the evolution of brain injury beyond the initial insult (*see for reviews:* [2,3]). Evolution of infarcts tends to differ according to the underlying vascular lesion and cerebral territories involved [4]. Non-malignant infarcts evolve approximately over 3–7 days post-stroke in rodents and become stable thereafter [5], while in humans infarct evolution takes days to weeks [6,7] with most stabilising between 1–3 months from stroke onset [8].

The importance of correctly diagnosing initial stroke severity and progression of injury relates to correct assignment of treatment options in stroke management since the initial size of a stroke lesion affects subsequent pathophysiological responses [9,10]. To this end, prognostic clinical approaches such as the use of the NIHSS (National Institutes of Health Stroke Scale) allow prediction of functional outcome and survival in stroke patients in order to support clinical management and to correctly stratify treatment groups in clinical trials aimed at achieving neuroprotection [11–13]. However with the development of treatment strategies that promote brain repair, a similar comprehensive evaluation of patients following stroke will be required to assist in defining patients more likely to respond to brain restoration treatments and rule out those that lack the biological factors required to achieve improved functional outcomes [14,15]. This highlights the need to further understand endogenous repair mechanisms and their response to different grades of stroke severity and subsequent damage.

Ischemic insults have now been shown to trigger neural progenitor cell proliferation and stem cell migration from the subventricular zone (SVZ) of the lateral ventricle to damaged regions of the brain [16,17] even in patients of advanced age [18]. Additionally, angiogenesis is one of the pivotal restorative mechanisms initiated after ischemic injury and involves the formation of new blood vessels from the damaged vascular networks [19,20]. Neurogenesis and angiogenesis are tightly coupled to one another and may influence brain remodelling and subsequent functional recovery in many patients following stroke [21–24]. The potential affect the size of the infarct has on the degree of angiogenesis has not been previously reported despite many studies focusing on the pathways involved in the induction of angiogenesis after ischemic brain injury. Likewise factors that influence the rate of neurogenesis remain to be defined. Here we investigate the effect of stroke severity on angiogenesis and SVZ cell proliferation and migration after cerebral ischemia using the endothelin-1 (ET-1) rat model of stroke, and correlate these findings with infarct volume, inflammation, scar formation and functional recovery.

Materials and Methods

Ethics Statement

All experiments were performed in strict accordance with the guidelines of the National Health & Medical Research Council of Australia Code of Practice for the Care and use of Animals for Experimental Purposes in Australia. The protocol was approved by the St Vincent's Hospital animal ethics committee (AEC009/09). All surgery was performed under general anaesthesia, and paracetamol (2 mg/kg in drinking water) was provided for 24 hr prior to and after surgery in order to minimize suffering and included monitoring each rat throughout the length of the study to ensure their wellbeing.

Surgical Preparation

A total of 37 adult male Hooded Wistar rats weighing 300–360 g (Laboratory Animal Services, University of Adelaide, Australia) were included in this study. Rats were group-housed (4 rats to a cage), until endothelin-1 induced middle cerebral artery constriction, whereupon they were housed in separate cages under diurnal lighting with ambient temperature maintained between 20 and 22°C. Rats were given free access to food and water. Rats were anaesthetised with a mixture of Ketamine/Xylazine (75 mg/kg: 10 mg/kg respectively i.p.) and maintained throughout surgery by inhalation of isoflurane (95% oxygen and 5% isoflurane). A 23-gauge stainless steel guide cannula was stereotaxically implanted into the cortex 2 mm dorsal to the right middle cerebral artery (MCA) (0.2 mm anterior, −5.9 mm lateral, −5.2 mm ventral) as in previous studies [5,14]. Rats were allowed to recover for 5 days prior to stroke induction.

Stroke Induction

Focal cerebral ischemia was induced in conscious rats by constriction of the right middle cerebral artery with perivascular administration of endothelin-1 (ET-1; American Peptide Company, Inc. CA, USA; 40 pmol in 2 μl of saline over 10 min) ($n = 34$) similar to previous studies [14]. Characteristic behavioural changes indicating stroke included clenching and dragging of the contralateral forepaw and continuous circling in an anti-clockwise direction. These behavioural changes observed during stroke induction were scored 1 to 5 for stroke severity (according to our previously established protocol) with 5 being the most severe [14]. Changes in behaviour occurred routinely over 2 to 60 minutes from initiation of ET-1 infusion and rats that did not display any behavioural change were considered not to have suffered a stroke and were excluded from further study. Sham-operated rats ($n = 3$) underwent cannula implantation without ET-1 delivery.

Assessment of Functional Outcome

Neurological assessments were conducted on all rats prior to any surgical procedures (pre-surgery), immediately prior to ET-1-induced stroke (pre-stroke) and 24, 48, 72 hrs, 7 and 14 days post-stroke. Animals were tested and scored for neurological abnormalities based on abnormal posture and hemiplegia as previously described [25,26]. Forelimb asymmetry between the contralateral and ipsilateral forepaws was evaluated using the sticky label test by measuring latency to touch and remove attached stimuli [27]. Neurological scores from each rat post-stroke were compared to pre-stroke scores, thus each rat acted as its own control.

Quantification of Ischemic Damage

Rats were decapitated 7 ($n = 15$) or 14 days ($n = 19$) after stroke, forebrains removed, frozen over liquid nitrogen, and stored at −80°C prior to processing. Coronal sections (16 μm thick) were prepared using a Leica cryostat (Leica Microsystems, Wetzlar, Germany) at eight pre-determined coronal planes throughout the brain from −3.2 to 6.8 mm relative to Bregma. The extent of brain injury following stroke was determined in triplicate unstained slide mounted sections using a micro computer imaging device (MCID M4 image analyser, Imaging Research Inc., St. Catharines, ON, Canada) according to the methods of Callaway and colleagues [28]. Total infarct volume was determined by integrating the cross-sectional area of damage at each stereotaxic level with the distances between levels [29]. The influence of oedema was corrected for by applying the following formula: (area of normal hemisphere/area of infarcted hemisphere) × area of infarct [30].

Immunohistochemistry

Immunohistochemical staining was performed in adjacent sections to those used to quantify damage in order to identify blood vessels, proliferating SVZ cells, migrating SVZ neuroblasts, radial glial cells, as well as inflammatory cells after stroke. Control experiments included either omission of each primary antibody from the protocol or the inclusion of the appropriate IgG control to verify the specificity of each antibody. All sections were analysed with an ABC detection kit (Elite Vectastain, Vector Labs, Burlingame, CA, USA) for 30 mins followed by washes in phosphate buffered saline (PBS 0.1 M pH 7.4; 3×5 min) and 5 min incubation with diaminobenzidine (DAB; Sigma, St. Louis, MO, USA). The resultant colour reaction was visualised with an Olympus microscope (Albertslund, Denmark).

Blood vessel detection. For detection of blood vessels, sections were first fixed with methanol (−20°C for 15 minutes) and then washed in PBS (0.1 M; pH 7.4) containing 0.05% Tween 20 detergent (PBT) (3×5 min) followed by a 30 min block in 10% normal goat serum in PBT prior to washes in PBS (0.1 M; 3×5 min). Sections were then incubated for 1 hour with rabbit anti-von Willebrand factor (vWF; 1:200, Millipore, Billerica, MA, USA) in PBT containing 5% NGS (0.1 M, pH 7.4) prior to washes in PBS (0.1 M; 3×5 min) and 30 min incubation with secondary antibody biotinylated goat anti-rabbit (1:200, Vector Labs, Burlingame, CA, USA). Sections were further analysed as described above.

SVZ cell proliferation. For the detection of proliferating cells within the SVZ sections were fixed in 4% paraformaldehyde (PFA in 0.1 M PBS, pH 7.4, for 15 min RT) and then washed in PBS (0.1 M; 3×5 min) prior to incubation in blocking solution containing 5% NGS and 0.3% Triton X-100. Sections were then incubated with rabbit anti-Ki67 (Ki67; 1:1000, Labvision Thermo Scientific, Fremont, CA, USA) for 1 hour in a mixture of PBS (0.1 M; pH 7.4) containing 5% NGS prior to PBS washes (0.1 M; 3×5 min) and incubation with secondary antibody biotinylated goat anti-rabbit (1:200, Vector Labs, Burlingame, CA, USA) for 30 min. Sections were further analysed as described above.

Immature migrating neurons within the SVZ. For the detection of migrating immature neurons or neuroblasts within the SVZ sections were fixed in 4% paraformaldehyde (PFA in 0.1 M PBS, pH 7.4, for 15 min RT) and then washed in PBS (0.1 M; 3×5 min) prior to antigen retrieval with 10% proteinase K (DAKO, Glostrup, Denmark) in 0.1 M PBS for 3 min following by incubation in 30% fetal calf serum to stop proteinase K activity for 30 min. Sections were washed in PBS (0.1 M; 3×5 min) followed by incubation in blocking solution containing 5% NGS in 0.1 M PBS for 30 min. Sections were then incubated with guinea-pig anti-doublecortin (DCX; 1:3000, Millipore, Billerica, MA, USA) for 1 hour in a mixture of PBS (0.1 M; pH 7.4) containing 5% NGS prior to PBS washes (0.1 M; 3×5 min) and incubated with secondary antibody biotinylated goat anti-guinea-pig (1:200, Vector Labs, Burlingame, CA, USA) for 30 min. Sections were further analysed as described above.

Microglia/macrophages. For detection of microglia/macrophages, sections were fixed by serial acetone dilutions (50:100×2 min each at RT) and washed in PBS (0.1 M; 3×5 min) prior to 30 min incubation in DAKO serum-free protein block (DAKO, Glostrup, Denmark). Sections were then incubated for 1 hour with mouse anti-OX42/CD11b (OX42; 1:100, Serotec, Raleigh, NC, USA) prior to washes in PBS (0.1 M; 3×5 min) and 30 min incubation with secondary biotinylated goat anti-mouse (1:200, DAKO, Glostrup, Denmark). Sections were further analysed as described above.

Astrocytes. For detection of astrocytes sections were fixed in 4% paraformaldehyde (PFA in 0.1 M PBS, pH 7.4, for 15 min RT) and washed in PBS (0.1 M; 3×5 min) prior to incubation in block solution containing 5% NGS and 0.3% Triton X-100 in PBS (0.1 M). Tissue sections were then incubated with mouse anti-glial fibrillary acidic protein (GFAP; 1:400, Millipore, Billerica, MA, USA) before washing in PBS (0.1 M; 3×5 min) and incubating for 30 min with secondary antibody biotinylated goat anti-mouse (1:200, DAKO, Glostrup, Denmark) and analysed as above.

Immunofluorescence

Adjacent sections to those used for immunohistochemical staining, were fixed in 4% PFA for 10 min and washed in PBS (0.1 M, pH 7.4, 3×5 min). Sections were then subjected to block with DAKO serum-free protein block (Glostrup, Denmark) for 30 min. Dual immunofluorescent techniques were employed where the primary antibody for vascular endothelial cells (vWF, 1:200) was incubated overnight at 4°C in a mixture of PBS (0.1 M, pH 7.4) containing 2% NDS, 2% NGS, 0.3% Triton X-100, together with either: mouse anti-OX42/CD11b (1:100) to detect microglia/macrophages; mouse anti-neuron specific nuclear protein (NeuN; 1:400, Millipore, Billerica, MA, USA) to identify neurons; or mouse anti-GFAP (1:400, Millipore, Billerica, MA, USA) to detect astrocytes.

For characterisation of cells within the SVZ, rabbit anti-Ki67 (Ki67; 1:2000, Labvision Thermo Scientific, Fremont, CA, USA) was co-incubated with either mouse anti-GFAP (1:400, Millipore, Billerica, MA, USA) or guinea-pig anti-doublecortin (DCX; 1:500, Millipore, Billerica, MA, USA); and mouse anti-Nestin (1:400, Cell Signalling Technology, Danvers, MA, USA) was co-incubated with and rabbit anti-GFAP (1:400, DAKO, Glostrup, Denmark) overnight at 4°C in a mixture of PBS (0.1 M, pH 7.4) containing 2% NGS and 0.3% Triton X-100.

Tissue sections were then washed in PBS (0.1 M, pH 7.4, 3×5 min) and transferred for incubation with an appropriate secondary antibody (1:500 for all) for 2.5 hr at room temperature; Alexa-568 goat anti-rabbit and Alexa-488 donkey anti-mouse (Invitrogen Life Technologies, Grand Island, NY, USA) for the detection of vWF with either OX42 or GFAP; or Alexa-568 goat anti-mouse and Alexa-488 donkey anti-rabbit for the detection of vWF with NeuN; or Alexa-568 goat anti-rabbit and Alexa-488 goat anti-mouse for detection of GFAP with either Nestin or Ki67; or Alexa-568 goat anti-rabbit and Alexa-488 goat anti-guinea pig for detection of Ki67 with DCX. Following incubation with secondary antibodies tissue sections were washed in PBS (0.1 M, pH 7.4, 3×5 min) and then cover-slipped with DAKO fluorescent mounting medium. In control experiments, primary antibodies were omitted or the appropriate IgG control was included to verify the specificity of each antibody. Resulting sections were examined with a fluorescence microscope equipped with a 578–603 nm filter set for detection of red fluorescence and 495–519 nm filter set for the detection of green fluorescence (ZeissAxioskop2, North Ryde, Australia).

Quantification of Immunohistochemistry

Resulting tissue sections were viewed using an Olympus BH-2 microscope (Albertslund, Denmark) under x20 magnification with at least three sections per region used for assessment. MCID generated images that were used to assess infarct were used as a reference and four common regions of interest where damage was routinely observed were identified in each section for assessment: the damaged cortex, damaged striatum, and the border region surrounding the damage for both the striatum and cortex. Each area used for analysis was then compared with the appropriate corresponding mirror region in the contralateral hemisphere, as well as to sham-operated controls, using exactly the same sample area (*see* figure 1J–L).

Blood vessels. Blood vessel quantification was assessed 14 days post-stroke in vWF-labelled sections at two anatomical levels (+0.2 mm and −0.84 mm relative to bregma) shown in previous studies to routinely result in damage. Using digital video imaging (TK C 1480E; JVC, Wayne, NJ, USA), an automated systematic random sampling point-counting system was applied with a Computer Assisted Stereological Toolbox (CAST System; Olympus) [31]. Sampling commenced randomly within each defined field and the number of points that overlay either blood vessels or where appropriate immuno-labelled cells, was scored and then divided by the total number of points counted in each field. The number of blood vessels detected in the ipsilateral sample region was then compared to the contralateral region and expressed as 100% control. For quantification of blood vessels a common area of interest within the cortex and striatum across all stroke rats was identified based on the appearance of both small and large vWF labelled microvessel and compared directly with the contralateral mirror image.

SVZ cell proliferation. Ki67 positive cells within the SVZ were quantified at both 7 and 14 days post-stroke in triplicate consecutive sections (+1.2 mm bregma) to ensure the same location within the SVZ was analysed for all animals. Cells within the ipsilateral SVZ and contralateral SVZ were quantified using the cell counter plugin tool for National Institute of Health ImageJ software (USA). Images were obtained using an Olympus microscope (Albertslund, Denmark) under x20 magnification (the same magnification utilised with CAST counts). Due to a small counting frame within the SVZ total cell numbers were quantified using standard stereological techniques and ImageJ. The total number of proliferating cells detected in the ipsilateral SVZ was then compared to the corresponding contralateral SVZ and expressed as 100% control.

SVZ radial glial cell proliferation. Proliferating radial glial cells (Ki67/GFAP positive) within the ipsilateral SVZ and contralateral SVZ were quantified using the cell counter plugin for National Institute of Health ImageJ software (USA). Qualitative images of immature astrocytes (Nestin/GFAP positive) observed extending from the SVZ toward penumbral regions was obtained. Images were obtained using a laser scanning inverted confocal imaging system (Nikon Instruments Inc., Melville, NY, USA) under x40 magnification (a higher magnification was required to achieve greater image resolution for cell counts). For quantification, images of the SVZ were presented as collapsed reconstructions of 10 optical sections captured every 0.5 μm on the z-axis, at a scan speed of 0.5 frame/sec, a resolution of 1024×1024 pixels with the line acquisition mode. Due to a small counting frame within the SVZ cell numbers were quantified using standard stereological techniques and ImageJ. The total number of proliferating radial glial cells detected in the ipsilateral SVZ was then compared to the corresponding contralateral SVZ and expressed as 100% control.

SVZ neuronal cell migration. Migrating immature neurons or neuroblasts (DCX positive) within the ipsilateral SVZ and contralateral SVZ were quantified using the cell counter plugin for National Institute of Health ImageJ software (USA). DCX positive cells within the ipsilateral SVZ and contralateral SVZ were quantified using the cell counter plugin for National Institute of Health ImageJ software (USA). Images were obtained using an Olympus microscope (Albertslund, Denmark) under x20 magnification (the same magnification utilised with CAST counts). Qualitative images of proliferating immature neurons (Ki67/DCX positive) observed within the SVZ were obtained using a laser scanning inverted confocal imaging system (Nikon Instruments Inc., Melville, NY, USA) under x40 magnification (a higher magnification was required to achieve greater image resolution for cell counts). Images were presented as collapsed reconstructions of 17 optical sections captured every 0.4 μm on the z-axis, at a scan speed of 0.5 frame/sec, a resolution of 1024×1024 pixels with the line acquisition mode. Due to a small counting frame within the SVZ cell numbers were quantified using standard stereological techniques and ImageJ. The total number of immature neurons in the ipsilateral SVZ was then compared to the corresponding contralateral SVZ and expressed as 100% control.

Activated microglia/macrophages. Quantification of inflammatory cells was assessed within the same brain regions of interest as assessed for blood vessel quantification using the automated systematic random sampling point-counting system. The number of OX42 positive cells that displayed an amoeboid morphology with reduced processes (indicative of activation) were counted and expressed as a percentage of the total number of counts (cross hairs) within the defined sample area within the ipsilateral or contralateral hemispheres. Resting microglia displaying morphologies of small cell bodies with highly ramified processes were excluded from counts.

Astrocytes. GFAP labelled reactive astrogliosis was assessed and quantified based on morphological stage of activation [32]. Different gradations of reactive astrogliosis and glial scar formation were identified based on cellular hypertrophy, and length and thickness of processes and classified as either activated astrocytes or diffuse astrocytes. Quantification of activated or diffuse astrocytes within the cortical and striatal core damage and border regions was also counted using the automated systematic random sampling point-counting system and expressed as a percentage of the total number of counts (cross hairs) within the defined sample area.

Statistical Analyses

All statistical analysis was conducted in consultation with a statistical consultant, Rachel Sore of the Statistical Consulting Centre with the University of Melbourne, Victoria, Australia. Neurological outcome data was analysed by Kruskal-Wallis non-parametric ANOVA followed by Dunn's post-test. Hemineglect data were analysed by repeated measures for two-way ANOVA (side×hr/days after stroke) to compare latencies in the ipsilateral and contralateral forepaws over time. Individual comparisons were made using Bonferroni multiple comparisons test for all analyses where ANOVA yielded a significant result or Mann Whitney test for comparisons between two data-sets. Values are presented as mean ± SEM unless stated otherwise. To test for correlation between infarct volume and either: angiogenesis, SVZ cell proliferation, migrating SVZ neuroblasts or inflammatory cell activation, the Pearson product-moment coefficient, r, for ordinal values was determined using GraphPad Prism, version 6 (GraphPad Software Inc., San Diego CA). *P*-values less than 0.05 were considered significant.

Results

Functional Outcome

Significant neurological deficits were observed 24 hrs to 7 days post-stroke when compared to pre-stroke scores ($P<0.0001$ $n=19$, non-parametric ANOVA; Figure 1A) but not beyond 7 days. Latency to touch and remove sticky labels from the stroke affected contralateral forepaw was also significantly increased when compared with the ipsilateral forelimb between 24 and 72 hrs after stroke ($P<0.05$, Two-way ANOVA; Figures 1B, C), but no significant deficits were detected after this time.

Infarct Analysis

Histopathology 14 days after stroke revealed damage in the frontal, parietal and insular cortex and the striatum. Rats assigned lower stroke ratings during induction of stroke (ET-1 infusion) displayed damage within the cortex whereas those assigned larger stroke ratings demonstrated damage within both the cortex and striatum (Figure 1J–L) as in previous studies [14]. Rats with higher stroke severity scores exhibited significantly greater infarct volumes in both 7 and 14 day recovery groups ($r=0.88$, $P<0.0001$, Figure 1D). A positive correlation between total infarct volume and neurological deficit score was also found 24 hr ($r=0.52$, $P<0.05$; Figure 1E), 48 hr ($r=0.70$, $P<0.001$; Figure 1F), 72 hr ($r=0.60$, $P<0.01$; Figure 1G), and 7 days ($r=0.54$, $P<0.05$; Figure 1H), but not at 14 days post-stroke ($r=0.16$; Figure 1I).

Angiogenesis and Infarct Correlation

vWF labelled blood vessels revealed regions of angiogenesis both within and around the core infarct of the cortex and where relevant in the damaged striatum. Both large and thin walled microvessels were point counted within a defined sample area (800 μm^2) from the same anatomical region for all rats and compared to the contralateral mirror image (undamaged tissue). Blood vessel counts were then correlated with the quantified infarct volume for each rat. Positive correlations between infarct size and blood vessel numbers were detected in the ipsilateral core cortex ($r=0.81$, $P<0.0001$; Figure 2A), surrounding border cortex ($r=0.66$, $P<0.005$; Figure 2B), core striatum ($r=0.91$, $P<0.005$; Figure 2C) and border striatum ($r=0.73$, $P<0.05$; Figure 2D), with larger infarcts correlating with increased vascular density. The number of blood vessels (vWF+) significantly increased within the ipsilateral core cortex ($P<0.0001$), border cortex ($P<0.01$), core striatum ($P<0.01$) and border striatum ($P<0.05$, Scatter plots,

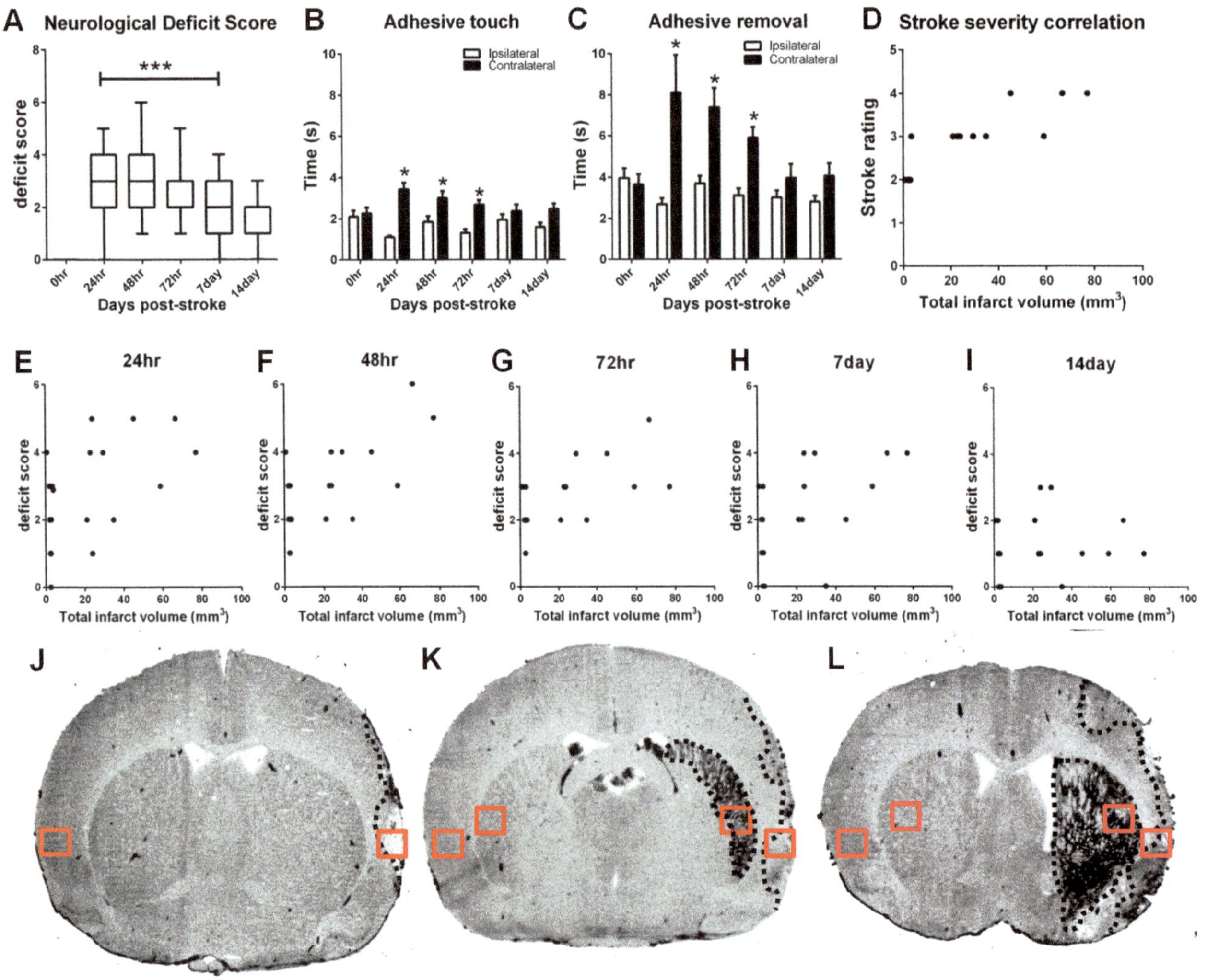

Figure 1. Neurological outcome 14 days after ET-1 induced stroke. Combined neurological deficit scores (A). Data presented as box plots include hinges extending from the 25th to 75th percentiles, the median line within the box and whiskers extending to the minimum and maximum values of the dataset. ***$P<0.0001$ vs 0 hr pre-stroke score ($n=19$, non-parametric ANOVA). Latency to touch (B) and remove an adhesive (C) on the contralateral (stroke affected) forelimb compared with the ipsilateral forelimb. Data presented as mean ± SEM, *$P<0.05$ compared with the ipsilateral forelimb at the same time measurement (ANOVA). Scatter plots depicting correlation between infarct volumes and stroke severity rating ($r=0.88$, $P<0.0001$; D) (Pearson product moment correlation coefficients). A significant correlation was found between total infarct volume and neurological deficit score at 24 ($r=0.52$, $P<0.05$; E), 48 ($r=0.70$, $P<0.001$; F), 72 hr ($r=0.60$, $P<0.01$; G), and 7 day ($r=0.54$, $P<0.05$; H) post-stroke but not thereafter ($r=0.16$; I) (Pearson product moment correlation coefficients). MCID images of coronal sections taken from three animals with stroke ratings ranging from low to high; stroke rating #2 (J), #3 (K), and #4 (L) displaying damage to varying degrees within the cortex and striatum marked by the black dotted line. Consistent regions used for quantification within the infarcted cortex and striatum can be visualised by the red boxes (J–L).

non-parametric ANOVA; Figure 3E–H) 14 days post-stroke when compared to the corresponding contralateral hemisphere or when compared to either hemisphere of sham-operated animals. No significant differences were observed between the contralateral hemisphere of ET-1 stroke affected animals and either hemisphere of sham-operated animals (Figure 3E–H). To confirm an association between damage after stroke and angiogenesis, immunofluorescent double labelling for neurons (NeuN) and blood vessels (vWF) confirmed that greater levels of angiogenesis occurred in regions where there was greatest neuronal loss (Figure 2I–K).

SVZ Cell Proliferation, Migration, Neural Differentiation and Infarct Correlation

In order to determine the effects of stroke on the neurogenic niche we first characterised cell proliferation within the SVZ. Ki67 positive cells were counted in both the ipsilateral and contralateral SVZ region from both 7 and 14 day recovery groups. The total number of proliferating cells within the SVZ significantly increased 7 days post-stroke compared to sham-operated animals ($P<0.05$, Scatter plots, non-parametric ANOVA; Figure 3A). This increase was no-longer detected 14 days post-stroke. At 7 days post-stroke a positive correlation was found between infarct volume and Ki67 labelled SVZ cells ($r=0.73$, $P<0.005$, $n=15$; Figure 3B), with larger infarcts associated with increased cell proliferation. No correlation between infarct volume and SVZ

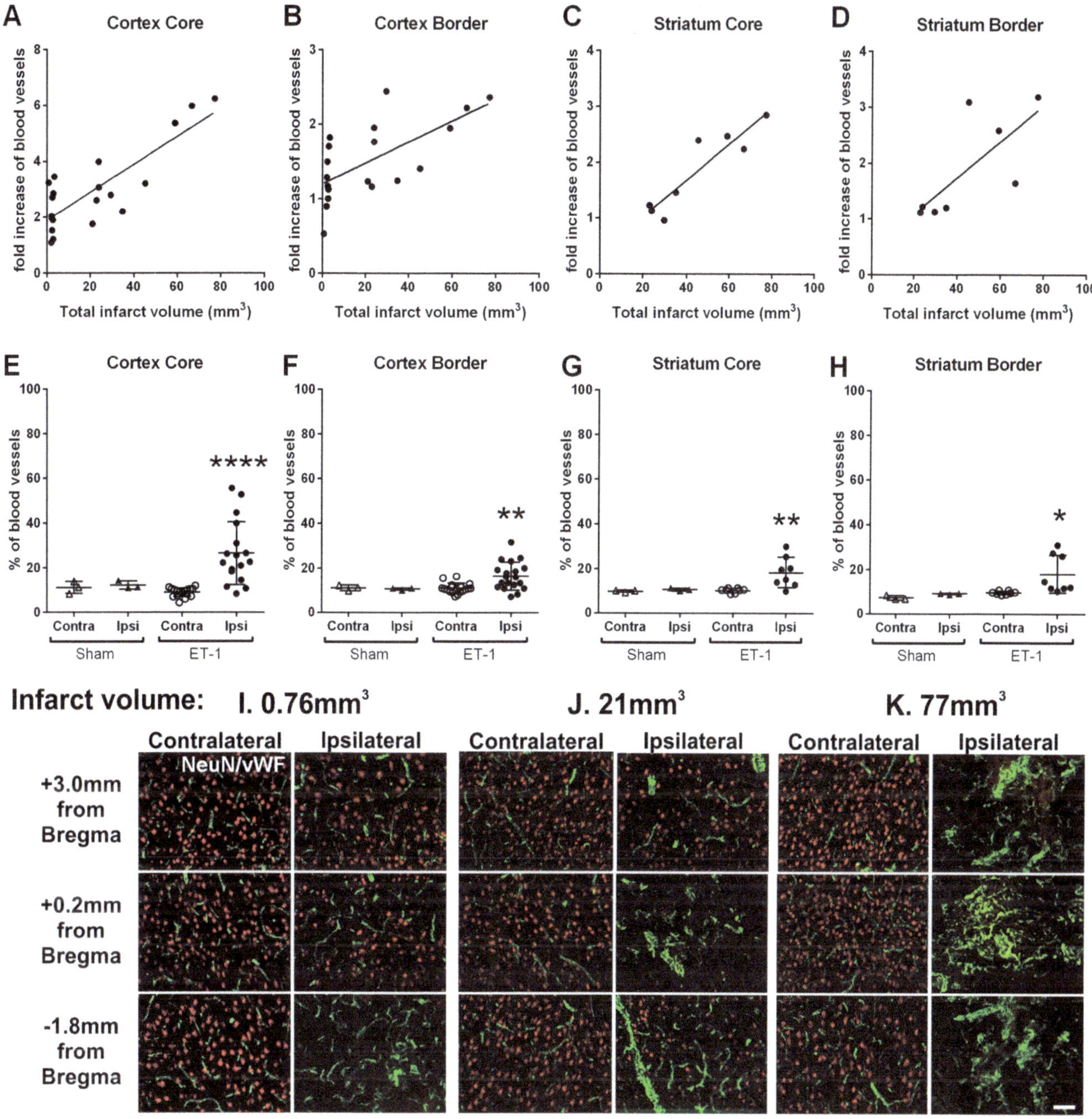

Figure 2. Angiogenesis and infarct volume 14 days post-stroke. Scatter plots depict a significant correlation found between degree of angiogenesis and infarct volume within cortex core (r = 0.81, $P<0.0001$, $n = 19$; A), cortex border (r = 0.66, $P<0.005$, $n = 19$; B), striatum core (r = 0.91, $P<0.005$, $n = 8$; C) and striatum border (r = 0.73, $P<0.05$, $n = 8$; D) (Pearson product moment correlation coefficients). Scatter plots of blood vessels (vWF+) from sham-operated ($n = 3$) and 14 day post-stroke animals ($n = 19$) revealed a significant increase in the number of blood vessels within the ipsilateral cortical and striatal core and border regions only (non-parametric ANOVA; E–H). Data presented as mean ± SEM, *$P<0.05$, **$P<0.01$, ****$P<0.0001$ compared with the contralateral hemisphere of ET-1 stroke affected animals and either hemisphere of sham-operated animals. No significant differences were observed between the contralateral hemisphere of ET-1 stroke affected animals and either hemisphere of sham-operated animals. Angiogenesis and neuronal loss within the stroke damaged brain (I–K). Immunohistochemical localisation of neurons (red) and blood vessels (green) in the cortex of stroke affected rat brains with total infarct volumes ranging from 0.76–77 mm^3. Increased angiogenesis is observed in regions with greatest neuronal loss (ipsilateral columns I, J and K). Scale bar: I–K 100 μm.

proliferation was found 14 days post-stroke (r = 0.07, $n = 19$; Figure 3C).

We then examined the effects of stroke on stem cell differentiation within the SVZ. We detected both Ki67/GFAP/Nestin positive radial glial cells as well as immature migrating neuronal cells identified as DCX staining. We therefore quantified Ki67/GFAP+ cells and DCX+ cells separately along the lateral ventricle in both the ipsilateral and contralateral SVZ 7 days post-stroke at the same anatomical level for all sections (+1.2 mm relative to bregma).

The number of proliferating radial glial cells (Ki67+/GFAP+) increased 7 days post-stroke compared to sham-operated animals

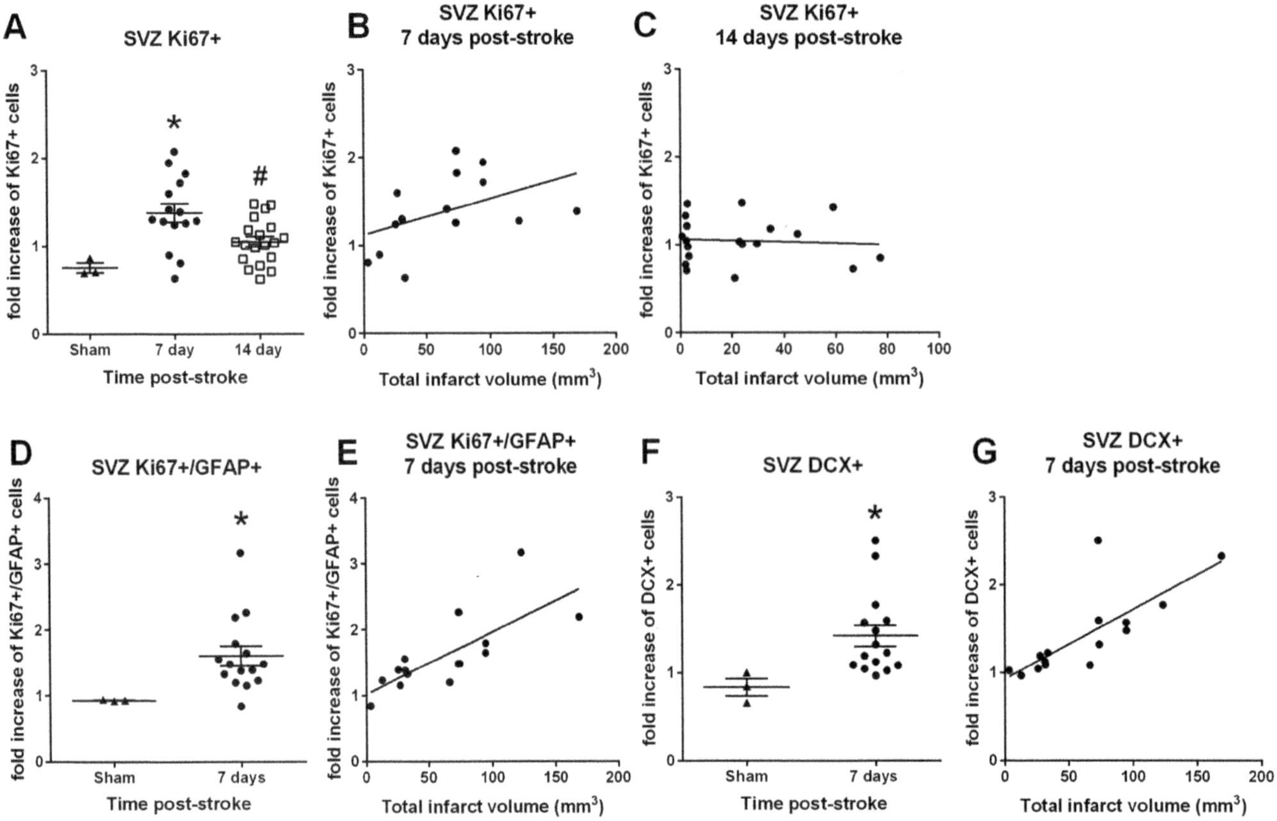

Figure 3. SVZ cell proliferation/migration, neural differentiation and infarct correlation 7 days post-stroke. Scatter plots of proliferating SVZ cells (Ki67+) from sham-operated ($n=3$), 7 day post-stroke ($n=15$) and 14 day post-stroke groups ($n=19$) revealed a significant increase in the number of proliferating SVZ cells 7 days post-stroke (non-parametric ANOVA; A). Data presented as mean ± SEM, *$P<0.05$ compared with sham-operated animals and #$P<0.05$ compared with 7 day post-stroke animals. A significant correlation was found between proliferating SVZ cells (Ki67+) and infarct volume 7 days post-stroke ($r=0.73$, $P<0.005$, $n=15$; B) but not at 14 days ($r=0.07$; C) (Pearson product moment correlation coefficients). Scatter plots depict a significant increase in proliferating radial glial cells within the SVZ at 7 days post-stroke (Mann Whitney test; D). Data presented as mean ± SEM, *$P<0.05$ compared with sham-operated animals. Within the SVZ, a positive correlation was observed between infarct volumes and the number of proliferating radial glial cells (Ki67+/GFAP+; $r=0.73$, $P<0.005$; E) 7 days post-stroke (Pearson product moment correlation coefficients). Scatter plots depict a significant increase in the number of immature neuronal cells within the SVZ at 7 days post-stroke (DCX+, Mann Whitney test; F). Data presented as mean ± SEM, *$P<0.05$ compared with sham-operated animals. Infarct volume significantly correlated with the number of immature neurons generated from the SVZ 7 days post-stroke (DCX+; $r=0.77$, $P<0.001$; G) (Pearson product moment correlation coefficients).

($P<0.05$, Scatter plots, Mann Whitney test; Figure 3D). There was also a significant correlation between infarct volume and the number of Ki67/GFAP co-labelled cells within SVZ ($r=0.73$, $P<0.005$, $n=15$; Figure 3E) 7 days post-stroke.

The number of DCX+ cells was also increased within and surrounding the SVZ 7 days post-stroke compared to sham-operated animals ($P<0.05$, Scatter plots, Mann Whitney test; Figure 3F). These DCX+ cells, did not stain with either Ki67 or GFAP and a significant correlation was also found between infarct volume and the number of DCX positive cells within the SVZ ($r=0.77$, $P<0.001$, $n=15$; Figure 3G) 7 days post-stroke.

Immunofluorescence staining revealed a greater number of Ki67 positive (Figure 4A–C) and DCX positive (Figure 4D–F) cells within the SVZ of animals with larger infarct volumes. Nestin/GFAP positive immunostaining revealed a large number of radial glial cells extending from the SVZ towards the cortical and striatal penumbral regions 7 days post-stroke, with many new activated Nestin+ astrocytes detected within the border zone contributing to glial scar formation at both 7 and 14 days post stroke (Figure 4G–L). The number of Nestin/GFAP positive astrocytes detected in the border zone also appeared increased with larger infarct volumes (Figure 4J–L).

Inflammatory Response and Infarct Correlation

Activated microglia/macrophages. OX42 labelling revealed both resting and activated microglia/macrophages in the contralateral and ipsilateral hemisphere respectively. Resting microglia were observed to have a ramified morphology with small cell bodies and long fine branched processes (Figure 5A) [33]. Activated microglia appeared more amoeboid in morphology with large cell bodies with retracted processes, similar in appearance to blood derived macrophages [34,35] (Figure 5B, C). Since reactive microglia can develop into a phagocytic phenotype that is indistinguishable from infiltrating blood borne macrophages and lack discriminating cellular markers [35–37] both activated microglia and blood borne macrophages were quantified together. A significant increase in the number of activated microglia/macrophages was detected in the ipsilateral hemisphere up to 14 days after stroke. A positive correlation was found between the number of activated microglia/macrophages and infarct volume within the ipsilateral core cortex ($r=0.88$, $P<0.0001$, $n=19$;

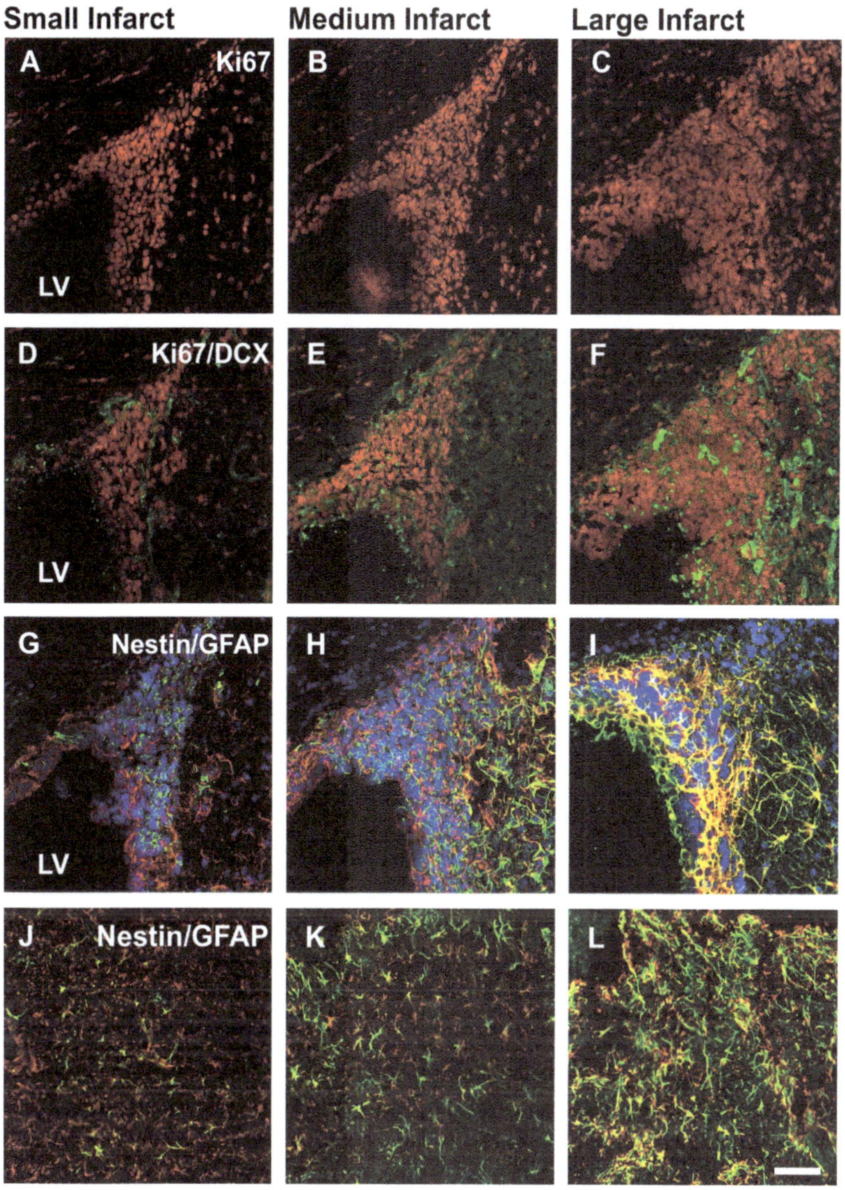

Figure 4. SVZ cell proliferation, migration, neural differentiation and scar formation across varied infarct volumes. Representative photomicrographs of proliferating cells (Ki67+; red; A–C) and non-proliferating immature neuronal cells (Ki67+/DCX+; red/green respectively; D–F) lining the ipsilateral SVZ, radial glial cells migrating from the ipsilateral SVZ (Nestin+/GFAP+; green/red respectively with co-expression giving a yellow appearance; G–I) and new activated astrocytes located within the cortical penumbra contributing to the glial scar (Nestin+/GFAP+; J–L). Images were taken from animals with small, medium and large infarcts. LV: Lateral ventricle. Scale bar: A–L 50 μm.

Figure 5D), border cortex (r = 0.70, $P<0.001$, $n = 19$; Figure 5E), core striatum (r = 0.86, $P<0.01$, $n = 8$; Figure 5F) and border striatum (r = 0.77, $P<0.05$, $n = 8$; Figure 5G) with larger infarcts containing more OX-42 positive cells within a consistent sample area. Contrastingly, within the contralateral hemisphere in regions that mirrored areas defined in the ipsilateral hemisphere, the number of activated microglia/macrophages negatively correlated with the size of infarct. This was observed within the core cortical (r = 0.81, $P<0.0001$, $n = 19$; Figure 5H), border cortex (r = 0.75, $P<0.0005$, $n = 19$; Figure 5I), core striatum (r = 0.75, $P<0.05$, $n = 8$; Figure 5J) and border striatum (r = 0.75, $P<0.05$, $n = 8$; Figure 5K). Activated microglia within the contralateral hemisphere were observed through the corpus callosum (Figure 5L–O) with increased state of activation observed closer to the site of damage.

Astrogliosis. Astrocytes were quantified based on morphological distinctions. Astrocytes of normal quiescent appearance were found in regions remote from the lesion site or within the contralateral hemisphere (Figure 6A) and were identified by low GFAP expression with long slender processes that did not overlap. Activated astrocytes were defined by an up-regulation of GFAP expression with cellular hypertrophy without pronounced overlap of processes (Figure 6B). Finally, severely diffuse astrocytes were identified based on pronounced up-regulation of GFAP expression, prominent cell body and process hypertrophy, with distinct process overlap and dense packing of cells to form a glial scar (Figure 6C). Within the core cortex, little or no activated astrocytes

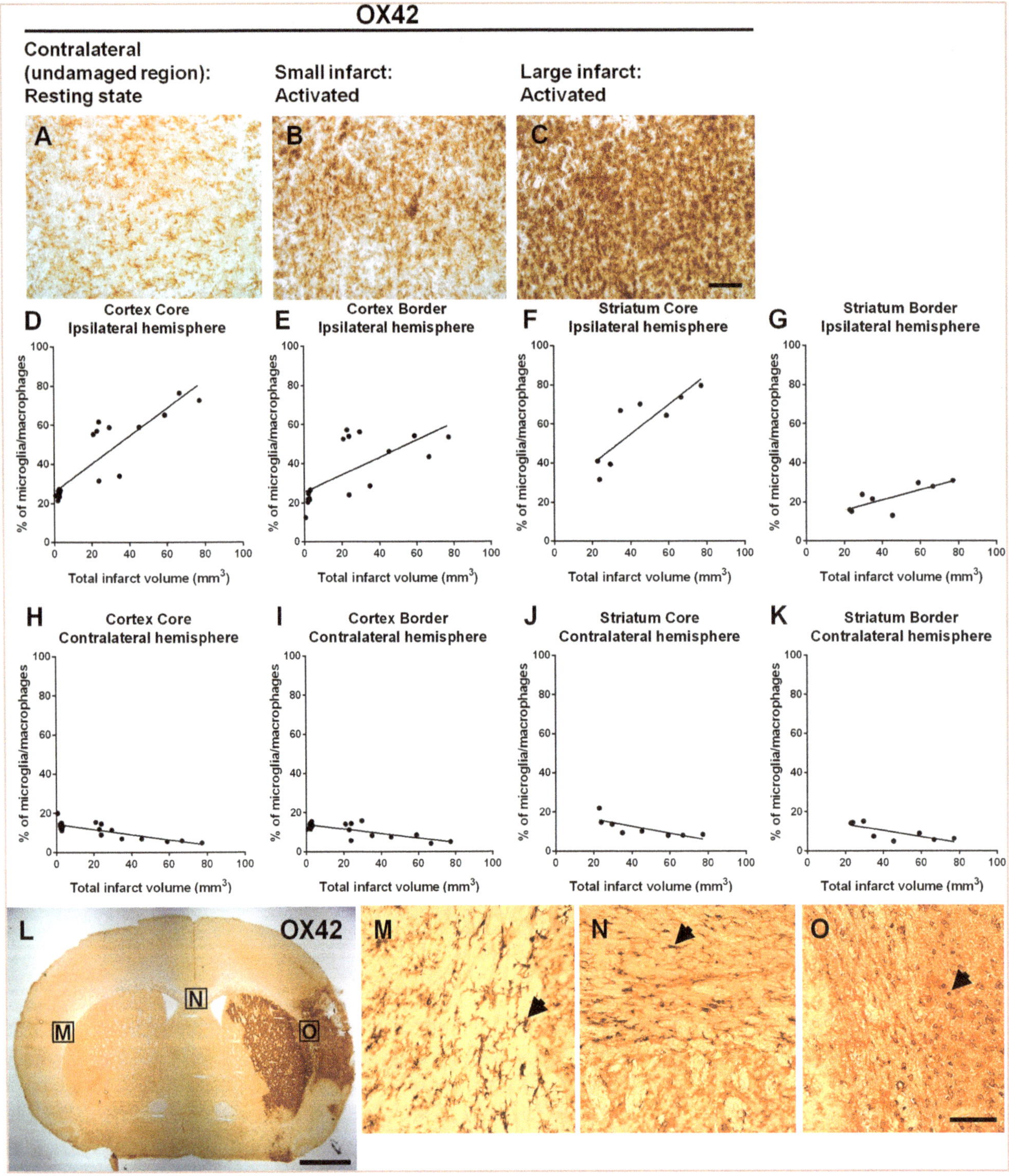

Figure 5. Immunohistochemical analysis of microglia and macrophages 14 days post-stroke. Immunohistochemical images of OX42 labelled microglia/macrophages within the contralateral undamaged hemisphere (A), ipsilateral core cortex of a small infarct (B) versus a large infarct (C). Within the ipsilateral hemisphere, a positive correlation was observed between infarct volume and the number of microglia and macrophages in the core cortex ($r=0.88$, $P<0.0001$, $n=19$; D), surrounding cortex ($r=0.70$, $P<0.001$, $n=19$; E), core striatum ($r=0.86$, $P<0.01$, $n=8$); F), and border striatum ($r=0.77$, $P<0.05$, $n=8$; G). In contrast, the number of microglia and macrophages in the mirror image areas on the contralateral side negatively correlated with infarct volumes within the core cortex ($r=0.81$, $P<0.0001$, $n=19$; H), border cortex ($r=0.75$, $P<0.0005$, $n=19$; I), core striatum ($r=0.75$, $P<0.05$, $n=8$; J), and border striatum ($r=0.75$, $P<0.05$, $n=8$; K) (Pearson product moment correlation coefficients). Activated microglia can be observed within the corpus callosum, and potentially represent microglia migrating from the contralateral undamaged hemisphere to sites of damage within the ipsilateral hemisphere (L). Magnified immunohistochemical images that correspond to boxes labelled (M to O) in (L) illustrate the possible migration pathway of microglia along the corpus callosum as indicated by the arrows. Scale bar: (A–C) 100 μm, (L) 2500 μm, (M–O) 50 μm.

were observed 14 days post-stroke (Figure 6D) and diffuse astrocytes were detected in very low numbers in this region (Figure 6E). Increased GFAP immunoreactivity was predominantly observed within the border zones of the infarct. In cortical regions surrounding the infarct (border zone), infarct volumes negatively correlated with the number of moderately activated astrocytes ($r = 0.87$, $P<0.0001$, $n = 19$; Figure 6F) but positively correlated with diffuse astrocytes ($r = 0.96$, $P<0.0001$, $n = 19$; Figure 6G). Little or no activated astrocytes were observed within the core striatum 14 days post-stroke (Figure 6H). A modest correlation was observed between infarct size and diffuse astrocytes within the core striatum ($r = 0.93$, $P<0.001$, $n = 8$; Figure 6I). Within the border zone surrounding the striatal infarct, lesion volume negatively correlated with activated astrocytes ($r = 0.85$, $P<0.01$, $n = 8$; Figure 6J) but positively correlated with diffuse astrocytes ($r = 0.89$, $P<0.005$, $n = 8$; Figure 6K). Larger infarct volumes were associated with greater glial scar formation encircling the damaged striatum and cortex.

Discussion

In the present study we confirm that the ET-1 model of stroke is a valuable tool for studying brain remodelling and long term recovery, specifically angiogenesis, microglia/macrophage activation, astrocytic morphological transition and SVZ cell proliferation, differentiation and migration. There is a positive correlation between lesion size and proliferation and differentiation of cells within the SVZ 7 days post-stroke, as well as between lesion size and the degree of angiogenesis, microglia activation and astrogliosis 14 days after stroke. This confirms and extends the initial report of Nagai *et al* [9] who showed pathological responses initiated by stroke affects the magnitude of the inflammatory response, and identifies the effect of stroke severity on subsequent repair mechanisms, important factors to consider when exploring treatment strategies that promote recovery of the injured brain.

Predictive Outcome and Long Term Recovery

Neurological deficit scores after stroke have commonly been used as a predictor of long term outcomes [38,39]. The current scales however, do not take into account spontaneous recovery of functions that occur weeks to months after stroke without change to the resulting brain infarct. None-the-less use of such scales has proven beneficial when assigning patients to treatment. We have previously reported the benefits of predicting stroke outcome using the ET-1 model of stroke in conscious rats, where variability in stroke severity reliably correlates with infarct volumes up to 3 day post-stroke [14]. To this end stroke outcomes using the ET-1 model allow clinically relevant assessments of stroke pathology since stroke in humans is highly variable: a large infarct can result following occlusion of a major artery such as the MCA or a small infarct can result due to occlusion of a single penetrating artery [40]. Predicting stroke outcome using rodent models has also been described where neurological deficits are tested upon recovery from anaesthesia [41]. In the present study we demonstrate that whilst a neurological scale at the time of stroke can be reliably used to predict histological outcome up to 14 days, it is not a reliable long-term predictor of neurological outcome, since recovery of deficits observed 14 days after stroke did not correlate with reduced lesion size.

Angiogenesis and Infarct Size

The potential for brain regeneration relies heavily on the surrounding microenvironment and for neuronal replacement to occur it requires supporting vasculature. Angiogenesis is a fundamental process occurring during development and in wound healing in adults, and previous studies using the MCA thread occlusion model have reported new vasculature develops mostly within the peri-infarct zone [19,42]. In contrast, we showed evidence of angiogenesis across the entire infarct in addition to the border zone [5], similar to that which occurs in humans where a significantly higher microvessel density is observed across the damaged region of the brain [20]. We now demonstrate that larger infarct volumes result in increased microvessel density within the core infarct as well as the peri-infarct zone, suggesting that even the most severely damaged brain might be capable of supporting neuronal replacement.

Previously the degree of angiogenesis, measured by increased cerebral blood flow and microvessel density, has been correlated with longer survival in stroke affected patients [20] suggesting that active angiogenesis may be beneficial to the damaged brain. Indeed we have previously reported that with spontaneous functional recovery newly formed vascular networks are detected within damaged regions [5]. One possible mechanism may be associated with the damage sustained to cerebral blood vessels themselves, such that a greater degree of vascular sprouting may result from an increased number of damaged vessels. Cerebral ischemia initially compromises blood vessels and may result in extensive damage to the vessel wall. In the present study we confirmed that a greater degree of angiogenesis occurs in regions associated with extensive neuronal loss and increased stroke severity. Thus increased vascular damage is associated with increased neuronal loss, resulting in increased angiogenesis.

The angiogenic process can improve the perfusion of oxygen and nutrients to ischemic and surrounding tissues where partially affected neurons that have the capability of surviving reside, which in turn may improve functional outcome following stroke [19]. Proliferation of endothelial cells within damaged brain regions are initiated within days after ischemic events [43,44] and the process of active angiogenesis may be beneficial for the ischemic brain. Interestingly, the correlation between angiogenesis and improved neurological outcome following stroke has been observed in both animal stroke models and human stroke patients [20,45,46]. Angiogenesis has also been linked directly with other endogenous recovery mechanisms including neurogenesis, synaptogenesis and neuronal and synaptic plasticity which are all events involved in the long-term repair and restoration process of the brain after stroke. If these repair processes are not achieved then vessel density may later regress. Clearly angiogenesis is a potential target for improved regenerative recovery after ischemic stroke.

Neurogenesis and Infarct Size

Ischemic insults to the brain have now been shown to trigger progenitor cell proliferation and stem cell migration from the SVZ of the lateral ventricle to damaged regions of the brain. We saw increased SVZ cell proliferation in the ipsilateral hemisphere 7 days post-stroke. Importantly, rats with larger infarcts were shown to have a greater degree of SVZ cell proliferation. Previous studies have shown proliferating SVZ stem cells increase as early as 2 days post-stoke, an effect that peaks by 7 days and returns to normal by 14 days [47,48]. Ours is the first study to show that this effect is initially amplified with increasing stroke severity, but is not sustained beyond this time.

The adult SVZ contains a heterogeneous population of cells including SVZ radial glial cells (type B cells), rapidly dividing transient amplifying cells (type C cells) and migratory neuroblasts (type A cells) [49,50]. Normally within the adult SVZ, newly generated stem cells migrate through the rostral migratory stream (RMS) into the olfactory bulb and differentiate into interneurons

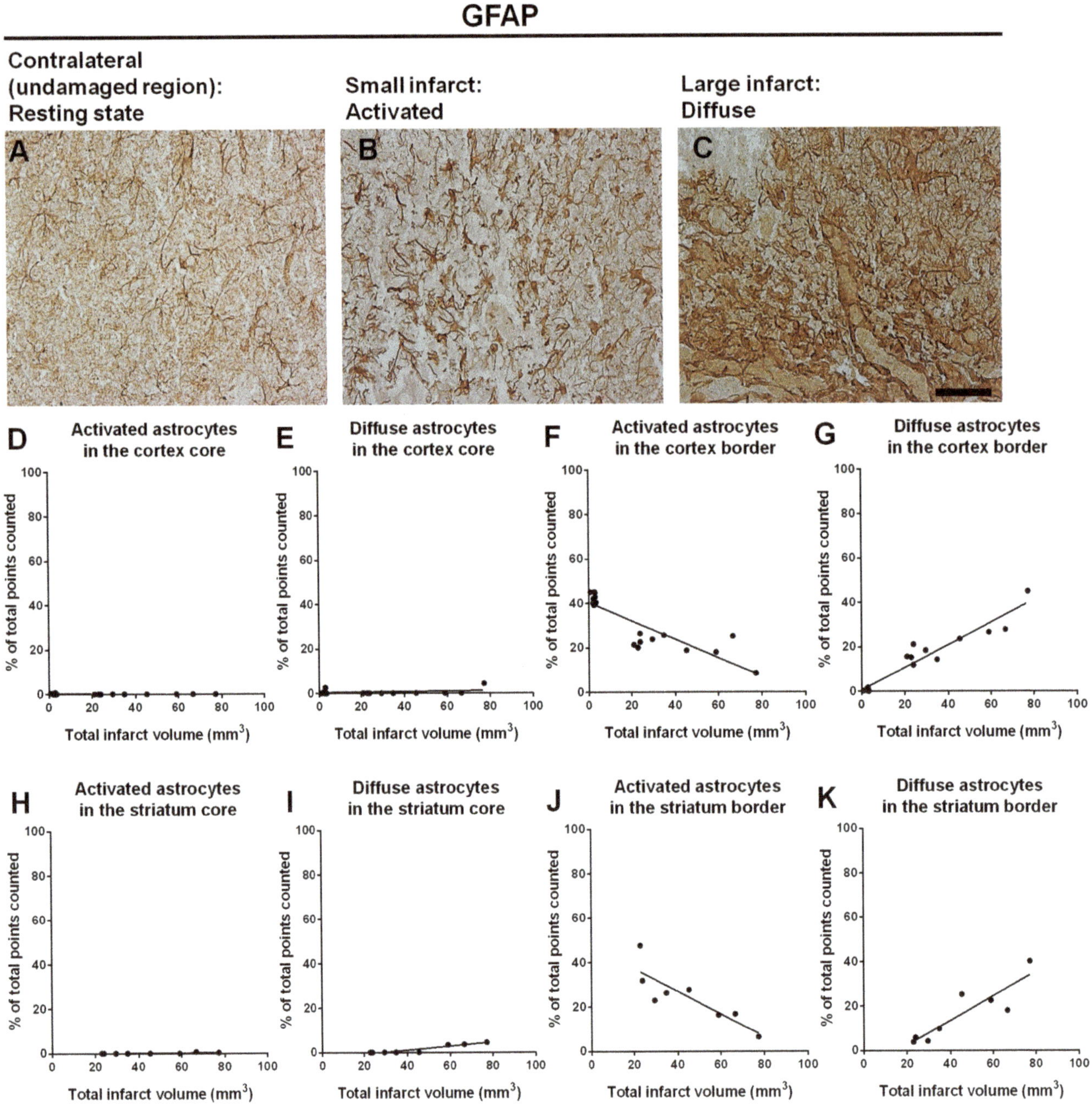

Figure 6. Analysis of activated and diffuse astrocytic morphologies 14 days post-stroke. Immunohistochemical images of GFAP positive astrocytes of a quiescent appearance found within the contralateral hemisphere (A), activated astrocytes surrounding a small infarct (B) and diffuse astrocytes bordering a large infarct (C). Within the core cortex, no activated astrocytes were found (D) and diffuse astrocytes were in very low numbers (E). In regions bordering the infarct, infarct volumes either negatively correlated with the number of activated astrocytes ($r = 0.87$, $P < 0.0001$, $n = 19$; F) or positively correlated with the number of diffuse astrocytes ($r = 0.96$, $P < 0.0001$, $n = 19$; G). No activated astrocytes were detected within the striatum core (H). A modest correlation was observed between infarct size and diffuse astrocytes within the core striatum ($r = 0.93$, $P < 0.001$, $n = 8$; I). In areas surrounding the striatum, infarct sizes either negatively correlated with activated astrocytes ($r = 0.85$, $P < 0.01$, $n = 8$; J) or positively correlated with diffuse astrocytes ($r = 0.89$, $P < 0.005$, $n = 8$; K) (Pearson product moment correlation coefficients). Scale bar: A–C 100 μm.

[51]. Cerebral ischemia alters the migration pathway and neuroblasts generated from the SVZ migrate to the injured brain regions instead, where only a few differentiate into new neurons (< 0.2%) [48]. In the present study rats with larger infarcts showed evidence of increased SVZ proliferation with a greater number of cells generated following a neuronal differentiation path as evidenced by increased DCX staining. DCX positive neuroblasts were not however evident within penumbral regions (Figure S1D–G), possibly suggesting a low survival rate of these new neurons with greater stroke severity. Arvidsson *et al.* [48] previously described the unfavourable hostile environment of severely ischemic tissue for newly formed neurons.

A notable loop of interactions between newly formed stem cells and blood vessels has been reported [24] and this interaction may be magnified with larger infarct volumes. Activated endothelial cells, injured and newly forming blood vessels release an array of trophic factors including vascular endothelial growth factor (VEGF) and brain-derived neurotrophic factor (BDNF) which can evoke neurogenesis, are chemotactic for progenitor cells and may enhance the survival and integration of neuroblasts into the brain tissue [18,22,52].

In the present study larger infarct volumes also correlated with an increase in the number of radial glial cells generated within the SVZ 7 days post-stroke. Radial glial cells retain neural stem cell-like properties and are capable of migrating from the SVZ towards the damaged brain where they can differentiate into either neurons or astrocytes based on the microenvironment [50,53,54]. Our results demonstrate that an increase in the number of SVZ derived radial glial cells 7 days post-stroke appear to be extending towards cortical and striatal penumbral regions of animals with larger infarcts (Figure S1A–C). By 14 days Nestin expressing reactive astrocytes are detected within the glial scar and possibly indicate a new cell population of reactive astrocytes that have migrated from the SVZ to the site of injury in response to stroke. These results indicate that without intervention, newly generated stem cells extend towards the damaged brain but have a greater propensity to become astrocytes that in turn contribute to glial scar formation that poses a major obstacle to brain repair.

Microglial Response to Lesion Size

Previous studies have reported a positive correlation between infarct size and microglia activation up to 7 days following discrete photochemically induced thrombotic lesions of the cerebral cortex [9]. We now show that this effect is also true for brain injury following focal ischemia using the ET-1 model with a 14 day recovery. Furthermore, we observed within the contralateral hemisphere a decrease in the percentage of activated microglia/macrophages in rats with larger infarcts. Microglia can become motile and actively move to the site of injury following chemotactic signals [55,56] and have also been found to migrate through the corpus callosum to arrive to their desired destination [57]. Indeed in the present study we observed in rats a reduction in the number of microglia in the contralateral hemisphere as well as graded changes in morphological activation throughout the corpus collasum, suggesting movement of microglia from uninjured brain regions to the infarcted hemisphere as described by others [55,56]. Therefore, the accumulation of microglia within the infarcted region at 14 days is likely to comprise of proliferating resident microglia as well as migrating microglia [58].

The accumulation of activated microglia/macrophages within ischemic regions occurs early after stroke with a peak response occurring at 7 days [59] when the inflammatory response peaks [5]. Our data now indicate a significant inflammatory response persists 14 days post-stroke where the size of the lesion still dictates the level of inflammatory cell activation. Persistent microglial activation can become maladaptive with the release of cytotoxic molecules [60,61] and pro-inflammatory cytokines that have been found to be neurotoxic [2,62,63]. In contrast, recent reports suggest that activated microglia may also play a role in brain repair. For it has been implicated in increasing neurogenesis *in vitro* [64] and *in vivo* [65] following stroke, and free radicals derived from activated microglia might also have a role in promoting angiogenesis [5]. Microglia may also exert neuroprotection by producing neurotrophic molecules such as brain-derived neurotrophic factor (BDNF), insulin-like growth factor 1 (IGF-1), and several other growth factors [66]. However the degree of injury may be an important stimulus for microglia, determining whether they play a detrimental or beneficial role. Establishing the microglia/macrophage response after an ischemic insult will assist in the understanding of endogenous processes occurring to highlight the positive and negative influences these inflammatory cells may have on endogenous repair mechanisms that support neuronal differentiation and survival of migrating neural progenitor cells.

Astrocytic Response to Varying Infarct Volumes

Positive correlations between lesion size and astrocytic activation has also been reported by Nagai *et al* [9]. Quantification of activated astrocytes according to morphological transition in correlation with infarct volume has not been previously reported. Astrogliosis following injury to the brain is not a simple all-or-none phenomenon, but a finely gradated continuum of morphological change that can either influence brain preservation or result in long-lasting scar formation and reorganisation of tissue structure [32,67]. We now confirm that larger infarct volumes contain an increased percentage of severely diffuse reactive astrocytes, and a decrease in the percentage of moderately activated astrocytes within border regions of the infarct.

Astrocytes with moderately activated morphologies have been thought to initially provide trophic and protective support to neurons [68] that may promote neuroprotection and could possibly create an environment conducive to facilitate neurite extension and axonal outgrowth to aid in regeneration [69]. If immediate restoration of blood flow after initial stroke insult is initiated, astrocytes of mild or moderately active morphologies have the potential to resolve and return to their appearance in healthy tissue once the triggering mechanism is resolved [70]. On the other hand if the insult continues to persist without resolution, astrocytes transition into severely diffuse reactive distinctions and may not revert to their previous morphological states [70]. These severely diffuse reactive astrocytes may no longer be beneficial to neurons and can instead majorly impede axonal regrowth through formation of the glial scar and secretion of extracellular matrix molecules that prevent axonal regeneration [67,71–73].

Based on our findings larger infarcts induce astrocytic transition to severely diffuse morphologies that could possibly contribute to the spread of damage as well as combining to form a physical barrier to brain remodelling and repair. Importantly we now show that increased cell proliferation within the SVZ of rats with larger infarcts contribute to increased glial scar formation since we observed a greater proportion of Nestin/GFAP positive cells extending from the SVZ as well as within the border zone. Much focus in developing treatment strategies that encourage brain repair has been to target increased proliferation and migration of neural progenitor cells from the SVZ after brain injury [74–78]. Treatments aimed towards up-regulating endogenous proliferation from either the SVZ or dentate gyrus of the hippocampus should also confirm the fate of the newly generated cells to appropriately assess the therapeutic benefit [79]. Given the results presented in the current study it is now clearly important to characterise the long term impact of these treatments across differing stroke severities. Particularly since increasing stem cell proliferation and migration may be counterproductive if the microenvironment supports conversion to astrocytes that accentuate the glial scar rather than conversion to new neurons.

Conclusion

The potential for brain regeneration relies heavily on the surrounding microenvironment and this includes the pathogenic contribution from inflammatory cells, angiogenesis and neural stem cells. Ours is the first study to demonstrate a positive correlation between stroke severity and the effects on pathological responses to brain recovery using a focal model of cerebral ischemia. In addition, our results have highlighted the importance of taking into consideration infarct size when developing therapies that are targeted towards promoting neurogenesis. Therapeutic strategies aimed at increasing cell proliferation and migration from the SVZ need to pay particular attention to the phenotypic transformation of neural progenitor cells following treatments to avoid unwanted additional scar formation. Understanding the endogenous pathways initiated after ischemic insult will enable us to design better therapies to augment the restorative power of the cerebral vasculature as well as improve brain remodelling for improved functional outcomes.

Supporting Information

Figure S1 SVZ cell extension towards infarct and neural differentiation. Photomicrographs of the contralateral (A) and ipsilateral (B) hemispheres depicting radial glial cells mainly within the ipsilateral hemisphere extending from the SVZ towards the cortical and striatal penumbral regions (Nestin+/GFAP+; green/red respectively with co-expression giving a yellow appearance). Core infarct regions are marked by a white dotted line. Merged immunofluorescent image of radial glial cells extending towards the penumbra from the SVZ as indicated by the arrows (Nestin/GFAP/DAPI; green/red/blue respectively with Nestin/GFAP co-expression giving a yellow appearance; C). Immunofluorescent images depicting immature neuronal cells (DAPI/DCX+; blue/green respectively; D–G) within the penumbra cortex (D) and SVZ of the ipsilateral hemisphere (E) and mirror images of the contralateral hemisphere (F, G). All images were taken from animals with large infarcts. LV: Lateral ventricle, Ctx: Cortex, Stm: Striatum. Scale bar: A,B 400 μm, C 40 μm, D, G 100 μm, E, F 50 μm.

Author Contributions

Conceived and designed the experiments: CLR GJD. Performed the experiments: HCSA LB CLR. Analyzed the data: HCSA. Contributed reagents/materials/analysis tools: CLR. Wrote the paper: HCSA CLR.

References

1. Lansberg MG, Straka M, Kemp S, Mlynash M, Wechsler LR, et al. (2012) MRI profile and response to endovascular reperfusion after stroke (DEFUSE 2): a prospective cohort study. Lancet Neurol 11: 860–867.
2. Dirnagl U, Iadecola C, Moskowitz MA (1999) Pathobiology of ischaemic stroke: an integrated view. Trends Neurosci 22: 391–397.
3. Lo EH, Dalkara T, Moskowitz MA (2003) Mechanisms, challenges and opportunities in stroke. Nat Rev Neurosci 4: 399–415.
4. Huang IJ, Chen CY, Chung HW, Chang DC, Lee CC, et al. (2001) Time course of cerebral infarction in the middle cerebral arterial territory: deep watershed versus territorial subtypes on diffusion-weighted MR images. Radiology 221: 35–42.
5. Taylor C, Weston RM, Dusting GJ, Roulston CL (2013) NADPH Oxidase and Angiogenesis Following Endothelin-1 Induced Stroke in Rats: Role for Nox2 in Brain Repair. Brain Sci 3: 294–317.
6. Schwamm LH, Koroshetz WJ, Sorensen AG, Wang B, Copen WA, et al. (1998) Time course of lesion development in patients with acute stroke: serial diffusion- and hemodynamic-weighted magnetic resonance imaging. Stroke 29: 2268–2276.
7. Saunders DE, Howe FA, van den Boogaart A, McLean MA, Griffiths JR, et al. (1995) Continuing ischemic damage after acute middle cerebral artery infarction in humans demonstrated by short-echo proton spectroscopy. Stroke 26: 1007–1013.
8. Brott T, Marler JR, Olinger CP, Adams HP Jr., Tomsick T, et al. (1989) Measurements of acute cerebral infarction: lesion size by computed tomography. Stroke 20: 871–875.
9. Nagai N, Kawao N, Okada K, Ishida C, Okumoto K, et al. (2010) Initial brain lesion size affects the extent of subsequent pathophysiological responses. Brain Res 1322: 109–117.
10. Cramer SC (2012) Stratifying patients with stroke in trials that target brain repair. Stroke 41: S114–116.
11. Goldstein LB, Samsa GP (1997) Reliability of the National Institutes of Health Stroke Scale. Extension to non-neurologists in the context of a clinical trial. Stroke 28: 307–310.
12. Leira EC, Adams HP Jr., Rosenthal GE, Torner JC (2008) Baseline NIH stroke scale responses estimate the probability of each particular stroke subtype. Cerebrovasc Dis 26: 573–577.
13. Counsell C, Dennis M, McDowall M, Warlow C (2002) Predicting outcome after acute and subacute stroke: development and validation of new prognostic models. Stroke 33: 1041–1047.
14. Roulston CL, Callaway JK, Jarrott B, Woodman OL, Dusting GJ (2008) Using behaviour to predict stroke severity in conscious rats: post-stroke treatment with 3′, 4′-dihydroxyflavonol improves recovery. Eur J Pharmacol 584: 100–110.
15. Cramer SC, Parrish TB, Levy RM, Stebbins GT, Ruland SD, et al. (2007) Predicting functional gains in a stroke trial. Stroke 38: 2108–2114.
16. Zhang R, Zhang Z, Wang L, Wang Y, Gousev A, et al. (2004) Activated neural stem cells contribute to stroke-induced neurogenesis and neuroblast migration toward the infarct boundary in adult rats. J Cereb Blood Flow Metab 24: 441–448.
17. Zhang RL, Zhang ZG, Chopp M (2008) Ischemic stroke and neurogenesis in the subventricular zone. Neuropharmacology 55: 345–352.
18. Minger SL, Ekonomou A, Carta EM, Chinoy A, Perry RH, et al. (2007) Endogenous neurogenesis in the human brain following cerebral infarction. Regen Med 2: 69–74.
19. Sbarbati A, Pietra C, Baldassarri AM, Guerrini U, Ziviani L, et al. (1996) The microvascular system in ischemic cortical lesions. Acta Neuropathol 92: 56–63.
20. Krupinski J, Kaluza J, Kumar P, Kumar S, Wang JM (1994) Role of angiogenesis in patients with cerebral ischemic stroke. Stroke 25: 1794–1798.
21. Gauthier LV, Taub E, Perkins C, Ortmann M, Mark VW, et al. (2008) Remodeling the brain: plastic structural brain changes produced by different motor therapies after stroke. Stroke 39: 1520–1525.
22. Leventhal C, Rafii S, Rafii D, Shahar A, Goldman SA (1999) Endothelial trophic support of neuronal production and recruitment from the adult mammalian subependyma. Mol Cell Neurosci 13: 450–464.
23. Palmer TD, Willhoite AR, Gage FH (2000) Vascular niche for adult hippocampal neurogenesis. J Comp Neurol 425: 479–494.
24. Ohab JJ, Fleming S, Blesch A, Carmichael ST (2006) A neurovascular niche for neurogenesis after stroke. J Neurosci 26: 13007–13016.
25. Yamamoto M, Tamura A, Kirino T, Shimizu M, Sano K (1988) Behavioral changes after focal cerebral ischemia by left middle cerebral artery occlusion in rats. Brain Res 452: 323–328.
26. De Ryck M, Van Reempts J, Borgers M, Wauquier A, Janssen PA (1989) Photochemical stroke model: flunarizine prevents sensorimotor deficits after neocortical infarcts in rats. Stroke 20: 1383–1390.
27. Callaway JK, Knight MJ, Watkins DJ, Beart PM, Jarrott B (1999) Delayed treatment with AM-36, a novel neuroprotective agent, reduces neuronal damage after endothelin-1-induced middle cerebral artery occlusion in conscious rats. Stroke 30: 2704–2712; discussion 2712.
28. Callaway JK, Knight MJ, Watkins DJ, Beart PM, Jarrott B, et al. (2000) A novel, rapid, computerized method for quantitation of neuronal damage in a rat model of stroke. J Neurosci Methods 102: 53–60.
29. Osborne KA, Shigeno T, Balarsky AM, Ford I, McCulloch J, et al. (1987) Quantitative assessment of early brain damage in a rat model of focal cerebral ischaemia. J Neurol Neurosurg Psychiatry 50: 402–410.
30. Leach MJ, Swan JH, Eisenthal D, Dopson M, Nobbs M (1993) BW619C89, a glutamate release inhibitor, protects against focal cerebral ischemic damage. Stroke 24: 1063–1067.
31. Lokmic Z, Mitchell GM (2011) Visualisation and stereological assessment of blood and lymphatic vessels. Histol Histopathol 26: 781–796.
32. Sofroniew MV, Vinters HV (2010) Astrocytes: biology and pathology. Acta Neuropathol 119: 7–35.
33. Kettenmann H, Hanisch UK, Noda M, Verkhratsky A (2011) Physiology of microglia. Physiol Rev 91: 461–553.
34. Tanaka R, Komine-Kobayashi M, Mochizuki H, Yamada M, Furuya T, et al. (2003) Migration of enhanced green fluorescent protein expressing bone marrow-derived microglia/macrophage into the mouse brain following permanent focal ischemia. Neuroscience 117: 531–539.
35. Schilling M, Besselmann M, Leonhard C, Mueller M, Ringelstein EB, et al. (2003) Microglial activation precedes and predominates over macrophage infiltration in transient focal cerebral ischemia: a study in green fluorescent protein transgenic bone marrow chimeric mice. Exp Neurol 183: 25–33.
36. Jin R, Yang G, Li G (2010) Inflammatory mechanisms in ischemic stroke: role of inflammatory cells. J Leukoc Biol 87: 779–789.
37. Schilling M, Besselmann M, Muller M, Strecker JK, Ringelstein EB, et al. (2005) Predominant phagocytic activity of resident microglia over hematogenous macrophages following transient focal cerebral ischemia: an investigation using

green fluorescent protein transgenic bone marrow chimeric mice. Exp Neurol 196: 290–297.
38. Jongbloed L (1986) Prediction of function after stroke: a critical review. Stroke 17: 765–776.
39. Konig IR, Ziegler A, Bluhmki E, Hacke W, Bath PM, et al. (2008) Predicting long-term outcome after acute ischemic stroke: a simple index works in patients from controlled clinical trials. Stroke 39: 1821–1826.
40. Arboix A, Marti-Vilalta JL (2009) Lacunar stroke. Expert Rev Neurother 9: 179–196.
41. Boyko M, Ohayon S, Goldsmith T, Novack L, Novack V, et al. (2011) Morphological and neuro-behavioral parallels in the rat model of stroke. Behav Brain Res 223: 17–23.
42. Bosomtwi A, Jiang Q, Ding GL, Zhang L, Zhang ZG, et al. (2008) Quantitative evaluation of microvascular density after stroke in rats using MRI. J Cereb Blood Flow Metab 28: 1978–1987.
43. Szpak GM, Lechowicz W, Lewandowska E, Bertrand E, Wierzba-Bobrowicz T, et al. (1999) Border zone neovascularization in cerebral ischemic infarct. Folia Neuropathol 37: 264–268.
44. Chen HH, Chien CH, Liu HM (1994) Correlation between angiogenesis and basic fibroblast growth factor expression in experimental brain infarct. Stroke 25: 1651–1657.
45. Liu XS, Zhang ZG, Zhang RL, Gregg S, Morris DC, et al. (2007) Stroke induces gene profile changes associated with neurogenesis and angiogenesis in adult subventricular zone progenitor cells. J Cereb Blood Flow Metab 27: 564–574.
46. Henderson RD, Eliasziw M, Fox AJ, Rothwell PM, Barnett HJ (2000) Angiographically defined collateral circulation and risk of stroke in patients with severe carotid artery stenosis. North American Symptomatic Carotid Endarterectomy Trial (NASCET) Group. Stroke 31: 128–132.
47. Zhang RL, Zhang ZG, Lu M, Wang Y, Yang JJ, et al. (2006) Reduction of the cell cycle length by decreasing G1 phase and cell cycle reentry expand neuronal progenitor cells in the subventricular zone of adult rat after stroke. J Cereb Blood Flow Metab 26: 857–863.
48. Arvidsson A, Collin T, Kirik D, Kokaia Z, Lindvall O (2002) Neuronal replacement from endogenous precursors in the adult brain after stroke. Nat Med 8: 963–970.
49. Doetsch F, Caille I, Lim DA, Garcia-Verdugo JM, Alvarez-Buylla A (1999) Subventricular zone astrocytes are neural stem cells in the adult mammalian brain. Cell 97: 703–716.
50. Gregg C, Weiss S (2003) Generation of functional radial glial cells by embryonic and adult forebrain neural stem cells. J Neurosci 23: 11587–11601.
51. Garcia-Verdugo JM, Doetsch F, Wichterle H, Lim DA, Alvarez-Buylla A (1998) Architecture and cell types of the adult subventricular zone: in search of the stem cells. J Neurobiol 36: 234–248.
52. Shen Q, Goderie SK, Jin L, Karanth N, Sun Y, et al. (2004) Endothelial cells stimulate self-renewal and expand neurogenesis of neural stem cells. Science 304: 1338–1340.
53. Merkle FT, Tramontin AD, Garcia-Verdugo JM, Alvarez-Buylla A (2004) Radial glia give rise to adult neural stem cells in the subventricular zone. Proc Natl Acad Sci USA 101: 17528–17532.
54. Zhang RL, Zhang ZG, Wang Y, LeTourneau Y, Liu XS, et al. (2007) Stroke induces ependymal cell transformation into radial glia in the subventricular zone of the adult rodent sbrain. J Cereb Blood Flow Metab 27: 1201–1212.
55. Brockhaus J, Moller T, Kettenmann H (1996) Phagocytozing ameboid microglial cells studied in a mouse corpus callosum slice preparation. Glia 16: 81–90.
56. Davalos D, Grutzendler J, Yang G, Kim JV, Zuo Y, et al. (2005) ATP mediates rapid microglial response to local brain injury in vivo. Nat Neurosci 8: 752–758.
57. Marks L, Carswell HV, Peters EE, Graham DI, Patterson J, et al. (2001) Characterization of the microglial response to cerebral ischemia in the stroke-prone spontaneously hypertensive rat. Hypertension 38: 116–122.
58. Schroeter M, Jander S, Witte OW, Stoll G (1999) Heterogeneity of the microglial response in photochemically induced focal ischemia of the rat cerebral cortex. Neuroscience 89: 1367–1377.
59. Ito D, Tanaka K, Suzuki S, Dembo T, Fukuuchi Y (2001) Enhanced expression of Iba1, ionized calcium-binding adapter molecule 1, after transient focal cerebral ischemia in rat brain. Stroke 32: 1208–1215.
60. Colton CA, Gilbert DL (1987) Production of superoxide anions by a CNS macrophage, the microglia. FEBS Lett 223: 284–288.
61. Moss DW, Bates TE (2001) Activation of murine microglial cell lines by lipopolysaccharide and interferon-gamma causes NO-mediated decreases in mitochondrial and cellular function. Eur J Neurosci 13: 529–538.
62. Raivich G, Jones LL, Werner A, Bluthmann H, Doetschmann T, et al. (1999) Molecular signals for glial activation: pro- and anti-inflammatory cytokines in the injured brain. Acta Neurochir Suppl 73: 21–30.
63. Hanisch UK (2002) Microglia as a source and target of cytokines. Glia 40: 140–155.
64. Walton NM, Sutter BM, Laywell ED, Levkoff LH, Kearns SM, et al. (2006) Microglia instruct subventricular zone neurogenesis. Glia 54: 815–825.
65. Thored P, Heldmann U, Gomes-Leal W, Gisler R, Darsalia V, et al. (2009) Long-term accumulation of microglia with proneurogenic phenotype concomitant with persistent neurogenesis in adult subventricular zone after stroke. Glia 57: 835–849.
66. Lucas SM, Rothwell NJ, Gibson RM (2006) The role of inflammation in CNS injury and disease. Br J Pharmacol 147 Suppl 1: S232–240.
67. McGraw J, Hiebert GW, Steeves JD (2001) Modulating astrogliosis after neurotrauma. J Neurosci Res 63: 109–115.
68. Rossi DJ, Brady JD, Mohr C (2007) Astrocyte metabolism and signaling during brain ischemia. Nat Neurosci 10: 1377–1386.
69. Cramer SC, Chopp M (2000) Recovery recapitulates ontogeny. Trends Neurosci 23: 265–271.
70. Sofroniew MV (2009) Molecular dissection of reactive astrogliosis and glial scar formation. Trends Neurosci 32: 638–647.
71. Ridet JL, Malhotra SK, Privat A, Gage FH (1997) Reactive astrocytes: cellular and molecular cues to biological function. Trends Neurosci 20: 570–577.
72. Costa S, Planchenault T, Charriere-Bertrand C, Mouchel Y, Fages C, et al. (2002) Astroglial permissivity for neuritic outgrowth in neuron-astrocyte cocultures depends on regulation of laminin bioavailability. Glia 37: 105–113.
73. Fawcett JW (2006) Overcoming inhibition in the damaged spinal cord. J Neurotrauma. 2006/04/25 ed. 371–383.
74. Chen J, Zhang ZG, Li Y, Wang Y, Wang L, et al. (2003) Statins induce angiogenesis, neurogenesis, and synaptogenesis after stroke. Ann Neurol 53: 743–751.
75. Zhang R, Wang Y, Zhang L, Zhang Z, Tsang W, et al. (2002) Sildenafil (Viagra) induces neurogenesis and promotes functional recovery after stroke in rats. Stroke 33: 2675–2680.
76. Chen J, Li Y, Katakowski M, Chen X, Wang L, et al. (2003) Intravenous bone marrow stromal cell therapy reduces apoptosis and promotes endogenous cell proliferation after stroke in female rat. J Neurosci Res 73: 778–786.
77. Kim YR, Kim HN, Ahn SM, Choi YH, Shin HK, et al. (2014) Electroacupuncture Promotes Post-Stroke Functional Recovery via Enhancing Endogenous Neurogenesis in Mouse Focal Cerebral Ischemia. PLoS One 9: e90000.
78. Yoo SW, Kim SS, Lee SY, Lee HS, Kim HS, et al. (2008) Mesenchymal stem cells promote proliferation of endogenous neural stem cells and survival of newborn cells in a rat stroke model. Exp Mol Med 40: 387–397.
79. Gonzalez FF, Larpthaveesarp A, McQuillen P, Derugin N, Wendland M, et al. (2013) Erythropoietin increases neurogenesis and oligodendrogliosis of subventricular zone precursor cells after neonatal stroke. Stroke 44: 753–758.

22

High Incidence of Ischemic Stroke Occurrence in Irradiated Lung Cancer Patients: A Population-Based Surgical Cohort Study

**Shih-Kai Hung[1,8], Moon-Sing Lee[1,8], Wen-Yen Chiou[1,8], Ching-Chih Lee[2,8], Yi-Chun Chen[3,8], Chun-Liang Lai[4,8], Nai-Chuan Chien[5,8], Wen-Lin Hsu[7,8], Dai-Wei Liu[7,8], Yu-Chieh Su[6,8], Szu-Chi Li[6,8], Hung-Chih Lai[6,8], Shiang-Jiun Tsai[1], Feng-Chun Hsu[1], Hon-Yi Lin[1,8,9]*

Departments of Radiation Oncology, Buddhist Dalin Tzu Chi Hospital, Taiwan, ROC, **2** Department of Otolaryngology, Buddhist Dalin Tzu Chi Hospital, Taiwan, ROC, **3** Division of Nephrology, Buddhist Dalin Tzu Chi Hospital, Taiwan, ROC, **4** Division of Chest Medicine, Buddhist Dalin Tzu Chi Hospital, Taiwan, ROC, **5** Division of Thoracic Surgery, Buddhist Dalin Tzu Chi Hospital, Taiwan, ROC, **6** Division of Hematology-Oncology, Buddhist Dalin Tzu Chi Hospital, Taiwan, ROC, **7** Department of Radiation Oncology, Buddhist Tzu Chi General Hospital, Hualien, Taiwan, ROC, **8** School of Medicine, Tzu Chi University, Hualien, Taiwan, ROC, **9** Institute of Molecular Biology, National Chung Cheng University, Min-Hsiung, Chia-Yi, Taiwan, ROC

Abstract

Background and Purpose: A high risk of stroke occurrence has been reported in several types of irradiated cancer patients. However, clinical data are lacking in irradiated lung cancer patients. The present study intended to explore a risk level of ischemic stroke occurrence in irradiated lung cancer patients.

Methods: A nationwide population-based database obtained from the Taiwan National Health Insurance was analyzed. Between 2003 and 2006, we recruited 560 resected lung cancer patients into two study groups: surgery-plus-irradiation ($n = 112$) and surgery-alone ($n = 448$). Patients treated with chemotherapy were excluded. Propensity score match was used for pairing cases with a ratio of 1:4. Two-year ischemic-stroke-free survival was defined as the primary endpoint.

Results: Three observations supported a high risk of ischemic stroke occurrence in patients with postoperative irradiation when compared with those patients with surgery alone: first, a high incidence per 1,000 person-year (22.3 versus 11.2, 1.99 folds); second, a low two-year ischemic-stroke-free survival rate (92.2% versus 98.1%, $P = 0.019$); and third, a high adjusted hazard ratio (HR, 4.19; 95% CI, 1.44–12.22; $P = 0.009$). More notably, the highest risk of ischemic stroke occurrence was found in irradiated patients who had diabetes mellitus (HR, 34.74; 95% CI, 6.35->100; $P<0.0001$).

Conclusions: A high incidence of ischemic stroke was observed in irradiated lung cancer patients, especially in those with diabetes mellitus. For these patients, close clinical surveillance and strict diabetes control should be considered. Further studies to define detail biological mechanisms are encouraged.

Editor: John D. Minna, Univesity of Texas Southwestern Medical Center at Dallas, United States of America

Funding: This study is supported by research grants of Buddhist Dalin Tzu Chi Hospital: DTCRD-99-I-12 and DTCRD-100(2)-I-14. The funders had no role in study design, data collection and analysis, decision to publish, or preparation of the manuscript.

Competing Interests: The authors have declared that no competing interests exist.

* E-mail: doc16021@gmail.com

Introduction

High risks of stroke occurrence have been observed in irradiated cancer patients

Stroke is a major disease burden worldwide – once occurred, it may result in significant morbidities and mortality [1]. In the literature, a high risk of stroke occurrence has been reported in several types of irradiated cancer patients, such as head and neck cancers [2], breast cancer [3], and Hodgkin's lymphoma [4]. In these irradiated patients, one treatment point is similar. That is, radiotherapy (RT) is given to cover primary and lymphatic-drainage areas, which include the neck and/or mediastinum [5,6]. In such a condition, ionizing radiation cannot be avoided to deliver on brain-supplied blood vessels [6,7]. As a result, late vascular damage and subsequent embolic events may occur [8].

Little is known about risk of stroke occurrence in irradiated lung cancer patients

Clinically, the mediastinum was irradiated in both lung cancer and Hodgkin's lymphoma patients. However, when compared with irradiated Hodgkin's lymphoma patients [4,9,10], reported evidence of stroke risk is largely lacking in irradiated lung cancer patients. From the literature, it is clear that RT-associated stroke is particularly noted in long-term survivors [11,12]. Thus, this data discrepancy may be partly due to a significant difference of patient survival in these two disease entities. In lung cancer patients, an

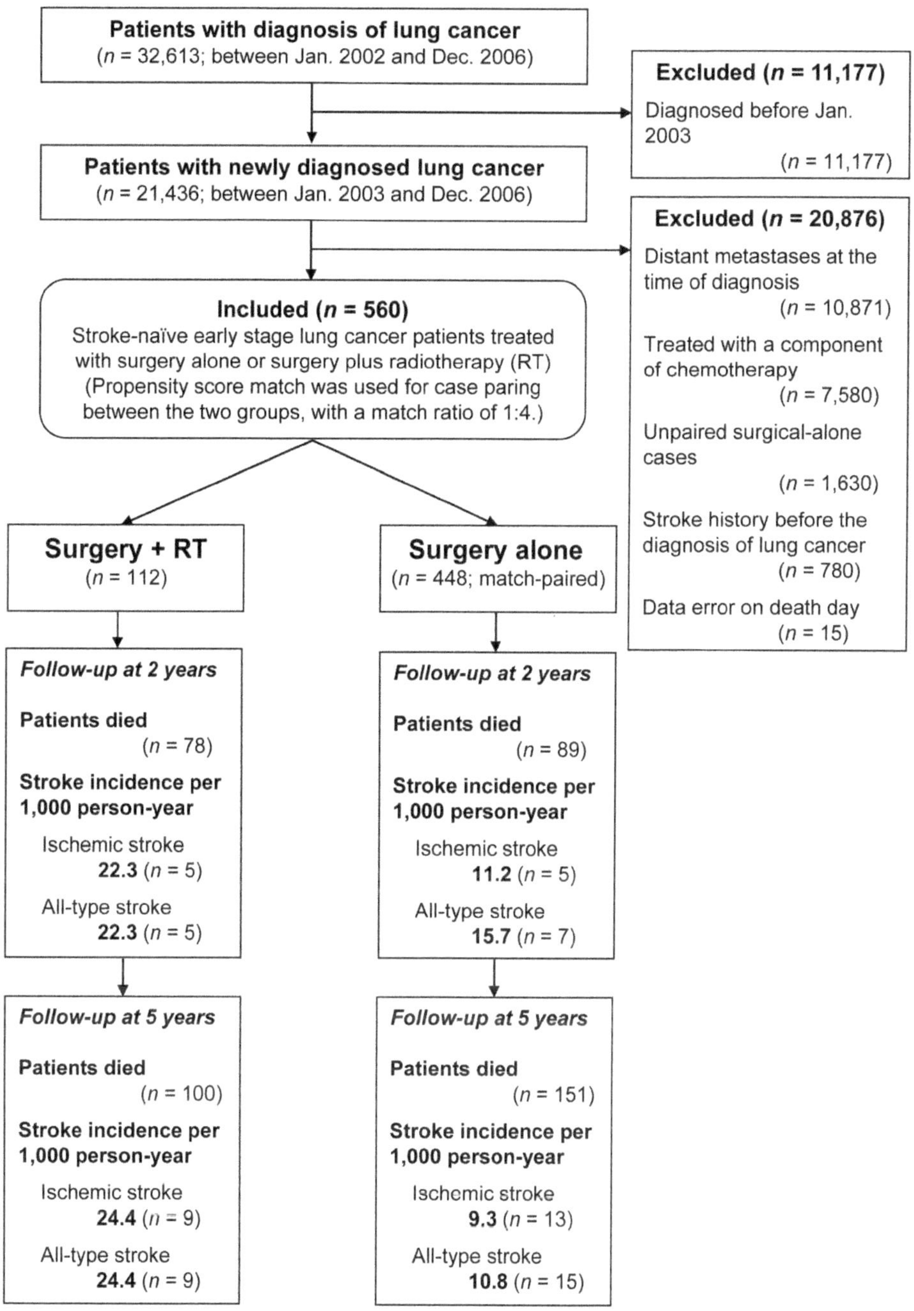

Figure 1. Flow chart of patient allocation. With respect to patients treated with surgery plus radiotherapy (RT), patients treated with surgery alone were match-paired by using a ratio of 1:4. **Note**: Data coded errors were validated by using the data subset of Registry for Catastrophe Illness.

average shorter survival may obscure an observation of stroke occurrence.

Recently, a high stroke risk has been reported in lung cancer patients. More notably, this risk effect can be early observed at a follow-up time of two years [13]. This finding sheds us a light to explore a potential risk of ischemic stroke occurrence in irradiated lung cancer patients.

Purpose of the present study

The present study intended to explore whether a risk of ischemic stroke occurrence is really high in irradiated lung cancer patients. Early stage lung cancer patients treated with surgery – but without a component of chemotherapy – were recruited. Of these, patients treated with postoperative radiotherapy were defined as the group of interesting. On the other hand, patients treated with surgery alone were match-paired as intra-cohort controls. Multivariate analysis confirmed a high risk association of ischemic stroke occurrence in irradiated lung cancer patients, especially in those patients with diabetes mellitus.

Table 1. Patient and demographic characteristics according to treatment groups.

	Treatment group, *n* (%)			Total, *n* (%)
	Surgery + RT	Surgery alone	*P* value	
Age			*0.999*	
≤65 years	77 (68.8)	308 (68.8)		385 (68.8)
>65 years	35 (31.5)	140 (31.3)		175 (31.3)
Gender			*0.766*	
Male	84 (75.0)	342 (76.3)		426 (76.1)
Female	28 (25.0)	106 (23.7)		134 (23.9)
Hypertension			*0.464*	
Yes	31 (27.7)	109 (24.3)		140 (25.0)
No	81 (72.3)	339 (75.7)		420 (75.0)
Diabetes mellitus			*0.819*	
Yes	19 (17.0)	72 (16.1)		91 (16.3)
No	93 (83.0)	376 (83.9)		469 (83.8)
CAD*			*0.341*	
Yes	11 (9.8)	32 (7.1)		43 (7.7)
No	101 (90.2)	416 (92.9)		517 (92.3)
Atrial fibrillation			*0.885*	
Yes	1 (0.9)	3 (0.7)		3 (0.5)
No	111 (99.1)	445 (99.3)		557 (99.5)
Geographic region			*0.926*	
Northern	44 (39.3)	187 (41.7)		231 (41.3)
Central	27 (24.1)	111 (24.8)		138 (24.6)
Southern	39 (34.8)	144 (32.1)		183 (32.7)
Eastern	2 (1.8)	6 (1.3)		8 (1.4)
Urbanization level			*0.776*	
Urban	26 (23.2)	109 (24.3)		135 (24.1)
Suburban	42 (37.5)	152 (33.9)		194 (34.6)
Rural	44 (39.3)	187 (41.7)		231 (41.3)
Total	112 (100.0)	448 (100.0)		560 (100.0)

Abbreviation: **RT**, radiotherapy; **CAD**, coronary artery disease.
Note 1: All above factors were used for propensity-score match to balance study groups.
Note 2: All *P* values were calculated by using chi-square test.

Methods

Database and ethic statement

The present study used a research database obtained from the Taiwan National Health Insurance (TNHI). This database covered medical care of more than 97% of Taiwanese [14,15]. The human experiments followed here were in accordance with the Helsinki Declaration and were approved by the Institution Review Board (IRB) of our institution, i.e. Buddhist Dalin Tzu Chi Hospital (approved number, B10001019). The IRB waived requirement for written informed consents from patients involved because researchers cannot contact with individual patients from this de-identified database [13,16].

Patient allocation and study groups

Between Jan. 2003 and Dec. 2006, we recruited 560 newly diagnosed early stage lung cancer patients into the following two groups: surgery plus radiotherapy ($n = 112$) and surgery alone ($n = 448$; Fig. 1 and table 1).

Fig. 1 shows flow chart of patient allocation. First, lung cancer patients were identified by using International Classification of Diseases, Ninth Revision, Clinical Modification (ICD-9-CM) code 162 ($n = 32{,}613$). Next, lung cancer diagnosis was validated by using a peer-confirmed data subset, i.e. Registry Data for Catastrophe Illness [13]. Then, we excluded patients with lung cancer history to identify newly diagnosed lung cancer patients ($n = 21{,}436$). Furthermore, we excluded 20,876 patients by using following criteria: distant metastases at the time of diagnosis ($n = 10{,}871$; ICD-9-CM codes, 196–199), chemotherapy used ($n = 7{,}580$), unpaired cases ($n = 1{,}630$), previous stroke ($n = 780$), and data error ($n = 15$).

Finally, we recruited 112 early stage lung cancer patients treated with surgery and postoperative radiotherapy into the surgery-plus-RT group. With a match ratio of 1:4, propensity score paired 448 patients treated with surgery alone into the surgical-alone group. All data were validated by two independent database-specific biostatisticians, i.e. Miss Tsai and Hsu.

Patients and Treatments

In clinical practice, postoperative chemotherapy was used in patients with positive mediastinum lymph nodes, i.e. pN1-3/stage II-III disease [17,18]. Moreover, chemotherapy itself has been reported to enhance a risk of thrombosis-related vascular events in lung cancer patients [19]. Thus, the present study excluded patients treated with a component of chemotherapy. As a result, all included patients were early stage lung cancer patients treated with surgery plus radiotherapy or surgery alone. According to requirement of the Taiwan Health Insurance, major thoracic surgeries and radiotherapy were conducted by board-certified thoracic surgeons and radiation oncologists, respectively. In radiotherapy, postoperative irradiation alone was given in patients with positive surgical margin. For these patients, bronchial stump and high risk nodal stations of the mediastinum were irradiating targets [6,17,20]. In conventional fractionation, the highest dose was ranged from 45 Gy to 64.8 Gy according to individual department guidelines. These department guidelines were regularly audited by Taiwan Cancer Center Accreditation [21].

Propensity score match: create comparable groups before analysis

In observation studies, it is crucial to reduce baseline imbalance before analysis. In this regard, we used propensity score match to pair cases [22]. Eight factors were match-paired before analysis: age [23], gender [23], hypertension [1], diabetes mellitus [24], coronary artery disease [25], atrial fibrillation [26], geographic region [27], and urbanization level [28]. With a ratio of 1:4, a total of 448 surgery-alone patients were match-paired with respect to 112 surgery-plus-RT patients (Fig. 1 and Table 1).

The primary endpoint and measurements

The present study defined two-year ischemic-stroke-free survival rate as the primary end point (ICD-9-CM codes, 433-438) [13]. All-type stroke-free survival rate was also calculated (ICD-9-CM codes, 430-438). Effective sizes of stroke occurrence were estimated by using univariate and multivariate analyses.

Urbanization level has been reported to affect incidence of stroke occurrence [14]. Thus, it was defined as one of independent

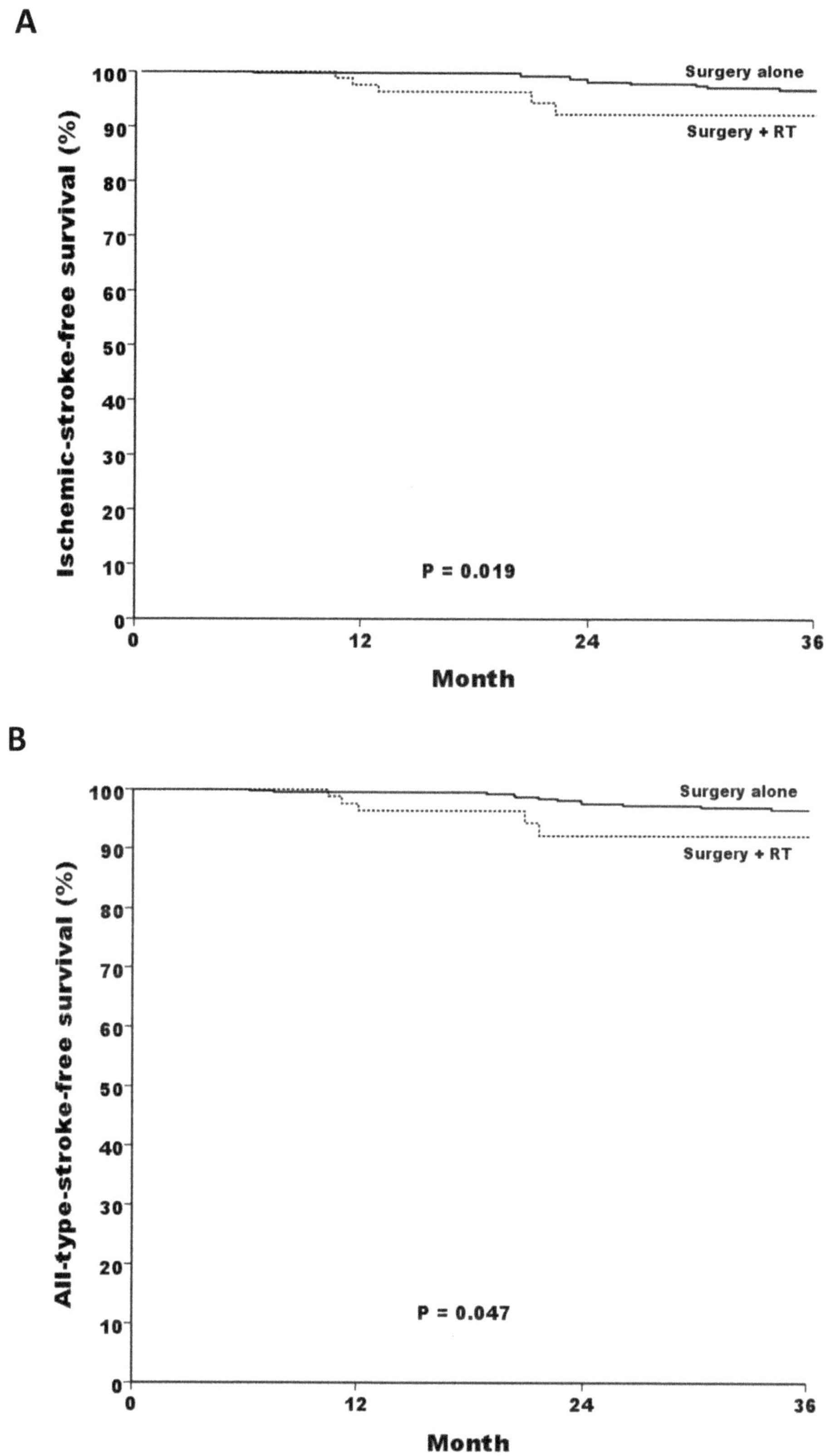

Figure 2. Kaplan-Meier estimates of 2-year stroke-free rates according to treatment groups (surgery-plus-RT versus surgery-alone). Panel 2A, ischemic-stroke-free rates: 92.2% versus 98.1%, $P = 0.019$; and **Panel 2B,** all-stroke-free rates, 92.2% versus 97.6%, $P = 0.047$.

Table 2. Hazard ratios for ischemic stroke occurrence according to predictive factors.

	HR (95% CI)	
	Univariate	**Multivariate**
Age (>65 vs. ≤65 years)	3.52 (1.38–8.94), $P=0.008$*	2.40 (0.89–6.47), $P=0.078$
Gender (male vs. female)	2.94 (0.67–12.80), $P=0.150$	NA
Hypertension (Yes vs. No)	5.37 (0.71–40.62), $P=0.103$	NA
Diabetes mellitus (Yes vs. No)	5.89 (2.33–14.85), $P<0.0001$**	5.02 (1.86–13.53), $P=0.001$**
CAD (Yes vs. No)	1.63 (0.37–7.12), $P=0.511$	NA
Atrial fibrillation (Yes vs. No)	1.86 (0.45–7.65), $P=0.387$	NA
Geographic region (4 categories)	1.16 (0.43–3.12), $P=0.767$	NA
Urbanization level (3 categories)	1.60 (0.51–5.05) $P=0.417$	NA
COPD (Yes vs. No)	1.07 (0.19–5.87) $P=0.933$	NA
Tuberculosis (Yes vs. No)	0.85 (0.28–2.59), $P=0.781$	NA
CHF (Yes vs. No)	2.38 (0.76–7.39) $P=0.133$	NA
CKD (Yes vs. No)	1.35 (0.87–2.09), $P=0.081$	1.48 (0.17–10.27), $P=0.58$
Post-OP RT (Yes vs. No)	3.28 (1.15–9.37), $P=0.026$*	4.19 (1.44–12.22), $P=0.009$**

Abbreviations: **HR**, hazard ratio; **95% CI**, 95% confidence interval; **vs.**, versus; **CAD**, coronary artery disease; **COPD**, chronic obstructive pulmonary disease; **CHF**, congestive heart failure; **CKD**, chronic kidney disease; OP, surgery; **RT**, radiotherapy; *, $P<0.05$; **, $P<0.01$.
Note: All *P* values were calculated by using Cox proportional hazard analysis.

variables. The following factors were used to determine urbanization level: population density, percentage of residents with a college or higher education, percentage of residents >65 years of age, percentage of residents who were agriculture workers, and number of physicians per 100,000 people. Radiation dose was estimated by using the charge code of external beam radiotherapy (code number: 36012B).

Statistical analysis

Analysis were conducted according to the CONSORT statement [29], and STROBE guideline [30]. Two statistical packages, i.e. SAS (version 9.2; SAS Institute, Inc., Cary, NC) and SPSS (version 12, SPSS Inc., Chicago, IL), were applied, accordingly. Following statistical methods were used: Kaplan-Meier analysis to estimate stroke-free survival; log-rank test to assess curve difference; chi-square test to evaluate differences between category variables; and, Cox proportional hazard regression to conduct univariate and multivariate analyses for time-to-event endpoint. Independent factors that identified by multivariate analysis were used for stratified sensitivity analysis. To estimate an effective size, hazard ratio (HR) was provided with a 95% confidence interval (95% CI) in addition to a conventional *P* value. All tests were two-tailed and considered to be statistically significant when $P<0.05$.

Results

Study groups and patients

With a match ratio of 1:4, a total of 560 patients were recruited into the following two study groups: surgery plus RT ($n=112$) and surgery alone ($n=448$; Fig. 1). All living patients were followed up for at least 2 years (median, 42.8 months; range, 24.8–72.8). Most patients were aged less than 65 years ($n=385$, 68.8%) and male gender ($n=426$; 76.1%). Propensity-score match balances eight baseline factors before analysis (Table 1).

The primary endpoint: to explore a risk level of ischemic stroke occurrence

Two observations supported a high incidence of ischemic stroke occurrence in surgery-plus-RT patients when compared with surgical-alone patients: first, a high ischemic-stroke incidence per 1,000 person-year at 2 years (22.3 versus 11.2, 1.99 folds) and at 5 years (24.4 versus 9.3, 2.62 folds; Fig. 1); and second, low 2-year ischemic-stroke-free and all-stroke-free survival rates, 92.2% versus 98.1% ($P=0.019$; Fig. 2A) and 92.2% versus 97.6% ($P=0.047$; Fig. 2B), respectively. In patients received radiotherapy, a higher estimated dose level seemly associated with a lower 2-year ischemic-stroke-free survival; however, log-rank test didn't support a statistical significance (89.8% versus 96.3%, $P=0.476$).

Multivariate analysis confirmed two independent risk factors

To explore risk level of ischemic stroke occurrence, univariate and multivariate analysis were conducted (Table 2). In univariate analysis, three factors showed a statistical significance ($P<0.05$): diabetes mellitus ($P<0.0001$), age (>65 vs. ≤65 years; $P=0.008$), and treatment (surgery plus RT vs. surgery alone; $P=0.026$). One factor demonstrated a statistical trend ($0.05<P<0.10$): chronic kidney disease (yes vs. no; $P=0.081$). These four factors were used in further multivariate analysis.

Multivariate analysis identified two independent risk factors: diabetes mellitus (adjusted HR, 5.02; 95% CI, 1.86–13.53; $P=0.001$); and, postoperative irradiation (adjusted HR, 4.19; 95% CI, 1.44–12.22; $P=0.009$; Table 2 and Fig. 3A–B).

Sensitivity analysis according to status of irradiation and diabetes

To further demarcate risk levels of ischemic stroke occurrence, we performed a stratified sensitivity analysis according to two independent risk factors: diabetes mellitus and postoperative irradiation. Table 3 shows a trend of increasing risk of ischemic

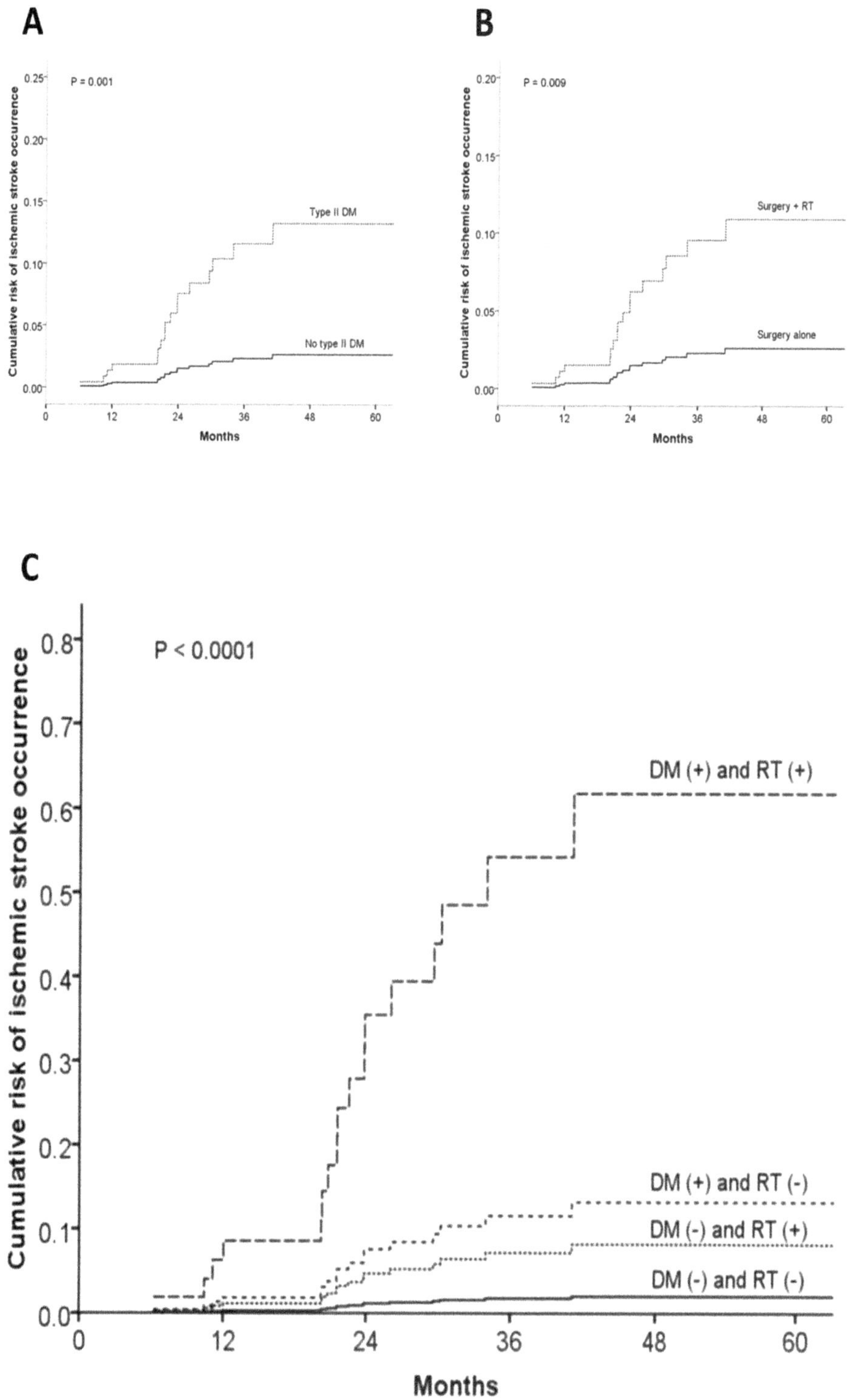

Figure 3. Cumulative risk estimates of ischemic stroke occurrence according to diabetes and irradiation. Panel 3A, adjusted HR in patients with type II diabetic mellitus (DM), 5.02 (95% CI 1.86–13.53; $P = 0.001$), when compared with those without type II DM; **Panel 3B**, adjusted HR in the surgery + RT group, 4.19 (95% CI 1.44–12.22; $P = 0.009$), when compared with the surgery alone group; and **Panel 3C**, the highest HR in patients with both DM and RT, 34.74 (95% CI 6.35–>100; $P < 0.0001$), when compared with patients with both of none (reference value = 1).

Table 3. Hazard ratios for stroke occurrence in lung cancer patients stratified by treatment groups and diabetes mellitus.

	HR (95% CI)			
	The surgery-plus-RT group (*n*=112)		**The surgery-alone group (*n*=448)**	
	Diabetes	**No Diabetes**	**Diabetes**	**No Diabetes**
All-type stroke	27.33 (5.25->100), *P*<0.0001	4.05 (1.38–11.89), *P*=0.010	4.90 (1.78–13.52), *P*=0.002	1
Ischemic stroke	34.74 (6.35->100), *P*<0.0001	3.95 (1.97–7.92), *P*=0.005	6.57 (2.21–19.54), *P*=0.001	1

Abbreviations: **HR**, hazard ratio; **95% CI**, 95% confidence interval; **RT**, radiotherapy.
Note 1: All adjusted hazard ratios were estimated by using Cox proportional hazard analysis.
Note 2: Patients in the surgery-alone group without diabetes were as the reference (value = 1).

stroke occurrence in the following four subgroups: non-diabetic and non-irradiated (HR, 1; as the reference); diabetic but non-irradiated (HR, 6.57; 95% CI, 2.21–19.54; *P*=0.001); non-diabetic but irradiated (HR, 3.95; 95% CI, 1.97–7.92; *P*=0.005); and most remarkably, both diabetic and irradiated (HR, 34.74; 95% CI, 6.35->100; *P*<0.0001). This observation may suggest an enhanced damage effect of irradiation on diabetic injured blood vessels (Fig. 3C).

Discussion

Study question and main finding: a high risk of ischemic stroke occurrence was observed in irradiated lung cancer patients

In the literature, a high risk of ischemic stroke has been reported in irradiated cancer patients [2–4]. However, available data are limited in irradiated lung cancer patients. Recently, a high risk of ischemic stroke has been reported in lung cancer patients when compared with non-cancer controls: incidence per 1,000 person-year, 21.8 versus 15.1; and HR, 1.43 (95% CI, 1.34–1.51). Remarkably, this risk effect can be observed at a follow-up of two years [13]. These lines of evidence inspired the present study to explore whether a risk of ischemic stroke occurrence is also high in irradiated lung cancer patients.

In the present study, three observations supported a high risk of ischemic stroke occurrence in irradiated lung cancer patients when compared with non-irradiated patients: first, a high incidence per 1,000 person-year (22.3 versus 11.2, 1.99 folds); second, a low ischemic-stroke-free survival rate (92.2% versus 98.1%, *P*=0.019); and third, a high adjusted hazard ratio (HR, 4.19; 95% CI, 1.44–12.22; *P*=0.009). More notably, the highest risk of ischemic stroke occurrence was observed in diabetic-and-then-irradiated lung cancer patients (HR, 34.74; 95% CI, 6.35->100; *P*<0.0001).

Biological reasoning: irradiation may further damage diabetic injured blood vessels

The present study generates a biological hypothesis: irradiation may further damage diabetic injured blood vessels and then increase a risk of embolic events in blood-supplied end organs.

Two lines of evidence supported this hypothesis. First, it is well known that diabetic vascular damages enhance a risk of thromboembolic events [24]. Second, clinical data suggested a rare but significant association of increasing ischemic stroke occurrence in irradiated cancer patients, such as head and neck cancers [2], breast cancer [3], and Hodgkin's lymphoma [4]. In these patients, regional nodal stations were irradiated, including the neck and/or mediastinum [5,6]. In such a condition, ionizing radiation cannot be avoided to deliver on brain-supplied blood vessels [6,7]. As a result, aberrant mural thrombosis may be generated, and a risk of brain stroke reasonably increased [31,32].

The mediastinum was irradiated in patients with lung cancer and Hodgkin's lymphoma [6]; however, clinical data are largely lacking in irradiated lung cancer patients. Herein, the present study provided a population-based observation that a high risk of ischemic stroke occurrence may be associated with irradiated lung cancer patients, at least in a surgical cohort. Some molecular factors may play a role for this association, such as activation of reactive oxygen species [33–35], and nuclear factor kappa-B [35,36]. However, detail biological interactions are largely unknown. Further studies are encouraged to investigate underpinning molecular mechanisms.

A population-based surgical cohort is suitable to explore a risk level of ischemic stroke occurrence in irradiated lung cancer patients

To explore stroke risk in irradiated lung cancer patients, it is suitable to select a surgical cohort as study population [17,37,38]. Several reasons supported this viewpoint. First, lung cancer patients treated surgically demonstrated a technically resectable and medically operable status. This cohort feature avoided confounding effects from poor performance status and massive medical comorbidities. Second, lung cancer itself may increase a risk of stroke occurrence [13,39,40]. Thus, for comparing stroke risk in lung cancer patients, intra-cohort controls are better than non-cancer controls. In this regard, patients treated with surgical alone can be recruited as suitable controls in a surgical cohort. More notably, third, resected lung cancer patients demonstrated a longer survival than that of unresectable patients – this pattern allows an observation of stroke occurrence more likely.

Study strength

Undoubtedly, randomized controlled trials are the gold standard in conducting clinical research [41]. However, population-based observation studies are useful in several conditions: first, to delineate what is achieved in the real medical world [42–44]; second, to explore an association of rare events [30,45,46]; and third, to approach issues that are difficult or infeasible to be investigated by using randomized controlled trials [43,44]. In this regard, the present study applied a population-based design to investigate whether a risk of ischemic stroke occurrence is really high in irradiated lung cancer patients.

In clinical studies, regression model is useful to adjust confounding effects among multiple covariates [22,47]; however, residual confounding may occur. Therefore, it is crucial to conduct an adequate case match before analyses. In this regard, propensity score match is recommended [43,47]. After match, intergroup balance, study quality, and inference cleanness were improved in the present study. Moreover, sensitivity analysis is useful in investigating unmeasured confounding and hazard effects [15,48]. The present study used a stratified sensitivity analysis according to independent risk factors. The highest risk of stroke occurrence was observed in diabetic-and-then-irradiated lung cancer patients. Further studies to investigate underlying biological mechanisms should be considered.

Study limitations

The present study has several limitations. First, all included patients are anonymous in our database. Researchers cannot contact with individual patients or institutions to collect additional information, such as smoking habits, cancer stage, radiotherapy details, and body mass index. Thus, for overcoming this problem, we used COPD as a surrogate variable to represent, in part, smoking habits [15,49]. Moreover, we excluded patients treated with chemotherapy. This exclusion omitted patients with positive mediastinum lymph nodes, i.e. those patients with pN1-3/stage II-III disease. Furthermore, we used radiotherapy charge code to estimate a radiation dose level.

Second, diagnosis is depended on ICD-9-CM codes in our database. Thus, the Taiwan Insurance Bureau regularly conducted external audits to maintain coding accuracy. Moreover, the present study used Registry Data for Catastrophe Illness for validation. Third, due to a limitation of case number, the present study cannot conduct full multilevel sensitivity analysis as that of a previously excellent study [15]. Instead, we performed a stratified sensitivity analysis according to independent factors. Fourth, patients taken with self-paid targeted therapies, such as Gefitinib (Iressa), cannot be identified. Although such cases were few during the study period, this may slightly affect our results.

Taken together, further prospective studies should be conducted to confirm our results. Nevertheless, the present study re-sheds us a light that population-based studies are useful in exploring a rare-event association and then to generate a biological hypothesis for further investigation.

Conclusion

In a population-based surgical cohort, a high risk of ischemic stroke occurrence was observed in irradiated lung cancer patients, especially in those patients with diabetes mellitus. For these patients, close clinical surveillance and strict diabetes control should be considered. Further studies to define detail biological mechanisms are encouraged.

Acknowledgments

This study utilizes pre-released de-identified data from the Taiwan National Health Insurance Research Database that provided by the Bureau of Taiwan National Health Insurance (TNHI), Department of Health, and managed by National Health Research Institutes (registry number 99029). The interpretation and conclusions contained herein are not those of the Bureau of National Health Insurance, Department of Health, or National Health Research Institutes.

Author Contributions

Conceived and designed the experiments: S-KH M-SL W-YC C-CL Y-CC H-YL. Performed the experiments: C-LL N-CC W-LH H-YL. Analyzed the data: D-WL Y-CS S-CL H-YL. Contributed reagents/materials/analysis tools: H-CL S-JT H-YL. Wrote the paper: F-CH H-YL.

References

1. Roger VL, Go AS, Lloyd-Jones DM, Adams RJ, Berry JD, et al. (2011) Heart disease and stroke statistics—2011 update: a report from the American Heart Association. Circulation 123: e18–e209.
2. Huang YS, Lee CC, Chang TS, Ho HC, Su YC, et al. (2011) Increased risk of stroke in young head and neck cancer patients treated with radiotherapy or chemotherapy. Oral Oncol 47: 1092–1097.
3. Stokes EL, Tyldesley S, Woods R, Wai E, Olivotto IA (2011) Effect of nodal irradiation and fraction size on cardiac and cerebrovascular mortality in women with breast cancer treated with local and locoregional radiotherapy. Int J Radiat Oncol Biol Phys 80: 403–409.
4. De Bruin ML, Dorresteijn LD, van't Veer MB, Krol AD, van der Pal HJ, et al. (2009) Increased risk of stroke and transient ischemic attack in 5-year survivors of Hodgkin lymphoma. J Natl Cancer Inst 101: 928–937.
5. Moore KL, Agur AMR, Dalley AF (2011) Essential clinical anatomy. Philadelphia, PA: Lippincott Williams & Wilkins. xxviii, 703 p. p.
6. Phillips TL, Hoppe RT, Roach M (2010) Leibel and Phillips Textbook of Radiation Oncology. Philadelphia: Saunders, an imprint of Elsevier Inc.
7. Agur AMR, Dalley AF (2009) Grant's atlas of anatomy. Philadelphia, Pa.; London: Lippincott Williams & Wilkins. xvi, 864 p. p.
8. Hall EJ, Giaccia AJ (2012) Radiobiology for the radiologist. Philadelphia: Wolters Kluwer Health/Lippincott Williams & Wilkins. ix, 546 p. p.
9. Moser EC, Noordijk EM, van Leeuwen FE, le Cessie S, Baars JW, et al. (2006) Long-term risk of cardiovascular disease after treatment for aggressive non-Hodgkin lymphoma. Blood 107: 2912–2919.
10. Dorresteijn LD, Stewart FA, Boogerd W (2006) Stroke as a late treatment effect of Hodgkin's disease. J Clin Oncol 24: 1480; author reply 1480–1481.
11. Mueller S, Sear K, Hills NK, Chettout N, Afghani S, et al. (2013) Risk of first and recurrent stroke in childhood cancer survivors treated with cranial and cervical radiation therapy. Int J Radiat Oncol Biol Phys 86: 643–648.
12. Mueller S, Fullerton HJ, Stratton K, Leisenring W, Weathers RE, et al. (2013) Radiation, atherosclerotic risk factors, and stroke risk in survivors of pediatric cancer: a report from the Childhood Cancer Survivor Study. Int J Radiat Oncol Biol Phys 86: 649–655.
13. Chen PC, Muo CH, Lee YT, Yu YH, Sung FC (2011) Lung cancer and incidence of stroke: a population-based cohort study. Stroke 42: 3034–3039.
14. Lee CC, Su YC, Ho HC, Hung SK, Lee MS, et al. (2011) Increased risk of ischemic stroke in young nasopharyngeal carcinoma patients. Int J Radiat Oncol Biol Phys 81: e833–838.
15. Tsan YT, Lee CH, Ho WC, Lin MH, Wang JD, et al. (2013) Statins and the risk of hepatocellular carcinoma in patients with hepatitis C virus infection. J Clin Oncol 31: 1514–1521.
16. Tsai SJ, Huang YS, Tung CH, Lee CC, Lee MS, et al. (2013) Increased risk of ischemic stroke in cervical cancer patients: a nationwide population-based study. Radiat Oncol 8: 41.
17. NCCN.org (2013) Clinical Practice Guidelines in Oncology: Non-small cell lung cancer. Version 2.2013 ed: NCCN.org. pp. (NCCN Guidelines).
18. Greene FL (2006) AJCC cancer staging atlas. New York, NY: Springer. ix, 352 p. p.
19. Numico G, Garrone O, Dongiovanni V, Silvestris N, Colantonio I, et al. (2005) Prospective evaluation of major vascular events in patients with nonsmall cell lung carcinoma treated with cisplatin and gemcitabine. Cancer 103: 994–999.
20. Rami-Porta R, Crowley JJ, Goldstraw P (2009) The revised TNM staging system for lung cancer. Ann Thorac Cardiovasc Surg 15: 4–9.
21. Institutes TNHR (2014) Taiwan Cancer Center Accreditation.
22. Katz MH (2010) Evaluating clinical and public health interventions: a practical guide to study design and statistics. Cambridge: Cambridge University Press. xii, 163 p. p.
23. Chien KL, Su TC, Hsu HC, Chang WT, Chen PC, et al. (2010) Constructing the prediction model for the risk of stroke in a Chinese population: report from a cohort study in Taiwan. Stroke 41: 1858–1864.
24. Cui R, Iso H, Yamagishi K, Saito I, Kokubo Y, et al. (2011) Diabetes mellitus and risk of stroke and its subtypes among Japanese: the Japan public health center study. Stroke 42: 2611–2614.
25. Schwartz F, Ruhil AV, Denham S, Shubrook J, Simpson C, et al. (2009) High self-reported prevalence of diabetes mellitus, heart disease, and stroke in 11 counties of rural Appalachian Ohio. J Rural Health 25: 226–230.
26. Walkey AJ, Wiener RS, Ghobrial JM, Curtis LH, Benjamin EJ (2011) Incident stroke and mortality associated with new-onset atrial fibrillation in patients hospitalized with severe sepsis. JAMA 306: 2248–2254.
27. Engstrom G, Jerntorp I, Pessah-Rasmussen H, Hedblad B, Berglund G, et al. (2001) Geographic distribution of stroke incidence within an urban population: relations to socioeconomic circumstances and prevalence of cardiovascular risk factors. Stroke 32: 1098–1103.
28. Lin HC, Lin YJ, Liu TC, Chen CS, Chiu WT (2007) Urbanization and stroke prevalence in Taiwan: analysis of a nationwide survey. J Urban Health 84: 604–614.

29. Schulz KF, Altman DG, Moher D (2010) CONSORT 2010 statement: updated guidelines for reporting parallel group randomized trials. Ann Intern Med 152: 726–732.
30. von Elm E, Altman DG, Egger M, Pocock SJ, Gotzsche PC, et al. (2007) The Strengthening the Reporting of Observational Studies in Epidemiology (STROBE) statement: guidelines for reporting observational studies. PLoS Med 4: e296.
31. Stewart FA, Hoving S, Russell NS (2010) Vascular damage as an underlying mechanism of cardiac and cerebral toxicity in irradiated cancer patients. Radiat Res 174: 865–869.
32. Dorresteijn LD, Kappelle AC, Scholz NM, Munneke M, Scholma JT, et al. (2005) Increased carotid wall thickening after radiotherapy on the neck. Eur J Cancer 41: 1026–1030.
33. Muhammad S, Bierhaus A, Schwaninger M (2009) Reactive oxygen species in diabetes-induced vascular damage, stroke, and Alzheimer's disease. J Alzheimers Dis 16: 775–785.
34. Fatehi-Hassanabad Z, Chan CB, Furman BL (2010) Reactive oxygen species and endothelial function in diabetes. Eur J Pharmacol 636: 8–17.
35. Halle M, Hall P, Tornvall P (2011) Cardiovascular disease associated with radiotherapy: activation of nuclear factor kappa-B. J Intern Med 269: 469–477.
36. Romzova M, Hohenadel D, Kolostova K, Pinterova D, Fojtikova M, et al. (2006) NFkappaB and its inhibitor IkappaB in relation to type 2 diabetes and its microvascular and atherosclerotic complications. Hum Immunol 67: 706–713.
37. Trodella L, Granone P, Valente S, Valentini V, Balducci M, et al. (2002) Adjuvant radiotherapy in non-small cell lung cancer with pathological stage I: definitive results of a phase III randomized trial. Radiother Oncol 62: 11–19.
38. Granone P, Trodella L, Margaritora S, Cesario A, Corbo GM, et al. (2000) Radiotherapy versus follow-up in the treatment of pathological stage Ia and Ib non-small cell lung cancer. Early stopped analysis of a randomized controlled study. Eur J Cardiothorac Surg 18: 418–424.
39. Lee EJ, Nah HW, Kwon JY, Kang DW, Kwon SU, et al. (2013) Ischemic stroke in patients with cancer: Is it different from usual strokes? Int J Stroke.
40. Zoller B, Ji J, Sundquist J, Sundquist K (2012) Risk of haemorrhagic and ischaemic stroke in patients with cancer: a nationwide follow-up study from Sweden. Eur J Cancer 48: 1875–1883.
41. Levitt SH, Aeppli D, Nierengarten MB (2003) Evidence-based medicine: its effect on treatment recommendations as illustrated by the changing role of postmastectomy irradiation to treat breast cancer. Int J Radiat Oncol Biol Phys 55: 645–650.
42. Owonikoko TK, Ragin C, Chen Z, Kim S, Behera M, et al. (2013) Real-World Effectiveness of Systemic Agents Approved for Advanced Non-Small Cell Lung Cancer: A SEER-Medicare Analysis. Oncologist.
43. Rosenbaum PR (2010) Design of observational studies. New York; London: Springer. xviii, 384 p. p.
44. Maruyama K, Kawahara N, Shin M, Tago M, Kishimoto J, et al. (2005) The risk of hemorrhage after radiosurgery for cerebral arteriovenous malformations. N Engl J Med 352: 146–153.
45. Lin HW, Tu YY, Lin SY, Su WJ, Lin WL, et al. (2011) Risk of ovarian cancer in women with pelvic inflammatory disease: a population-based study. Lancet Oncol 12: 900–904.
46. Lee CC, Ho HC, Hsiao SH, Huang TT, Lin HY, et al. (2012) Infectious complications in head and neck cancer patients treated with cetuximab: propensity score and instrumental variable analysis. PLoS One 7: e50163.
47. Steyerberg EW (2009) Clinical prediction models: a practical approach to development, validation, and updating. New York; London: Springer. xxviii, 497 p. p.
48. VanderWeele TJ (2013) Unmeasured confounding and hazard scales: sensitivity analysis for total, direct, and indirect effects. Eur J Epidemiol 28: 113–117.
49. Stang P, Lydick E, Silberman C, Kempel A, Keating ET (2000) The prevalence of COPD: using smoking rates to estimate disease frequency in the general population. Chest 117: 354S–359S.

23

Mechanism of Protection by Soluble Epoxide Hydrolase Inhibition in Type 2 Diabetic Stroke

Kristen L. Zuloaga[1], Stephanie M. Krasnow[2], Xinxia Zhu[2], Wenri Zhang[1], Sari A. Jouihan[1], Robert E. Shangraw[1], Nabil J. Alkayed[1], Daniel L. Marks[2]*

1 The Knight Cardiovascular Institute, Department of Anesthesiology & Perioperative Medicine, Oregon Health & Science University, Portland, Oregon, United States of America, **2** Papé Family Pediatric Research Institute, Department of Pediatrics, Oregon Health and Science University, Portland, Oregon, United States of America

Abstract

Inhibition of soluble epoxide hydrolase (sEH) is a potential target of therapy for ischemic injury. sEH metabolizes neuroprotective epoxyeicosatrienoic acids (EETs). We recently demonstrated that sEH inhibition reduces infarct size after middle cerebral artery occlusion (MCAO) in type 1 diabetic mice. We hypothesized that inhibition of sEH would protect against ischemic injury in type 2 diabetic mice. Type 2 diabetes was produced by combined high-fat diet, nicotinamide and streptozotocin in male mice. Diabetic and control mice were treated with vehicle or the sEH inhibitor t-AUCB then subjected to 60-min MCAO. Compared to chow-fed mice, high fat diet-fed mice exhibited an upregulation of sEH mRNA and protein in brain, but no differences in brain EETs levels were observed between groups. Type 2 diabetic mice had increased blood glucose levels at baseline and throughout ischemia, decreased laser-Doppler perfusion of the MCA territory after reperfusion, and sustained larger cortical infarcts compared to control mice. t-AUCB decreased fasting glucose levels at baseline and throughout ischemia, improved cortical perfusion after MCAO and significantly reduced infarct size in diabetic mice. We conclude that sEH inhibition, as a preventative treatment, improves glycemic status, post-ischemic reperfusion in the ischemic territory, and stroke outcome in type 2 diabetic mice.

Editor: Jens Minnerup, University of Münster, Germany

Funding: This work was supported, in part, by the National Institute of Neurological Disorders and Stroke (R01NS044313 and R01NS070837 to Dr. Alkayed and F32NS082017-01 to Dr. Zuloaga) and the National Institute of Diabetes and Digestive and Kidney Diseases (R01DK70333 to Dr. Marks). The funders had no role in study design, data collection and analysis, decision to publish, or preparation of the manuscript.

Competing Interests: The authors have declared that no competing interests exist.

* E-mail: marksd@ohsu.edu

Introduction

Individuals with diabetes have more than twice the risk for stroke compared to non-diabetic individuals [1]. Hyperglycemia is also associated with poor stroke outcome in both humans [2–4] and in several rodent models of stroke [5–10]. Approximately 40% of ischemic stroke patients are hyperglycemic upon admission to the hospital [4]. Clinically, blood glucose levels correlate with both infarct size and degree of disability [4]. However, tight glycemic control in hyperglycemic patients has failed to protect against stroke incidence or improve outcome in clinical trials [11–16]. Since tight glycemic control has failed to protect hyperglycemic patients from increased stroke risk and worse stroke outcome, the goal of the current study was to determine if inhibition of soluble epoxide hydrolase (sEH) would protect against ischemic injury in type 2 diabetic mice. sEH is a potential mediator of ischemic injury via its metabolism of neuroprotective epoxyeicosatrienoic acids (EETs). sEH is expressed in a variety of cells in the brain including cerebrovascular endothelium, vascular smooth muscle cells, neurons, oligodendrocytes, and astrocytes [17].

Using a rodent model of type 1 diabetes, we have recently shown that hyperglycemia decreases brain EETs concentrations and increases infarct size after MCAO [8]. Furthermore, we showed that sEH inhibition could restore brain EETs concentrations and reduce infarct size in type 1 diabetic mice [8]. While both type 1 and 2 diabetes mellitus are characterized by hyperglycemia, the two diseases are metabolically quite distinct. Type 1 diabetes results in hyperglycemia due to destruction of pancreatic beta cells leading to absolute insulin deficiency. In contrast type 2 diabetes results in hyperglycemia due to insulin resistance or relative insulin deficiency, and is commonly associated with obesity, dyslipidemia, and hypertension [18]. In the current study, we wanted to determine whether the protective effect of sEH inhibition would extend to the setting of type 2 diabetes, a much more prevalent and complex hyperglycemic disease. In addition, we utilized a rodent model of pre-diabetes to determine if sEH is upregulated before development of overt type 2 diabetes. We hypothesized that inhibition of sEH, as a preventative treatment, would protect against ischemic injury in type 2 diabetic mice.

Materials and Methods

Ethics Statement

Our study was conducted in accordance with National Institutes of Health guidelines for care and use of animals in research and conformed to the Association for Assessment and Accreditation of Laboratory Animal Care AAALAC Accreditation and the Office of Laboratory Animal Welfare (OLAW Assurance #A3304-01, approved June 2012). All protocols were approved by the

Institutional Animal Care and Use Committee of Oregon Health & Science University (Portland, OR).

High Fat Diet Model of Pre-diabetes in Mice

Long-term high fat diet is a model of pre-diabetes in mice, leading to elevated body weight and impaired glucose tolerance without causing overt hyperglycemia [19]. Five-week old male C57BL/6J mice (JAX) were acclimatized to the animal facility and then placed on a high fat (60% fat) diet (D12492, Research Diets, Inc., New Brunswick, NJ) or normal chow (13% fat) diet (LabDiet 5001; Nestle Purina, St. Louis, MO) for 15 weeks. Weight was tracked biweekly. At 20 weeks of age, mice were fasted overnight then subjected to a glucose tolerance test (GTT). For the GTT, blood glucose was measured just prior to injection of glucose (2 g/kg, i.p.), and once every 15–30 minutes for 2 hrs after the injection. Insulin levels were measured by radioimmunoassay using a Rat Insulin RIA Kit (Millipore, Billerica, MA). Measurements were run in duplicate and performed according to the manufacturer's instructions. The intra-assay coefficient of variation was 5.7%.

High Fat Diet, Streptozotocin and Nicotinamide (HFD+STZ/NA) Model of Type 2 Diabetes in Mice

Five-week old male C57BL/6J mice (JAX) were acclimatized to the animal facility and placed on a high fat (60% fat) diet (D12492, Research Diets, Inc., New Brunswick, NJ) or normal chow (13% fat) diet (LabDiet 5001; Nestle Purina, St. Louis, MO) for 4 wks. After 4 wks on the high fat diet, mice were fasted overnight and treated with nicotinamide (NA; 240 mg/kg, i.p.) and streptozotocin (STZ; 100 mg/kg, i.p.) 15 min later. Chow-fed controls received equal volume of saline (i.p.) followed by 50 mM citric acid buffer (i.p) 15 min later. Two days later, the mice were again fasted and treated with either NA/STZ or saline/citric acid buffer. Nakamura et al. [1] demonstrated that with STZ treatment alone (type 1 diabetes model) pancreatic beta cells are lost, but that STZ-induced beta cell damage is attenuated by NA in a dose-dependent manner [20]. After 6 weeks on their diets, mice were fasted and glycemia in saphenous vein blood was measured by glucometer (Breeze 2, Bayer, Tarrytown, NY) to confirm hyperglycemia in type 2 diabetic mice. This model of type 2 diabetes has been well characterized and has been shown to cause insulin resistance [20].

Inhibition of Soluble Epoxide Hydrolase (sEH) Activity

In vivo sEH activity was inhibited with trans-4-[4-(3-Adamantan-1-yl-ureido) -cyclohexyloxy]-benzoic acid (t-AUCB), developed and generously provided by Dr. Bruce Hammock, University of California, Davis, CA [21]. Mice received 1 mg/kg or 2 mg/kg t-AUCB or saline vehicle i.p. daily for the final 6 days before cerebral ischemia, with the final t-AUCB dose administered immediately after reperfusion.

Middle Cerebral Artery Occlusion (MCAO)

MCAO was performed 2 weeks after completion of STZ/NA treatment or vehicle for corresponding controls. Transient (60-min) focal cerebral ischemia was induced in overnight-fasted mice using an intraluminal MCAO technique described previously [22]. Briefly, isoflurane-anesthetized mice were instrumented with a laser-Doppler probe and rectal temperature probe and MCAO ischemia induced via insertion of a silicone-coated 6-0 nylon monofilament into the right internal carotid artery until MCA flow was <20% of baseline. The occluding filament was subsequently withdrawn for reperfusion. Mice were allowed to recover and observed for 1 day, after which they were anesthetized with isoflurane, blood collected, and either sacrificed by decapitation and brains removed for infarct size measurement, or perfused with heparinized ice-cold saline for brain collection for qPCR, and Western blot. Insulin levels were measured in serum by radioimmunoassay using a Rat Insulin RIA Kit (Millipore, Billerica, MA). Measurements were run in duplicate and performed according to the manufacturer's instructions. The intra-assay coefficient of variation was 5.7%.

Brain Infarct Size

Infarct size in cerebral cortex, caudate putamen and total hemisphere was measured at 24 h after MCAO in 2-mm thick coronal brain sections using 2,3,5-triphenyltetrazolium chloride (TTC) staining and digital image analysis (SigmaScan Pro 5.0, Aspire Software, Ashburn, VA) as previously described [22]. To account for edema, infarcted area was estimated by subtracting the uninfarcted region in ipsilateral hemisphere from the contralateral hemisphere, and expressing infarct volume as a percentage of the contralateral hemisphere.

Real-time Quantitative PCR

Levels of EPHX2 (sEH gene) mRNA were determined as previously described [8]. In brief, RNA was isolated using a commercial kit (RNAqueous-Micro, Ambion, Austin, TX), contaminant genomic DNA removed by DNase treatment, and RNA reverse transcribed using a commercial high capacity cDNA archive kit (Applied Biosystems, Carlsbad, CA). Resulting cDNA was amplified using TaqMan Universal PCR amplification in a commercial sequence detection system (ABI Prism 7000, Applied Biosystems, Carlsbad, CA). Quantitative PCR was performed in a 96-well plate using 50 µl total volume, in triplicate. PCR was concurrently run on controls without template to assess DNA contamination and primer-dimer formation. Remaining RNA not reverse transcribed was included to control for genomic DNA amplification. 18S was measured as an internal control using an 18S mRNA control kit (FAM-TAMRA, Eurogentec, Seraing, BEL). EPHX2 primers were purchased as a TaqMan Gene Expression Assay (Invitrogen, Catalog #4351372). All final EPHX2 mRNA levels were normalized to 18S.

Western Blot

sEH protein expression was measured as previously described [8]. In brief, mice were perfused with ice-cold heparinized saline to remove blood, and brains were collected. Brains were homogenized in lysis buffer, centrifuged, and supernatant collected. Protein samples (40 µg) were separated by gel electrophoresis and then transferred to Polyvinylidene Difluoride (PVDF) membranes. Blots were blocked in 5% dry milk, and incubated at 4°C overnight with a primary rabbit polyclonal antibody against murine sEH (1:500; Cayman Chemical, Ann Arbor, MI). The signal was visualized using a horseradish peroxidase-linked (HRP) rabbit secondary antibody (1:1,000; GE Healthcare, Piscataway, NJ) followed by detection using Supersignal chemiluminescent reagents (Thermo Fisher Scientific, Waltham, MA) with a FluorChem FC2 (Protein Simple, Santa Clara, CA). Blots were stripped using Restore Western Blot Stripping Buffer (Thermo Fisher Scientific) and re-probed for beta actin (1:2,000; Sigma-Aldrich) and followed by HRP mouse secondary antibody (1:1,000; GE Healthcare) and re-imaged. Densitometry was quantified with AlphaView software (Protein Simple) and sEH protein was normalized relative to beta actin as expressed as a ratio compared to chow-fed mice.

Statistical Analysis

Data are expressed as mean ± SEM. Groups were compared by t-test for two groups or two-way ANOVA with post hoc Newman-Keuls test for multiple measures with multiple groups using GraphPad Prism (GraphPad Software, Inc, La Jolla, CA). Differences were considered significant at $p<0.05$.

Results

High Fat Diet Increases sEH mRNA and Protein Expression in Brain

Using a rodent model of pre-diabetes, we aimed to determine if sEH expression is altered in the pre-diabetic state, before development of overt type 2 diabetes. The HFD model of pre-diabetes causes impaired glucose tolerance and insulin resistance, without producing the overt hyperglycemia pathognomonic of type 2 diabetes mellitus [19]. Long-term treatment (15 weeks) with a high fat (60% fat) diet caused an increase in body weight (**Fig. 1A**), an increase in insulin levels (**Fig. 1B**) and a decrease in glucose tolerance (**Fig. 1C–D**) in high fat-fed compared to chow-fed mice ($p<0.001$). **Fig. 2A** shows that, compared to chow-fed mice, high fat diet-fed mice exhibited a 1.7 fold upregulation of EPHX2 (gene encoding for sEH) mRNA in cortex ($p<0.05$). **Fig. 2B** shows that sEH protein expression was also 20% higher in brains of high fat-diet fed mice compared to chow-fed mice ($p<0.01$). Despite changes in sEH expression, we did not detect differences in EETs levels, measured via liquid chromatography-tandem mass spectrometry [23], in brains of high fat diet-fed mice compared to chow-fed mice (515+/−62 pg/10 mg wet weight in high fat diet group vs. 399+/−13 pg/10 mg wet weight in chow group, n = 4–5 per group).

sEH Inhibition Attenuates Increases in Baseline Fasting Blood Glucose Levels in Type 2 Diabetic Mice

HFD+STZ/NA was used to model type 2 diabetes. The main endpoint diagnostic criterion for diabetes (either type 1 or type 2) is hyperglycemia [24]. STZ alone induces type 1 diabetes by destroying the pancreatic beta cells, causing insulinopenia and consequent hyperglycemia, and this treatment may also cause a decrease in body weight [20]. Co-administration of NA with STZ attenuates the beta cell injury and prevents overt hyperglycemia [20]. However, if STZ/NA are administered to mice on a high fat diet, the NA is less able to protect the beta cells, resulting in the constellation of hyperglycemia, insulin resistance, and impaired glucose tolerance [20]. This triad is the hallmark of type 2 diabetes [24]. Notably, these treated mice also exhibit hyperlipidemia [20], which is common in type 2 diabetic individuals. **Table 1** shows characteristics of study mice prior to MCAO, which did not differ among groups in age, body weight, or temperature. HFD+STZ/NA mice had increased fasting blood glucose levels compared to control mice at baseline ($p<0.001$, **Fig. 3A**). The sEH inhibitor t-AUCB reduced fasting blood glucose levels in HFD+STZ/NA mice ($p<0.05$) but not in control mice (**Fig. 3B**). In addition to baseline blood glucose levels, we also monitored blood glucose levels throughout the MCAO surgery and measured insulin levels 24 h after ischemia. There were no differences in serum insulin levels between groups (**Fig. 3C**). HFD+STZ/NA mice had increased blood glucose levels compared to control mice before MCAO, during the occlusion, and during reperfusion ($p<0.001$ vs. Control Vehicle, **Fig. 4**). Furthermore, t-AUCB treated HFD+STZ/NA mice had decreased blood glucose levels compared to vehicle-treated HFD+STZ/NA mice at each time point ($p<0.01$ vs. HFD+STZ/NA Vehicle, **Fig. 4**).

Cerebral Blood Flow during Reperfusion is Decreased in Type 2 Diabetic Mice and Rescued with sEH Inhibition

Fig. 5 shows that relative perfusion, measured by laser Doppler probe, of the MCA territory after reperfusion was decreased in HFD+STZ/NA mice compared to controls ($p<0.001$ vs. Control Vehicle). Furthermore, sEH inhibition with t-AUCB prevented the perfusion deficit of the MCA territory during reperfusion in HFD+STZ/NA mice ($p<0.01$ vs. HFD+STZ/NA Vehicle).

sEH Inhibition Prevented Type 2 Diabetes-induced Increases in Infarct Size following MCAO

Fig. 6 shows that HFD+STZ/NA vehicle-treated mice sustained a 66% larger cortical infarct size and 55% larger total hemisphere infarct size than control vehicle-treated mice ($p<0.05$). To test whether inhibition of sEH in HFD+STZ/NA-treated mice might decrease vulnerability to stroke, we blocked sEH activity using the specific antagonist t-AUCB during the week before MCAO. As stated above, treatment with t-AUCB decreased fasting glucose levels at baseline and throughout ischemia and improved reperfusion in the MCA territory in HFD+STZ/NA mice. In line with these improvements in glycemic status and cerebral perfusion, t-AUCB reduced cortical infarct size by 29% and total hemisphere infarct size by 31% in HFD+STZ/NA mice ($p<0.05$ vs. HFD+STZ/NA Vehicle, **Fig. 6**). Although the 1 mg/kg t-AUCB dose was not sufficient to reduce infarct size in control mice, a 2 mg/kg t-AUCB dose did decrease infarct size in control mice compared to vehicle treated control mice in the cortex, the striatum, and the total hemisphere ($p<0.05$ vs. HFD+STZ/NA Vehicle, **Fig. 7**).

Discussion

The goal of this study was to determine if sEH inhibition, used as a preventative treatment, could provide protection against ischemic brain injury in type 2 diabetic mice. Previous studies have shown that several animal models of diabetes increase infarct size following cerebral ischemia [7–10], as we also observed in the present study. Using a long-term high fat diet rodent model of pre-diabetes, our data show that pre-diabetes increases expression of sEH mRNA and protein in brain, but does not significantly alter EETs levels in brain. Using a rodent model of type 2 diabetes that combines high fat diet with STZ/NA treatment, we further demonstrated that sEH inhibition with t-AUCB decreases blood glucose levels, increases cerebral perfusion, and decreases infarct size in type 2 diabetic mice. Our findings show that sEH inhibition, used as a preventative treatment, improves glycemic status, post-ischemic reperfusion in the ischemic territory, and stroke outcome in the setting of type 2 diabetes. However, based on the current study we cannot determine the relative contribution, if any, of improvements glycemic status and cerebral perfusion on stroke outcome. Future studies will address this issue by experimentally controlling for blood glucose levels between groups by co-administering t-AUCB with Metformin.

The current data support a novel role for sEH in both pre-diabetes and type 2 diabetes. We have previously shown that hyperglycemia, caused by beta cell destruction with STZ, increases EPHX2 expression in cerebral vessels and decreases EETs levels in brain [8]. However, it was unclear if this effect could be elicited by factors involved in the etiology of type 2 diabetes, other than hyperglycemia. We used a long-term high fat diet to model pre-diabetes, a diet which increases body weight and impairs glucose tolerance in the absence of overt resting hyperglycemia [19]. The HFD mice exhibited hyperinsulinemia, which likely preserved euglycemia in the absence of a glucose challenge. A similar

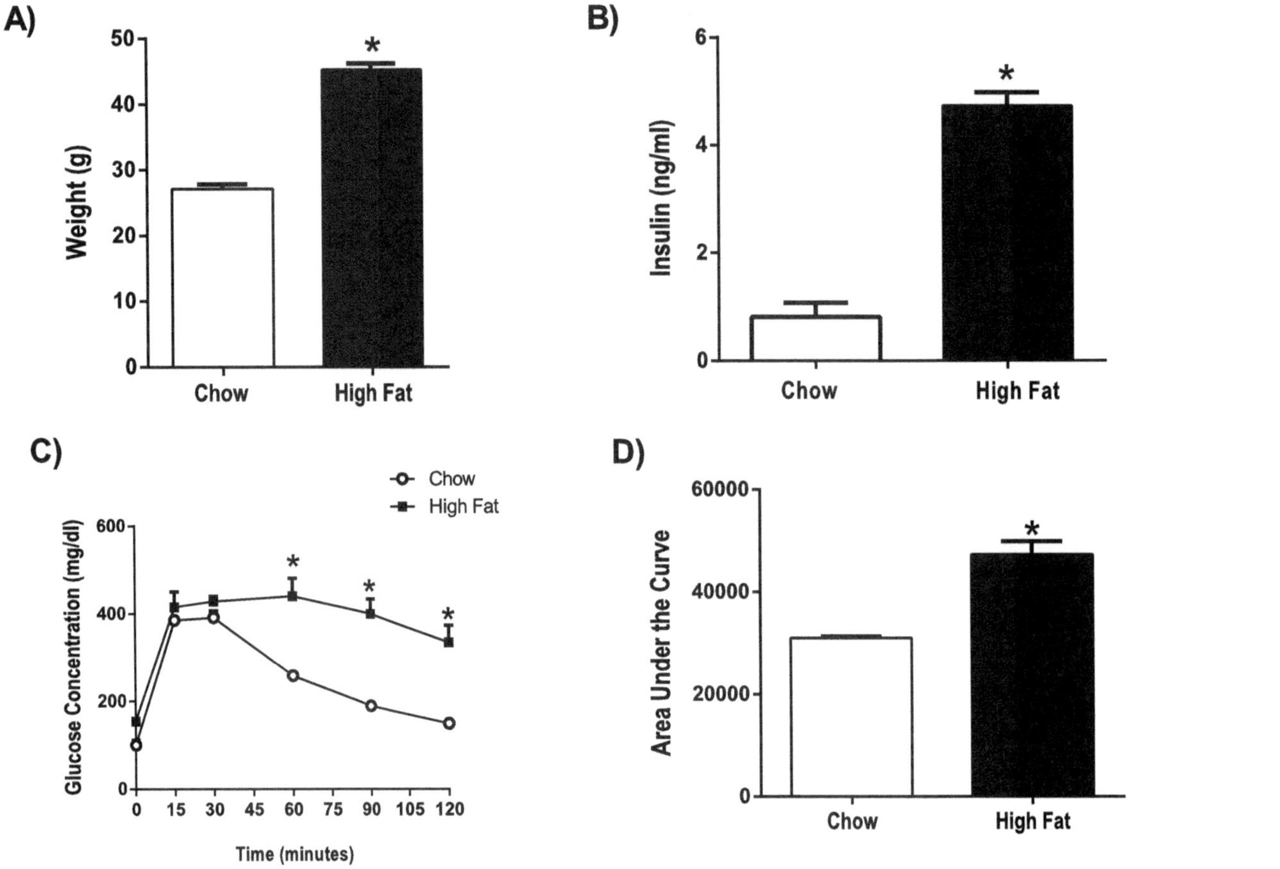

Figure 1. Pre-diabetic mice have increased body weight, increased insulin levels and decreased glucose tolerance. A) Body weight B) serum insulin levels, and C) blood glucose during i.p. glucose tolerance test (GTT) were measured in mice fed a low fat (Chow; n = 5) or high fat (n = 4) diet for 15 weeks. Mice were fasted overnight prior to the GTT. Glucose (2 g/kg body weight) was injected i.p. at time 0. D) Area under the curve from GTT test results was calculated for each treatment group. *p<0.001 vs. Chow.

phenomenon is observed clinically in patients with pre-diabetes. The first stage of pre-diabetes involves a long period of insulin resistance accompanied by a compensatory increase in pancreatic insulin secretion and increased beta cell mass [25]. During this phase, fasting glycemic status is normal, yet glucose intolerance can be unmasked in these patients with a glucose tolerance test

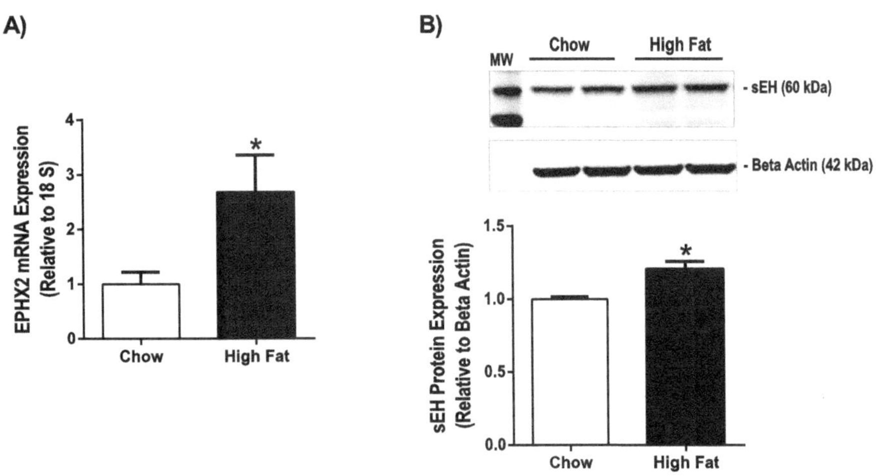

Figure 2. High fat diet increases sEH expression in brain. Mice were treated with a high fat (60% fat) or chow diet (13% fat) for 15 weeks. A) EPHX2 mRNA expression was measured via qPCR in cortex. EPHX2 expression was normalized to 18S expression. *p<0.05 vs. Chow, n = 7 per group. B) sEH protein expression was measured via Western blot in brain. sEH protein expression was normalized to beta actin protein expression. *p<0.01 vs. Chow, n = 4 per group.

Table 1. Baseline Characteristics of Type 2 Diabetic Mice and Controls.

	Control Vehicle	Control t-AUCB	HFD+STZ/NA Vehicle	HFD+STZ/NA t-AUCB
Age (weeks)	16±0.5	16±0.5	16±0.5	16±0.5
Weight (g)	26.0±0.8	25.6±0.8	26.8±0.9	25.7±0.8
Temp (°C)	36.5±0.5	36.5±0.5	36.5±0.5	36.5±0.5

Age, weight, and body temperature, monitored via rectal temperature probe, were measured in control and HFD+STZ/NA mice treated with vehicle or t-AUCB treatment (n = 11–16 mice per group).

(GTT). As the disease progresses, the increased insulin secretion progressively fails to compensate for the insulin resistance and hyperglycemia ensues over time. Eventually, the beta cells cannot produce enough insulin and hyperglycemia (type 2 diabetes) results [25]. Using the HFD model, we show that pre-diabetes causes increased EPHX2 gene expression as well as increased sEH protein expression in brain. These data indicate that sEH is elevated before the onset of type 2 diabetes. Surprisingly, despite increased mRNA and protein levels of sEH, we did not detect a statistically significant difference in EETs levels between chow and HFD fed mice. In fact, there was a trend for higher EETs in mice on HFD vs. normal chow. Because the level of EETs is regulated both by their synthesis via P450 epoxygenase and their metabolism via sEH, it is possible that EETs synthesis was increased to compensate for an increase in sEH expression. In a similar model, De Taeve et al. found that sEH mRNA and protein levels did not differ, but sEH activity was higher in adipose tissue from obese mice on "western-style" vs. regular diet [26]. If so, increased vulnerability to stroke injury in rodents fed a high fat diet, either in the presence (as we have observed) or absence of STZ/NA (as others have observed [27]), may not necessarily be the result of lower brain EETs, but rather to differences in insulin resistance and glycemic status. It is important to note that our model of pre-diabetes included impaired glucose tolerance. Clinical studies in pre-diabetic patients with impaired glucose tolerance show that these patients are at increased risk for stroke, while studies that do not include impaired glucose tolerance in their definition of pre-diabetes show less of an association [28].

Individuals with diabetes have more than twice the risk for stroke compared to non-diabetic individuals [1]. The mechanisms underlying increased ischemic sensitivity during the evolution of type 2 diabetes are poorly understood and no therapeutic options are currently available to reduce risk, other than weight reduction and glycemic control. Although hyperglycemia is associated with poor stroke outcome in both humans [2–4] and rodents [5–10], tight glycemic control in hyperglycemic patients has failed to

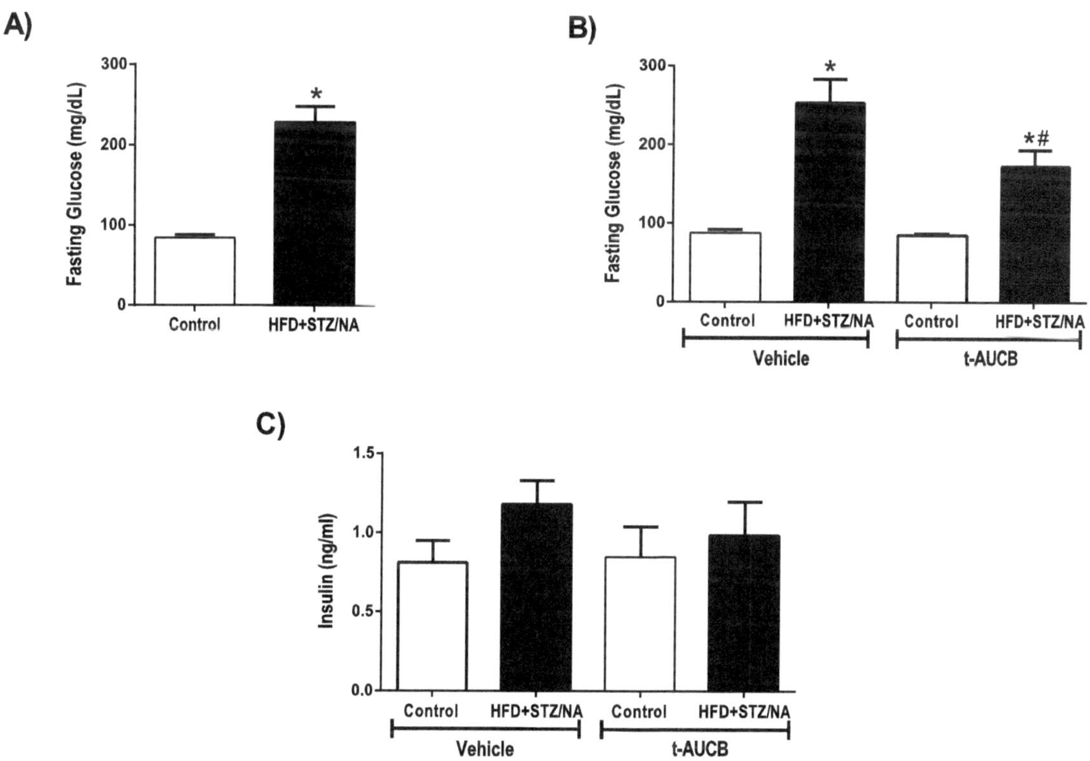

Figure 3. sEH inhibition decreased fasting glucose levels in type 2 diabetic mice. Fasting blood glucose levels were obtained from control and HFD+STZ/NA mice before (A) and after (B) treatment with the sEH inhibitor t-AUCB (1 mg/kg i.p. daily, 7 days) or vehicle. C) Serum insulin levels were also measured in t-AUCB or vehicle treated mice 24 h after ischemia. *$p<0.001$ vs. Control Vehicle, #$p<0.05$ vs. HFD+STZ/NA Vehicle. A) n = 20–22 per group. B) n = 5–8 per group. C) n = 2–6 per group.

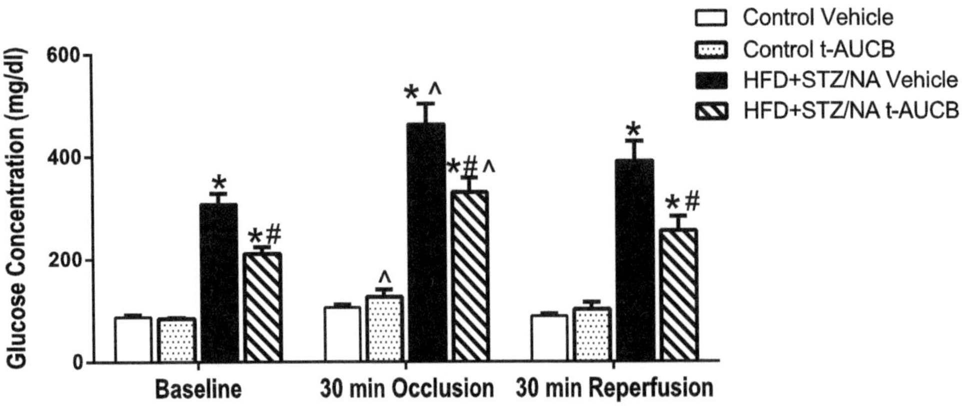

Figure 4. sEH inhibition decreased glucose levels in type 2 diabetic mice before, during, and after ischemia. Control and HFD+STZ/NA mice were treated with the sEH inhibitor t-AUCB (1 mg/kg i.p. daily, 7 days) or vehicle and subjected to middle cerebral artery occlusion (60 min). Blood glucose levels were measured at baseline, 30 min into the occlusion, and 30 min post-reperfusion. *$p<0.001$ vs. Control Vehicle, #$p<0.01$ vs. HFD+STZ/NA Vehicle. ^$p<0.05$ vs. baseline of same treatment group. N = 4–5 per group.

protect against stroke incidence or improve outcome in clinical trials [11–16]. Therefore, the goal the current study was determine if sEH inhibition is a potential therapeutic target for type 2 diabetic stroke.

Our current data confirm that type 2 diabetes, induced by high fat diet combined with STZ/NA treatment, enhances ischemic injury in multiple brain regions. In addition we show that type 2 diabetes also causes a decrease in perfusion to the ischemic territory following MCAO, suggesting that vascular mechanisms are contributing to the enhanced susceptibility to ischemic injury in the context of type 2 diabetes. This is in contrast to our previous findings using a model of type 1 diabetes, induced by STZ, in which we found that CBF and cortical perfusion were unaltered in type 1 diabetic mice [8] compared to controls. In contrast to our previous type 1 diabetes model in which STZ is administered alone, in the current study nicotinamide, a B3 vitamin and precursor to NAD+, was used to reduce the toxicity of STZ and prevent large reductions in beta cell mass in mice fed a high fat diet to more closely model type 2 diabetes[20]. The HFD+STZ/NA mice did not exhibit a difference in circulating insulin concentration compared to controls, most likely due to pancreatic beta cell damage, as indicated by their relative hyperglycemia compared to controls. Nakamura et al. have shown that insulinemia is not altered by STZ/NA [20]. A similar phenomenon is observed clinically in many type 2 diabetic patients, in which the pancreatic beta cells progressively fail to secrete adequate insulin to maintain normal glycemic status, at which time circulating insulin concentration is not elevated [24,25]. However, it should be noted that nicotinamide alone could also have had neuroprotective effects through multiple mechanisms. Nicotinamide has been shown to cross the blood brain barrier and to improve mitochondrial function/ATP synthesis following ischemia by acting as a PARP inhibitor [29]. Furthermore, nicotinamide has also been shown to protect against ischemic damage through the sirtuin-1 pathway [30]. However, these effects are unlikely to have contributed substantially to ischemic outcome

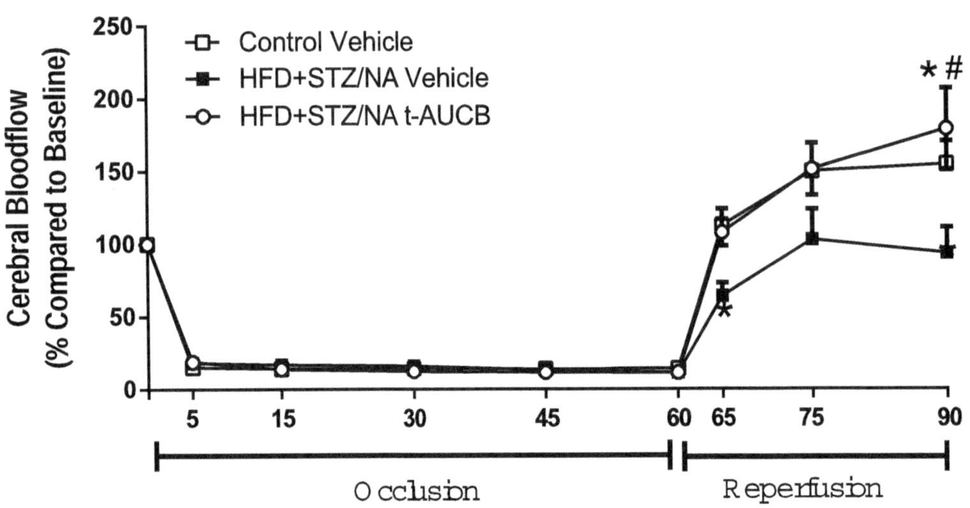

Figure 5. Cerebral Blood Flow during Reperfusion is Decreased in Diabetic Mice and Rescued with sEH Inhibition. Control and HFD+STZ/NA mice were treated with the sEH inhibitor t-AUCB (1 mg/kg i.p. daily, 7 days) or vehicle and subjected to middle cerebral artery occlusion (60 min). Relative perfusion, measured by laser Doppler probe, of the MCA territory measured continuously (averages of 5–15 min intervals are shown) at baseline, during the occlusion, and during 30 min post-reperfusion. *$p<0.001$ vs. Control Vehicle, #$p<0.01$ vs. HFD+STZ/NA Vehicle. N = 4–5 per group.

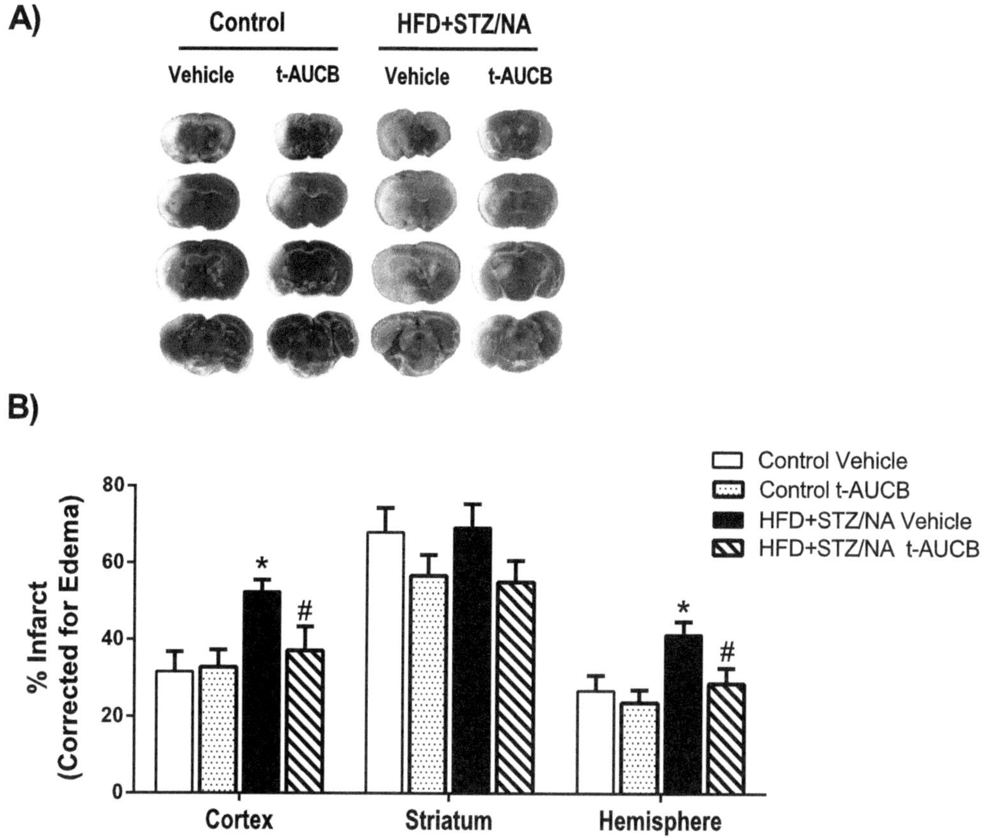

Figure 6. sEH inhibition prevented type 2 diabetic-induced increases in infarct size following MCAO. Control and HFD+STZ/NA mice were treated with the sEH inhibitor t-AUCB (1 mg/kg i.p. daily, 7 days) or vehicle and subjected to middle cerebral artery occlusion (60 min). Brains were harvested at 24 h post-MCAO, and infarct size measured by TTC staining and corrected for edema as described in methods. A) Representative images of infarct size in each treatment group. B) Infarct size is shown for separately for cortex, striatum, and total hemisphere. *$p<0.05$ vs. Control Vehicle, #$p<0.05$ vs. HFD+STZ/NA Vehicle, N = 8–10 per group.

in the current study, as the nicotinamide was administered two weeks prior to ischemia and the STZ/NA group had larger, not smaller, infarct size compared to controls. Nevertheless, important differences underlying etiology of type 1 and type 2 diabetic stroke may exist and warrant further investigation.

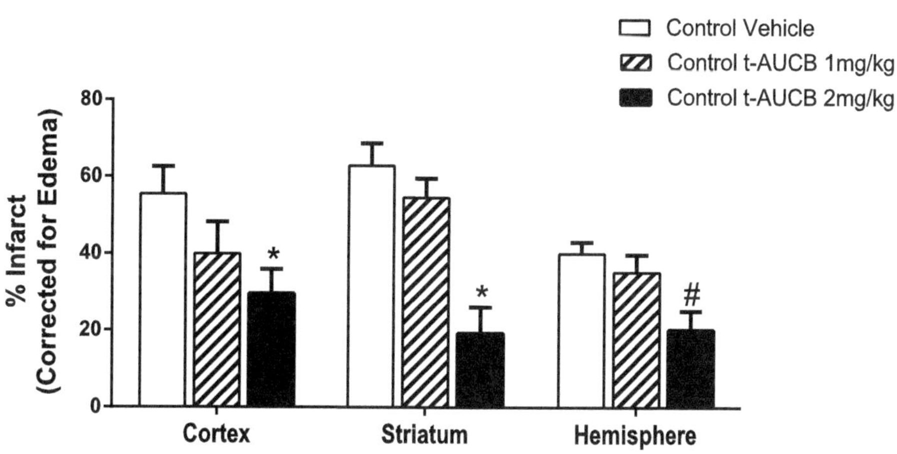

Figure 7. 2 mg/kg t-AUCB prevented reduced infarct size in control mice following MCAO. Control mice were treated with the sEH inhibitor t-AUCB (1 mg/kg or 2 mg/kg i.p. daily, 7 days) or vehicle and subjected to middle cerebral artery occlusion (60 min). Brains were harvested at 24 h post-MCAO, and infarct size measured by TTC staining and corrected for edema as described in methods. Infarct size is shown for separately for cortex, striatum, and total hemisphere. *$p<0.05$ vs. Control Vehicle of same brain region via 2-way ANOVA post-hoc test, #$p<0.01$ vs. Control Vehicle Hemisphere via t-test only, N = 7 per group.

Other studies support our finding that vascular mechanisms may contribute to enhanced injury in type 2 diabetic mice. For example, using the db/db genetic model for type 2 diabetes, it was found that diabetic male mice have decreased cerebrovascular diameter, arteriolar density, and decreased blood brain barrier function in the ischemic brain compared to wild type mice [31]. Using the Goto Kakaizaki rat model for type 2 diabetes, it has also been shown that diabetes decreases vascular volume in the ischemic cortex and striatum [32]. Taken together, these data provide evidence that type 2 diabetic rodents have enhanced injury after stroke that is mediated, in part, by vascular dysfunction.

We have previously shown that sEH inhibition protects the brain from ischemic injury by a mechanism linked to preservation of EETs in non-diabetic mice [22], and more recently in type 1 diabetic mice [8]. Our current data show that sEH inhibition also reduces infarct size in type 2 diabetic mice. Interestingly, t-AUCB reduced infarct size in type 2 diabetic mice at a lower dose (1 mg/kg) than the dose that was needed in control mice (2 mg/kg) to elicit the same protective effect, suggesting that diabetic mice may be more sensitive to the protective effects of sEH inhibition. However, since we did not monitor serum levels of t-AUCB in either cohort, a difference in pharmacokinetics between groups cannot be ruled out. Another limitation of the current study is that we did not assess functional outcomes of sEH inhibition following stroke. In a previous study [22], we have shown that another sEH inhibitor, AUDA-BE, was effective in reducing infarct when administered after stroke. In the current study, sEH inhibitor was administered before stroke, which has limited value as a stroke therapy, but is ideal for determining the role of sEH in the exacerbation of stroke injury in brains of type 2 diabetic mice, which was the goal of the current study. Based on previous studies in non-diabetic mice, it is possible that sEH inhibitors could also attenuate neurological deficits following stroke [33], and we intend to address this possibility in future studies. Nevertheless, we show that sEH inhibition improves both glycemic status and cerebral perfusion in the ischemic territory in type 2 diabetic mice when administered as a pre-treatment. This is in contrast to our findings in type 1 diabetic mice, in which sEH inhibition protected against ischemic damage without altering glycemic status or early (5 min) re-perfusion to the ischemic territory [8]. Therefore, sEH inhibition appears to protect against type 1 and type 2 diabetic stroke, at least in part, through different mechanisms. EETs can provide neuroprotection by multiple mechanisms including: enhancing vasodilation [17], inhibiting of platelet adhesion [34], reducing inflammation [35], reducing of oxygen free radicals [36], reducing apoptosis, or activating protective signal transduction [17,37]. In line with this, we have previously shown that sEH knockout mice are protected against ischemic injury in part due to enhanced cerebral blood flow after MCAO [38]. It has also been shown that EETs reduce ischemic injury by improving cerebrovascular structure and increasing microvascular density in spontaneously hypertensive rats [33].

In addition to the protective effects of EETs outlined above, EETs may have additional protective effects specifically in the context of diabetes. Although we did not observe differences in brain EETs levels in mice fed a high fat diet, sEH inhibition could still be more protective in type 2 diabetic mice than control mice because it could increase EETs in tissues other than the brain, especially the pancreas, which as previously reported by Luria et al. [39], would improve beta cell survival, insulin secretion and glycemic status. In line with this, we observed improvements in glycemic status consequent to sEH inhibition that could possibly have contributed to reductions in infarct size and cerebral perfusion. Since hyperglycemia is associated with poor stroke outcome in both humans [2–4] and rodents [5–10], any reduction in blood glucose levels may have also contributed to a reduction in infarct size. Furthermore, hyperglycemia has been shown to negatively affect cerebral vascular function and cerebral blood flow after ischemia [40,41] in some studies, although others have shown no effect [42,43]. Nevertheless, randomized prospective clinical trials have consistently failed to demonstrate that tight glycemic status improves outcome from stroke [12–16]. Similar to the reduction in blood glucose levels, in the HFD+STZ/NA mice, t-AUCB caused a 17% reduction in post-ischemic insulin levels compared to vehicle-treated HFD+STZ/NA, although this effect was not statistically significant. Likewise, enhancing EETs has been shown to enhance insulin signaling and improve insulin sensitivity [39,44–46]. Luo et al. showed that either deletion of the sEH-coding gene or pharmacological inhibition of sEH attenuated hyperglycemia in STZ-treated mice, a model for type 1 diabetes [46]. They found that sEH inhibition improved STZ hyperglycemia by directly limiting STZ-mediated damage to pancreatic β-cells [46]. Luria et al. demonstrated that either sEH inhibition or sEH gene deletion reduces the severity of insulin resistance in mice fed a HFD [39]. Specifically, they found that sEH inhibition/gene deletion increased insulin receptor signaling, pancreatic islet size and vascularization, glucose clearance during a glucose tolerance test (GTT), and insulin sensitivity during an insulin tolerance test. Thus, both the availability of insulin and the peripheral tissue response to the insulin were both improved by limiting the influence of sEH. They further showed that sEH gene deletion or sEH inhibition yielded fasting glycemia that was lower during a high-fat diet when compared to control animals on the same diet. All of these effects occurred without a reduction in body mass or adiposity, indicating that these are primary effects [39]. This improvement in glucose homeostasis plays a role in the ability of EETs to protect against diabetic cardiomyopathy [45]. Furthermore, glycemic control can improve vascularization, which is needed for brain repair, in the ischemic cortex and striatum in type 2 diabetic mice and enhance sensorimotor and cognitive function recovery [32]. Future studies will determine if the ability of sEH inhibition to improve glycemic control translates to enhanced repair and recovery following cerebral ischemia via vascular mechanisms, such as enhanced vascularization in the ischemic territory.

In summary, we found that 1) pre-diabetes, induced by long-term high fat diet, increases expression of sEH mRNA and protein but not EETs levels in brain, 2) type 2 diabetes, induced by a combination of high fat diet and STZ/NA, exacerbates cerebral infarct size after MCAO in mice, and 3) sEH inhibition with t-AUCB, when administered prior to the ischemic event, improves glycemic status, increases cerebral perfusion, and reduces brain infarct size after MCAO. These findings indicate sEH inhibition improves stroke outcome, glycemic status, and post-ischemic perfusion in the ischemic territory in setting of type 2 diabetes. This data suggest that sEH inhibition may be a potential preventative therapeutic target for improving stroke outcome in individuals with type 2 diabetes who are at increased risk for stroke [1].

Acknowledgments

The authors would like to thank the OHSU Bioanalytical Shared Resource/Pharmacokinetics Core for performing the EETs assay.

Author Contributions

Conceived and designed the experiments: KLZ SMK RES NJA DLM. Performed the experiments: KLZ SMK XZ WZ SAJ. Analyzed the data: KLZ SMK XZ WZ SAJ. Contributed reagents/materials/analysis tools: NJA DLM. Wrote the paper: KLZ RES NJA DLM.

References

1. Sarwar N, Gao P, Seshasai SR, Gobin R, Kaptoge S, et al. (2010) Diabetes mellitus, fasting blood glucose concentration, and risk of vascular disease: a collaborative meta-analysis of 102 prospective studies. Lancet 375: 2215–2222.
2. Megherbi SE, Milan C, Minier D, Couvreur G, Osseby GV, et al. (2003) Association between diabetes and stroke subtype on survival and functional outcome 3 months after stroke: data from the European BIOMED Stroke Project. Stroke 34: 688–694.
3. Pulsinelli WA, Levy DE, Sigsbee B, Scherer P, Plum F (1983) Increased damage after ischemic stroke in patients with hyperglycemia with or without established diabetes mellitus. Am J Med 74: 540–544.
4. Baird TA, Parsons MW, Phanh T, Butcher KS, Desmond PM, et al. (2003) Persistent poststroke hyperglycemia is independently associated with infarct expansion and worse clinical outcome. Stroke 34: 2208–2214.
5. Warner DS, Todd MM, Dexter F, Ludwig P, McAllister AM (1995) Temporal thresholds for hyperglycemia-augmented ischemic brain damage in rats. Stroke 26: 655–660.
6. Pulsinelli WA, Waldman S, Rawlinson D, Plum F (1982) Moderate hyperglycemia augments ischemic brain damage: a neuropathologic study in the rat. Neurology 32: 1239–1246.
7. Ning R, Chopp M, Yan T, Zacharek A, Zhang C, et al. (2012) Tissue plasminogen activator treatment of stroke in type-1 diabetes rats. Neuroscience 222: 326–332.
8. Jouihan SA, Zuloaga KL, Zhang W, Shangraw RE, Krasnow SM, et al. (2013) Role of soluble epoxide hydrolase in exacerbation of stroke by streptozotocin-induced type 1 diabetes mellitus. J Cereb Blood Flow Metab.
9. Tureyen K, Bowen K, Liang J, Dempsey RJ, Vemuganti R (2011) Exacerbated brain damage, edema and inflammation in type-2 diabetic mice subjected to focal ischemia. Journal of Neurochemistry 116: 499–507.
10. Dave KR, Tamariz J, Desai KM, Brand FJ, Liu A, et al. (2011) Recurrent Hypoglycemia Exacerbates Cerebral Ischemic Damage in Streptozotocin-Induced Diabetic Rats. Stroke 42: 1404–1411.
11. Finfer S, Chittock DR, Su SY, Blair D, Foster D, et al. (2009) Intensive versus conventional glucose control in critically ill patients. N Engl J Med 360: 1283–1297.
12. Patel A, MacMahon S, Chalmers J, Neal B, Billot L, et al. (2008) Intensive blood glucose control and vascular outcomes in patients with type 2 diabetes. N Engl J Med 358: 2560–2572.
13. Duckworth W, Abraira C, Moritz T, Reda D, Emanuele N, et al. (2009) Glucose control and vascular complications in veterans with type 2 diabetes. N Engl J Med 360: 129–139.
14. Gerstein HC, Miller ME, Byington RP, Goff DC Jr, Bigger JT, et al. (2008) Effects of intensive glucose lowering in type 2 diabetes. N Engl J Med 358: 2545–2559.
15. Gray CS, Hildreth AJ, Sandercock PA, O'Connell JE, Johnston DE, et al. (2007) Glucose-potassium insulin infusions in the management of post-stroke hyperglycaemia: the UK Glucose Insulin in Stroke Trial (GIST-UK). Lancet Neurol 6: 397–406.
16. Ntaios G, Papavasileiou V, Bargiota A, Makaritsis K, Michel P (2013) Intravenous insulin treatment in acute stroke: a systematic review and meta-analysis of randomized controlled trials. Int J Stroke.
17. Iliff JJ, Jia J, Nelson J, Goyagi T, Klaus J, et al. (2010) Epoxyeicosanoid signaling in CNS function and disease. Prostaglandins Other Lipid Mediat 91: 68–84.
18. McCrimmon RJ, Ryan CM, Frier BM (2012) Diabetes and cognitive dysfunction. Lancet 379: 2291–2299.
19. Obrosova IG, Ilnytska O, Lyzogubov VV, Pavlov IA, Mashtalir N, et al. (2007) High-Fat Diet Induced Neuropathy of Pre-Diabetes and Obesity: Effects of "Healthy" Diet and Aldose Reductase Inhibition. Diabetes 56: 2598–2608.
20. Nakamura T, Terajima T, Ogata T, Ueno K, Hashimoto N, et al. (2006) Establishment and pathophysiological characterization of type 2 diabetic mouse model produced by streptozotocin and nicotinamide. Biol Pharm Bull 29: 1167–1174.
21. Liu JY, Tsai HJ, Hwang SH, Jones PD, Morisseau C, et al. (2009) Pharmacokinetic optimization of four soluble epoxide hydrolase inhibitors for use in a murine model of inflammation. Br J Pharmacol 156: 284–296.
22. Zhang W, Koerner IP, Noppens R, Grafe M, Tsai H-J, et al. (2007) Soluble epoxide hydrolase: a novel therapeutic target in stroke. J Cereb Blood Flow Metab 27: 1931–1940.
23. Iliff JJ, Fairbanks SL, Balkowiec A, Alkayed NJ (2010) Epoxyeicosatrienoic acids are endogenous regulators of vasoactive neuropeptide release from trigeminal ganglion neurons. J Neurochem 115: 1530–1542.
24. AmericanDiabetesAssociation (2010) Diagnosis and classification of diabetes mellitus. Diabetes Care 33 Suppl 1: S62–69.
25. Bergman M (2013) Pathophysiology of prediabetes and treatment implications for the prevention of type 2 diabetes mellitus. Endocrine 43: 504–513.
26. De Taeye BM, Morisseau C, Coyle J, Covington JW, Luria A, et al. (2010) Expression and regulation of soluble epoxide hydrolase in adipose tissue. Obesity (Silver Spring) 18: 489–498.
27. Deutsch C, Portik-Dobos V, Smith AD, Ergul A, Dorrance AM (2009) Diet-induced obesity causes cerebral vessel remodeling and increases the damage caused by ischemic stroke. Microvasc Res 78: 100–106.
28. Meng L, Jeffrey LS, Keun-Sik H, Sarah S, Kuo-Hsuan C, et al. (2012) Effect of pre-diabetes on future risk of stroke: meta-analysis. BMJ 344.
29. Klaidman L, Morales M, Kem S, Yang J, Chang ML, et al. (2003) Nicotinamide Offers Multiple Protective Mechanisms in Stroke as a Precursor for NAD+, as a PARP Inhibitor and by Partial Restoration of Mitochondrial Function. Pharmacology 69: 150–157.
30. Wang P, Xu T-Y, Guan Y-F, Tian W-W, Viollet B, et al. (2011) Nicotinamide phosphoribosyltransferase protects against ischemic stroke through SIRT1-dependent adenosine monophosphate–activated kinase pathway. Annals of Neurology 69: 360–374.
31. Cui X, Chopp M, Zacharek A, Ye X, Roberts C, et al. (2011) Angiopoietin/Tie2 pathway mediates type 2 diabetes induced vascular damage after cerebral stroke. Neurobiol Dis 43: 285–292.
32. Prakash R, Li W, Qu Z, Johnson MA, Fagan SC, et al. (2013) Vascularization Pattern After Ischemic Stroke is Different in Control Versus Diabetic Rats: Relevance to Stroke Recovery. Stroke.
33. Simpkins AN, Rudic RD, Schreihofer DA, Roy S, Manhiani M, et al. (2009) Soluble Epoxide Inhibition Is Protective Against Cerebral Ischemia via Vascular and Neural Protection. The American Journal of Pathology 174: 2086–2095.
34. Heizer ML, McKinney JS, Ellis EF (1991) 14,15-Epoxyeicosatrienoic acid inhibits platelet aggregation in mouse cerebral arterioles. Stroke 22: 1389–1393.
35. Spector AA, Norris AW (2007) Action of epoxyeicosatrienoic acids on cellular function. Am J Physiol Cell Physiol 292: C996–1012.
36. Yang B, Graham L, Dikalov S, Mason RP, Falck JR, et al. (2001) Overexpression of cytochrome P450 CYP2J2 protects against hypoxia-reoxygenation injury in cultured bovine aortic endothelial cells. Mol Pharmacol 60: 310–320.
37. Merkel MJ, Liu L, Cao Z, Packwood W, Young J, et al. (2010) Inhibition of soluble epoxide hydrolase preserves cardiomyocytes: role of STAT3 signaling. Am J Physiol Heart Circ Physiol 298: H679–687.
38. Zhang W, Iliff JJ, Campbell CJ, Wang RK, Hurn PD, et al. (2009) Role of soluble epoxide hydrolase in the sex-specific vascular response to cerebral ischemia. J Cereb Blood Flow Metab 29: 1475–1481.
39. Luria A, Bettaieb A, Xi Y, Shieh GJ, Liu HC, et al. (2011) Soluble epoxide hydrolase deficiency alters pancreatic islet size and improves glucose homeostasis in a model of insulin resistance. Proc Natl Acad Sci USA 108: 9038–9043.
40. Fabian RH, Kent TA (2012) Hyperglycemia accentuates persistent "functional uncoupling" of cerebral microvascular nitric oxide and superoxide following focal ischemia/reperfusion in rats. Transl Stroke Res 3: 482–490.
41. Wang Z, Luo W, Li P, Qiu J, Luo Q (2008) Acute hyperglycemia compromises cerebral blood flow following cortical spreading depression in rats monitored by laser speckle imaging. J Biomed Opt 13: 064023.
42. Cipolla MJ, Godfrey JA (2010) Effect of hyperglycemia on brain penetrating arterioles and cerebral blood flow before and after ischemia/reperfusion. Transl Stroke Res 1: 127–134.
43. Luitse MJ, van Seeters T, Horsch AD, Kool HA, Velthuis BK, et al. (2013) Admission hyperglycaemia and cerebral perfusion deficits in acute ischaemic stroke. Cerebrovasc Dis 35: 163–167.
44. Xu X, Zhao CX, Wang L, Tu L, Fang X, et al. (2010) Increased CYP2J3 expression reduces insulin resistance in fructose-treated rats and db/db mice. Diabetes 59: 997–1005.
45. Ma B, Xiong X, Chen C, Li H, Xu X, et al. (2013) Cardiac-Specific Overexpression of CYP2J2 Attenuates Diabetic Cardiomyopathy in Male Streptozotocin-Induced Diabetic Mice. Endocrinology 154: 2843–2856.
46. Luo P, Chang HH, Zhou Y, Zhang S, Hwang SH, et al. (2010) Inhibition or deletion of soluble epoxide hydrolase prevents hyperglycemia, promotes insulin secretion, and reduces islet apoptosis. J Pharmacol Exp Ther 334: 430–438.

Effects of Comprehensive Stroke Care Capabilities on In-Hospital Mortality of Patients with Ischemic and Hemorrhagic Stroke: J-ASPECT Study

Koji Iihara[1]*, Kunihiro Nishimura[2], Akiko Kada[3], Jyoji Nakagawara[4], Kuniaki Ogasawara[5], Junichi Ono[6], Yoshiaki Shiokawa[7], Toru Aruga[8], Shigeru Miyachi[9], Izumi Nagata[10], Kazunori Toyoda[11], Shinya Matsuda[12], Yoshihiro Miyamoto[2], Akifumi Suzuki[13], Koichi B. Ishikawa[14], Hiroharu Kataoka[15], Fumiaki Nakamura[16], Satoru Kamitani[16]

1 Department of Neurosurgery, Graduate School of Medical Sciences, Kyushu University, Fukuoka, Japan, **2** Department of Preventive Medicine and Epidemiologic Informatics, National Cerebral and Cardiovascular Center, Suita, Japan, **3** Clinical Research Center, National Hospital Organization, Nagoya Medical Center, Nagoya, Japan, **4** Integrative Stroke Imaging Center, National Cerebral and Cardiovascular Center, Suita, Japan, **5** Department of Neurosurgery, Iwate Medical University, Morioka, Japan, **6** Chiba Cardiovascular Center, Ichihara, Japan, **7** Department of Neurosurgery, Kyorin University, Mitaka, Japan, **8** Showa University Hospital, Tokyo, Japan, **9** Department of Neurosurgery, Nagoya University, Nagoya, Japan, **10** Department of Neurosurgery, Nagasaki University, Nagasaki, Japan, **11** Department of Cerebrovascular Medicine, National Cerebral and Cardiovascular Center, Suita, Japan, **12** Department of Preventive Medicine and Community Health, University of Occupational and Environmental Health, Kita-Kyushu, Japan, **13** Research Institute for Brain and Blood Vessels, Akita, Japan, **14** Center for Cancer Control and Information Services, National Cancer Center, Tokyo, Japan, **15** Department of Neurosurgery, National Cerebral and Cardiovascular Center, Suita, Japan, **16** Department of Public Health, The University of Tokyo, Tokyo, Japan

Abstract

Background: The effectiveness of comprehensive stroke center (CSC) capabilities on stroke mortality remains uncertain. We performed a nationwide study to examine whether CSC capabilities influenced in-hospital mortality of patients with ischemic and hemorrhagic stroke.

Methods and Results: Of the 1,369 certified training institutions in Japan, 749 hospitals responded to a questionnaire survey regarding CSC capabilities that queried the availability of personnel, diagnostic techniques, specific expertise, infrastructure, and educational components recommended for CSCs. Among the institutions that responded, data on patients hospitalized for stroke between April 1, 2010 and March 31, 2011 were obtained from the Japanese Diagnosis Procedure Combination database. In-hospital mortality was analyzed using hierarchical logistic regression analysis adjusted for age, sex, level of consciousness on admission, comorbidities, and the number of fulfilled CSC items in each component and in total. Data from 265 institutions and 53,170 emergency-hospitalized patients were analyzed. Mortality rates were 7.8% for patients with ischemic stroke, 16.8% for patients with intracerebral hemorrhage (ICH), and 28.1% for patients with subarachnoid hemorrhage (SAH). Mortality adjusted for age, sex, and level of consciousness was significantly correlated with personnel, infrastructural, educational, and total CSC scores in patients with ischemic stroke. Mortality was significantly correlated with diagnostic, educational, and total CSC scores in patients with ICH and with specific expertise, infrastructural, educational, and total CSC scores in patients with SAH.

Conclusions: CSC capabilities were associated with reduced in-hospital mortality rates, and relevant aspects of care were found to be dependent on stroke type.

Editor: Hooman Kamel, Weill Cornell Medical College, United States of America

Funding: This study was supported by Grants-in-Aid from the Ministry of Health, Labour, and Welfare of Japan (Principal Investigator: Koji Iihara). The funders had no role in study design, data collection and analysis, decision to publish, or preparation of the manuscript.

Competing Interests: Ube Industries, Ltd., Central Hospital participated in this study by providing survey data.

* E-mail: kiihara@ns.med.kyushu-u.ac.jp

Introduction

In Japan, stroke is the third-leading cause of death, as well as a leading cause of long-term disability. Almost 270,000 individuals in Japan have a new or recurrent stroke each year, and nearly 120,000 individuals die following a stroke [1]. In 2000, the Brain Attack Coalition discussed the concept of stroke centers and proposed two types of centers: comprehensive [2] and primary [3]. Most patients with stroke can be appropriately treated at a primary stroke center (PSC), and the Joint Commission has established programs for certifying PSCs and measuring their performance [4]. The concept and recommended key components of comprehensive stroke centers (CSCs) enable intensive care and specialized techniques that are not available at most PSCs [2,5].

Table 1. Number and percentage of participating hospitals (n = 265) with the recommended items of comprehensive stroke care capabilities.

Components	Items	*n*	%
Personnel	Neurologists	143	54.0
	Neurosurgeons	251	94.7
	Endovascular physicians	118	44.5
	Critical care medicine	65	24.5
	Physical medicine and rehabilitation	42	15.8
	Rehabilitation therapy	265	100
	Stroke rehabilitation nurses	38	14.6
Diagnostic techniques	CT	264	99.6
	MRI with diffusion	237	89.4
	Digital cerebral angiography	226	85.6
	CT angiography	234	88.3
	Carotid duplex ultrasound	102	38.5
	TCD	53	20.2
Specific expertise	Carotid endarterectomy	231	87.2
	Clipping of intracranial aneurysm	250	94.3
	Hematoma removal/draining	253	95.5
	Coiling of intracranial aneurysm	153	57.7
	Intra-arterial reperfusion therapy	199	75.1
Infrastructure	Stroke unit	55	20.8
	Intensive care unit	169	63.8
	Operating room staffed 24/7	185	70.0
	Interventional services coverage 24/7	122	46.0
	Stroke registry	109	41.8
Education	Community education	147	55.7
	Professional education	171	64.8

CT, computed tomography; MRI, magnetic resonance imaging; TCD, transcranial Doppler.

Although stroke performance measures have been developed to monitor and improve quality of care, a substantial proportion of patients do not receive effective treatments, and population-based studies have been called for to evaluate the successful translation of evidence-based medicine into clinical practice [4] Organized stroke unit care is a form of in-hospital care provided by nurses, doctors, and therapists who work as a coordinated team specialized in caring for patients with stroke [6]. The effectiveness of organized stroke care has been reported for different ischemic stroke subtypes in the organized care index (OCI) using data from the Registry of the Canadian Stroke Network [7,8]. However, the effectiveness of CSC capabilities on the mortality of patients with ischemic and hemorrhagic stroke remains uncertain. In this study, we examined whether CSC capabilities influence in-hospital mortality for all types of stroke in a real-world setting by using data from the J-ASPECT nationwide stroke registry (obtained from the Japanese Diagnosis Procedure Combination [DPC]-based Payment System) [9].

Methods

Of the 1,369 certified training institutions of the Japan Neurosurgical Society, the Japanese Society of Neurology, and/or the Japan Stroke Society, 749 hospitals responded to a questionnaire survey regarding CSC capabilities. The CSC capabilities were assessed using 25 items specifically recommended for CSCs [2] that were divided into 5 components regarding (1) personnel (seven items: board-certified neurologists, board-certified neurosurgeons, board-certified endovascular physicians, board-certified physicians in critical care medicine, board-certified physicians in physical medicine and rehabilitation, personnel in rehabilitation therapy, and stroke rehabilitation nurses), (2) diagnostic techniques (six items: 24 hours/day, 7 days/week [24/7] availability of computed tomography [CT], magnetic resonance imaging [MRI] with diffusion-weighted imaging, digital cerebral angiography, CT angiography, carotid duplex ultrasound, and transcranial Doppler), (3) specific expertise (five items: carotid endarterectomy, clipping of intracranial aneurysms [IAs], removal of intracerebral hemorrhage [ICH], coiling of IAs, and intra-arterial reperfusion therapy), (4) infrastructure (five items: stroke unit, intensive care unit, operating room staffed 24/7, interventional services coverage 24/7, and stroke registry), and (5) educational components (two items: community education and professional education). A score of 1 point was assigned if the hospital met each recommended item, yielding a total CSC score of up to 25. The scores were also summed for each component (subcategory CSC score). The impact of specific aspects of acute stroke care (monitoring, early rehabilitation, admission to stroke care unit [SCU], acute stroke team, the organized stroke care index [7], existence of a tissue plasminogen activator [t-PA]

Table 2. Demographics of the study cohort according to the Diagnosis Procedure Combination (DPC) discharge database study in a comparison of hospitals that agreed to participate in the present study and those that did not.

	Participating hp (n = 265)	Non-participating hp (n = 484)	P value#
Hospital characteristics (CSC scores)			
Total score (25 items)	15.4±4.2	13.5±4.6	<0.001
Personnel (7 items)	3.5±1.2	3.1±1.3	<0.001
Diagnostic techniques (6 items)	4.2±1.2	3.9±1.3	0.002
Specific expertise (5 items)	4.0±1.4	3.6±1.6	<0.001
Infrastructure (5 items)	2.4±1.4	1.9±1.4	<0.001
Education (2 items)	1.2±0.8	1.0±0.8	0.002
Number of beds, n (%)			
20–49	3 (1.1)	13 (2.7)	<0.001
50–99	9 (3.4)	21 (4.3)	
100–299	66 (24.9)	166 (34.3)	
300–499	97 (36.6)	163 (33.7)	
500–	90 (34.0)	117 (24.2)	
Annual stroke cases, n (%)			
0–49	8 (3.0)	43 (8.9)	0.003
50–99	31 (11.7)	47 (9.7)	
100–199	56 (21.1)	143 (29.5)	
200–299	67 (25.3)	88 (18.2)	
300–	92 (34.7)	136 (28.1)	
Annual volume of t-PA infusion	8.3	6.4	0.002

#Wilcoxon rank-sum test.
CSC, comprehensive stroke center.
Hp, hospital.

protocol, number of t-PA cases/year, and number of acute stroke cases/year) on stroke mortality was also examined. This survey was completed by neurosurgeons or neurologists in the responding hospitals and returned by mail. Any incomplete answers were completed in follow-up phone interviews with the neurosurgeons or neurologists of the study group. The English version of the survey is shown in File S1.

This cross-sectional survey used the DPC discharge database from participating institutions in the J-ASPECT Study. The DPC is a mixed case patient classification system that was launched in 2002 by the Ministry of Health, Labor, and Welfare of Japan and was linked with a lump-sum payment system [9]. Of the 749 hospitals that responded to the institutional survey regarding CSC capabilities, 265 agreed to participate in the DPC discharge database study (File S2). Computer software was developed to identify patients hospitalized because of acute stroke from the annual de-identified discharge database by using the International Classification of Diseases (ICD)-10 diagnosis codes related to ischemic stroke (I63.0-9), nontraumatic ICH (ICH: I61.0-9, I62.0-1, and I62.9), and subarachnoid hemorrhage (SAH: I60.0-9). Because of major differences in their typical prognosis, patients with transient ischemic attack were excluded. Patients hospitalized because of ischemic and hemorrhagic stroke between April 1, 2010 and March 31, 2011 were included; however, patients with scheduled admissions were excluded from analysis. The following data were collected from the database: unique identifiers of hospitals, patients' age and sex, diagnoses, comorbidities at admission, in-hospital use of medications (antihypertensive agents, oral hypoglycemic agents, insulin, antihyperlipidemic agents, statins, anticoagulant agents, or antiplatelet agents), smoking, arrival by ambulance or not, level of consciousness at admission according to the Japan Coma Scale [10], and discharge status. The Japan Coma Scale [11] was originally published in 1974, the same year as the Glasgow Coma Scale (GCS) [12], and it remains one of the most popular grading scales for assessing impaired consciousness among health care professionals and personnel for emergency medical services in Japan. Grading with the 1-, 2-, and 3-digit codes corresponds to the following statuses: 1) the patient is awake in the absence of any stimulation, 2) the patient can be aroused but reverts to the previous state after the cessation of stimulation, and 3) the patient cannot be aroused even by forceful mechanical stimulation. Each specific digit status is further subdivided into three levels: 1-digit code into 1, 2, and 3; 2-digit code into 10, 20, and 30; and 3-digit code into 100, 200, and 300 (Table S1). In addition to these nine grades, a normal level of consciousness is graded as zero. Consciousness level on admission was determined by the physician and data on all medication use was collected electronically from the claim data. Comorbidity was determined primarily from the ICD-10 code, but was also checked against what medications and procedures the patient was receiving/undergoing, to see if these were compatible with the code data. Smoking was defined by the physician's record, which rated patients as active or inactive smokers. In-hospital mortality, defined as death by the time of discharge from the hospital, was analyzed with the total and subcategory CSC scores using hierarchical logistic regression analysis adjusted for age, sex,

Table 3. Demographics of the patient study cohort at the time of diagnosis and hospital characteristics according to stroke type.

	Total (n=53,170)	Ischemic Stroke (n=32,671)	Intracerebral hemorrhage (n=15,699)	Subarachnoid hemorrhage (n=4,934)
Male, n (%)	29,353 (55.2)	18,816 (57.6)	9,030 (57.5)	1,584 (32.1)
Age, mean years ±SD	72.5±13.1	74.4±12.2	70.7±13.5	64.7±14.8
Hypertension, n (%)	39,918 (75.1)	22,531 (69.0)	13,281 (84.6)	4,229 (85.7)
Diabetes Mellitus, n (%)	13,725 (25.8)	9,318 (28.5)	3,278 (20.9)	1,174 (23.8)
Hyperlipidemia, n (%)	15,015 (28.2)	11,104 (34.0)	2,529 (16.1)	1,412 (28.6)
Smoking (n=4,4842)	12,761 (24.0)	8,188 (25.1)	3,540 (22.5)	1,074 (21.8)
Medications during hospitalization				
Antihypertensive agent	34,136 (64.2)	17,694 (54.2)	12,537 (79.9)	4,019 (81.5)
Anti-renin-angiotensin system agent	19,881 (37.4)	10,262 (31.4)	8,280 (52.7)	1,410 (28.6)
Ca channel antagonist	25,984 (48.9)	10,469 (32.0)	11,719 (74.6)	3,903 (79.1)
Sympathetic antagonist	6,334 (11.9)	3,821 (11.7)	2,172 (13.8)	364 (7.4)
*β-blocker, α,β-blocker	4,357 (8.2)	3,048 (9.3)	1,133 (7.2)	188 (3.8)
α-blocker	2,374 (4.5)	953 (2.9)	1,232 (7.8)	200 (4.1)
Diuretic agent	9,950 (18.7)	5,860 (17.9)	3,074 (19.6)	1,049 (21.3)
Loop diuretic	7,434 (14.0)	4,609 (14.1)	1,912 (12.2)	940 (19.1)
Other diuretic	4,425 (8.3)	2,527 (7.7)	1,653 (10.5)	255 (5.2)
Antidiabetic agent	10,295 (19.4)	6,784 (20.8)	2,473 (15.8)	1,075 (21.8)
Insulin	7,654 (14.4)	4,597 (14.1)	2,044 (13.0)	1,046 (21.2)
Oral antidiabetic agent	5,749 (10.8)	4,459 (13.6)	1,110 (7.1)	197 (4.0)
Antihyperlipidemic agent	12,387 (23.3)	9,264 (28.4)	1,839 (11.7)	1,310 (26.6)
Statin	10,099 (19.0)	7,840 (24.0)	1,366 (8.7)	912 (18.5)
Antiplatelet agent	23,635 (44.5)	21,746 (66.6)	625 (4.0)	1,298 (26.3)
Aspirin	11,929 (22.4)	11,119 (34.0)	378 (2.4)	447 (9.1)
Japan Coma Scale				
0, n (%)	19,635 (36.9)	15,027 (46.0)	3,620 (23.1)	1,024 (20.8)
1-digit code, n (%)	19,371 (36.4)	12,375 (37.9)	5,934 (37.8)	1,117 (22.6)
2-digit code, n (%)	6,937 (13.0)	3,396 (10.4)	2,705 (17.2)	852 (17.3)
3-digit code, n (%)	7,227 (13.6)	1,873 (5.7)	3,440 (21.9)	1,941 (39.3)
Emergency admission by ambulance, n (%)	31,995 (60.2)	17,336 (53.1)	10,909 (69.5)	3,830 (77.6)
Average days in hospital (range)	21 (11–40)	20 (12–38)	22 (10–43)	30 (12–54)
Hospital characteristics (CSC scores)				
Total score (25 items)		16.7±3.8	16.8±3.4	17.1±3.4
Personnel (7 items)		3.7±1.2	3.7±1.2	3.8±1.2
Diagnostic techniques (6 items)		4.4±1.1	4.5±1.0	4.5±1.0
Specific expertise (5 items)		4.4±1.0	4.4±0.9	4.5±0.8
Infrastructure (5 items)		2.8±1.3	2.9±1.3	2.9±1.3
Education (2 items)		1.4±0.8	1.4±0.8	1.4±0.8

CSC, comprehensive stroke center.
*A composite variable with a pure beta antagonist and a mixed alpha/beta adrenergic antagonist (e.g., labetalol).

Japan Coma Scale score, comorbidities, and institutional difference.

Ethics Statement

This research plan was designed by the authors and approved by the Institutional Review Board of the National Cerebral and Cardiovascular Center, which waived the requirement for individual informed consent.

Statistical Analysis

We used hierarchical logistic regression models [13,14] to estimate odds ratios (ORs) for in-hospital mortality. Each model had two levels of hierarchy (hospital and patient) while considering the random effects of hospital variation, as well as fixed effects of CSC score and patient effects of age, sex, and level of consciousness. The total score and each subcategory score were analyzed separately. We also divided CSC score into quintiles and analyzed the trend with the Cochran-Armitage trend test. The

Table 4. The impact of total comprehensive stroke care (CSC) score on in-hospital mortality after ischemic stroke, adjusted by age, sex, and level of consciousness at admission according to the Japan Coma Scale (JCS).

Factor	OR	95% CI	P value
Male	1.23	1.12–1.35	<0.001
Age	1.40	1.34–1.47	<0.001
CSC total score	0.97	0.96–0.99	0.001
JCS			
normal	1		
one-digit code	2.40	2.11–2.74	<0.001
two-digit code	7.46	6.47–8.60	<0.001
three-digit code	21.62	18.69–25.02	<0.001

CI, confidence interval; CSC, comprehensive stroke care; JCS, Japan Coma Scale; OR, odds ratio.

difference between participating and non-participating hospitals in the DPC discharge study was determined by Wilcoxon rank-sum test. The analyses were performed using SAS version 9.2 (SAS Institute Inc., Cary, NC, USA) and STATA version 12 (STATA Corp, College Station, TX, USA).

Results

A total of 265 hospitals participated in this study. The number and percentage of the participating hospitals with the recommended items of CSC capabilities are shown in Table 1. The distribution of total CSC scores ranged from 1 to 23 (mean: 15.4, median: 14 standard deviation [SD]: 4.2, interquartile range [IQR]: 11–18). Because we initially sent the CSC questionnaire to 749 hospitals, we sought to determine whether there was a selection bias in stroke care capabilities that could have impacted which hospitals returned the questionnaire. We found that such a bias did exist; in fact, the total CSC scores, subcategory CSC scores and annual volume of t-PA infusion, with the exception of the diagnostic techniques and education/research subcategories, were significantly higher for the participating hospitals than for the non-participating hospitals (Table 2).

Data from 265 institutions and 53,170 emergency-hospitalized patients (age in years, mean ±SD: 72.5±13.1; male: 55.2%) were analyzed. Patient demographics according to stroke type at the time of diagnosis are shown in Table 3. The study cohort included 32,671 patients with ischemic stroke (age: 74.4±12.2 years; male: 57.6%), 15,699 with ICH (age: 70.7±13.5 years; male: 57.5%), and 4,934 with SAH (age: 64.7±14.8 years; male: 32.1%). Use of antihypertensive agents, antidiabetic agents, antihyperlipidemic agents, and antiplatelet agents is also shown in Table 3. Almost 60% of the patients arrived by ambulance, with the incidence ranging from 77.6% for SAH to 53.1% for ischemic stroke. These rates of arrival by ambulance based on stroke type were in accordance with different degrees of stroke severity, as reflected by level of consciousness. Hospital characteristics shown by total and subcategory CSC scores did not reveal any significant differences with respect to stroke type.

Overall, mortality rates were 7.8% for ischemic stroke, 16.8% for ICH, and 28.1% for SAH. Table 4–6 show the results of a hierarchical logistic regression analysis of these data. Mortality of patients with ischemic stroke was significantly correlated with male sex (OR = 1.23), age (10 incremental years, OR = 1.4), and level of consciousness (1-digit code: OR = 2.4, 2-digit code: OR = 7.46, 3-digit code: OR = 21.62, versus zero [normal consciousness {control}]) as patient characteristics, and total CSC score (OR = 0.97) adjusted for age, sex, and level of consciousness as a hospital characteristic (Table 4). Mortality of patients with ICH was also significantly correlated with male sex (OR = 1.72), age (10 incremental years, OR = 1.36), and level of consciousness (1-digit code: OR = 1.45, 2-digit code: OR = 4.22, 3-digit code: OR = 49.59, versus zero as control) as patient characteristics and total CSC score (OR = 0.97) adjusted for age, sex, and level of consciousness as a hospital characteristic (Table 5). Mortality of

Table 5. The impact of total comprehensive stroke care (CSC) score on in-hospital mortality after intracerebral hemorrhage, adjusted by age, sex, and level of consciousness at admission according to the Japan Coma Scale (JCS).

Factor	OR	95% CI	P value
Male	1.72	1.54–1.92	<0.001
Age	1.36	1.30–1.42	<0.001
CSC total score	0.97	0.95–0.99	0.003
JCS			
normal	1		
one-digit code	1.45	1.14–1.83	0.002
two-digit code	4.22	3.34–5.33	<0.001
three-digit code	49.59	40.12–61.27	<0.001

CI, confidence interval; CSC, comprehensive stroke care; JCS, Japan Coma Scale; OR, odds ratio.

Table 6. The impact of total comprehensive stroke care (CSC) score on in-hospital mortality after subarachnoid hemorrhage, adjusted by age, sex, and level of consciousness at admission according to the Japan Coma Scale (JCS).

Factor	OR	95%CI	P value
Male	1.39	1.17–1.65	<0.001
Age	1.37	1.29–1.45	<0.001
CSC total score	0.95	0.93–0.98	<0.001
JCS			
normal	1		
one-digit code	1.05	0.75–1.46	0.785
two-digit code	2.01	1.46–2.77	<0.001
three-digit code	17.13	13.14–22.35	<0.001

CI, confidence interval; CSC, comprehensive stroke care; JCS, Japan Coma Scale; OR, odds ratio.

patients with SAH was likewise significantly correlated with male sex (OR = 1.39), age (10 incremental years, OR = 1.37), and level of consciousness (2-digit code: OR = 2.01, 3-digit code: OR = 17.12, versus zero as control) as patient characteristics and total CSC score (OR = 0.95) adjusted for age, sex, and level of consciousness as a hospital characteristic. Therefore, total CSC score was independently associated with in-hospital mortality for all stroke types after adjusting for age, sex, and stroke severity (Table 6). The impact of total CSC score on in-hospital mortality for ischemic stroke and ICH remained significant after adjustment for age, sex, severity of stroke, and existence of comorbid conditions (hypertension, diabetes mellitus, and hyperlipidemia) (Table S2–S4).

Table 7–9 show the correlations between CSC subcategory scores and in-hospital mortality adjusted for age, sex, and level of consciousness depending on the different stroke types: mortality of patients with ischemic stroke was significantly correlated with subcategory scores in personnel (OR = 0.93), infrastructure (OR = 0.94), and education (OR = 0.89) (Table 7). Mortality of patients with ICH was significantly correlated with subcategory scores in diagnostic technique (OR = 0.91), infrastructure (OR = 0.92), and education (OR = 0.91) (Table 8). Mortality of patients with SAH was significantly associated with subcategory scores in personnel (OR = 0.91) specific expertise (OR = 0.83), infrastructure (OR = 0.89), and education (OR = 0.84) (Table 9). We found that while infrastructure and education subcategory CSC scores significantly impacted outcomes for all types of stroke, other subcategory CSC scores were differentially associated with in-hospital mortality depending on stroke type.

Figure 1 shows the impact of total CSC score classified into quintiles (Q1: 4–12, Q2: 13–14, Q3: 15–17, Q4: 18, Q5: 19–23) on the in-hospital mortality of patients with all types of stroke (a), ischemic stroke (b), ICH (c), and SAH (d) after adjusting for age, sex and level of consciousness. There was a significant association between total CSC score and in-hospital mortality in all types of stroke (all P<0.001) (Table 4–6). Figure 2 illustrates the impact of total CSC score on the in-hospital mortality of patients with all types of stroke (a), ischemic stroke (b), ICH (c), and SAH (d) after adjustment for age; sex; level of consciousness; and incidence of hypertension, hyperlipidemia, and diabetes mellitus. The association between total CSC score and in-hospital mortality in patients after all types of stroke (a), ischemic stroke (b), and ICH (c) remained significant after adjustment for age; sex; level of consciousness; and incidence of hypertension, hyperlipidemia, and diabetes mellitus. This same association was not evident in patients with SAH (P = 0.601) (Table 10).

Hospitals with higher CSC scores were also more likely to provide early rehabilitation, improved monitoring, the possibility of admission to an SCU, presence of an acute stroke care team, existence of a t-PA protocol, greater numbers of t-PA cases/year, and higher scores on the organized stroke care index. In addition to the CSC score, the processes of acute stroke care, such as admission to SCU, presence of an acute stroke team, the organized stroke care index [7], and number of acute stroke cases/staff physician significantly impacted in-hospital mortality after all types of acute stroke, although in some cases, to a greater or lesser degree for the different types of stroke (Table 11–14).

Discussion

Using the nationwide discharge data obtained from the Japanese DPC-based Payment System, we evaluated the effect of

Table 7. The impact of subcategory CSC score on in-hospital mortality after ischemic stroke adjusted by age, sex and JCS.

Component	OR	95% CI	P value
Personnel	0.93	0.88–0.98	0.008
Diagnostic techniques	0.95	0.90–1.01	0.090
Specific expertise	0.96	0.90–1.01	0.136
Infrastructure	0.94	0.90–0.99	0.014
Education/research	0.89	0.83–0.96	0.003

CI, confidence interval; CSC, comprehensive stroke care; JCS, Japan Coma Scale; OR, odds ratio.

Table 8. The impact of subcategory CSC score on in-hospital mortality after intracerebral hemorrhage adjusted by age, sex and JCS.

Component	OR	95% CI	P value
Personnel	0.98	0.92–1.04	0.523
Diagnostic techniques	0.91	0.85–0.98	0.012
Specific expertise	0.93	0.86–1.00	0.055
Infrastructure	0.92	0.87–0.98	0.005
Education/research	0.91	0.83–1.00	0.047

CI, confidence interval; CSC, comprehensive stroke care; JCS, Japan Coma Scale; OR, odds ratio.

hospital characteristics based on the recommended components of CSCs [2] on the in-hospital mortality of patients with acute ischemic and hemorrhagic stroke treated between April 1, 2010 and March 31, 2011. We found that the total CSC score was significantly associated with in-hospital mortality rates irrespective of stroke type after adjustment for age, sex, and initial level of consciousness according to the Japan Coma Scale. However, the subcategory scores that were significantly associated with in-hospital mortality differed among stroke type. Importantly, the association between total CSC scores and in-hospital mortality remained significant after adjustment for age; sex; initial level of consciousness according to the Japan Coma Scale; and incidence of hypertension, diabetes mellitus and hyperlipidemia for all types of stroke except SAH. These findings highlight the importance of CSC capabilities for optimal treatment of ischemic and hemorrhagic stroke and will enable health care professionals and policy makers to focus their efforts on improving specific aspects of CSC capabilities for different types of stroke.

Increasing attention has been given to defining the quality and value of health care through the reporting of process and outcome measures. Following the original proposal to establish CSCs [2], detailed metrics for measuring quality of care in CSCs have been reported [5]. The so-called "drip-and-ship" model has emerged as a paradigm for emergency departments that are able to diagnose acute ischemic stroke and administer intravenous (IV) recombinant t-PA (rt-PA) but lack the infrastructure to provide intensive monitoring for patients after rt-PA administration [15,16]. A recent study demonstrated that despite having more severe strokes on arrival at the CSC, transfer-in patients with acute ischemic stroke had in-hospital mortality similar to that of front door patients and were more likely to be discharged to rehabilitation. These findings lend support to the concept of regionalized stroke care and directing patients with greater disability to more advanced stroke centers [17]. At present, no official certification of stroke centers in Japan has been launched, and the current study indicates that patients with acute ischemic stroke or hemorrhagic stroke are being admitted on an emergent basis to hospitals with similar CSC total and subcategory scores.

In the present study, stroke severity was adjusted by baseline level of consciousness according to the Japan Coma Scale [10,11]. The Get With the Guidelines-Stroke (GWTG-Stroke) risk model was recently developed to predict in-hospital ischemic stroke mortality, suggesting that the National Institutes of Health Stroke Scale (NIHSS) score provides substantial incremental information on a patient's mortality risk [18], emphasizing the importance of adjustment of stroke severity to develop a hospital risk model for mortality [19]. Previous prospective multicenter study has demonstrated that the development of a decreased level of consciousness within the initial hours after stroke onset, as evaluated by a simple six-point scale, is a powerful independent predictor of mortality after a major ischemic stroke of the anterior vasculature [20]. In hemorrhagic stroke, the degree of impaired consciousness at admission was also included in the various proposed ICH scores to predict functional outcome and mortality [21,22]. This study demonstrated that the level of consciousness at admission, as measured by the Japan Coma Scale, is a powerful independent predictor of mortality after ischemic and hemorrhagic stroke. Determining an individual patient's risk of mortality at admission could improve clinical care by providing valuable information to patients and their family members and by identifying those at high risk for poor outcomes who may require more intensive resources.

Health care quality of CSCs in the present study was scored on the basis of the results of a questionnaire referring to 25 items originally recommended by the Brain Attack Coalition. Although there is now increasingly good evidence from initiatives like GWTG-Stroke [23] that a process based on the systematic collection and evaluation of stroke performance measures can

Table 9. The impact of subcategory CSC score on in-hospital mortality after subarachnoid hemorrhage adjusted by age, sex and JCS.

Component	OR	95% CI	P value
Personnel	0.91	0.84–0.98	0.016
Diagnostic techniques	1.01	0.92–1.11	0.896
Specific expertise	0.83	0.75–0.93	<0.001
Infrastructure	0.89	0.83–0.96	0.002
Education/research	0.84	0.75–0.95	0.005

CI, confidence interval; CSC, comprehensive stroke care; JCS, Japan Coma Scale; OR, odds ratio.

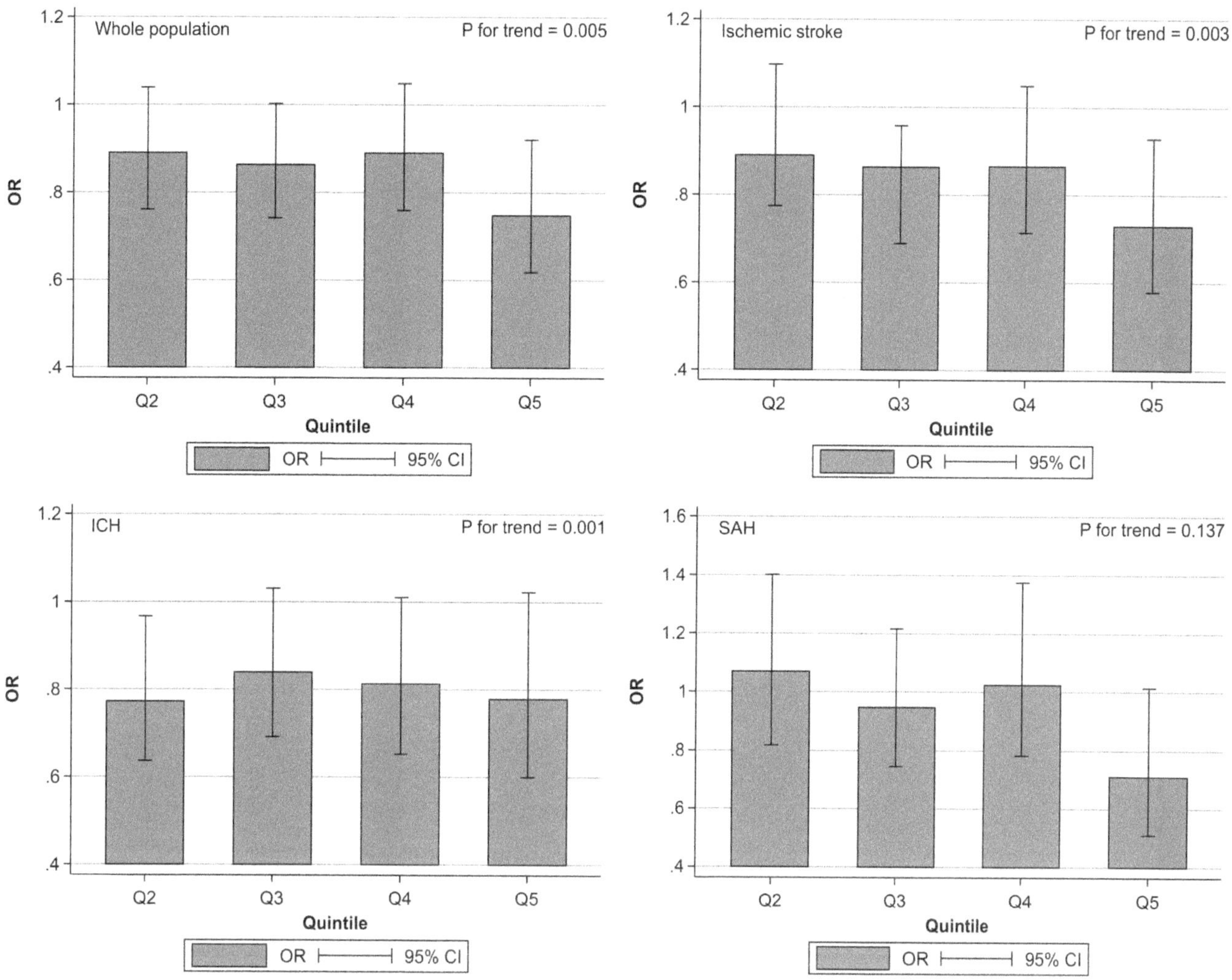

Figure 1. Associations between total comprehensive stroke care (CSC) scores separated into quintiles (Q1: 4–12, Q2: 13–14, Q3: 15–17, Q4: 18, Q5: 19–23) and in-hospital mortality of patients after all types of stroke (a), ischemic stroke (b), intracerebral hemorrhage (ICH) (c), and subarachnoid hemorrhage (SAH) (d), after adjustment for age and sex. Odds ratios (ORs) and 95% confidence intervals (CIs) of in-hospital mortality of each total CSC score quintile are depicted compared with that of Q1 as control.

rapidly improve the quality of stroke care delivered by hospitals, current metrics are mostly limited to process measures that address the care of patients with ischemic stroke in acute hospital-based settings [4]. In addition, there is a pressing need to demonstrate a direct link between better adherence to stroke performance measures and improved patient-oriented outcomes [4,24].

One potential issue with the interpretation of this study could be the lack of a control group. Although there is currently no clear consensus regarding the recommended criteria for CSCs in Japan, the present study distinctly shows that the CSC scores widely distributed in Figure 1 and classified into quintiles were significantly associated with in-hospital mortality for all types of stroke; in fact, mortality after all types of stroke markedly decreased, for example, in ischemic stroke cases by about 40% in hospitals in the highest quintile compared with those in the lowest quintile.

In the present study, our questionnaire was primarily based on the American definition of CSCs. However, according to the definitions derived from a European survey of experts in the field [25], facilities that meet the criteria for CSCs should include the capability to conduct sophisticated monitoring, such as automated electrocardiography (ECG) monitoring at bedside and automated monitoring of pulse oximetry, in addition to the numerous aspects of care capability indexed by the American definition of CSCs used in this study. According to the European approach, to meet the criteria for CSCs, hospitals should have the availability of at least 80% of the components rated as absolutely necessary by at least 50% of experts who participated in the previous expert survey; moreover, these components must be present in each of 6 categories and include the 19 components rated as absolutely necessary by >75% of experts. Based on the present results and an additional ongoing study using a validation cohort in Japan, the criteria for the designation of CSCs in Japan should be determined after further thorough discussion among Japanese stroke experts.

The present study demonstrated the feasibility and impact of using nationwide discharge data with hierarchical logistic regression analysis to examine the random effects that vary among hospitals, as well as the fixed effects of CSC score and patient effects of age, sex, and level of consciousness. We used unique hospital ID in random-intercept hierarchical regression models to assess the association between CSC score and mortality, adjusting

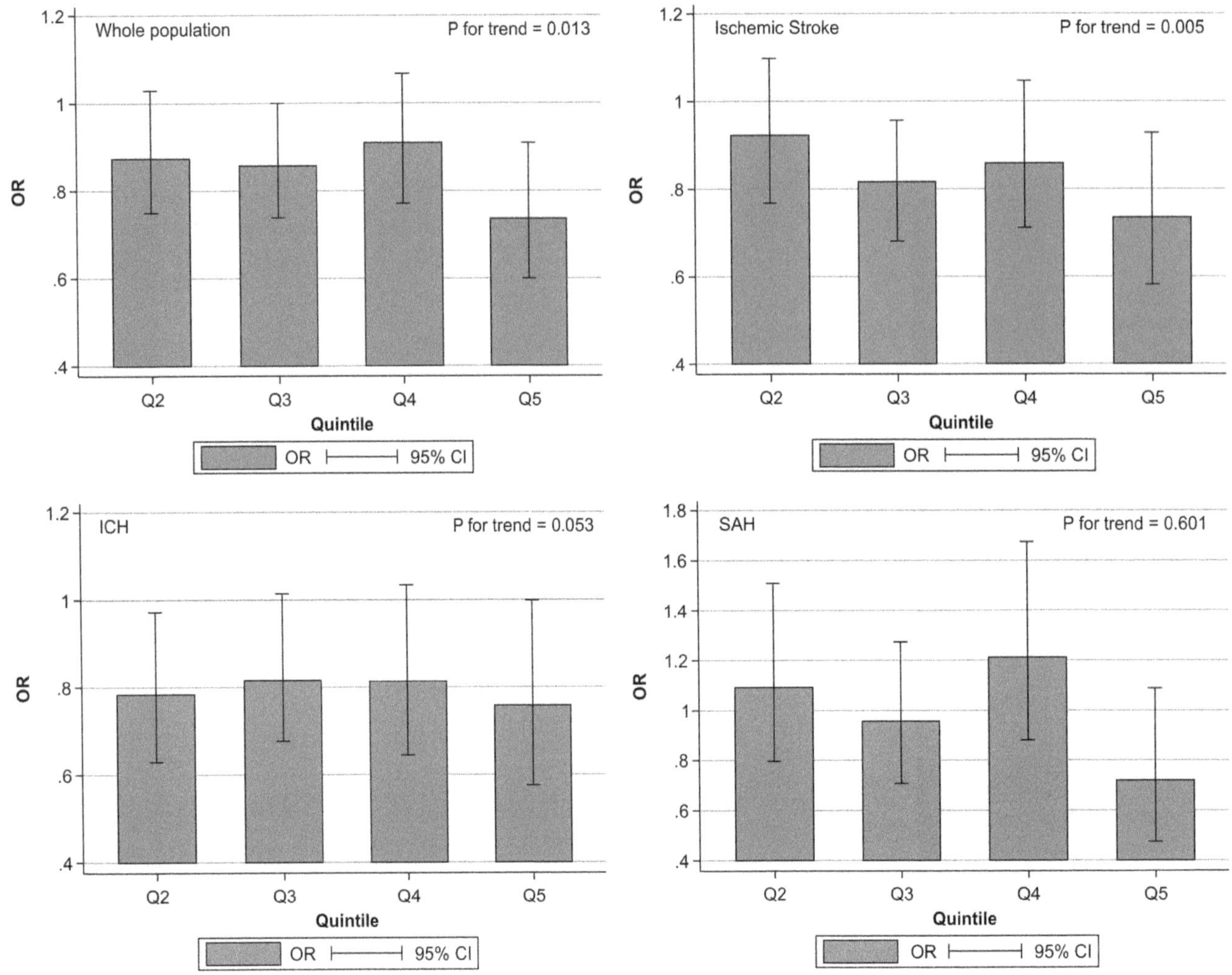

Figure 2. Associations between total comprehensive stroke care (CSC) scores separated into quintiles (Q1: 4–12, Q2: 13–14, Q3: 15–17, Q4: 18, Q5: 19–23) and in-hospital mortality of patients after all types of stroke (a), ischemic stroke (b), intracerebral hemorrhage (ICH) (c), and subarachnoid hemorrhage (SAH) (d), after adjustment for age; sex; initial level of consciousness; and incidence of hypertension, hyperlipidemia, and diabetes mellitus. Odds ratios (ORs) and 95% confidence intervals (CIs) of the in-hospital mortality of each total CSC score quintile are depicted compared with that of Q1 as control.

for patient characteristics and the hospital where a patient was treated.

This model adjusts for hospital-level effects that arise from factors such as geographical location and ageing of the local population. After adjustment, we can isolate the pure CSC score effects on mortality by hospital, as discussed by Localio et al. [26]. If the CSC score is no longer significant after accounting for hospital-level variation, the differences in mortality can be assumed to arise from differences among hospitals. This approach enabled us to elucidate the impact of various CSC metrics on in-hospital mortality of patients with different stroke types. By expanding the scope of performance measures to include all types of stroke, the present study was able to direct links between specific recommended items of CSC capacities and in-hospital mortality after both hemorrhagic and ischemic stroke. While previous reports [7] showed that aspects of acute stroke care, such as admission to an SCU, the presence of an acute stroke team, and the organized stroke care index, were significantly associated with effects on in-hospital mortality after acute stroke, the present study clearly shows that the same is true for the CSC score based on the items recommended by the American Stroke Association.

Finally, one could argue that there really is no concept of 3/4 CSCs, but rather only CSCs or PSCs. In light of the existing evidence regarding the impact of the recommended CSC items on stroke outcomes, we advocate a CSC scoring system to examine the impact of availability of the recommended items on in-hospital mortality for all types of stroke. Considering the marked impact of the CSC score on outcome after all types of stroke, the differential impacts of CSC subcategory scores for different stroke types may make a single simple and effective CSC criterion unrealistic as a tool to produce a nationwide reduction in stroke mortality. In our opinion, it may be a more viable option to employ CSC scores in a more limited fashion, that is, to benchmark the state of care currently provided by medical centers treating stroke patients.

Limitations

First, the questionnaire used in this study is new and has not undergone pilot testing or systematic analysis; thus, its validity and reliability are uncertain. The current set of CSC score items does

Table 10. Associations between total comprehensive stroke care (CSC) scores separated into quintiles (Q1: 4–12, Q2: 13–14, Q3: 15–17, Q4: 18, Q5: 19–23) and in-hospital mortality of patients after all types of stroke (a), ischemic stroke (b), intracerebral hemorrhage (ICH) (c), and subarachnoid hemorrhage (SAH) (d), model 1: after adjustment for age, sex, and initial level of consciousness; and model 2: after adjustment for age, sex, initial level of consciousness, and incidence of hypertension, hyperlipidemia, and diabetes mellitus.

		Model 1					Model 2				
Type of Stroke	**Quintile**	**OR**	**P value**	**95% CI**		**P for trend**	**OR**	**P value**	**95% CI**		**P for trend**
Whole Population (n = 53,170)	Q2	0.87	0.077	0.74	1.02	0.005	0.88	0.119	0.75	1.03	0.013
	Q3	0.84	0.023	0.72	0.98		0.86	0.045	0.74	1.00	
	Q4	0.87	0.115	0.74	1.03		0.91	0.254	0.77	1.07	
	Q5	0.73	0.003	0.60	0.90		0.74	0.004	0.60	0.91	
Ischemic Stroke (n = 32,671)	Q2	0.90	0.278	0.75	1.08	0.003	0.92	0.356	0.77	1.10	0.005
	Q3	0.79	0.008	0.66	0.94		0.81	0.015	0.68	0.96	
	Q4	0.84	0.097	0.69	1.03		0.86	0.131	0.71	1.05	
	Q5	0.71	0.006	0.56	0.91		0.73	0.01	0.58	0.93	
ICH (n = 15,699)	Q2	0.76	0.015	0.62	0.95	<0.001	0.79	0.034	0.63	0.98	0.053
	Q3	0.82	0.058	0.67	1.01		0.83	0.083	0.68	1.02	
	Q4	0.79	0.039	0.63	0.99		0.82	0.099	0.65	1.04	
	Q5	0.76	0.050	0.58	1.00		0.76	0.051	0.58	1.00	
SAH (n = 4,934)	Q2	1.04	0.814	0.78	1.38	0.137	1.10	0.568	0.80	1.51	0.601
	Q3	0.92	0.524	0.71	1.19		0.96	0.767	0.71	1.28	
	Q4	1.00	0.975	0.75	1.34		1.22	0.232	0.88	1.68	
	Q5	0.68	0.043	0.47	0.99		0.73	0.126	0.48	1.09	

ICH, intracerebral hemorrhage; SAH, subarachnoid hemorrhage.

not include all worthwhile items related to CSC. These items were appropriately modified from the original American version [2] in consideration of the medical, social, and logistical differences between the U.S. and Japan. For example, most cerebrovascular surgeries, including carotid endarterectomy and neurointervention, are performed by neurosurgeons rather than vascular surgeons or neuroradiologists. At the beginning of this project, a survey including the 25 components recommended by the Brain Attack Coalition in 2005 was created after a review of the literature on comprehensive stroke centers and a thorough discussion by an expert panel. Some recommended items such as availability of ventriculostomy were excluded from our questionnaire merely for simplicity, and thus to increase the response rate of the survey, since they seemed to be identical to recommendations of the board-certified neurosurgeons of Japan. On the other hand, some items such as transesophageal echocardiography were excluded because of the expected very low usage of this examination. According to the Japanese Stroke Databank 2009, for example, transesophageal echocardiography was performed for only 5.4% of the 34,417 acute ischemic stroke

Table 11. Impact of processes of stroke care on in-hospital mortality after all types of stroke.

	OR	**P value**	**95% CI**
Monitoring (%)	1.04	0.53	0.92–1.17
Early rehabilitation (%)	1.15	0.352	0.86–1.52
Admission to SCU (%)	0.87	0.039	0.76–0.99
Acute stroke team	0.88	0.029	0.79–0.99
Organized care index*	0.93	0.031	0.86–0.99
Existence of t-PA protocol (%)	0.88	0.295	0.69–1.12
Number of t-PA cases/year (mean)	1.00	0.203	0.99–1.00
Number of acute stroke patients/staff physician (mean)	0.999	0.012	0.998–1.000

*The organized stroke care index was created to represent different levels of access to organized stroke care ranging from 0 to 3 as determined by the presence of early rehabilitation, acute stroke team assessment, and admission to a stroke unit based on the report of Saposnik et al. (2009).
SCU, stroke care unit; t-PA, tissue plasminogen activator.

Table 12. Impact of processes of stroke care on in-hospital mortality after ischemic stroke.

	OR	P value	95% CI
Monitoring (%)	0.98	0.738	0.85–1.12
Early rehabilitation (%)	1.09	0.615	0.78–1.52
Admission to SCU (%)	0.91	0.218	0.78–1.06
Acute stroke team	0.85	0.016	0.74–0.97
Organized care index*	0.92	0.055	0.85–1.00
Existence of t-PA protocol (%)	0.82	0.158	0.61–1.08
Number of t-PA cases/year (mean)	0.99	0.132	0.98–1.00
Number of acute stroke patients/staff physician (mean)	0.999	0.047	0.998–1.000

*The organized stroke care index was created to represent different levels of access to organized stroke care ranging from 0 to 3 as determined by the presence of early rehabilitation, acute stroke team assessment, and admission to a stroke unit based on the report of Saposnik et al. (2009).
SCU, stroke care unit; t-PA, tissue plasminogen activator.

Table 13. Impact of processes of stroke care on in-hospital mortality after intracerebral hemorrhage.

	OR	P value	95% CI
Monitoring (%)	1.12	0.177	0.95–1.32
Early rehabilitation (%)	1.39	0.091	0.95–2.03
Hospitalization for SCU (%)	0.84	0.048	0.70–1.00
Acute stroke team	0.90	0.194	0.77–1.05
Organized care index*	0.93	0.163	0.85–1.03
Existence of t-PA protocol (%)	0.84	0.314	0.60–1.18
Number of t-PA cases/year (mean)	1.00	0.313	0.99–1.00
Number of acute stroke patients/staff physician (mean)	0.999	0.043	0.998–1.000

*The organized stroke care index was created to represent different levels of access to organized stroke care ranging from 0 to 3 as determined by the presence of early rehabilitation, acute stroke team assessment, and admission to a stroke unit based on the report of Saposnik et al. (2009).
SCU, stroke care unit; t-PA, tissue plasminogen activator.

Table 14. Impact of processes of stroke care on in-hospital mortality after subarachnoid hemorrhage.

	OR	P value	95% CI
Monitoring (%)	1.04	0.737	0.84–1.28
Early rehabilitation (%)	1.02	0.945	0.63–1.64
Admission to SCU (%)	0.79	0.039	0.63–0.99
Acute stroke team	0.85	0.101	0.69–1.03
Organized care index*	0.88	0.034	0.78–0.99
Existence of t-PA protocol (%)	1.09	0.732	0.66–1.81
Number of t-PA cases/year (mean)	1.00	0.456	0.98–1.01
Number of acute stroke patients/staff physician (mean)	0.998	0.006	0.997–1.000

*The organized stroke care index was created to represent different levels of access to organized stroke care ranging from 0 to 3 as determined by the presence of early rehabilitation, acute stroke team assessment, and admission to a stroke unit based on the report of Saposnik et al. (2009).
SCU, stroke care unit; t-PA, tissue plasminogen activator.

patients in a real-world situation. The impact of this examination on the mortality rates of this study would be difficult to evaluate because of low usage. All 25 components of the questionnaire are shown in the appendix. Second, discharge data obtained from the Japanese DPC-based Payment System lacks important information, such as post-discharge data and an NIHSS or GCS score as an index of stroke severity at admission. Although the Japan Coma Scale proved to be a powerful independent predictor of mortality after all types of stroke, further study is necessary to validate the results of the present study with another indicator of stroke severity, such as the NIHSS or GCS. This can be done separately or in combination with a validation data set (the estimated data volume in the J-ASPECT 2013 is more than 80,000 cases that will be available in 2013). Third, there is an inherent risk of information bias when evaluating data obtained by self-assessment. Moreover, hospitals actively working to improve stroke care may have been more likely to respond to the questionnaire. Admittedly, the participation rate of DPC data collection of the J-ASPECT study was relatively low. The participation rates were 19.4% of the 1,369 certified training institutions of the Japan Neurosurgical Society, and 35.4% of the 749 hospitals that responded to the institutional survey. However, the institutes that participated in the present study tended to have more beds and more stroke cases than average. This suggests that the hospitals that were more active in stroke care and potentially eligible for CSC participated in this study. Therefore, the present results may not generalize to non-participating hospitals. External validation greatly increases the reliability of self-assessment data. Accordingly, we plan to validate the information regarding hospital characteristics and outcomes by using a small sample set from the 2010 validation cohort of the present study. Since the number of participating hospitals in this study is increasing every year, we are planning to evaluate how the validity and reliability of the CSC score in predicting stroke patient mortality changes when weighting factors are applied to the recommended items, stroke type, and severity. Through annual evaluations, we aim to achieve higher predictive validity and responsiveness to establish the usefulness of the CSC score. Fourth, we assigned 1 point if the hospital met each recommended item for CSC. However, this equal weight assumption is probably not valid since some components were not significant on subgroup analysis. Although some associations between individual CSC components and mortality achieved significance, several did not but were very close to significant, based on the confidence intervals. These non-significant trends are telling and suggest that the subgroup component analyses were underpowered and thus prone to type 2 error. In addition, we performed multiple comparisons for each stroke type, and therefore, some of the secondary analyses, particularly those that evaluated the impact of stroke care procedures on in-hospital mortality, are prone to type 1 error. We need a larger sample size to validate each recommended item and appropriately weight the subscores.

Conclusions

Although patient demographics and stroke severity are important predictors of in-hospital mortality of patients with all types of stroke, CSC capacities were associated with reduced in-hospital mortality rates, with relevant aspects of care dependent on stroke type.

Supporting Information

File S1 English translation of the survey.

File S2 List of the participating hospitals (J-ASPECT Study).

Table S1 Japan Coma Scale for grading impaired consciousness.

Table S2 The impact of total comprehensive stroke care (CSC) score on in-hospital mortality after ischemic stroke adjusted by age, sex, level of consciousness at admission, and incidence of hypertension (HTN), diabetes mellitus(DM), and hyperlipidemia(HPL).

Table S3 The impact of total comprehensive stroke care (CSC) score on in-hospital mortality after intracerebral hemorrhage adjusted by age, sex, level of consciousness at admission, and incidence of hypertension (HTN), diabetes mellitus(DM), and hyperlipidemia(HPL).

Table S4 The impact of total comprehensive stroke care (CSC) score on in-hospital mortality after subarachnoid hemorrhage adjusted by age, sex, level of consciousness at admission, and incidence of hypertension (HTN), diabetes mellitus(DM), and hyperlipidemia(HPL).

Acknowledgments

The names of the participating 265 hospitals are listed in the File S2. We thank Drs. Manabu Hasegawa, Shunichi Fukuhara, Hisae Mori, Takuro Nakae, and Noriaki Iwata for their helpful discussions and Ms. Arisa Ishitoko and Ai Shigemura for secretarial assistance.

Author Contributions

Conceived and designed the experiments: KI KN AK. Analyzed the data: KI KN AK. Wrote the paper: KI KN AK. Collection of data: JN KO JO YS TA S. Miyachi IN KT S. Matsuda YM AS KBI HK FN SK.

References

1. The vital statistics of Japan (2011). Available: http://www.e-stat.go.jp/SG1/estat/ListE.do?lid=000001101881. Accessed 2013 Nov 22.
2. Alberts MJ, Latchaw RE, Selman WR, Shephard T, Hadley MN, et al. (2005) Recommendations for comprehensive stroke centers: A consensus statement from the Brain Attack Coalition. Stroke 36: 1597–1616.
3. Alberts MJ, Hademenos G, Latchaw RE, Jagoda A, Marler JR, et al. (2000) Recommendations for the establishment of primary stroke centers. Brain Attack Coalition. JAMA. 283: 3102–3109.
4. Reeves MJ, Parker C, Fonarow GC, Smith EE, Schwamm LH (2010) Development of stroke performance measures: Definitions, methods, and current measures. Stroke 41: 1573–1578.
5. Leifer D, Bravata DM, Connors JJ 3rd, Hinchey JA, Jauch EC, et al. (2011) Metrics for measuring quality of care in comprehensive stroke centers: Detailed follow-up to Brain Attack Coalition comprehensive stroke center recommendations: A statement for healthcare professionals from the American Heart Association/American Stroke Association. Stroke 42: 849–877.
6. Stroke Unit Trialists' Collaboration (2007) Organised inpatient (stroke unit) care for stroke. Cochrane Database Syst Rev 4: CD000197.
7. Saposnik G, Kapral MK, Coutts SB, Fang J, Demchuk AM, et al. (2009) Do all age groups benefit from organized inpatient stroke care? Stroke 40: 3321–3327.
8. Smith EE, Hassan KA, Fang J, Selchen D, Kapral MK, et al. (2010) Do all ischemic stroke subtypes benefit from organized inpatient stroke care? Neurology 75: 456–462.
9. Yasunaga H, Ide H, Imamura T, Ohe K (2005) Impact of the Japanese Diagnosis Procedure Combination-based Payment System on cardiovascular medicine-related costs. Int Heart J 46: 855–866.
10. Ohta T, Kikuchi H, Hashi K, Kudo Y (1986) Nizofenone administration in the acute stage following subarachnoid hemorrhage. Results of a multi-center controlled double-blind clinical study. J Neurosurg 64: 420–426.

11. Ohta T, Waga S, Handa W, Saito I, Takeuchi K (1974) [new grading of level of disordered consiousness (author's transl)]. No Shinkei Geka 2: 623–627.
12. Teasdale G, Jennett B (1974) Assessment of coma and impaired consciousness. A practical scale. Lancet 2: 81–84.
13. Shahian DM, Normand SL (2008) Comparison of "risk-adjusted" hospital outcomes. Circulation 117: 1955–1963.
14. Seghieri C, Mimmi S, Lenzi J, Fantini MP (2012) 30-day in-hospital mortality after acute myocardial infarction in Tuscany (Italy): An observational study using hospital discharge data. BMC Med Res Methodol 12: 170.
15. Cramer SC, Stradling D, Brown DM, Carrillo-Nunez IM, Ciabarra A, et al. (2012) Organization of a United States county system for comprehensive acute stroke care. Stroke 43: 1089–1093.
16. Qureshi AI, Chaudhry SA, Rodriguez GJ, Suri MF, Lakshminarayan K, et al. (2012) Outcome of the 'drip-and-ship' paradigm among patients with acute ischemic stroke: Results of a statewide study. Cerebrovasc Dis Extra 2: 1-8.
17. Ali SF, Singhal AB, Viswanathan A, Rost NS, Schwamm LH (2013) Characteristics and outcomes among patients transferred to a regional comprehensive stroke center for tertiary care. Stroke 44: 3148–3153.
18. Smith EE, Shobha N, Dai D, Olson DM, Reeves MJ, et al. (2010) Risk score for in-hospital ischemic stroke mortality derived and validated within the Get With the Guidelines-Stroke Program. Circulation 122: 1496–1504.
19. Fonarow GC, Pan W, Saver JL, Smith EE, Reeves MJ, et al. (2012) Comparison of 30-day mortality models for profiling hospital performance in acute ischemic stroke with vs without adjustment for stroke severity. JAMA 308: 257–264.
20. Cucchiara BL, Kasner SE, Wolk DA, Lyden PD, Knappertz VA, et al. (2004) Early impairment in consciousness predicts mortality after hemispheric ischemic stroke. Crit Care Med 32: 241–245.
21. Hemphill JC 3rd, Farrant M, Neill TA Jr (2009) Prospective validation of the ICH Score for 12-month functional outcome. Neurology 73: 1088–1094.
22. Weimar C, Benemann J, Diener HC, German Stroke Study Collaboration (2006) Development and validation of the Essen Intracerebral Haemorrhage Score. J Neurol Neurosurg Psychiatry 77: 601–605.
23. Schwamm LH, Fonarow GC, Reeves MJ, Pan W, Frankel MR, et al. (2009) Get With the Guidelines-Stroke is associated with sustained improvement in care for patients hospitalized with acute stroke or transient ischemic attack. Circulation 119: 107–115.
24. Qureshi AI, Majidi S, Chaudhry SA, Qureshi MH, Suri MF (2013) Validation of intracerebral hemorrhage-specific intensity of care quality metrics. J Stroke Cerebrovasc Dis 22: 661–667.
25. Leys D, Ringelstein EB, Kaste M, Hacke W, Executive Committee of the European Stroke Initiative (2007) Facilities available in European hospitals treating stroke patients. Stroke 38: 2985–2991.
26. Localio AR, Berlin JA, Ten Have TR, Kimmel SE (2001) Adjustments for center in multicenter studies: an overview. Ann Intern Med 135: 112–123.

Permissions

All chapters in this book were first published in PLOS ONE, by The Public Library of Science; hereby published with permission under the Creative Commons Attribution License or equivalent. Every chapter published in this book has been scrutinized by our experts. Their significance has been extensively debated. The topics covered herein carry significant findings which will fuel the growth of the discipline. They may even be implemented as practical applications or may be referred to as a beginning point for another development.

The contributors of this book come from diverse backgrounds, making this book a truly international effort. This book will bring forth new frontiers with its revolutionizing research information and detailed analysis of the nascent developments around the world.

We would like to thank all the contributing authors for lending their expertise to make the book truly unique. They have played a crucial role in the development of this book. Without their invaluable contributions this book wouldn't have been possible. They have made vital efforts to compile up to date information on the varied aspects of this subject to make this book a valuable addition to the collection of many professionals and students.

This book was conceptualized with the vision of imparting up-to-date information and advanced data in this field. To ensure the same, a matchless editorial board was set up. Every individual on the board went through rigorous rounds of assessment to prove their worth. After which they invested a large part of their time researching and compiling the most relevant data for our readers.

The editorial board has been involved in producing this book since its inception. They have spent rigorous hours researching and exploring the diverse topics which have resulted in the successful publishing of this book. They have passed on their knowledge of decades through this book. To expedite this challenging task, the publisher supported the team at every step. A small team of assistant editors was also appointed to further simplify the editing procedure and attain best results for the readers.

Apart from the editorial board, the designing team has also invested a significant amount of their time in understanding the subject and creating the most relevant covers. They scrutinized every image to scout for the most suitable representation of the subject and create an appropriate cover for the book.

The publishing team has been an ardent support to the editorial, designing and production team. Their endless efforts to recruit the best for this project, has resulted in the accomplishment of this book. They are a veteran in the field of academics and their pool of knowledge is as vast as their experience in printing. Their expertise and guidance has proved useful at every step. Their uncompromising quality standards have made this book an exceptional effort. Their encouragement from time to time has been an inspiration for everyone.

The publisher and the editorial board hope that this book will prove to be a valuable piece of knowledge for researchers, students, practitioners and scholars across the globe.

List of Contributors

Mohammed Iqbal Hossain and David Ian Stapleton
Department of Physiology, St. Vincent's Campus, The University of Melbourne, Melbourne, Victoria, Australia

Carli Lorraine Roulston
Department of Medicine, St. Vincent's Campus, The University of Melbourne, Melbourne, Victoria, Australia

Zhen-Ni Guo, Shuo Yan, Cunling Lv, Hang Jin and Yi Yang
Neuroscience Center, Department of Neurology, the First Norman Bethune Hospital of Jilin University, Chang Chun, China

Jia Liu
Shenzhen Institutes of Advanced Technology, Chinese Academy of Sciences, Xueyuan Avenue, Shenzhen University Town, Shenzhen, China

Yingqi Xing
Center for Neurovascular ultrasound, the First Norman Bethune Hospital of Jilin University, Chang Chun, China

Gu Gong, Ling Hu, Wei Wu, Lin Cai and Liang Yin
Department of Anaesthesiology, General Hospital of the People's Liberation Army, Chengdu, Sichuan, China

Lei Xiang
Department of Neurology, Tianjin Huanhu Hospital, Tianjin, China

Libang Yuan and Hailong Dong
Department of Anaesthesiology, Xijing Hospital, Fourth Military Medical University, Xi'an, Shaanxi, China

Lili Luo
Department of Pediatrics, West China Second University Hospital, Sichuan University, Sichuan, China
Key Laboratory of Obstetric & Gynecologic and Pediatric Diseases and Birth Defects of Ministry of Education, Sichuan University, Sichuan, China
Department of Emergency, West China Second University Hospital, Sichuan University, Sichuan, China

Dapeng Chen and Jinlin Wu
Department of Pediatrics, West China Second University Hospital, Sichuan University, Sichuan, China

Yi Qu and Dezhi Mu
Department of Pediatrics, West China Second University Hospital, Sichuan University, Sichuan, China
Key Laboratory of Obstetric & Gynecologic and Pediatric Diseases and Birth Defects of Ministry of Education, Sichuan University, Sichuan, China

Xihong Li
Department of Emergency, West China Second University Hospital, Sichuan University, Sichuan, China

Xiaoqing Ni
Department of Geriatrics, 107th Hospital of Chinese People's Liberation Army, Binzhou Medical University, Yantai, Shandong, People's Republic of China

Jiawei Zhang
Department of Urology, 107th Hospital of Chinese People's Liberation Army, Binzhou Medical University, Yantai, Shandong, People's Republic of China

Hongxuan Wang , Yamei Tang , Xiaoming Rong, Hui Li, Rui Pan, Yidong Wang and Ying Peng
Department of Neurology, Sun Yat-sen Memorial Hospital, Sun Yat-sen University, Guangzhou, Guangdong Province, China

Dileep R. Yavagal
Cerebral Vascular Disease Research Laboratories, Leonard M. Miller School of Medicine, University of Miami, Miami, Florida, United States of America

Department of Neurology, Leonard M. Miller School of Medicine, University of Miami, Miami, Florida, United States of America
Interdisciplinary Stem Cell Institute, Leonard M. Miller School of Medicine, University of Miami, Miami, Florida, United States of America

Baowan Lin and Philip S. Garza
Cerebral Vascular Disease Research Laboratories, Leonard M. Miller School of Medicine, University of Miami, Miami, Florida, United States of America

Ami P. Raval and Miguel Perez-Pinzon
Cerebral Vascular Disease Research Laboratories, Leonard M. Miller School of Medicine, University of Miami, Miami, Florida, United States of America, Department of Neurology, Leonard M. Miller School of Medicine, University of Miami, Miami, Florida, United States of America

Chuanhui Dong, Weizhao Zhao, Tatjana Rundek and Ralph L. Sacco
Department of Neurology, Leonard M. Miller School of Medicine, University of Miami, Miami, Florida, United States of America

Erika B. Rangel and Ian McNiece
Interdisciplinary Stem Cell Institute, Leonard M. Miller School of Medicine, University of Miami, Miami, Florida, United States of America

Joshua M. Hare
Interdisciplinary Stem Cell Institute, Leonard M. Miller School of Medicine, University of Miami, Miami, Florida, United States of America
The Department of Medicine, Leonard M. Miller School of Medicine, University of Miami, Miami, Florida, United States of America

Sheng-Kai Wu
Institute of Biomedical Engineering, College of Medicine and College of Engineering, National Taiwan University, Taipei, Taiwan

Ming-Tao Yang
Institute of Pharmacology, College of Medicine, National Taiwan University, Taipei, Taiwan
Department of Pediatrics, Far Eastern Memorial Hospital, New Taipei City, Taiwan

Kai-Hsiang Kang, Houng-Chi Liou, Dai-Hua Lu and Wen-Mei Fu
Institute of Pharmacology, College of Medicine, National Taiwan University, Taipei, Taiwan

Win-Li Lin
Institute of Biomedical Engineering, College of Medicine and College of Engineering, National Taiwan University, Taipei, Taiwan
Division of Medical Engineering Research, National Health Research Institutes, Miaoli, Taiwan

Chia-Wei Lin and Yu-Tsun Ho
Department of Physical Medicine and Rehabilitation, National Taiwan University Hospital, Taipei, Taiwan

Ya-Ping Huang
Department of Physical Medicine and Rehabilitation, National Taiwan University Hospital Yu-Lin Branch, Yunlin, Taiwan

Yueh-Hsia Chiu
Department and Graduate Institute of Health Care Management, Chang Gung University, Tao-Yuan, Taiwan

Shin-Liang Pan
Department of Physical Medicine and Rehabilitation, National Taiwan University Hospital, Taipei, Taiwan
Department of Physical Medicine and Rehabilitation, National Taiwan University College of Medicine, Taipei, Taiwan

Xiao-ying Yang
Department of Clinical Laboratory, Shanghai Jiao Tong University, Affiliated the Sixth People Hospital Fengxian Branch, Shanghai, P. R. China

Shan Gao, Yan Chen, Xing-sheng Zhou and Jing-E Wang
Department of Neurology, Shanghai Jiao Tong University, Affiliated the Sixth People Hospital Fengxian Branch, Shanghai, P. R. China

Jie Ding
Department of Neurology, Tianjin Union Medicine Center, Tianjin, P. R. China

Mateusz G. Adamski
Department of Neurology, SUNY Downstate Medical Center, Brooklyn, New York, United States of America
Department of Neurology, Jagiellonian University Medical College, Krakow, Poland

Yan Li, Erin Wagner, Hua Yu, Chloe Seales-Bailey, Qing Hao and Alison E. Baird
Department of Neurology, SUNY Downstate Medical Center, Brooklyn, New York, United States of America

Helen Durkin
Department of Pathology, SUNY Downstate Medical Center, Brooklyn, New York, United States of America

Steven A. Soper
University of North Carolina, Chapel Hill, North Carolina, United States of America

Michael Murphy
Louisiana State University, Baton Rouge, Louisiana, United States of America

Jen-Yu Wang and Cheng-Yi Wang
Department of Internal Medicine, Cardinal Tien Hospital, School of Medicine, Fu-Jen Catholic University, New Taipei City, Taiwan

Yung-Sung Huang
Division of Neurology, Department of Internal Medicine, Buddhist Dalin Tzu Chi General Hospital, Chiayi, Taiwan

Pin-Fan Chen
Division of Metabolism and Endocrinology, Department of Internal Medicine, Buddhist Dalin Tzu Chi General Hospital, Chiayi, Taiwan

Kuang-Yung Huang
School of Medicine, Tzu Chi University, Hualian, Taiwan
Division of Allergy, Immunology, and Rheumatology, Department of Internal Medicine, Buddhist Dalin Tzu Chi General Hospital, Chiayi, Taiwan

Pesus Chou
Community Medicine Research Center and Institute of Public Health, National Yang-Ming University, Taipei, Taiwan

Wei-Cheng Lian
Division of Metabolism and Endocrinology, Department of Internal Medicine, Buddhist Dalin Tzu Chi General Hospital, Chiayi, Taiwan
School of Medicine, Tzu Chi University, Hualian, Taiwan

Ching-Chih Lee
School of Medicine, Tzu Chi University, Hualian, Taiwan
Community Medicine Research Center and Institute of Public Health, National Yang-Ming University, Taipei, Taiwan
Department of Otolaryngology, Buddhist Dalin Tzu Chi General Hospital, Chiayi, Taiwan
Department of Education, Buddhist Dalin Tzu Chi General Hospital, Chiayi, Taiwan
Center for Clinical Epidemiology and Biostatistics, Buddhist Dalin Tzu Chi General Hospital, Chiayi, Taiwan

Joon-Tae Kim
Department of Neurology, Cerebrovascular Center, Chonnam National University Hospital, Gwangju, Korea
Biomedical Research Institute, Chonnam National University Hospital, Gwangju, Korea

Suk-Hee Heo
Department of Radiology, Chonnam National University Hwasun Hospital, Hwasun, Jeonnam, Korea

Man-Seok Park, Jane Chang, Kang-Ho Choi, Ki-Hyun Cho
Department of Neurology, Cerebrovascular Center, Chonnam National University Hospital, Gwangju, Korea

Zamir Merali
Physiology and Experimental Medicine, The Hospital For Sick Children, Toronto, Ontario, Canada

Meah MingYang Gao and Tim Bowes
Department of Medical Imaging, University of Toronto, Toronto, Ontario, Canada

Jian Chen and Kenneth Evans
Ontario Cancer Biomarker Network, Toronto, Ontario Canada

Andrea Kassner
Department of Medical Imaging, University of Toronto, Toronto, Ontario, Canada
Physiology and Experimental Medicine, The Hospital For Sick Children, Toronto, Ontario, Canada

Arja Helin-Salmivaara
Department of Pharmacology, Drug Development and Therapeutics, University of Turku, Turku, Finland Unit of Primary Health Care, Hospital District of Helsinki and Uusimaa, Helsinki, Finland

Piia Lavikainen
Department of Pharmacology, Drug Development and Therapeutics, University of Turku, Turku, Finland

Emma Aarnio
Department of Clinical Pharmacology, Tykslab, Turku University Hospital, Turku, Finland, School of Pharmacy, University of Eastern Finland, Kuopio, Finland

Risto Huupponen
Department of Pharmacology, Drug Development and Therapeutics, University of Turku, Turku, Finland
Department of Clinical Pharmacology, Tykslab, Turku University Hospital, Turku, Finland

Maarit Jaana Korhonen
Department of Pharmacology, Drug Development and Therapeutics, University of Turku, Turku, Finland
Department of Public Health, University of Turku, Turku, Finland

Jiunn-Tay Lee and Giia-Sheun Peng
Department of Neurology, Tri-Service General Hospital, National Defense Medical Center, Taipei, Taiwan, Republic of China

Wen Ting Chung
Graduate Institute of Clinical Medicine, Taipei Medical University, Taipei, Taiwan, Republic of China

Jin-Ding Lin
School of Public Health, National Defense Medical Center, Taipei, Taiwan, Republic of China

Chih-Hsin Muo
Department of Public Health, China Medical University Hospital, Taichung, Taiwan, Republic of China
Management Office for Health Data, China Medical University Hospital, Taichung, Taiwan, Republic of China

Che-Chen Lin
Management Office for Health Data, China Medical University Hospital, Taichung, Taiwan, Republic of China

Chi-Pang Wen
Institute of Population Health Sciences, National Health Research Institutes, Zhunan, Taiwan, Republic of China

I-Kuan Wang
Graduate Institute of Clinical Medical Science, China Medical University, Taichung, Taiwan, Republic of China
Department of Internal Medicine, College of Medicine, China Medical University, Taichung, Taiwan, Republic of China
Division of Kidney Disease, China Medical University Hospital, Taichung, Taiwan, Republic of China

Chun-Hung Tseng
Department of Internal Medicine, College of Medicine, China Medical University, Taichung, Taiwan, Republic of China
Department of Neurology, China Medical University Hospital, Taichung, Taiwan, Republic of China

Chia-Hung Kao
Graduate Institute of Clinical Medicine Science and School of Medicine, College of Medicine, China Medical University, Taichung, Taiwan, Republic of China
Department of Nuclear Medicine and PET Center, China Medical University Hospital, Taichung, Taiwan, Republic of China

Chung Y. Hsu
Graduate Institute of Clinical Medical Science, China Medical University, Taichung, Taiwan, Republic of China

Kuo-Lun Huang, Yeu-Jhy Chang, Ting-Yu Chang, Chi-Hung Liu and Tsong-Hai Lee
Stroke Center and Department of Neurology, Linkou Chang Gung Memorial Hospital, Taoyuan, Taiwan
College of Medicine, Chang Gung University, Taoyuan, Taiwan

Chien-Hung Chang
Stroke Center and Department of Neurology, Linkou Chang Gung Memorial Hospital, Taoyuan, Taiwan

College of Medicine, Chang Gung University, Taoyuan, Taiwan
Department of Electrical Engineering, Chang Gung University, Taoyuan, Taiwan

IChang Hsieh
College of Medicine, Chang Gung University, Taoyuan, Taiwan
Department of Internal Medicine, Section of Cardiology, Linkou Chang Gung Memorial Hospital, Taoyuan, Taiwan

Ho-Fai Wong and Yau-Yau Wai
College of Medicine, Chang Gung University, Taoyuan, Taiwan
Department of Medical Imaging and Intervention, Linkou Chang Gung Memorial Hospital, Taoyuan, Taiwan

Yu-Wei Chen
Department of Neurology, Landseed Hospital, Taoyuan, Taiwan
Department of Neurology, National Taiwan University Hospital, Taipei City, Taiwan
Department of Computer Science and Information Engineering, National Central University, Zhongli City, Taiwan

Bak-Sau Yip
Department of Neurology, National Taiwan University Hospital Hsinchu Branch, Hsinchu, Taiwan

Yan Yun, Chi Ma and XiaoChun Ma
School of Medicine, Shandong University, Ji'nan, Shandong, People's Republic of China

Judith Kooiman, Bas Spaans, Koen A. J. van Beers, Jonna R. Bank, Wilke R. van
de Peppel, Frederikus A. Klok and Menno V. Huisman
Department of Thrombosis and Hemostasis, Leiden University Medical Center, Leiden, The Netherlands

Nienke van Rein
Department of Thrombosis and Hemostasis, Leiden University Medical Center, Leiden, The Netherlands
Einthoven Laboratory of Experimental Vascular Medicine, Leiden University Medical Center, Leiden, The Netherlands

Antonio Iglesias del Sol
Department of Internal Medicine, Rijnland Hospital, Leiderdorp, The Netherlands

Suzanne C. Cannegieter
Department of Clinical Epidemiology, Leiden University Medical Center, Leiden, The Netherlands

Ton J. Rabelink
Department of Nephrology, Leiden University Medical Center, Leiden, The Netherlands

Gregory Y. H. Lip
Haemostasis, Thrombosis, and Vascular Biology Unit, University of Birmingham Centre for Cardiovascular Sciences, City Hospital, Birmingham, United Kingdom

Navjot Kaur, Avaneesh Pandey, Harish Negi, Nusrat Shafiq and Samir Malhotra
Department of Pharmacology, Post Graduate Institute of Medical Education & Research, Chandigarh, India

Srinivas Reddy
Department of Cardiology, Post Graduate Institute of Medical Education & Research, Chandigarh, India

Harpreet Kaur
ICMR- Advanced centre for evidence based child health, Advance Paediatric Centre, Post Graduate Institute of Medical Education & Research, Chandigarh, India

Neelima Chadha
Dr. Tulsi Das Library, Post Graduate Institute of Medical Education & Research, Chandigarh, India

Hima C. S. Abeysinghe
Department of Surgery, St Vincent's Campus, University of Melbourne, Victoria, Australia

Laita Bokhari
Neurotrauma Research team, Department of Medicine, St Vincent's Campus, University of Melbourne, Victoria, Australia
Department of Biochemistry and Molecular Biology, Bio21 Molecular Science and Biotechnology Institute, University of Melbourne, Victoria, Australia

Gregory J. Dusting
Cytoprotection Pharmacology Program, Centre for Eye Research, The Royal Eye and Ear Hospital Melbourne, Victoria, Australia
Department of Opthamology, Faculty of Medicine, University of Melbourne, Victoria, Australia

Carli L. Roulston
Neurotrauma Research team, Department of Medicine, St Vincent's Campus, University of Melbourne, Victoria, Australia

Shih-Kai Hung, Moon-Sing Lee and Wen-Yen Chiou
Departments of Radiation Oncology, Buddhist Dalin Tzu Chi Hospital, Taiwan, ROC
School of Medicine, Tzu Chi University, Hualien, Taiwan, ROC

Ching-Chih Lee
Department of Otolaryngology, Buddhist Dalin Tzu Chi Hospital, Taiwan, ROC
School of Medicine, Tzu Chi University, Hualien, Taiwan, ROC

Yi-Chun Chen
Division of Nephrology, Buddhist Dalin Tzu Chi Hospital, Taiwan, ROC
School of Medicine, Tzu Chi University, Hualien, Taiwan, ROC

Chun-Liang Lai
Division of Chest Medicine, Buddhist Dalin Tzu Chi Hospital, Taiwan, ROC
School of Medicine, Tzu Chi University, Hualien, Taiwan, ROC

Nai-Chuan Chien
Division of Thoracic Surgery, Buddhist Dalin Tzu Chi Hospital, Taiwan, ROC
School of Medicine, Tzu Chi University, Hualien, Taiwan, ROC

Wen-Lin Hsu and Dai-Wei Liu
Department of Radiation Oncology, Buddhist Tzu Chi General Hospital, Hualien, Taiwan, ROC
School of Medicine, Tzu Chi University, Hualien, Taiwan, ROC

Yu-Chieh Su, Szu-Chi Li and Hung-Chih Lai
Division of Hematology-Oncology, Buddhist Dalin Tzu Chi Hospital, Taiwan, ROC
School of Medicine, Tzu Chi University, Hualien, Taiwan, ROC

Shiang-Jiun Tsai and Feng-Chun Hsu
Departments of Radiation Oncology, Buddhist Dalin Tzu Chi Hospital, Taiwan, ROC

Hon-Yi Lin
Departments of Radiation Oncology, Buddhist Dalin Tzu Chi Hospital, Taiwan, ROC
School of Medicine, Tzu Chi University, Hualien, Taiwan, ROC
Institute of Molecular Biology, National Chung Cheng University, Min-Hsiung, Chia-Yi, Taiwan, ROC

Kristen L. Zuloaga, Wenri Zhang, Sari A. Jouihan, Robert E. Shangraw and Nabil J. Alkayed
The Knight Cardiovascular Institute, Department of Anesthesiology & Perioperative Medicine, Oregon Health & Science University, Portland, Oregon, United States of America

Stephanie M. Krasnow, Xinxia Zhu and Daniel L. Marks
Papé Family Pediatric Research Institute, Department of Pediatrics, Oregon Health and Science University, Portland, Oregon, United States of America

Koji Iihara
Department of Neurosurgery, Graduate School of Medical Sciences, Kyushu University, Fukuoka, Japan

Kunihiro Nishimura and Yoshihiro Miyamoto
Department of Preventive Medicine and Epidemiologic Informatics, National Cerebral and Cardiovascular Center, Suita, Japan

Akiko Kada
Clinical Research Center, National Hospital Organization, Nagoya Medical Center, Nagoya, Japan

Jyoji Nakagawara
Integrative Stroke Imaging Center, National Cerebral and Cardiovascular Center, Suita, Japan

Kuniaki Ogasawara
Department of Neurosurgery, Iwate Medical University, Morioka, Japan

Junichi Ono
Chiba Cardiovascular Center, Ichihara, Japan

Yoshiaki Shiokawa
Department of Neurosurgery, Kyorin University, Mitaka, Japan

Toru Aruga
Showa University Hospital, Tokyo, Japan

Shigeru Miyachi
Department of Neurosurgery, Nagoya University, Nagoya, Japan

Izumi Nagata
Department of Neurosurgery, Nagasaki University, Nagasaki, Japan

Kazunori Toyoda
Department of Cerebrovascular Medicine, National Cerebral and Cardiovascular Center, Suita, Japan

Shinya Matsuda
Department of Preventive Medicine and Community Health, University of Occupational and Environmental Health, Kita-Kyushu, Japan

Akifumi Suzuki
Research Institute for Brain and Blood Vessels, Akita, Japan

Koichi B. Ishikawa
Center for Cancer Control and Information Services, National Cancer Center, Tokyo, Japan

Hiroharu Kataoka
Department of Neurosurgery, National Cerebral and Cardiovascular Center, Suita, Japan

Fumiaki Nakamura and Satoru Kamitani
Department of Public Health, The University of Tokyo, Tokyo, Japan

Index